Medical Imaging: Clinical Applications

Medical Imaging: Clinical Applications

Editor: Kenneth Washington

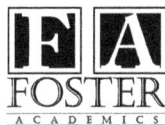

FA
FOSTER
ACADEMICS

www.fosteracademics.com

www.fosteracademics.com

F A
FOSTER
A C A D E M I C S

Cataloging-in-Publication Data

Medical imaging : clinical applications / edited by Kenneth Washington.
   p. cm.
Includes bibliographical references and index.
ISBN 978-1-63242-624-6
   1. Diagnostic imaging. 2. Imaging systems in medicine. 3. Radiography, Medical.
I. Washington, Kenneth.
RC78.7.D53 M43 2019
616.075 4--dc23

Foster Academics,
118-35 Queens Blvd., Suite 400,
Forest Hills, NY 11375, USA

ISBN 978-1-63242-624-6 (Hardback)

Contents

Permissions

List of Contributors

Index

Preface

The world is advancing at a fast pace like never before. Therefore, the need is to keep up with the latest developments. This book was an idea that came to fruition when the specialists in the area realized the need to coordinate together and document essential themes in the subject. That's when I was requested to be the editor. Editing this book has been an honour as it brings together diverse authors researching on different streams of the field. The book collates essential materials contributed by veterans in the area which can be utilized by students and researchers alike.

The visual representation of the interior of the human body for the purpose of clinical analysis and for the diagnosis and treatment of diseases is achieved through medical imaging. It also allows the understanding of normal physiology and anatomy. Some medical imaging techniques are magnetic resonance imaging (MRI), endoscopy, positron emission tomography (PET), medical ultrasonography, etc. Volume rendering techniques are used to provide a 3D visualization of the body or region of the body under study. Imaging techniques such as MRI and PET are typically used in neuroscience and oncology. Medical imaging may be used also to gain insight into complications in pregnancy, routine prenatal care and intercurrent diseases. Medical imaging is also a major tool in clinical trials as it allows quick visualization and assessment. The topics covered in this extensive book deal with the clinical applications of medical imaging. It aims to present researches that have transformed this discipline and aided its advancement. This book is a vital tool for all researching or studying this discipline as it gives incredible insights into emerging trends and concepts.

Each chapter is a sole-standing publication that reflects each author's interpretation. Thus, the book displays a multi-facetted picture of our current understanding of application, resources and aspects of the field. I would like to thank the contributors of this book and my family for their endless support.

Editor

A comparison of the quality of image acquisition between the incident dark field and sidestream dark field video-microscopes

Edward Gilbert-Kawai[1*], Jonny Coppel[1], Vassiliki Bountziouka[2], Can Ince[3], Daniel Martin[1,4] and for the Caudwell Xtreme Everest and Xtreme Everest 2 Research Groups

Abstract

Background: The 'Cytocam' is a third generation video-microscope, which enables real time visualisation of the *in vivo* microcirculation. Based upon the principle of incident dark field (IDF) illumination, this hand held computer-controlled device was designed to address the technical limitations of its predecessors, orthogonal polarization spectroscopy and sidestream dark field (SDF) imaging. In this manuscript, we aimed to compare the quality of sublingual microcirculatory image acquisition between the IDF and SDF devices.

Methods: Using the microcirculatory image quality scoring (MIQS) system, (six categories scored as either 0 = optimal, 1 = acceptable, or 10 = unacceptable), two independent raters compared 30 films acquired using the Cytocam IDF video-microscope, to an equal number obtained with an SDF device. Blinded to the origin of the films, the raters were therefore able to score between 0 and 60 for each film analysed. The scores' distributions between the two techniques were compared.

Results: The median MIQS (95 % CI) given to the SDF camera was 7 (1.5–12), as compared to 1 (0.5–1.0) for the IDF device ($p < 0.0001$). Of the six categories assessed by the MIQS, nearly one fifth of the SDF videos were scored as unacceptable for pressure (20 %), content (20 %), and stability (17 %), with focus scoring deficiently 13 % of the time. High agreement between the two raters scoring values was evident, with an intra-class correlation coefficient (ICC) of 0.96 (95 % CI: 0.94, 0.98).

Conclusions: These results demonstrate that the quality of sublingual microcirculatory image acquisition is superior in the Cytocam IDF video-microscope, as compared to the SDF video-microscope.

Keywords: Microcirculation, Microscopy, Validation, Capillary

Background

Incident dark field (IDF) imaging is an important technique that allows real time visualisation of the microcirculation [1]. Based upon the illumination of microvessels covered by a thin epithelial layer, it may be thought of as the successor to both orthogonal polarization spectroscopy (OPS) [2], and more recently, sidestream dark field (SDF) imaging [3]. Introduced in 2012, this third generation hand-held camera

known as the Cytocam IDF video-microscope (Braedius Medical, Huizen, The Netherlands), was developed in an attempt to overcome many of the previous generations devices technical limitations [1]. These included; i) the limitations imposed by analogue video cameras, ii) the inability to achieve automatic microcirculation analysis, iii) pressure-induced microcirculatory alterations (predominantly caused by the heavy weight of the devices (SDF camera weight 320 g), iv) the requirement for hand operated focussing, and v) poor quality of image acquisition [4].

The Cytocam is a lightweight (120 g), fully digitalised pen-like device (length 220 mm, diameter 23 mm) that applies the principle of incident dark field microscopy introduced by Sherman and Cook in 1971 [5]. Blood

* Correspondence: e.gilbert@ucl.ac.uk
[1]University College London Centre for Altitude Space and Extreme Environment Medicine, UCLH NIHR Biomedical Research Centre, Institute of Sport and Exercise Health, 170 Tottenham Court Road, London W1T 7HA, UK
Full list of author information is available at the end of the article

vessels <100 μm in diameter, and <1000 μm below the surface of an organ or mucosal surface, are visualised in a two-dimensional plane through the process of epi-illumination [5]. Highly illuminating light emitting diodes (LEDs) enable suitable tissue penetration, and to avoid motion induced blurring secondary to fast moving erythrocytes [6], a very short LED pulse time of two milliseconds is utilised. Image delineation is optimised using a 3.5 megapixel high-resolution sensor, an optical magnification factor of four times, and an optical resolution of more than 300 lines/mm - an improvement of 50 % over SDF devices. This is further enhanced with an effective field of view (FOV) almost three times as large as earlier devices (1.55 × 1.16 mm, FOV area = 1.79 mm^2), which may be magnified by a factor of 211 times on the display monitor [1]. Improved focussing is achieved through an integrated distance measurement system, which through the means of a manually adjusting the piezo linear motor via the computer interface, can alter the sensor position in steps of two microns. This novel quantitative focusing mechanism results in an accurate and repeatable focus distance, without having to repeatedly adjust the focus depth for every subsequent measurement. Finally, the IDF video-microscope has the capabilities for direct microcirculation analysis where the images are recorded digitally and analysed automatically. Specialised software automatically detects and quantitatively assesses

the vessels' diameters, and the flow velocity of erythrocytes within visualised vessels. Previously analysis of SDF videos required their conversion from analogue to digital images, with subsequent off-line analysis using specialised image processing software [7].

Although the IDF device should have significant superiority, in terms of image quality, over previous technologies this requires confirmation. We therefore set out to directly compare IDF and SDF images in a formalised manner.

Methods

Thirty films of human sublingual microcirculation obtained using an SDF video-microscope (MicroVision Medical, Amsterdam, Netherlands), were compared to thirty comparable films obtained using the Cytocam IDF video-microscope. The films were picked at random from a database of over 800 SDF and IDF films, all of which were obtained from healthy adult volunteers who had given informed consent. Ethical approval for the study had been obtained from University College London Research and Ethics Committee. Two raters (EGK, JC), blinded to the device on which the video was generated, independently graded the films using the Microcirculation image quality score (MISQ) system [8]. In 2007 a consensus statement that outlined five key principles for optimal image acquisition [9]. These were:

Table 1 The Microcirculation image quality score

Category	Brief description	Optimal (0)	Acceptable (1)	Unacceptable (10)
Illumination	Brightness and contrast of video	Even illumination across the entire field of view. Contrast sufficient to see small vessels against a background of tissue.	The video borders on being too dark or bright to distinguish vessels from tissue but the vessels are still identifiable.	The video is oversaturated/too bright or too dark to make out analysable features. Insufficient contrast to resolve flow rate.
Duration	Number of frames in the video clip and how it represents the actual pathology	Analysable video segment is ≥5 s long (>150 frames)	Analysable video segment is 3–5 s (between 90 and 150 frames)	Analysable video segment <3 s (90 frames)
Focus	Image sharpness in region of interest	Good focus for all vessels (small and large) in the entire field of view. Plasma gaps and red blood cells are visible.	<1/2 field of view is out of focus or edges of the vessels are slightly out of focus.	Video is completely out of focus such that no small vessel can be seen.
Content	Determination of the types of vessels and/or presence of occluding artefacts in the image.	Video is free of occlusions. Good distribution of large and small vessels. Less than 30 % of the vessels are looped upon themselves	Video may have a few artefacts. Acceptable distribution of large and small vessels. About 30–50 % of the vessels are looped.	Most of the field of view has occluding artefacts such as saliva or bubbles. More that 50 % vessels are looped upon themselves.
Stability	Frame motion that can be adequately stabilised without motion blur	Movement is within ¼ of the field of view. No motion blur.	Movement is within ½ field of view. No motion blur.	Movement is greater than ½ of the field of view and/or motion blur in frame
Pressure	Iatrogenic mechanical pressure causing misrepresentation of flow	Flow is constant throughout the entire movie. No obvious signs of artificially sluggish or stopped flow. Good flow in the largest vessels.	Signs of pressure (localised sluggish flow in a specific large vessel), but flow appears to be unimpeded based on good flow in most large vessels.	Obvious pressure artefacts associated with probe movement, and/or flow that starts and stops, reversal of flow. Poor or changing flow in larger venules.

Adapted from: 'Quality Scoring Metrics: The microcirculation image quality score: development and preliminary evaluation of a proposed approach to grading quality of image acquisition for bedside videomicroscopy' [8]

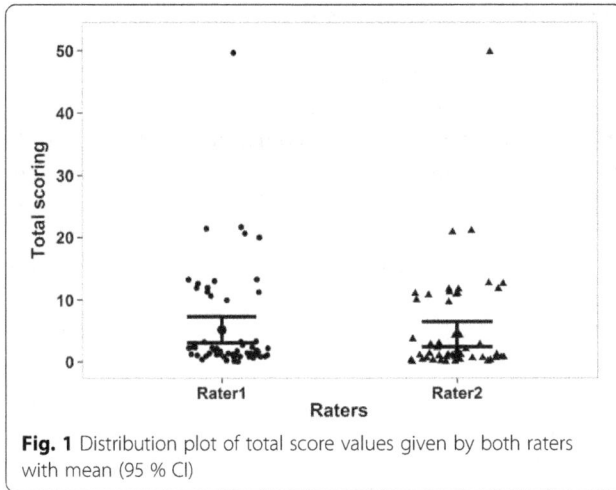

Fig. 1 Distribution plot of total score values given by both raters with mean (95 % CI)

1. Five separate image sites per organ
2. Avoidance of pressure artefacts
3. Elimination of secretions
4. Adequate focus and contrast adjustment
5. High quality recording

In 2013, a more formal approach to grading the quality of image acquisition prior to analysis was described, thereby giving a semi-objective measure of its suitability to be entered for computer analysis and quantification [8]. Six key characteristics of image capture were identified and encompassed within the 'Microcirculation Image Quality Score' (MIQS) (Table 1).

Each of the six categories is graded as 0 (optimal), 1 (acceptable) or 10 (unacceptable). If the total of the six categories is >10, then the video is unsuitable for Table 1 analysis and discarded. This somewhat peculiar scoring system is used, for if any one category is designated as unacceptable, it enforces that the video is not used [8].

The agreement between the two raters was assessed using the intra-class correlation coefficient and Bland and Altman limits of agreement. Over the range of scores given, Spearman's correlation coefficient was used to assess the degree of over- or under- estimation of the score by either rater. The Mann–Whitney U-test was used to compare the score's distribution between the two techniques. The two-tailed significance level was set at 0.05, and R (version 3.1.0) was used for the analyses.

Results

All 60 videos were analysed by both raters and no problems were encountered. The distribution of the individual total scores by rater is shown in Fig. 1.

Very good agreement between raters' total scores are evident with an intra-class correlation coefficient of 0.96 (95 % CI: 0.94, 0.98). In addition, good agreement is evident in Fig. 2 (mean difference (rater2 – rater1): –0.75), and whilst some individual variation may exist as indicated by the slightly wide limits of agreement (–4.86; 3.36), no over- or under- estimation trend by either rater was demonstrated (rho = –0.165, $p = 0.21$). For each device, the breakdown percentages of films scored as optimal, acceptable or unacceptable is presented in Table 2. When comparing the tools, the median score (95 % CI) given to the SDF video-microscope was 7 (1.5; 12), as opposed to 1 (0.5; 1.0) for the IDF video-microscope ($p < 0.0001$). The distribution of these values may be seen in Fig. 3. Examples of images taken with the Incident Dark Field imaging

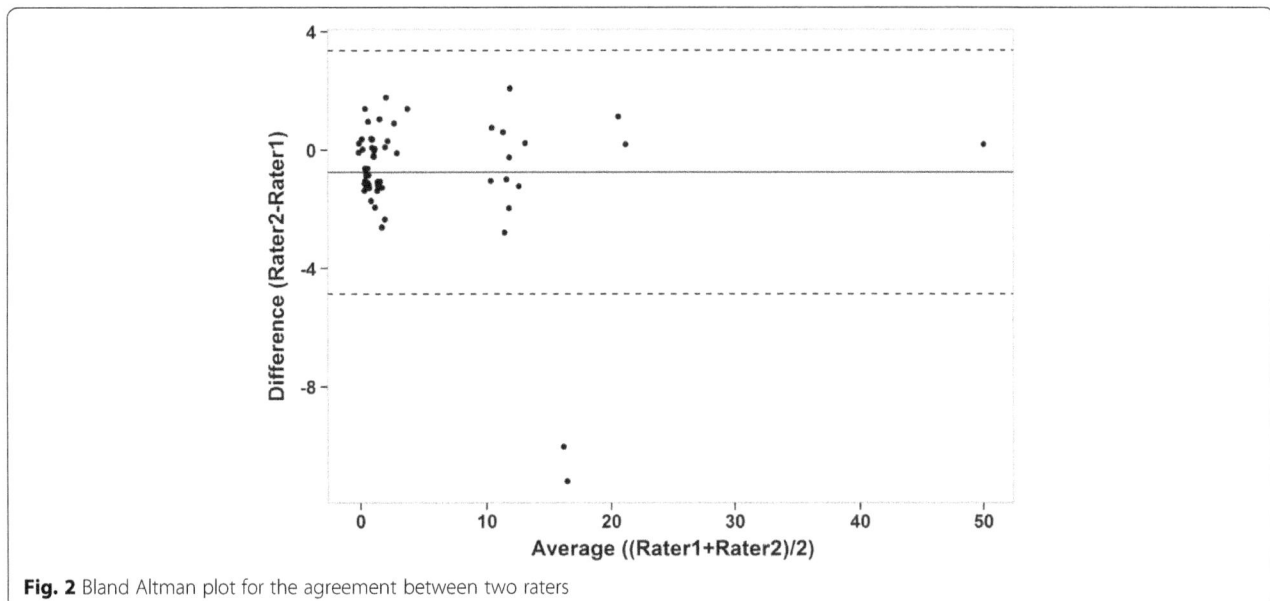

Fig. 2 Bland Altman plot for the agreement between two raters

Table 2 Percentage (%) of IDF and SDF films scored as optimal, acceptable, or unacceptable

Category	Optimal (Score = 0)		Acceptable (Score = 1)		Unacceptable (Score = 10)	
	IDF	SDF	IDF	SDF	IDF	SDF
Stability	68	50	32	33	0	17
Pressure	73	67	27	13	0	20
Illumination	92	67	8	30	0	3
Duration[a]	100	100	0	0	0	0
Focus	98	43	15	43	0	13
Content	88	65	12	15	0	20

[a]Images were all cut to 150 frames in length prior to analysis, hence both IDF and SDF demonstrate optimal scores for this category

camera, and Sidestream Dark Field imaging camera can be seen in Additional files 1 and 2.

Discussion

These results demonstrate for the first time, that the Cytocam IDF video-microscope is superior to the SDF video-microscope in terms of the quality of sublingual microcirculatory image acquisition.

High agreement between the two raters scoring values was demonstrated, and whilst it is evident from the Bland Altman plot that some individual variation existed between raters, neither individual demonstrated a trend in over- or under-estimating the score as the total values increased. Using the total score value to determine if an image was deemed suitable for analysis, (i.e. if given a total score ≥10 renders the video as unacceptable), there was 100 % exact agreement (95 % CI: 94 %; 100 %) between the two raters.

As to whether the IDF video-microscope was superior to the SDF video-microscope in terms of providing acceptable images for analysis, the median score of 7 given to the SDF images, as opposed to 1 for the IDF videos, indicates that the SDF camera is more prone to produce

unacceptable results. In this instance, 100 % of the images obtained using the IDF video-microscope were judged to be acceptable for data analysis, as opposed to only 50 % of these data collected using the SDF device. Table 2 demonstrates how the individual components of the MIQS system were scored for both cameras. From this we are able to see which categories SDF scored particularly poorly for as compared to IDF. The IDF video-microscope did not receive any scores of 10 from either rater, however nearly a fifth of the SDF videos were scored as unacceptable for stability (17 %), pressure (20 %), and content (20 %), with focus scoring deficiently 13 % of the time. This indicates superior IDF image acquisition for multiple categories, as opposed to in only one area of data capture.

Although 60 films chosen at random from a large database of images were analysed (30 for each device), a weakness in this manuscript was that no power calculation was performed prior to commencing. This said, the strong statistical significance supports the belief that it was adequately powered. Additionally, as the MIQS still relies on observer input to grade images, it is thus subjective in its film assessment. Nevertheless, it is the most formal approach to image grading we have to date, and the high ICC supports its use.

Conclusion

In conclusion, these data demonstrate that the IDF video-microscope provides improved image acquisition of human sublingual microcirculation when compared to the SDF video-microscope. Superior in five out of the six categories comprising the MIQS, the use of IDF offers an advanced insight into the clinical evaluation of the microvasculature.

Abbreviations
FOV: Field of view; IDF: Incident dark field; LED: Light emitting diode; MIQS: Microcirculation image quality score; OPS: Orthogonal polarization spectroscopy; SDF: Sidestream dark field.

Competing interest
Can Ince has developed SDF imaging and is listed as inventor on related patents commercialized by MicroVision Medical (MVM) under a license from the Academic Medical Center (AMC). He has been a consultant for MVM in the past, but has not been involved with this company for more than 5 years now, except that he still holds shares. Braedius Medical, a company owned by a relative of Can Ince, has developed and designed a hand held microscope called CytoCam-IDF imaging. Dr Ince has no financial relation with Braedius Medical of any sort; he had never owned shares, or received consultancy or speaker fees from Braedius Medical. The authors declare that they had no competing interests.

Authors' contributions
E G-K: Design of study, conduct of study, analysis of data, writing manuscript. JC: Conduct of study, analysis of data, writing manuscript. VB: Analysis of data, writing manuscript. CI: Design of study, writing manuscript. DM: Analysis of data, writing manuscript. All authors read and approved the final manuscript.

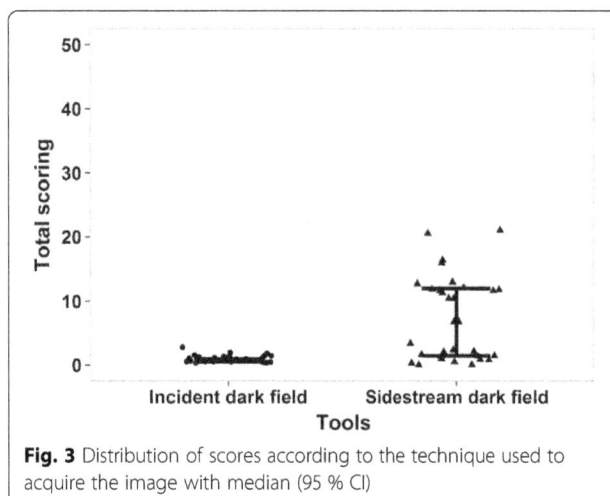

Fig. 3 Distribution of scores according to the technique used to acquire the image with median (95 % CI)

A comparison of the quality of image acquisition between the incident dark field and sidestream dark field...

5

Acknowledgements

The members of the Caudwell Xtreme Everest Research Group are as follows:
V. Ahuja, G. Aref-Adib, R. Burnham, A. Chisholm, K. Clarke, D. Coates, M.
Coates, D. Cook, M. Cox, S. Dhillon, C. Dougall, P. Doyle, P. Duncan, M. Edsell,
L. Edwards, L. Evans, P. Gardiner, M. Grocott, P. Gunning, N. Hart, J. Harrington, J.
Harvey, C. Holloway, D. Howard, D. Hurlbut, C. Imray, C. Ince, M. Jonas, J. van der
Kaaij, M. Khosravi, N. Kolfschoten, D. Levett, H. Luery, A. Luks, D. Martin, R.
McMorrow, P. Meale, K. Mitchell, H. Montgomery, G. Morgan, J. Morgan, A.
Murray, M. Mythen, S. Newman, M. O'Dwyer, J. Pate, T. Plant, M. Pun, P.
Richards, A. Richardson, G. Rodway, J. Simpson, C. Stroud, M. Stroud, J. Stygal, B.
Symons, P. Szawarski, A. Van Tulleken, C. Van Tulleken, A. Vercueil, L. Wandrag,
M. Wilson, J. Windsor.
Scientific Advisory Group: B. Basnyat, C. Clarke, T. Hornbein, J. Milledge, J. West.
Members of the Xtreme Everest 2 Research Group are as follows:
S Abraham, T Adams, W Anseeuw, R Astin, B Basnyat, O Burdall, J Carroll, A
Cobb, J Coppel, O Couppis, J Court, A Cumptsey, T Davies, S Dhillon, N
Diamond, C Dougall, T Geliot, E Gilbert-Kawai, G Gilbert-Kawai, E Gnaiger, M
Grocott, C Haldane, P Hennis, J Horscroft, D Howard, S Jack, B Jarvis, W Jenner,
G Jones, J van der Kaaij, J Kenth, A Kotwica, R Kumar BC, J Lacey, V Laner, D
Levett, D Martin, P Meale, K Mitchell, Z Mahomed, J Moonie, A Murray, M
Mythen, P Mythen, K O'Brien, I. Ruggles-Brice, K Salmon, A Sheperdigian, T
Smedley, B Symons, C Tomlinson, A Vercueil, L Wandrag, S Ward, A Wight, C
Wilkinson, S Wythe.
Scientific Advisory Board: M Feelisch, E Gilbert-Kawai, M Grocott (chair), M
Hanson, D Levett, D Martin, K Mitchell, H Montgomery, R Moon, A Murray,
M Mythen, M Peters.

Author details

[1]University College London Centre for Altitude Space and Extreme
Environment Medicine, UCLH NIHR Biomedical Research Centre, Institute of
Sport and Exercise Health, 170 Tottenham Court Road, London W1T 7HA, UK.
[2]Statistical Support Service, Population, Policy and Practice Programme,
Institute of Child Health, University College London, London, England.
[3]Department of Intensive Care, Erasmus MC University Hospital Rotterdam,
3000 Rotterdam, The Netherlands. [4]Division of Neonatology, Erasmus
MC-Sophia Children's Hospital, Wytemaweg 80, P.O. Box 2060, 3000 CB
Rotterdam, Netherlands.

References

1. Aykut G IY, Ince C.: A new generation computer controlled imaging sensor based hand held microscope for quantifying bedside microcirculatory alterations. In Annual update in Intensive Care and Emergency Medicine 2014 Edited by Vincent JL. Springer; 2014:pp. 367-pp. 385.
2. Groner W, Winkelman JW, Harris AG, Ince C, Bouma GJ, Messmer K, et al. Orthogonal polarization spectral imaging: a new method for study of the microcirculation. Nat Med. 1999;5:1209–12.
3. Goedhart PT, Khalilzada M, Bezemer R, Merza J, Ince C. Sidestream Dark Field (SDF) imaging: a novel stroboscopic LED ring-based imaging modality for clinical assessment of the microcirculation. Opt Express. 2007;15:15101–14.
4. Mik EG, Johannes T, Fries M. Clinical microvascular monitoring: a bright future without a future? Crit Care Med. 2009;37:2980–1.
5. Sherman H, Klausner S, Cook WA. Incident dark-field illumination: a new method for microcirculatory study. Angiology. 1971;22:295–303.
6. Cerny V. Sublingual microcirculation. Appl Cardiopulm Pathophysiol. 2012;16:229–48.
7. Dobbe JSG, Atasever B, Van Zijderveld R, Ince C. Measurement of functional microcirculatory geometry and velocity distributions using automated image analysis. Med Biol Eng Comput. 2008;46:659–70.
8. Massey MJ, Larochelle E, Najarro G, Karmacharla A, Arnold R, Trzeciak S, et al. The microcirculation image quality score: development and preliminary evaluation of a proposed approach to grading quality of image acquisition for bedside videomicroscopy. J Crit Care. 2013;28:913–7.
9. De Backer D, Hollenberg S, Boerma C, Goedhart P, Buchele G, Ospina-Tascon G, et al. How to evaluate the microcirculation: report of a round table conference. Crit Care. 2007;11:R101.

2

Ultrasonographic prevalence and characteristics of non-palpable thyroid incidentalomas in a hospital-based population in a sub-Saharan country

Boniface Moifo[1,2]* iD, Jean Roger Moulion Tapouh[1,3], Sylviane Dongmo Fomekong[1], François Djomou[1,3] and Emmanuella Manka'a Wankie[4]

Abstract

Background: Thyroid incidentalomas (TI) are highly prevalent asymptomatic thyroid nodules with ultrasound as the best imaging modality for their detection and characterization. Although they are mostly benign, potential for malignancy is up to 10–15%.

In sub-Saharan Africa little data exists on the prevalence and risk categorization of TI. The aim of this study was to determine the prevalence and ultrasound characteristics of non-palpable thyroid incidentalomas among adults in sub-Saharan setting.

Methods: A cross sectional study was carried out between March and August 2015, at two university teaching hospitals. Sampling was consecutive and included all adults aged $\geq$ 16 years, presenting for any ultrasound other than for the thyroid, with no history or clinical signs of thyroid disease, and no palpable thyroid lesion. Ultrasound was done using 4 to 11 MHz linear probes. Subjects with diffuse thyroid abnormalities were excluded. Variables studied were age, gender, thyroid volume, ultrasound characteristics of thyroid nodules, TIRADS scores. Differences were considered statistically significant for p-value < 0.05.

Results: The prevalence of TI was 28.3% (126 persons with TI /446 examined). This prevalence was 46.2% in population $\geq$ 61-year-old; 6.3% in population $\leq$ 20-year-old; 33.3% for females and 18.4% for males (p < 0.001). Of the 241 TI found, 49.4% were cysts, 33.6% solid, 17.0% mixed; 37.8% <5 mm and 22% >10 mm. Solid TI were mainly hyperechoic (42.0%), 3/81 were markedly hypoechoic. Sixty-nine out of 126 persons with TI (54.8%) had at least two nodules. Solitary nodules were predominant in the age group $\leq$20 years. Of 241 TI, 129 (53.5%) were classified TIRADS 2, 81 (33.6%) TIRADS 3, 25 (10.4%) TIRADS 4A, 6 (2.5%) TIRADS 4B, and none TIRADS 5. Characteristics associated with increased risk of malignancy where mostly founded on solid nodules (p < 0.000) and nodules larger than 15 mm (p < 0.001).

Conclusion: Thyroid incidentalomas were very frequent with a prevalence of 28.3% and potential risk of malignancy in 12.9%. Prevalence had a tendency to increase with age and in female. Cystic nodules were the most prevalent. Potential for malignancy would be increased for larger and solid nodules.

Keywords: Thyroid incidentaloma, Thyroid nodule, TIRADS, Prevalence, Sub-Saharan country

* Correspondence: bmoifo@yahoo.fr
[1]Department of Radiology and Radiation Oncology, Faculty of Medicine and Biomedical Sciences, The University of Yaounde 1, Yaounde, Cameroon
[2]Radiology Department YGOPH, Yaounde Gynaeco-Obstetric and Pediatric Hospital, PO Box 4362, Yaounde, Cameroon
Full list of author information is available at the end of the article

Background

Thyroid incidentalomas (TIs) are asymptomatic nodules discovered accidentally during imaging studies indicated for other reasons [1]. Ultrasound is the best imaging modality for the detection and characterization of these nodules [2, 3]. Various studies have reported a prevalence between 50 and 67% [2, 4–7]. They are mostly benign. However, there is a potential for malignancy in less than 10–15% [1, 2, 8], depending on the method of sampling and the characteristics of nodules.

TIs therefore represent a clinical challenge and a source of anxiety to patients. The clinician needs to correctly access the risk of each nodule, in order to correctly determine if and what further investigation is necessary. The TIRADS (Thyroid Imaging Reporting and Data System) permits this classification with recommendations on the need for cytologic verification or ultrasound surveillance [6, 7, 9, 10].

In sub-Saharan Africa little data exists on the prevalence and risk categorization of TI [11]. The aim of this study was therefore, to determine their prevalence in the adult population, and describe their ultrasound characteristics based on TIRADS.

Methods

A cross-sectional study was carried out in two university teaching hospitals from March to August 2015.

Study population

Persons aged ≥ 16 years, referred to the diagnostic imaging department for ultrasound scans other than that of the thyroid, who accepted freely to participate in the study were included. They had no history, palpable or other clinical signs of thyroid disease. A consecutive non-probabilistic sample was taken. Patients with diffuse thyroid disease were excluded. Verbal informed consent from participants was required.

Thyroid ultrasound procedure and image interpretation

The ultrasound was done free of charge using the routine procedure [12], with linear probes of 4–11 MHz frequency. The machines used were *Prosound alpha 6* (Hitachi Medical Europe, France) 2015 and *SSI-8000* (Sonoscape Co Ltd, China) *2013*. Images were stored in the hard drive of each machine. An initial interpretation was done by the operator during the course of the scan. A second reading was done later by the operator and two radiologists with at least five years' experience in thyroid sonography. Nodules were classified by consensus according to TIRADS (Table 1), as proposed by Russ and al [9, 13].

Table 1 TIRADS classification according to Russ and al [9, 13]

TIRADS	Signification	Ultrasonographic characteristics	Malignancy risk (%)
TIRADS 1	Normal thyroid	• Normal thyroid US	-
TIRADS 2	Benign aspects	• Simple cyst • Spongiform nodule • 'White knight' aspect • Isolated macrocalcification • Typical sub-acute thyroiditis	0.0
TIRADS 3	Probably benign aspects	• None of the high suspicious aspect • Isoechogenic • Hyperechogenic	0.25
TIRADS 4A	Low suspicious aspect	• None of the high suspicious aspect • Moderately hypoechogenic	6.0
TIRADS 4B	High suspicious aspects with 1 or 2 signs and no adenopathy	• Taller-than-wide shape • Irregular or microlobulated margins • Microcalcifications • Marked hypoechogenicity	69.0
TIRADS 5	High suspicious aspects with ≥ 3 signs and/or adenopathy	• Taller-than-wide shape • Irregular or microlobulated margins • Microcalcifications • Marked hypoechogenicity	100

A preconceived data collection form was filled out for each subject. Variables studied included: age, gender, thyroid volume, ultrasound characteristics of any nodules found (echogenicity, calcifications, borders, height/breadth in transverse plane), and TIRADS score for each TI. The CSPro 5.1 software was used to create the data entry mask anonymously. Stata version 11 and SPSS version 18 software enabled the analysis of the data. The chi square test assessed the association between the TIRADS score and various socio-demographic and sonographic characteristics. The comparison of the prevalences were performed using the Fisher exact test. Results were expressed in numbers and percentages for categorical variables. Differences were considered statistically significant for $p < 0.05$.

Table 2 Prevalence of thyroid incidentalomas (TIs) with respect to age and gender

TIs Age (years)	Female		Male		Total	
	Population	n (%)	Population	n (%)	Population	n (%)
≤20	13	1 (7.7)	3	0 (0.0)	16	1 (6.3)
21–40	163	35 (21.5)	54	2 (3.7)	217	37 (17.1)
41–60	90	43 (47.8)	71	21 (29.6)	161	64 (39.8)
≥ 61	28	19 (67.9)	24	5 (20.8)	52	24 (46.2)
Total	294	98 (33.3)	152	28 (18.4)	446	126 (28.3)

($p < 0.001$)

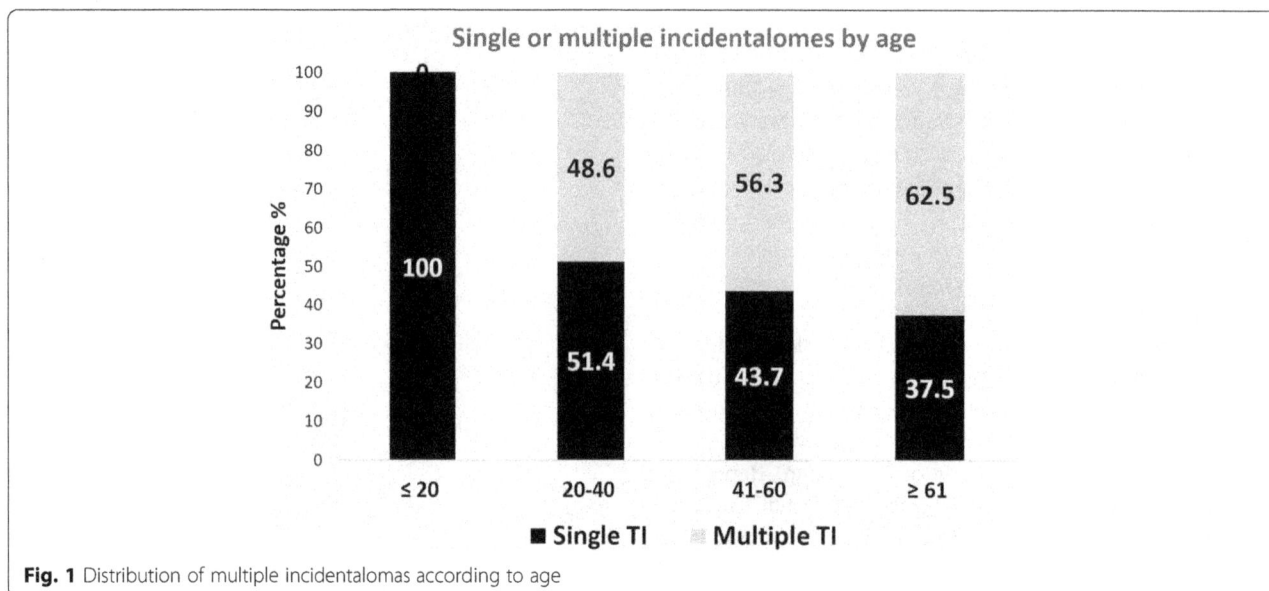

Fig. 1 Distribution of multiple incidentalomas according to age

Results

Four hundred and forty six subjects aged 16 to 89 were included, with 294 females (65.9%; sex ratio F/H = 1.9). The most frequent age groups was 21–40 years with 48.7% (Table 2).

Of the 446 individuals included, 126 had thyroid incidentalomas giving a prevalence of TIs of 28.3%. This prevalence was 33.3% among women ($p < 0.001$) and 46.6% in individuals aged more than 60 years (Table 2).

Characteristics of incidentalomas

The 126 subjects with TI cumulated a total of 241 TIs with 69 individuals (54.8%) having two or more TI (Fig. 1). Multiple TI was found in 57.2% of females and 42.2% of males.

The location of TI was 54.0% (130/241) in the right lobe and 3.7% in the isthmus (9 cases). Most were inferiorly (base) located 38.2% (92/241), followed by location within the corpus (31.1%).

Of the 241 TIs, cystic nodules accounted for 49.4%; solid nodules for 33.6%; mixed (cystic and solid) for

17.0%. According to size 37.8% TIs were <5 mm and 22% >10 mm (Table 3).

In regard to solid nodules (81/241), 42.0% were hyperechoic, 29.6% isoechoic, 24.7% with moderate hypoechogenicity and 3.7% were markedly hypoechoic. 39 solid TIs had a peripheral hypoechoic ring.

Solid and mixed incidentalomas had well defined borders in 91.0% of cases; ten nodules (8.2%) had indistinct borders. Eight nodules had macrocalcifications, two had microcalcifications. Half of them did not show any form of vascularization on Doppler examination (pulse and power). Peripheral vascularization was seen in 39.3% of cases (48/122). Only one nodule presented predominantly central vascularization.

TIRADS classification of TIs

Of 241 TIs, 129 (53.5%) were classified TIRADS 2 (Fig. 2), 81 (33.6%) TIRADS 3 (Fig. 3), 25 (10.4%) TIRADS 4A, 6 (2.5%) TIRADS 4B (Fig. 4), and none TIRADS 5.

Of the 31 TIRADS 4 thyroid incidentalomas, 77.4% were solid and 22.6% mixed ($p < 0.000$). None was cystic (Table 4); 14.3% of TIRADS 4 nodules were 10–15 mm, 22% were > 15 mm.

There was no significantly strong association between age, gender and TIRADS score. Prevalence of potentially malignant nodules (TIRADS 4) increased with size ($p < 0.001$): Table 5.

Discussion

The aim of this study was to determine the prevalence and ultrasound characteristics of thyroid incidentalomas, amongst adult in a hospital based setting.

Table 3 Distribution of incidentalomas with respect to size and tissue structure

Thyroid incidentalomas	Cystic	Solid	Mixed	Total
Largest diameter	n (%)	n (%)	n (%)	n (%)
< 5 mm	67 (73.6)	11 (12.1)	13 (14.3)	91 (37.8)
5–9	41 (42.3)	36 (37.1)	20 (20.6)	97 (40.3)
10–14	8 (22.9)	23 (65.7)	4 (11.4)	35 (14.5)
≥ 15	3 (16.7)	11 (61.1)	4 (22.2)	18 (7.5)
Total	119 (49.4)	81 (33.6)	41 (17.0)	241 (100)

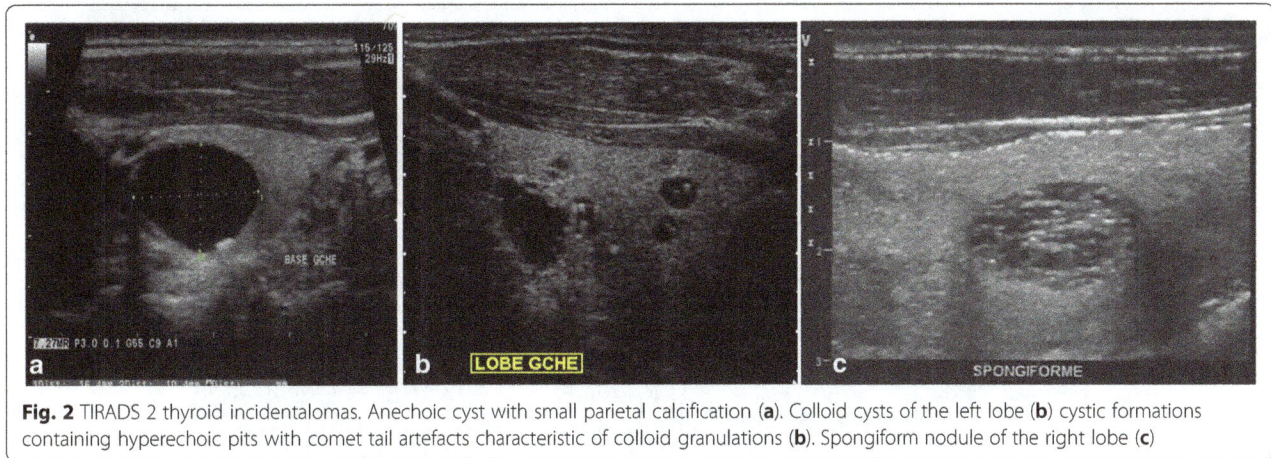

Fig. 2 TIRADS 2 thyroid incidentalomas. Anechoic cyst with small parietal calcification (**a**). Colloid cysts of the left lobe (**b**) cystic formations containing hyperechoic pits with comet tail artefacts characteristic of colloid granulations (**b**). Spongiform nodule of the right lobe (**c**)

The prevalence of TIs was 28.3% with 49.4% being cysts, and 87.1% classified TIRADS 2 or 3.

Population

Our population is comparable to those studied by Papini and al in Italy [2] and by Kim and al in Seoul [14], with female predominance. In our study women represented more than 2/3 of the population. This could be explained by the higher proportion of women referred to the imaging department, as well as in the general population in our setting.

The mean age in our study was 42 years. Papini and Kim [2, 14] had higher mean ages of 47.8 and 49.2 respectively.

Prevalence of thyroid incidentalomas on ultrasound examination

In our series, the prevalence of TIs was estimated at 28.3% compared to 27% in southern Finland [15]. This is slightly higher than the 22.4% reported by Olusola-Bello in Nigeria [11] and 21% by Kamran and al in Karachi, Pakistan [16], both in 2014. In 2009, in Germany, Guth and al [17] reported 68% prevalence with 53% < 5 mm. The prevalence therefore varies with age, sex, technology available (operator, probe frequency), the minimum size of nodules, and the presence or absence of iodine deficiency in the population. High resolution machines now permit the detection of much smaller nodules, a few millimeters in size [12].

Prevalence of TIs was significantly higher in females (33.3%; $p < 0.001$), than males (18.4%). This has been also reported by authors in Nigeria [11], Pakistan [16] and Iran [18]. It is generally known that the prevalence of TIs amongst females is four times that of males [10]. This prevalence increases with age, with maximum prevalence in persons > 60 years. TIs are considered as part of the physiologic aging process of the thyroid gland [10, 11, 15, 16]. This might also explain the increase in prevalence with age in our population.

Ultrasound characteristics of thyroid incidentalomas

The locations of TIs had a tendency to be in the right lobe (54%). This result was similar to the previous reports [2, 11, 16]. It might be explained by the difference of the native sizes between right and left lobes, that the right lobe was supposed to be 1.2 folds larger than the left [19–21].

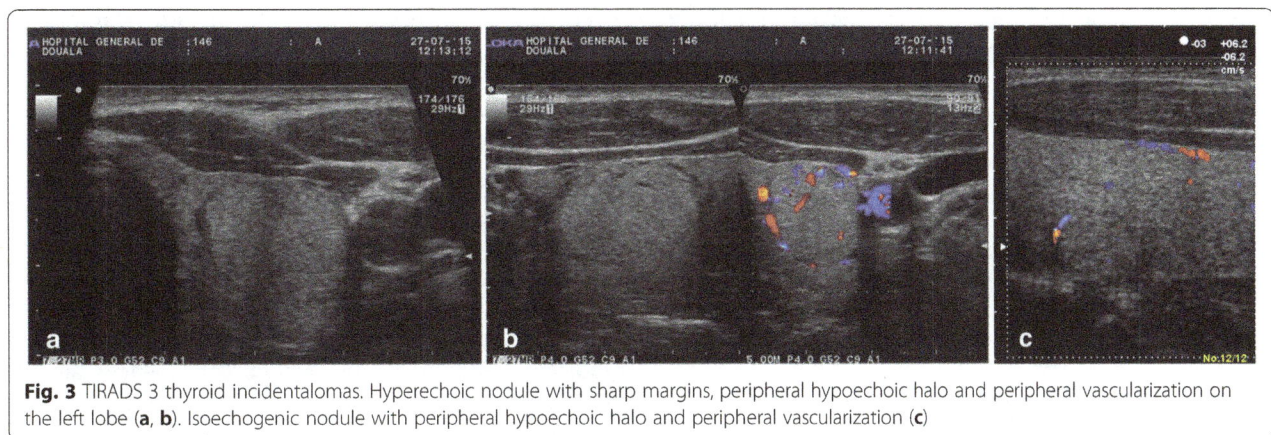

Fig. 3 TIRADS 3 thyroid incidentalomas. Hyperechoic nodule with sharp margins, peripheral hypoechoic halo and peripheral vascularization on the left lobe (**a**, **b**). Isoechogenic nodule with peripheral hypoechoic halo and peripheral vascularization (**c**)

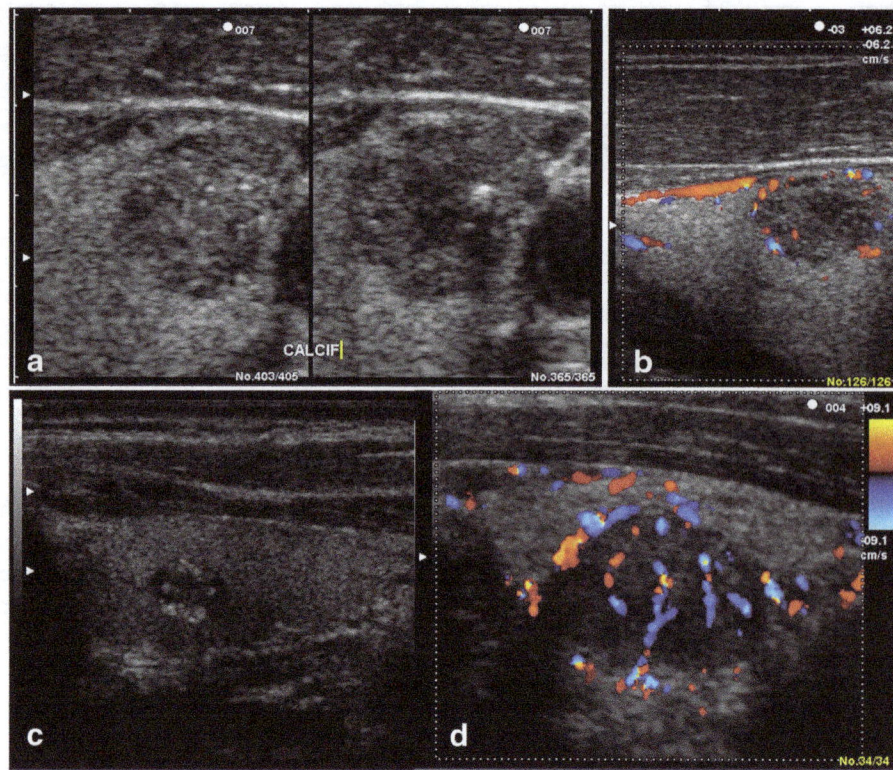

Fig. 4 TIRADS 4 incidentalomas. TIRADS 4A: a moderately hypoechoic solid nodule of sharp margins (**a**) with peripheral vascularization (**b**). TIRADS 4B: hypoechoic nodule with microcalcifications (**c**) and marked hypoechoic nodule with mixed vascularization (**d**)

Almost half of TIs were cystic in nature (49.4%) in line with other studies [7, 10, 11]. Solid nodules (33.61%) were mainly hyperechoic (42.0%). Other authors found a predominance of isoechoic or hyperechoic nodules too [2, 7, 14, 18, 22]. Characteristics to indicate malignant potentials were rare in our series (one case with lobulated margins, two cases with microcalcifications). Liebeskind and al [23] had similar findings. Different studies showed marked variability in the size of nodules. We found 22% of nodules ≥ 10 mm in our series, compared to 43% by Kamran and al [16] and 66.5% by Kim and al [14]. Fine needle aspiration is usually recommended for nodules ≥ 10 mm; those < 5 mm are usually transitory, difficult to characterize and to aspirate.

Table 4 TIRADS classification of thyroid incidentalomas with respect to tissue structure

Thyroid incidentalomas Classification	Cystic n (%)	Solid n (%)	Mixed n (%)	Total n (%)
TIRADS 2	116 (48.1)	1 (0.4)	12 (5.0)	129 (53.5)
TIRADS 3	3 (1.3)	56 (23.2)	22 (9.1)	81 (33.6)
TIRADS 4A	0 (0.0)	20 (8.3)	5 (2.1)	25 (10.4)
TIRADS 4B	0 (0.0)	4 (1.7)	2 (0.8)	6 (2.5)
Total	119 (49.4)	81 (33.6)	41 (17.0)	241 (100.0)

$(p < 0.001)$

TIRADS classification (Table 1) of thyroid incidentalomas

We had similar prevalence of TIRADS 2 nodules (54.5%) as Olusola-Bello and al (54.0%) in Nigeria [11]; these two populations share similar characteristics. The risk of malignancy in our series was 12.9%, which falls within the range of 7–15% described in existing literature [2, 3, 9, 14]. There was a significant association between risk of malignancy and solidity of nodules ($p < 0.000$): of the 31 nodules classified TIRADS 4, 77.4% were solid and 22.6% of mixed echogenicity. Solidity of nodules is considered suspicious of malignancy in the TIRADS classification, as opposed to purely cystic and spongiform nodules. There is also an association between size and risk of malignancy ($p < 0.001$), the prevalence of potentially malignant nodules increases with size (14.3% of TIRADS 4 nodules were 10–15 mm, 22% were > 15 mm). This reiterates the need for cytological examination of nodules > 10 mm whereas those < 5 mm do not need this [10, 14].

We did not find an association between the TIRADS score and age or sex. Capelli and al did not find a significant difference in the prevalence of malignant nodules among the two sexes [22]. Kim and al [14] reported a significantly higher prevalence among females who however represented 4/5 of their study population.

Table 5 Prevalence of TIRADS 4 thyroid incidentalomas with respect to size

Size	< 5 mm	5–9 mm	10–15 mm	>15 mm	Total
n (TIRADS 2, 3 and 4)	91	97	35	18	241
TIRADS 4A	8	11	3	3	25
TIRADS 4B	1	2	2	1	6
Malignant potential (4A + 4B)	9.9%	13.4%	14.3%	22.2%	12.9%

($P < 0.001$)

There were some limitations in this study: first this study was conducted in a hospital-based setting; and second no cytological analysis of nodules was performed because participants were either reticent to do so, or lost to follow up. A community based study may better determine the true prevalence of thyroid incidentalomas in the general population.

Conclusion

Thyroid incidentalomas were very frequent with a prevalence of 28.3% and a potential risk of malignancy in 12.9%. Prevalence had a tendency to be increased with age and female sex. Purely cystic nodules are the most frequent. Risks of malignancy would be increased for a larger size and would be higher for TIs of solid components.

Abbreviations
TI: Thyroid incidentalomas; TIRADS: Thyroid imaging reporting and data system

Acknowledgements
The authors wish to thank Dr Martine TCHUEM TCHUENTE for helping with the patients' selection and records.

Funding
None. The authors have no funding source to disclose.

Authors' contributions
BM conceived the study and participated in its design, data collection, statistical analysis and drafting of the manuscript. JRMT participated in the study design, review of the images and statistical analysis. SDF participated in data collection, the review of the images, statistical analysis and the drafting of the manuscript. FD participated in data collection and proof-reading of the manuscript. EMW participated in data collection and proof-reading of the manuscript. All authors read and approved the final version of the manuscript.

Competing interests
The authors declare that they have no competing interests.

Author details
[1]Department of Radiology and Radiation Oncology, Faculty of Medicine and Biomedical Sciences, The University of Yaounde 1, Yaounde, Cameroon. [2]Radiology Department YGOPH, Yaounde Gynaeco-Obstetric and Pediatric Hospital, PO Box 4362, Yaounde, Cameroon. [3]Yaounde University Teaching Hospital, Yaounde, Cameroon. [4]Douala General Hospital, Douala, Cameroon.

References
1. Wilhelm S. Evaluation of thyroid incidentaloma. Surg Clin North Am. 2014;94(3):485–97.
2. Papini E, Guglielmi R, Bianchini A, Crescenzi A, Taccogna S, Nardi F, et al. Risk of malignancy in nonpalpable thyroid nodules: predictive value of ultrasound and color-Doppler features. J Clin Endocrinol Metab. 2002;87(5):1941–6.
3. Kang HW, No JH, Chung JH, Min Y-K, Lee M-S, Lee M-K, et al. Prevalence, clinical and ultrasonographic characteristics of thyroid incidentalomas. Thyroid Off J Am Thyroid Assoc. 2004;14(1):29–33.
4. Hoang JK, Lee WK, Lee M, Johnson D, Farrell S. US Features of Thyroid Malignancy: Pearls and Pitfalls. RadioGraphics. 2007;27(3):847–60.
5. Kim KM, Park JB, Kang SJ, Bae KS. Ultrasonographic guideline for thyroid nodules cytology: single institute experience. J Korean Surg Soc. 2013;84(2):73–9.
6. Kwak JY, Han KH, Yoon JH, Moon HJ, Son EJ, Park SH, et al. Thyroid imaging reporting and data system for US features of nodules: a step in establishing better stratification of cancer risk. Radiology. 2011;260(3):892–9.
7. Russ G, Leboulleux S, Leenhardt L, Hegedüs L. Thyroid Incidentalomas: Epidemiology, Risk Stratification with Ultrasound and Workup. Eur Thyroid J. 2014;3(3):154–63.
8. Koike E, Noguchi S, Yamashita H, et al. Ultrasonographic characteristics of thyroid nodules: Prediction of malignancy. Arch Surg. 2001;136(3):334–7.
9. Moifo B, Takoeta EO, Tambe J, Blanc F, Fotsin JG. Reliability of Thyroid Imaging Reporting and Data System (TIRADS) Classification in Differentiating Benign from Malignant Thyroid Nodules. Open J Radiol. 2013;3(3):103–7.
10. Tramalloni J, Wémeau JL. Consensus français sur la prise en charge du nodule thyroïdien : ce que le radiologue doit connaître. EMC Radiol Imag Médicale Cardiovasc Thorac Cervicale. 2012;7(4):1–18.
11. Olusola-Bello MA, Agunloye AM, Adeyinka AO. Ultrasound prevalence and characteristics of incidental thyroid lesions in Nigerian adults. Afr J Med Med Sci. 2013;42(2):125–30.
12. Tramalloni J, Monpeyssen H. Échographie de la thyroïde. 01/2013 (2ème édition). ELSEVIER / MASSON; 2013. 191 p.
13. Russ G, Bigorgne C, Royer B, Rouxel A, Bienvenu-Perrard M. Le système TIRADS en échographie thyroïdienne. J Radiol. 2011;92(7–8):701–13.
14. Kim D-L, Song K-H, Kim SK. High prevalence of carcinoma in ultrasonography-guided fine needle aspiration cytology of thyroid nodules. Endocr J. 2008;55(1):135–42.
15. Karaszewski B, Wilkowski M, Tomasiuk T, Szramkowska M, Klasa A, Obołończyk L, et al. The prevalence of incidentaloma–asymptomatic thyroid nodules in the Tricity (Gdansk, Sopot, Gdynia) population. Endokrynol Pol. 2006;57(3):196–200.
16. Kamran M, Hassan N, Ali M, Ahmad F, Shahzad S, Zehra N. Frequency of thyroid incidentalomas in Karachi population. Pak J Med Sci. 2014;30(4):793–7.
17. Guth S, Theune U, Aberle J, Galach A, Bamberger CM. Very high prevalence of thyroid nodules detected by high frequency (13 MHz) ultrasound examination. Eur J Clin Invest. 2009;39(8):699–706.
18. Mohammadi A, Amirazodi E, Masudi S, Pedram A. Ultrasonographic Prevalence of Thyroid Incidentaloma in Bushehr, Southern Iran. Iran J Radiol. 2009;6(2):65–8.
19. Şahin E, Elboğa U, Kalender E. Regional reference values of thyroid gland volume in Turkish Adults. Srp Arh Celok Lek. 2015;143(3–4):141–5.
20. Müller-Leisse C, Tröger J, Khabirpour F, Pöckler C. Normal values of thyroid gland volume. Ultrasound measurements in schoolchildren 7 to 20 years of age. Dtsch Med Wochenschr 1946. 1988;113(48):1872–5.
21. Moifo B, Djomou F, Dongmo Fomekong S, Tapouh Jr M, Manka'a Wankie E, Bola A, Ndjolo A, Gonsu Fotsin J. Ultrasound biometrics of normal thyroid gland of Cameroonian adults. J Afr Imag Med. 2016;8(3):102–6.
22. Cappelli C, Castellano M, Pirola I, Cumetti D, Agosti B, Gandossi E, et al. The predictive value of ultrasound findings in the management of thyroid nodules. QJM. 2006;100(1):29–35.
23. Liebeskind A, Sikora AG, Komisar A, Slavit D, Fried K. Rates of malignancy in incidentally discovered thyroid nodules evaluated with sonography and fine-needle aspiration. J Ultrasound Med. 2005;24(5):629–34.

3

Evaluation of energy spectrum CT for the measurement of thyroid iodine content

Weiguang Shao[†], Jingang Liu[†] and Dianmei Liu[*]

Abstract

Background: This study aims to provide a reference for the diagnosis of iodine deficiency disorder by evaluating the normal thyroid iodine content by energy spectrum computed tomography (CT) and calculating the iodine content ratio of thyroid to sternocleidomastoid.

Methods: The thyroid glands of 226 patients were scanned by energy spectrum CT, and the images were analyzed using the GSI Viewer software. Based on the imaging findings, the iodine levels of the thyroid lobes as well as the bilateral sternocleidomastoids were evaluated, and their iodine content ratios were calculated.

Results: No statistically significant difference was found in the thyroid iodine content between the left and right thyroid lobes ($p > 0.05$). However, there was a significant difference in the thyroid iodine content between men and women ($p < 0.01$). Additionally, the thyroid iodine content was found to decrease gradually with age. The iodine content ratio of thyroid to sternocleidomastoid was 96.6271 ± 33.2442.

Conclusion: Gemstone energy spectrum CT can be used for the measurement of thyroid iodine content in the human body. It can play a significant role in the diagnosis of iodine deficiency disorder.

Keywords: Energy spectrum CT imaging, Thyroid, Iodine content

Background

Iodine, an essential trace element for the human body, is closely related to the thyroid and is essential for the synthesis of the thyroid hormones. Iodine deficiency or excess iodine can cause thyroid dysfunction [1, 2], leading to abnormal iodine content in the thyroid tissues, which results in disorders of the thyroid and other organs of the body [3–5]. The iodine intake levels of the thyroid and *in vivo* storage concentrations can be evaluated by measurement of the iodine content of the thyroid tissue. These values can be used to determine whether the thyroid dysfunction is caused by iodine deficiency or excess, which is clinically significant in the diagnosis of thyroid diseases [6]. Previously, the iodine content of the body was indirectly determined by the measurement of urine iodine levels [7, 8] and thyroid iodine absorption rates [9]. However, the iodine content of the thyroid glands cannot be measured by these methods. Thyroid iodine content can be determined by

the conversion of thyroid CT values; however, X-rays, which are used to achieve excitation in this process, have a limited spectral energy range, which inevitably leads to inaccuracies in the CT values, thus affecting the results of quantitative diagnosis [10, 11]. Gemstone energy spectrum CT is based on the differences in the X-ray attenuation coefficients of different materials. This technique can be used to obtain not only monoergic images, but also substance-separation images [12, 13]. Iodine-based substance separation images are very sensitive to iodine deposition and exhibit good resolution of tissues such as the thyroid gland; they can, therefore, be used for the quantification of the thyroid iodine content. In the present study, the possibility of energy spectrum CT iodine-based substance-separation imaging completely or partly replacing the previous methods for the measurement of thyroid iodine content was evaluated.

Methods

Subjects

Patients who underwent cervical and thyroid CT imaging between October 2010 and May 2011 were enrolled in this

* Correspondence: dianmeiliu@163.com
[†]Equal contributors
Department of Imaging Center, the Affiliated Hospital of Weifang Medical University, Weifang 261031, China

study. All of the patients had undergone energy spectrum CT imaging of the thyroid and sternocleidomastoid. None of the patients had received thyroid preparations, iodine products, or special foods such as laver, kelp, or seaweed. Patients with cysts, adenoma, calcifications, inflammation, and other disorders and/or dysfunctions of the thyroid were excluded. A total of 226 subjects between the ages of 18 and 77 years (mean age, 46 ± 17 years), including 119 male and 107 female patients were enrolled. This study was approved by the ethics committee of an affiliated hospital of the Weifang Medical College, and informed written consent had been obtained from all of the patients.

Computed tomography scanning and post-processing

Energy spectrum CT scanning was performed using the Discovery CT750 high definition (HD) scanner (GE Healthcare, Milwaukee, WI, USA), with the following scanning parameters: section thickness, 5.0 mm, with 5.0-mm intervals; thread interval, 0.984:1; speed, 39.37 mm/rotation; and rotation time, 0.8 s. The imaging data were reconstructed at a reconstruction thickness and interval of 0.625 mm and transmitted to AW4.4 workstations, where they were analyzed using the GSI viewer software. Monoergic images with optimal thyroid contrast-to-noise ratios (CNRs) were obtained from the energy spectrum curve. On the iodine-based substance-separation images, the largest thyroid layer was selected for the measurement of iodine content in the right and left thyroid lobes within 50 mm^2 circular areas. The iodine content was measured at two or three points on the upper pole of each lobe, and the mean value of these measurements was calculated. The iodine content in the bilateral sternocleidomastoids was also measured, and the iodine content ratio of thyroid to sternocleidomastoid was determined.

Statistical analysis

The data were recorded as the mean values ± standard deviations (SD) and analyzed using the SSPS v13.0 (Chicago IL, USA) software. Comparison of the thyroid iodine content between the male and female patients was performed using the t-test, while comparison of the thyroid iodine content among different age groups was performed by analysis of variance (F-test). Pairwise comparisons between the groups were performed using the SNK q-test. The level of significance of the test was determined at $\alpha = 0.05$, and statistical significance was determined at $p < 0.05$.

Results

Thyroid iodine content in the right and left lobes

A total of 226 right and 225 left thyroid lobes (because of one patient with an absent left lobe) were evaluated.

The mean iodine content in the left lobe was 1.5230 ± 0.4271 mg/cm^3 and that in the right lobe was 1.5236 ± 0.4365 mg/cm^3 (Table 1). The difference in iodine content between the right and left lobes was not statistically significant ($t = 0.0084$; $p > 0.05$).

Thyroid iodine content in male and female patients and iodine content ratio of thyroid to sternocleidomastoid

The mean value of the total iodine content in the thyroid glands was 1.5233 ± 0.4318 mg/cm^3. The difference in iodine content between the male and female patients was statistically significant ($t = 3.4743$; $p < 0.01$; Fig. 1 and Table 2). The iodine content ratio of thyroid to sternocleidomastoid (0.0161 ± 0.0615 mg/cm^3) was 96.6271 ± 33.2442, and it showed no statistically significant differences between the male and female patients ($t = 0.3817$; $p > 0.3817$; Fig. 1 and Table 2).

Optimal CNR of the thyroid glands

Monoergic images with optimal CNR of the thyroid glands against the sternocleidomastoid were achieved at 57.0167 ± 2.7647 keV (Fig. 2).

Thyroid iodine content in different age groups

The thyroid iodine content showed significant differences among the different age groups evaluated in the present study ($F = 9.66$; $p < 0.01$). Patients below 40 years of age had markedly higher thyroid iodine content than patients between the ages of 40 and 60 years and those above 60 years of age ($q = 5.6195$ and 5.6195, respectively; $p < 0.01$, both; Table 3). However, the difference in thyroid iodine content between patients between the ages of 40 and 60 years and those above 60 years of age was not statistically significant ($q = 0.3166$; $p > 0.3166$; Table 3).

Discussion
Characteristics of energy spectrum CT

Energy spectrum imaging was first studied in the 1970s [14]. This was followed by the clinical application of this research in dual energy imaging [15]. In the 2000s, it was almost possible to achieve substance separation with the dual-energy subtraction technique by means of CT scanning [16]. Using the instantaneous double kVp technique, it was possible to acquire a series of monoergic images at specific energy levels by means of energy spectrum CT in order to effectively avoid the beam

Table 1 Comparisons of the thyroid iodine content between the right and left lobes

	No. of cases	Iodine content (mg/cc)	t value	P value
Left lobe	225	1.5230 ± 0.4271	0.0084	0.9933
Right lobe	226	1.5236 ± 0.4365		

Data were shown as mean ± SD

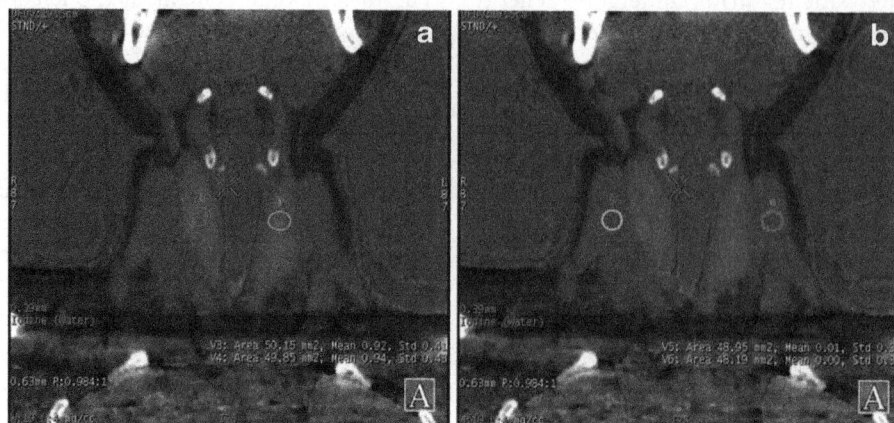

Fig. 1 a Was iodine-based image for determining the iodine content in thyroid glands. **b** was iodine-based image for determining the iodine content in bilateral sternocleidomastoids

hardening effect and improve the CNR of the images, thus obtaining stable and precise CT values. These advances resulted in the replacement of conventional CT, which is based on the variation of a single parameter, as the diagnostic modality of choice with energy and multi-parameter-based CT evaluation [17]. Image acquisition by CT is based on the attenuation of X-rays in the objects of interest. Each material has its own characteristic curve correlating the changes of the mass absorption coefficient with energy. Because of the inherent differences in their energy attenuation coefficients, different materials in an object can be identified and quantified by excitation at two different energy levels. This is the physical basis of substance-separation imaging [18]. By means of substance-separation imaging, each structure can be broken down into separate substances with different X-ray attenuation coefficients, following which, contrast images of these substances can be acquired and used for the qualitative analysis of the contents. Since iodine-based substance-separation imaging exhibits high sensitivity in the imaging of iodine deposits, it aids in better visualization of iodine-rich tissues such as the thyroid glands. Therefore, iodine-based thyroid density images can be used for the quantitative analysis of the iodine content of the thyroid glands.

Limitations of the previous evaluation methods

Thyroid iodine content accounts for about 20–50 % of the total iodine content of the human body. It has been reported that excessive iodine intake as well as its deficiency can lead to thyroid dysfunction, which exhibits a U-shaped relationship with iodine intake [19, 20]. Measurement of iodine content can reveal the amount of iodine reserve *in vivo* as well as the recent iodine intake levels. Previous determination methods mostly focused on the measurement of either urine iodine [7, 8] or the rate of thyroid iodine absorption [9]. However, the results obtained by such methods can be affected by the iodine content contributed by food and renal and gastrointestinal functions. The iodine content of the thyroid can also be analyzed by measurement of the CT values using a specific formula; however, the spectral range of X-rays is limited. Moreover, conventional CT image acquisition cannot effectively avoid the beam hardening effect in order to obtain stable and accurate CT values; this leads to inaccuracies in quantitative analysis [10, 11].

Advantages and clinical value of energy spectrum CT for the measurement of thyroid iodine content

Gemstone energy spectrum CT can be used to effectively determine the iodine content of the thyroid using iodine-based substance-separation images transformed from the X-ray attenuation curve. Errors due to inaccuracies of the CT values can be avoided, and accurate measurements of the iodine levels in the body can be obtained. Based on the results of specimen imaging studies by Li et al. [21], dual-energy CT can be considered

Table 2 Iodine content in thyroid and sternocleidomastoid of men and women

Groups	No. of cases	Iodine content (mg/cm^3)		Iodine ratio of thyroid to sternocleidomastoid
		Thyroid glands	Sternocleidomastoid	
Men	119	1.6395 ± 0.4105*	0.0175 ± 0.0635	94.6250 ± 37.3621
Women	107	1.4238 ± 0.3832	0.0145 ± 0.0613	98.0000 ± 29.0737

Data were shown as mean ± SD. *$P < 0.01$, compared with women

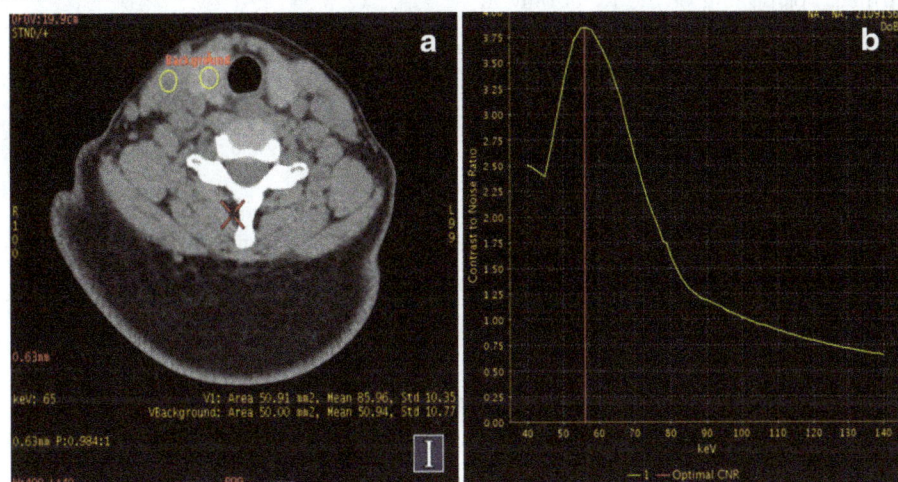

Fig. 2 a. Two ROIs were drawn in right thyroid gland and ipsilateral sternocleidomastoid respectively. **b**. Using the ipsilateral sternocleidomastoid as a contrast, the right thyroid gland had the best contrast to noise ratio (57 kev) to the surrounding tissues

as a promising quantitative approach for the differentiation of malignant and benign thyroid nodules. In the present study, the results of analysis of normal thyroid glands revealed no statistically significant differences in iodine content between the left and right thyroid lobes; however, significant differences in thyroid iodine content were observed between the male and female subjects, which might be associated with the differences in endocrine hormonal levels between the two sexes. We also found a gradual decline in the thyroid iodine content with increasing age, which suggests that thyroid function, including iodine reserve and uptake, exhibits a tendency to decline with age. The results of comparison among the different age groups revealed no significant differences in thyroid iodine content between patients between the ages of 40 and 60 years and those above 60 years of age. However, the thyroid iodine content of the patients of both groups was lower compared to that of the patients below 40 years of age, which indicates that thyroid function might start to decline from the age of 40. However, the relationship between age and thyroid function needs verification by further studies with larger sample sizes.

The iodine content ratio of thyroid to other tissues, which is normally about 100:1, is an important index in the diagnosis of iodine deficiency disorders; this ratio has been reported to be high as 400:1 in patients with iodine deficiency disorders [5]. In cases where the ratio is higher than 100:1, the concentration of iodine absorbed

should be evaluated. In cases where the ratio is close to 400:1, the patients are considered as exhibiting serious iodine deficiency. In the present study, the iodine content ratio of thyroid to sternocleidomastoid was 96.6271 ± 33.2442. Therefore, this value can be used as the reference for the diagnosis of iodine deficiency disorders by measurement of the thyroid iodine content by energy spectrum CT. Gemstone energy spectrum CT can be used not only to accurately measure the iodine content of the thyroid glands and determine the iodine content ratio of thyroid to sternocleidomastoid, but also to determine the volume of the thyroid glands and evaluate any complications because of other thyroid diseases. Thus, energy spectrum CT is more advantageous than conventional CT in the evaluation of thyroid function and morphology.

Limitations of this study

First, the sample size in the present study was too small, which resulted in the inclusion of subjects of a wide range of ages. Moreover, because of the small sample size, the age groups could not be evaluated in terms of sex-specific differences in thyroid iodine content. Further studies with larger sample sizes including higher numbers of subjects of each age group are required for obtaining more reliable results. Second, we positioned the ROIs only in the upper poles of the thyroid glands; however, whether the distribution of iodine is consistent across the entire thyroid gland

Table 3 Comparisons of thyroid iodine content among different age groups

Age groups	No. of cases	Iodine content (mg/cm^3)		q value	P value
<40 years (a)	59	1.7256 ± 0.4631	a vs. b	5.6195	<0.01
40 to 60 years (b)	96	1.4517 ± 0.3643	a vs. c	5.4158	<0.01
>60 years (c)	71	1.4368 ± 0.3465	b vs. c	0.3166	>0.05

has yet to be confirmed. Positioning of the ROIs only in the upper or lower poles of the thyroid gland might lead to inconsistency in the results. Third, the equipment used was expensive and involved the use of radioactive imaging agents. Therefore, its application in the routine screening of abnormal thyroid function might be challenging.

Conclusion

Gemstone energy spectrum CT can be used for the evaluation of thyroid iodine content in the human body. In the present study, imaging by this method revealed a gradual decrease in thyroid iodine content with age. Therefore, gemstone energy spectrum CT is a promising tool for the diagnosis of iodine deficiency disorder.

Abbreviations
CT, computed tomography; HD, high definition; CNR, contrast to noise ratio; SD, standard deviation.

Authors' contributions
DL designed and performed the study. She also reviewed and edited the manuscript; WS and JL acquired and analyzed the data and wrote the paper; all authors read and approved the final manuscript.

Competing interests
The authors declare that they have no competing interests.

References
1. Tan L, Sang Z, Shen J, Liu H, Chen W, Zhao N, et al. Prevalence of thyroid dysfunction with adequate and excessive iodine intake in Hebei Province, People's Republic of China. Public Health Nutr. 2014;17:1–6.
2. Yan YR, Liu Y, Huang H, Lv QG, Gao XL, Jiang J, et al. Iodine nutrition and thyroid diseases in Chengdu, China: an epidemiological study. QJM. 2014 [Epub ahead of print]
3. Sun X, Shan Z, Teng W. Effects of increased iodine intake on thyroid disorders. Endocrinol Metab (Seoul). 2014;29:240–7.
4. Hetzel BS. The development of a global program for the elimination of brain damage due to iodine deficiency. Asia Pac J Clin Nutr. 2012;21:164–70.
5. Chen ZP, Hetzel BS. Cretinism revisited. Best Pract Res Clin Endocrinol Metab. 2010;24:39–50.
6. Bürgi H. Iodine excess. J Best Pract Res Clin Endocrinol Metab. 2010;24:107–15.
7. World Health Organinzation, United Nations Children's Fund, International Council for Control of Iodine Deficiency Disorders. Assessment of iodine deficiency disorders and monitoring their elimination: a guide for programme managers. 3rd ed. Geneva: World Health Organinzation; 2007. p. 37–54.
8. Boasquevisque PC, Jarske RD, Dias CC, Quintaes IP, Santos MC, Musso C. Correlation between iodine urinary levels and pathological changes in thyroid glands. Arq Bras Endocrinol Metabol. 2013;57:727–32.
9. Narumi S, Nagasaki K, Ishii T, Muroya K, Asakura Y, Adachi M, et al. Nonclassic TSH resistance: TSHR mutation carriers with discrepantly high thyroidal iodine uptake. J Clin Endocrinol Metab. 2011;96:E1340–5.
10. Goodsitt MM, Christodoulou EG, Larson SC. Accuracies of the synthesized monochromatic CT numbers and effective atomic numbers obtained with a rapid kVp switching dual energy CT scanner. Med Phys. 2011;38:2222–32.
11. Wang L, Liu B, Wu XW, Wang J, Zhou Y, Wang WQ, et al. Correlation between CT attenuation value and iodine concentration in vitro: discrepancy between gemstone spectral imaging on single-source dual-energy CT and traditional polychromatic X-ray imaging. J Med Imaging Radiat Oncol. 2012;56:379–83.
12. Duan X, Wang J, Yu L, Leng S, McCollough CH. CT scanner x-ray spectrum estimation from transmission measurements. Med Phys. 2011;38:993–7.
13. Ascenti G, Siragusa C, Racchiusa S, Ielo I, Privitera G, Midili F, et al. Stone-targeted dual-energy CT: a new diagnostic approach to urinary calculosis. AJR Am J Roentgenol. 2010;195:953–8.
14. Chiro GD, Brooks RA, Kessler RM, Johnston GS, Jones AE, Herdt JR, et al. Tissue signatures with dual-energy computed tomography. Radiology. 1979;131:521–3.
15. Kalender WA, Klotz E, Suess C. Vertebral bone mineral analysis: an integrated approach with CT. Radiology. 1987;164:419–23.
16. Flohr TG, McCollough CH, Bruder H, Petersilka M, Gruber K, Süss C, et al. First performance evaluation of a dual-source CT (DSCT) system. Eur Radiol. 2006;16:256–68.
17. Zhang D, Li X, Liu B. Objective characterization of GE discovery CT750 HD scanner: gemstone spectral imaging mode. Med Phys. 2011;38:1178–88.
18. Anderson NG, Butler AP, Scott NJ, Cook NJ, Butzer JS, Schleich N, et al. Spectroscopic (multi-energy) CT distinguishes iodine and barium contrast material in MICE. Eur Radiol. 2010;20:2126–34.
19. Markou K, Georgopoulos N, Kyriazopoulou V, Vagenakis AG. Iodine-induced hypothyroidism. Thyroid. 2001;11:501–10.
20. Roti E, Uberti ED. Iodine excessive and hyperthyroidism. Thyroid. 2001;11:493–500.
21. Li M, Zheng XP, Li JY, Yang YL, Lu C, Xu H, et al. Dual-energy computed tomography imaging of thyroid nodule specimens: comparison with pathologic findings. Invest Radiol. 2012;47(1):58–64.

4

Characterization of ten white matter tracts in a representative sample of Cuban population

D. Góngora[1,2]*, M. Domínguez[3] and M. A. Bobes[1,2]

Abstract

Background: The diffusion tensor imaging technique (DTI) combined with tractography methods, has achieved the tridimensional reconstruction of white matter tracts in the brain. It allows their characterization in vivo in a non-invasive way. However, one of the largest sources of variability originates from the location of regions of interest, is therefore necessary schemes which make it possible to establish a protocol to be insensitive to variations in drawing thereof. The purpose of this paper is to stablish a reliable protocol to reconstruct ten prominent tracts of white matter and characterize them according to volume, fractional anisotropy and mean diffusivity. Also we explored the relationship among these factors with gender and hemispheric symmetry.

Methods: This study aims to characterize ten prominent tracts of white matter in a representative sample of Cuban population using this technique, including 84 healthy subjects. Diffusion tensors and subsequently fractional anisotropy and mean diffusivity maps were calculated from each subject's DTI scans. The trajectory of ten brain tracts was estimated by using deterministic tractography methods of fiber tracking. In such tracts, the volume, the FA and MD were calculated, creating a reference for their study in the Cuban population. The interactions between these variables with age, cerebral hemispheres and gender factors were explored using Repeated Measure Analysis of Variance.

Results: The volume values showed that a most part of tracts have bigger volume in left hemisphere. Also, the data showed bigger values of MD for males than females in all the tracts, an inverse behavior than FA values.

Conclusions: This work showed that is possible reconstruct white matter tracts using a unique region of interest scheme defined from standard to native space. Also, this study indicates differing developmental trajectories in white matter for males and females and the importance of taking gender into account in developmental DTI studies and in underlie gender-related cognitive differences.

Keywords: Diffusion tensor imaging, Volume, Fractional anisotropy, Mean diffusivity, White matter tracts

Background

The ability to identify and characterize the nerve fiber tracts that connect nodes (functional areas) is crucial to advance the understanding of brain function in both normal and pathological conditions. Nuclear Magnetic Resonance conventional techniques are able to distinguish specific white matter tracts only in small and restricted areas of the brain [1, 2]. However, using Diffusion Tensor Images (DTI) and processing techniques developed for the layout of the fibers, it has been possible to delineate and reconstruct three-dimensional fiber tracts of white matter, with a good agreement with anatomical data [3, 4]. This procedure, known as tractography, has opened a new window on the important topic of brain connectivity [5].

Based on DTI and applying a deterministic method dubbed Fiber Assignment by Continuous Tracking (FACT), the tractography allows the approximated reconstruction of white matter fibers, advancing from voxel by voxel, according to an estimate of the local

* Correspondence: daylin.gongora@gmail.com
[1]Key Laboratory for NeuroInformation of Ministry of Education, Center for Information in Medicine, University of Electronic Science and Technology of China, 2006, Xiyuan Ave, West Hi-Tech Zone, Chengdu 61000, China
[2]Cuban Neuroscience Center, 190th Ave between 25th and 27th Ave, Havana 11300, Cuba
Full list of author information is available at the end of the article

orientation of nerve fibers [4]. Here, the aforementioned estimation of the fiber path stops when it reaches the outer volume limits, a region where fractional anisotropy or some index of inter-voxel coherence is less than certain threshold values for which the uncertainty is considered high by taking a direction to follow, or up to a pre-selected region of interest [6].

The FACT method allows a good characterization of white matter tracts. In healthy subjects, this characterization is required to permit patterns analysis of brain connectivity, and to make comparisons with pathological conditions. The main white matter tracts have been successfully reconstructed in healthy subjects. However, it was used small samples (less than 30 subjects), mostly Caucasian populations without emphasis in variables that characterize the peculiarities of each tract [7–9].

In tractography, one of the largest sources of variability originates from the location of regions of interest (ROIs). ROIs are defined a priori as anatomical regions from which identify specific tracts [10]. It is therefore necessary ROIs schemes which make it possible to establish a protocol to be insensitive to variations in drawing thereof. This problem has been addressed in previous studies that have defined a set of tract-specific ROIs allowing the reproducible reconstruction of white matter tracts [7–9].

Practical applications of tractography have unquestionable value, for example in case of neurosurgery, where it provides guidance in preoperative planning [11, 12]. In this regard, to establish and validate reconstruction procedures of trajectories of white matter tracts in humans, reproducible between subjects, is crucial to allow an understandable use of this technique.

Given this background and the fact that there are variations in brain anatomy in terms of factors such as hemispheric symmetry, gender and studied population [13], the purpose of this paper is to reconstruct ten prominent tracts of white matter and characterize them according to volume, Fractional Anisotropy (FA) and Mean Diffusivity (MD). Also we explored the relationship among these factors with gender and hemispheric symmetry.

Methods
Sample
The sample included 84 healthy subjects who are part of the Cuban Project of Human Brain Mapping. This sample was made up of randomly selected subjects of the population of the municipality of La Lisa, Havana. This population is considered representative in terms of ethnic and gender distribution of the Cuban population. Participants were included in the study after reading,

accepting and sign an informed consent, in accordance with the ethical standards of the Declaration of Helsinki [14], and the experimental protocols were approved by the Ethics Committee of Cuban Neuroscience Center. A statistical description of the sample is presented in Table 1.

The total sample consisted of right handed subjects with an intelligence quotient (IQ) within the range reported as normal. IQ was obtained for each subject using the Spanish language version of the Wechsler Adult Intelligence III Scale [15].

Each subject underwent an interview and medical examination with Neurology and Psychiatry specialists, in order to rule out any pathology of the nervous system to invalidate their participation in the study. Neurological examination was performed following the procedure described in guidelines published by the Department of Health and Human Services U.S. in 2003. Mini-International Psychiatric Interview was used for psychiatric evaluation [16].

Acquisition of images
Using a scanner Siemens Symphony 1.5 T (Erlangen, Germany) was acquired for each subject a T1 anatomical image of high resolution 3D, and a standard scheme of diffusion gradients. The T1 anatomical image was recorded with the following characteristics: 160 contiguous sagittal slices 1 mm thick, field of view (FOV) = 256 × 256 mm^2, corresponding to a resolution in sagittal plane of 1×1 mm^2, echo time (ET) = 3.93 ms, repetition time (RT) = 3000 ms. Using a single echo planar imaging (EPI) sequence, twelve diffusion-weighted images were obtained (b = 1200 s/mm^2) and a reference T2 weighted image (b0 image) with no diffusion weighting (b = 0 s/mm^2). The acquisition parameters were: FOV = 256 × 256 mm^2, acquired matrix = 128 × 128, corresponding to a resolution in the axial plane of 2×2 mm^2, ET/RT = 160/7000 ms. The slice number was adapted to cover the whole brain with a slice thickness of 3 mm. The acquisition scheme was repeated 5 times to average the corresponding images and thus improving the signal/noise ratio.

In order to correct the distortions caused by magnetic field inhomogeneities in the series of diffusion-weighted images, phase and magnitude maps were obtained. The parameters used were: voxel size of 3.5 mm; ET_1 = 7.71 ms, ET_2 = 12.47 ms and RT = 672 ms.

Table 1 Statistical description of the sample

	Subjects (n)	School level[a]	Age[a]	Intelligence quotient[a]
Women	44	12.44 ± 2.46	38.75 ± 9.95	91.14 ± 11.87
Men	40	11.78 ± 2.44	31.00 ± 8.97	90.72 ± 11.44
Total	84	12.12 ± 2.46	35.06 ± 10.21	90.94 ± 11.60

[a]Mean values ± standard deviation

Processing diffusion weighted images

On b0 images was detected the presence of Gibbs artifacts around the ventricles. To correct these artifacts a Hanning filter was applied to these images. Then, Eddy currents correction was made by linear recording of weighted images to b0. Using the images of magnitude and phase, and Unwarping package of SPM5 program (http://www.fil.ion.ucl.ac.uk/spm/) the effects of main magnetic field inhomogeneities were corrected [17].

Estimation of the diffusion tensor and fiber tracking

The toolbox DTI & Fiber Tools v.3.0 [18] was utilized to estimate at each voxel the six elements of the diffusion tensor as formulated by Basser et al. [19]. After tensor diagonalization, three eigenvalues and eigenvectors were obtained and calculated FA and MD maps.

Three-dimensional reconstruction of the tracts was performed using FACT, a deterministic tractography method [4]. The parameters used in tracts reconstruction were for the beginning of traced FA threshold = 0.15 and Trace = 0.0016, and as a stop criteria FA = 0.10, Trace = 0.002 and maximum bending angle of 53.1 °.

The fiber tracking was performed in all brain voxels, and fibers that penetrated the previously defined ROIs were assigned to specific tracts associated with them. ROIs were defined for the following tracts: anterior thalamic radiation (ATR), cingulate gyrus associated cingulum (CGC), hippocampal gyrus associated cingulum (CGH), cortico-spinal tract (CST), inferior fronto-occipital fasciculus (IFOF), inferior longitudinal fasciculus (ILF), superior longitudinal fasciculus (SLF), uncinate fasciculus (UNC), forceps major (Fmj) and forceps minor (Fmn). The resulting path of these tracts were visually inspected and corrected in cases where necessary, by the exclusion of fibers that do not belongs anatomically to tracts.

Definition of ROIs in standard space and space transformation procedure to each subject anatomical space

Definition of ROIs for studied tracts was made by replicating a set of predefined ROI by Mori et al. [8] that was employed successfully in subsequent work [7, 9, 20, 21]. These ROIs were drawn using the program MRIcron (http://www.mccauslandcenter.sc.edu/crnl/mricron/) on a reference anatomical image with spatial resolution of $1 \times 1 \times 1$ mm^3 in stereotactic space of the Montreal Neurological Institute (MNI) [22]. The ROIs were then transformed to each individual brain space automatically, using a programmed routine in MatLab v.7.7 (MathWorks, Inc.).

Parameter estimation

Voxels that conformed each one of the estimated tracts were extracted. The volume of each tract was estimated by multiplication of the total number of voxels of each tract by a voxel volume (0.012 cm^3). The FA and MD was obtained as an estimate of the average in each tract, which resulted from the superposition of the specific coordinates for each tract on the corresponding maps of FA and MD.

Statistical analysis

The tracts were explored according to volume, FA and MD values using the Statistica software v.10.0 (StatSoft, Inc.) and was considered a level of significance of $\alpha = 0.05$ in all cases. The differences between hemispheres and gender were assessed using the General Lineal Model (GLM) for Repeated Measure Analysis of Variance (rmANOVA), considering the factors Gender, Age, Tracts and Hemisphere; the last two factors were used as within effects, Gender as categorical predictor and Age as continuous predictor. A Greenhouse and Geisser [23] correction was applied. Planned comparisons were performed subsequently by specific contrasts. The inter-hemispheric tracts (Fmj and Fmn) were excluded from hemispheric asymmetries analysis.

Results

Reconstruction of the tracts of interest

The reconstruction of the tracts of interest was possible using the deterministic method FACT and ROIs obtained for each subject by the transformation proceeding of reconstruction of the trajectory proposed for ten tracts of interest in each of the 84 subjects enrolled in the study. These tracts were classified for description in four functional categories: brainstem fibers and projection, association fibers, tracts of the limbic system and commissural fibers (See Additional file 1).

Characterization of reconstructed tracts

White matter tracts were characterized anatomically estimating the volume, FA and MD for each tract. The mean values in each tract are presented in Table 2. The average volume of studied tracts ranged from 5 to 38 cm^3, in correspondence with the anatomical characteristics of each one. The FA values in the sample ranged from 0.34 to 0.58. The MD, meanwhile, it was distributed in a range of values from 0.54×10^{-3} to 0.7×10^{-3} mm^{2}s^{-1}.

Gender differences and hemispheric asymmetries

In this paper we assessed if volume, FA and MD values had the same statistical behavior regarding hemisphere and gender using the GLM for rmANOVA, also the age was used as continuous predictor. However, no effect of

Table 2 Statistical description of Volume, FA and MD in the sample

		Volume (cm³)[a]	FA[a]	MD (×10⁻³mm²s⁻¹)[a]
Anterior thalamic radiation (ATR)	Left	16.18 ± 6.04	0.44 ± 0.07	0.63 ± 0.14
	Right	11.93 ± 4.43	0.48 ± 0.08	0.59 ± 0.15
Cingulate gyrus associated cingulum (CGC)	Left	6.62 ± 3.00	0.42 ± 0.07	0.58 ± 0.16
	Right	5.42 ± 2.97	0.40 ± 0.05	0.60 ± 0.14
Hippocampal gyrus associated cingulum (CGH)	Left	5.69 ± 3.11	0.36 ± 0.09	0.68 ± 0.21
	Right	6.52 ± 4.30	0.35 ± 0.08	0.70 ± 0.19
Cortico-spinal tract (CST)	Left	5.93 ± 3.39	0.56 ± 0.08	0.64 ± 0.15
	Right	5.13 ± 3.07	0.58 ± 0.10	0.62 ± 0.18
Forceps major (Fmj)		22.98 ± 9.89	0.52 ± 0.06	0.61 ± 0.16
Forceps minor (Fmn)		38.27 ± 10.90	0.45 ± 0.07	0.62 ± 0.17
Inferior fronto-occipital fasciculus (IFOF)	Left	23.88 ± 8.59	0.48 ± 0.09	0.58 ± 0.16
	Right	26.96 ± 8.18	0.45 ± 0.07	0.60 ± 0.15
Inferior longitudinal fasciculus (ILF)	Left	12.59 ± 5.54	0.47 ± 0.09	0.59 ± 0.17
	Right	9.97 ± 4.57	0.46 ± 0.09	0.60 ± 0.15
Superior longitudinal fasciculus (SLF)	Left	16.87 ± 5.79	0.47 ± 0.09	0.54 ± 0.16
	Right	12.40 ± 6.22	0.46 ± 0.08	0.55 ± 0.15
Uncinate fasciculus (UNC)	Left	7.81 ± 3.37	0.37 ± 0.08	0.62 ± 0.17
	Right	7.11 ± 3.74	0.38 ± 0.07	0.63 ± 0.17

[a]Mean values ± standard deviation

age was found in the analysis. Subsequently, multiple comparisons were performed across specific contrasts of significant parameters in the model.

Volume

The GLM Repeated Measure ANOVA using Tracts volume as repeated measures, Gender as categorical predictor and Age as continuous predictor showed that exist a main effect of Tracts volume ($F = 26.40$, df = 17, $p < 0.001$, $\varepsilon = 0.425$) and Gender ($F = 11.98$, df = 1, $p = 0.001$) (Fig. 1). The double interaction Tracts x Gender was significant ($F = 5.929$, df = 17, $p < 0.001$, $\varepsilon = 0.425$). The planned comparison analysis showed that the volume in female are significant larger than males for left ATR ($F(1,81) = 22.366$; $p < 0.001$), right ATR ($F(1,81) = 7.958$; $p = 0.006$), right CGH ($F(1,81) = 5.609$; $p = 0.020$), Fmj ($F(1,81) = 21.654$; $p < 0.001$) and Fmn ($F(1,81) = 12.896$; $p < 0.001$). The remaining tracts had larger volumes in females than males with no significant differences, with the exception of right CST and right UNC which presented larger volume for males (Fig. 1).

Excluding the commissural tracts, Fmj and Fmn, hemispheric asymmetries in volume were assessed by GLM Repeated Measure ANOVA using Tracts volume and Hemisphere as repeated measures, Gender as categorical predictor and Age as continuous predictor, showed that exist a main effect of Tracts ($F = 19.69$, df = 7, $p < 0.001$, $\varepsilon = 0.618$) and Hemisphere ($F = 11.9$,

df = 1, $p < 0.001$). The double interaction Tracts x Hemisphere ($F = 2.041$, df = 7, $p < 0.05$) were significant. Planned comparison showed that the volume in the left hemisphere is larger than the right in both genders for the following tracts: ATR ($F(1,81) = 52.461$; $p < 0.001$), CGC ($F(1,81) = 15.28$; $p < 0.001$), CST ($F(1,81) = 4.608$; $p = 0.035$), ILF ($F(1,81) = 18.968$; $p < 0,001$) and SLF ($F(1,81) = 34.558$; $p < 0.001$).On the contrary, the volume in the right hemisphere was larger in CGH ($F(1,81) = 5.624$, $p = 0.02$) and the IFOF ($F(1,81) = 12.377$; $p < 0,001$). No significant differences between hemispheres in the volume of UNC were founded.

Fractional anisotropy

The GLM Repeated Measure ANOVA using FA values (of each tract) as repeated measures, Gender as categorical predictor and Age as continuous predictor (Fig. 2) showed that exist a main effect of FA values ($F = 10.489$, df = 17, $p < 0.001$, $\varepsilon = 0.562$) and Gender ($F = 47.31$, df = 1, $p < 0.001$), with a significant interaction FA values x Gender ($F = 4.15$, df = 17, $p < 0.001$, $\varepsilon = 0.569$). The data showed bigger values of FA for females than males in all the tracts. By planned comparison analysis were found significant differences for left ATR ($F(1,80) = 39.628$; $p < 0.001$) and right ATR ($F(1,80) = 33.143$, $p < 0.001$), left CGC ($F(1,80) = 38.909$; $p < 0.001$) and right CGC ($F(1,80) = 24.015$; $p < 0.001$), left CGH ($F(1,80) = 30.044$; $p < 0.001$) and right CGH ($F(1,80) = 31.322$; $p < 0.001$),

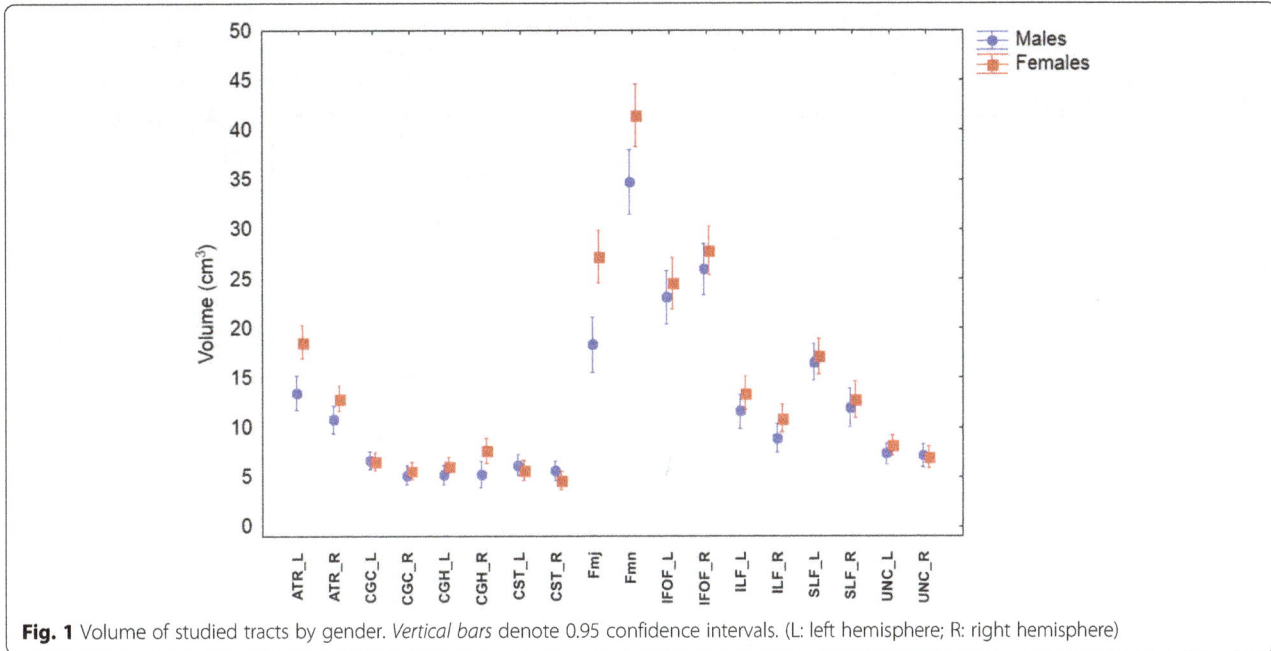

Fig. 1 Volume of studied tracts by gender. *Vertical bars* denote 0.95 confidence intervals. (L: left hemisphere; R: right hemisphere)

left CST (F(1,80) = 30.110; $p < 0.001$) and right CST (F(1,80) = 24.472; $p < 0.001$), Fmj (F(1,80) = 38.574; $p < 0.001$) and Fmn (F(1,80) = 40.929; $p < 0.001$), left IFOF (F(1,80) = 44.069; $p < 0.001$) and right IFOF (F(1,80) = 41.909; $p < 0.001$), left ILF (F(1,80) = 39.534; $p < 0,001$) and right ILF (F(1,80) = 34.545; $p < 0.001$), left SLF (F(1,80) = 45.333; $p < 0.001$) and right SLF (F(1,80) = 48.343; $p < 0,001$), left UNC (F(1,80) = 47.514; $p < 0.001$) and right UNC (F(1,80) = 46.738; $p < 0.001$) (Fig. 2).

Excluding the commissural tracts, Fmj and Fmn, hemispheric asymmetries in FA values were assessed by

GLM Repeated Measure ANOVA using FA values (of each tract) and Hemisphere as repeated measures, Gender as categorical predictor and Age as continuous predictor showed that exist a main effect of FA ($F = 28.629$, df = 7, $p < 0.001$, $\varepsilon = 0.769$) and no effect for Hemisphere ($F = 0.134$, df = 1, $p = 0.516$, $\varepsilon = 1$); however, de double interaction FA values x Hemisphere was significant ($F = 4.787$, df = 7, $p < 0.001$, $\varepsilon = 0.709$). Planned comparison showed that CGC (F(1,80) = 8.237, $p < 0.005$), CGH (F(1,80) = 7.916; $p < 0.005$), IFOF (F(1,80) = 92.369; $p < 0.001$), ILF (F(1,80) = 7.492; $p < 0.005$) have a left

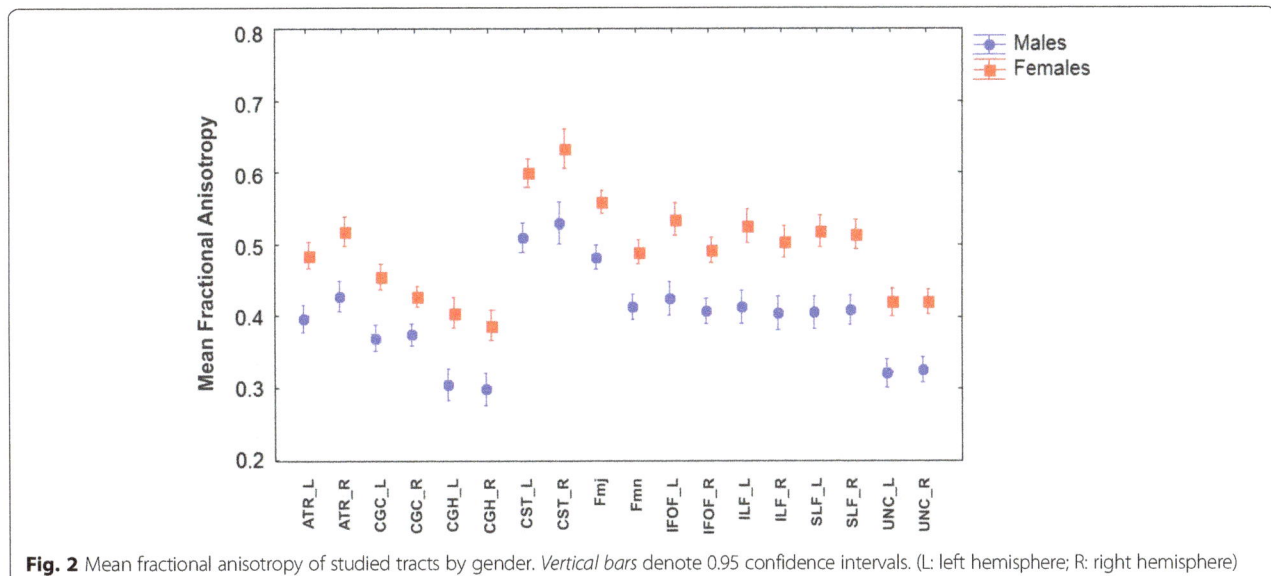

Fig. 2 Mean fractional anisotropy of studied tracts by gender. *Vertical bars* denote 0.95 confidence intervals. (L: left hemisphere; R: right hemisphere)

asymmetry (FA in left hemisphere > FA in the right hemisphere). On the contrary ATR (F(1,80) = 115.629; $p < 0.001$) and CST (F(1,80) = 20.621; $p < 0.001$) showed a right asymmetry. No significant differences between hemispheres in the FA values of SLF and UNC were founded.

Mean diffusivity

The GLM Repeated Measure ANOVA using MD values (of each tract) as repeated measures, Gender as categorical predictor and Age as continuous predictor (Fig. 3) showed that exist a main showed that exist a main effect of MD values ($F = 10.069$, df = 17, $p < 0.001$, $\varepsilon = 0.382$) and Gender ($F = 55.40$, df = 1, $p < 0.001$) with a significant interaction MD values x Gender ($F = 9.000$, df = 17, $p < 0.001$, $\varepsilon = 0.382$). The data showed bigger values of MD for males than females in all the tracts.

By planned comparison analysis were found significant differences for left ATR (F(1,80) = 48.650; p <0.001) and right ATR (F(1,80) = 50.375; $p < 0.001$), left CGC (F(1,80) = 54.193; $p < 0.001$) and right CGC (F(1,80) = 50.140; $p < 0.001$), left CGH (F(1,80) = 50.333; $p < 0.001$) and right CGH (F(1,80) = 43.136; $p < 0.001$), left CST (F(1,80) = 42.762; $p < 0.001$) and right CST (F(1,80) = 41.220; $p < 0.001$), Fmj (F(1,80) = 56.279; $p < 0.001$) and Fmn (F(1,80) = 57.800; $p < 0.001$), left IFOF (F(1,80) = 55.654; $p < 0.001$) and right IFOF (F(1,80) = 56.077; $p < 0.001$), left ILF (F(1,80) = 51.929; $p < 0.001$) and right ILF (F(1,80) = 59.954; $p < 0.001$), left SLF (F(1,80) = 57.911; $p < 0.001$) and right SLF (F(1,80) = 61.; $p < 0.001$), left UNC (F(1,80) = 61.483; $p < 0.001$) and right UNC (F(1,80) = 57.729; $p < 0.001$) (Fig. 3).

Excluding the commissural tracts, Fmj and Fmn, hemispheric asymmetries in MD values were assessed by GLM Repeated Measure ANOVA using MD values (of each tract) and Hemisphere as repeated measures showed that exist a main effect of MD values ($F = 14.643$, df = 7, $p < 0.001$, $\varepsilon = 0.476$) and no effect for Hemisphere ($F = 0.805$, df = 1, $p = 0.372$, $\varepsilon = 1$); however, de double interaction FA values x Hemisphere was significant ($F = 4.175$, df = 7, $p < 0.001$, $\varepsilon = 0.599$).

Planned comparison showed that CGC (F(1,80) = 31.748; $p < 0.001$), CGH (F(1,80) = 15.253; $p < 0.001$), IFOF (F(1,80) = 97.012; $p < 0.001$), ILF (F(1,80) = 5.320; $p < 0.023$) have a right asymmetry (MD in the right hemisphere > MD in left hemisphere). No significant differences between hemispheres in the MD values, SLF and UNC were founded despite of their right asymmetry. On the contrary ATR (F(1,80) = 122.194; $p < 0.001$) and CST (F(1,80) = 7.333; $p = 0.008$) showed a left asymmetry.

Discussion

Reconstruction of the tracts of interest

The tridimensional reconstruction of ten tracts of white matter was achieved in a representative sample of Cuban population. The protocol included ROIs in a native space of each individual and the tractography method known as FACT. The trajectories obtained agree with neuro-anatomic descriptions derivate from post-morten and other tractographic studies [8, 21, 24, 25].

The ROIs that defined tracts's trajectories were drawn on anatomical reference image from MNI steoreotaxic space according to the anatomical description reported for Mori et al. [8] and validated for Wakana et al. [7, 21]. Our data probed their reliability. These authors drawn the ROIs on each individual brain; however, we drawn the ROIs on MNI space and automatically were transformed to native space of each individual allowing the optimization of ROIs procedure and diminish the time needed for their analysis and the inter-subject variability.

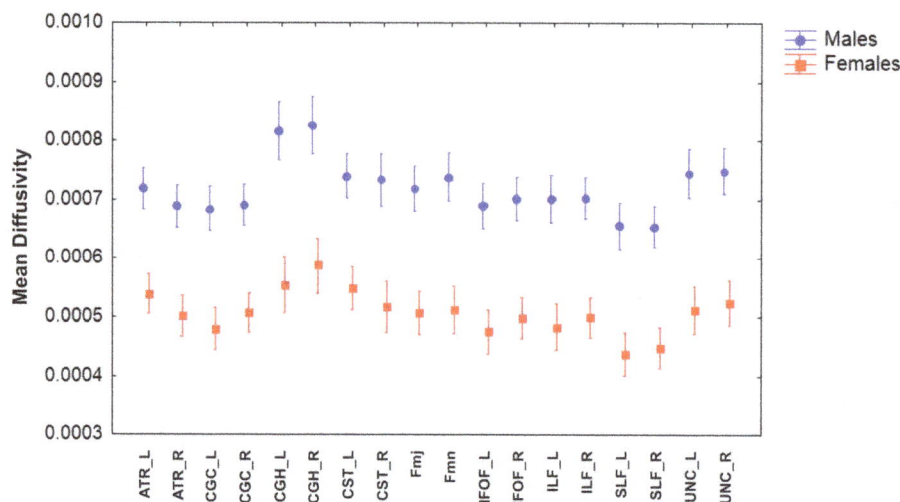

Fig. 3 Mean diffusivity of studied tracts by gender. *Vertical bars* denote 0.95 confidence intervals. (L: left hemisphere; R: right hemisphere)

Also this analysis begins from the total tracking of the all brain, and posteriorly the tracts were select using the ROIs. This approach produces a nice balance of fibers density [26] along the resultant tract giving reliability to the results.

The tracking method used (FACT) has been previously validated in several studies but they mostly use this algorithm as a tool for study white matter tracts in pathological conditions (e.g. [27–29]). Only a few reports have been dedicated to standardize and reproduce a methodology using this method for study many tracts at the same time and in healthy subjects [7–9, 21]. In cases where this kind of study was made, the sample used was small (less than 30 subjects). In this work it was achieve to replicate the reconstruction of several white matter tracts in a wide sample of healthy subjects ($n = 84$).

Characterization of reconstructed tracts

Previously, the parameters volume, FA and MD have been used to characterize white matter tracts [21, 30], being this paper a reference of these parameters in Cuban population.

The volume of studied tracts include a wide range of values (from five to 38 cm^3) as has been describe anteriorly [31]. The values of FA can vary widely according to register parameters and methodology applied, however the values of this study (0.34 FA 0.58) agree with the range of values reported for this variable in white matter tracts reconstructed by Wakana et al. [21] (0.42 FA 0.60). The values of MD varied between 18×10^{-5} and 23×10^{-5}, also were included in reported values [32].

All the reconstructed tracts show an inverse relationship pattern between FA and MD. This situation is not a trivial issue due to the MD value is similar between white matter of high anisotropy and gray matter of low anisotropy [33] moving into a narrow range of values. Only in case of cerebrospinal fluid take high values [34, 35] due to isotropic diffusion and free of barriers, producing high autovalues of diffusion tensor in all directions of water molecules [36, 37]; this phenomenon does not occur in gray matter where the water is restricted because of tissue properties. However, in white matter, the diffusion is anisotropic because of the packing of fibers and myelin presence [5], remaining MD low due to the small diffusion values in the perpendicular axis to the fiber directionality compensate that high diffusion in parallel axis to the fiber directionality. In this way, the mean of the autovalues of diffusion tensor remains low in white matter, because of that the MD can be used as a measure of presence of tissue. Otherwise, tracts constituted for fiber without an orientation pattern, myelin or packing structure will have low FA and high MD favoring the free diffusion. The unified using of FA and MD can be used as diagnostic tools in assess micro and meso-structural characteristic of brain tissue [38].

The tractography method FACT has some restrictions such as the acceptable angle between one voxel and the next one for a fiber trajectory, that can produce an underestimation in curved tracts (e.g. SLF and UNC) affecting the volume values. Also the volume estimation can be affected in fibers with bifurcation areas (e.g. IFOF) because the method can fail in estimate the way of the fibers. A presence of partial volume effects could affect the diffusion index due to mix of different kind of tissue in a voxel.

Gender differences and hemispheric asymmetries
Volume

Several studies have demonstrated the existence of differences in hemispheric symmetry of the volume of gray matter structures and gender differences in the adult population [39–41]; however, there are limited studies that have addressed these issues to the white matter [21, 42].

Statistical analysis showed gender differences with larger volume in females than males for left and right ATR, right CGH, Fmj and Fmn, and right ILF. However, previously studies described a higher volume of white matter in males than females [43, 44]. In these studies, were compared the segmentations of white matter from T1 images and not the specific tract volume, therefore the differences in white matter volume between gender seems to be heterogeneous along each tracts of brain. Because of that, the study of specific tracts using DTI can be a more accurately approach to this matter. On the other hand, a global analysis of white matter volume shows bigger values in males [41], using correction for total intracranial volume, although was founded a paralleled slope for grey and white matter with cranial volume, whereas in women the increase in white matter as a function of cranial volume was at a lower rate. However, voxel-based morphometry studies revealed significant main effects of sex but no significant effects of brain size in white and gray matter analysis [45]. In spite of the fact that we did not find gender differences for SLF, there is a report about left asymmetry in males while in females this tract has a more bilateral distribution [46].

A decrement in commissural tracts (Fmj and Fmn) has been associated to a diminished interhemispheric connectivity with brain size, which can explain the less volume in males. This hypothesis is supported by studies of delay of information conduction and cellular cost of the process [47].

A left asymmetry was detected for ATR, CGC, CST, ILF and SLF; while CGH and IFOF showed a right one. The fact that a great number of tracts have bigger volume in left hemisphere agree with left dominance is expected in our right-handed sample. Our data showed a left asymmentry for tracts involve in motor control (CST) and language (SLF) [48–51]. This left asymmetry for CST has been previously reported by Rademacher et al. [52] and Thiebaut de Schotten et al. [46] and confirmed by post-mortem studies [31], but White et al. [53] suggest that there is not such asymmetry. Also, left asymmetry in volume of SLF [46, 54], CGC and ILF [21] has been reported previously. On the contrary, there is evidence of no significant differences for ATR between hemispheres [21]. Moreover, have been described a right lateralization for CGH [21] and IFOF [21, 46] as same in our results. These facts suggest that right hemisphere seems to be specialized in more general functions that require integration of information, such as visual-spatial processing [55]. Specifically, CGH is involve in memory associative learning and episodic processing [56], while IFOF connects functional areas of visuo-spatial processing [57]. The UNC did not show differences between hemispheres, however in literature there are conflicting reports. Highley et al. [58] found that this fasciculus had bigger volume in right hemisphere, while Wakanana et al. [21] described left asymmetry. This inconsistency in the results may be due to different methodologies employed or small samples ($N < 30$).

In our analysis we included age as continuous predictor but we did not find any effect of that factor, probably because of the sample age is very homogenous and included mostly young adults. Nevertheless, several reports evince a global white matter volume increase from childhood to adultness [59, 60], and a further declination after maturation [61]. Generally, aging is associated with a reduction in white matter volume [62, 63] that seems to be more pervasive at times than even the gray matter decline [64], and generally involve a reduction in the integrity of white matter tracts [65, 66]. Also, it has been reported that males had more prominent age-related gray matter decreases and white matter volume and corpus callosal area increases compared with females what suggest that there are age-related sex differences in brain maturational processes [67].

Fractional anisotropy and mean diffusivity
In previous studies have been described differences by gender in FA in specific tracts [21, 30, 32], meanwhile our data exhibited greater values of FA for all tracts in females. Sexual dimorphism has been demonstrated in microstructural white matter organization in precentral, cingulate, and anterior temporal areas, but reporting lower values for females [68]. In specific tracts in females such as CST, which is involved in motor function, have been reported highest values, while males may undergo relatively more microstructural change in

projection and association fibers [69]. In another hand, Schmithorst et al. [70] had reported greater FA values in females for Fmj and Fmn, however when the entire corpus callosum has been studied the males happen to have the greatest values.

The FA showed significant left asymmetries for CGC, CGH, IFOF and ILF. Greater values of FA on lefts hemisphere have been describe previously for CGC [21], IFOF [21, 30, 71], ILF [21, 71], while CGH reported significant right asymmetry [21]. This lateralization was associated with higher microstructural integrity on the left side of limbic tracts (CGC and CGH) [72]. The ATR and CST had right asymmetries, which means in the ipsilateral hemisphere to handedness. That is an unexpected find because does not agree with postulation that right handed subject must have greater values of FA in contralateral hemisphere [49, 50], where have been observed better packing and arrangement of fibers that are involve in voluntary control of movement in contralateral hemisphere [40]. However the values are include in reported data for this index [30].

The data showed bigger values of MD for males than females in all the tracts, an inverse behavior than FA values. This higher MD values for females have been reported since adolescence for ILF and Fmj [69] and for CST in males [70]. However, in a study performed by Eluvathingal et al. [71] was not found gender effect over MD for any tracts except ILF, where girls had it lower values than males. The MD showed significant right asymmetries for CGC, CGH, IFOF and ILF, that means MD values have an inverse pattern than FA according to hemispheric asymmetries, besides gender asymmetry. The CGC and CGH have been previously reported with right-greater-than-left MD values, which remain for CGC even after normalization procedure [72]. Also data from IFOF and ILF have been reported with this asymmetry [71]. Besides the variety of reports some studies analyzing MD have revealed that it is a sensitive measure when were compared controls and pathological subjects [73]. No difference between hemispheres or gender for SLF and UNC were found, either FA or MD measures. This does not agree with previous results were a right-higher-than-left anisotropic asymmetry was found [74] for these tracts, however Büchel et al. [40] reported a left asymmetry for SLF. Also Kitamura et al. [75] had detected gender difference in the FA values for the right UNC.

As well as in statistical analysis of volume, neither FA or MD showed any effect of age probably due to the age of the sample is around young adultness. However, these index have been used to explain the changes in white matter integrity that occurs across life spam. Previous reports of DTI studies have shown an increased FA [76] throughout brain white matter during childhood, adolescence, and young adulthood [71, 77–79] and later elderly adults have displayed a significant decline in several white matter tracts [80]. On the other hand, Inano et al. [81] suggest there are no sex differences in the aging process of the white matter in a sample with an age range from 24.9 to 84.8 years.

Limitations

The resolution is limited due to the voxel size employed in diffusion imaging series. Also it is possible the modification of diffusion indexes by noise, partial volume effect and crossing fibers regions, which can miss estimate the parameters.

The tract volume was not normalized according to intracranial volume. However, is postulated that differences in hemispheric symmetry and gender are not modified for normalization procedure [21, 82].

Conclusions

Our work shows that is possible reconstruct white matter tracts using a unique ROIs scheme defined on a standard space, that can be transformed automatically to individual anatomy, minimizing the effect of investigator's manipulation. Also, allows the creation of a database of volume and diffusion parameters in Cuban population that can be used as normative sample in others studies. The volume values showed that a most part of tracts have bigger volume in left hemisphere. The data showed bigger values of MD for males than females in all the tracts, an inverse behavior than FA values. These results indicate differing developmental trajectories in white matter for males and females and the importance of taking gender into account in developmental DTI studies and in underlie gender-related cognitive differences. This study will provide the opportunity to analyze gender-specific nature of brain diseases supported by a control sample that allows the comparison between normal and pathological status.

Abbreviations

ATR: Anterior thalamic radiation; CGC: Cingulate gyrus associated cingulum; CGH: Hippocampal gyrus associated cingulum; CST: Corticospinal tract; DTI: Diffusion tensor imaging; EPI: Echo planar Imaging; ET: Echo time; FA: Fractional anisotropy; FACT: Fast assignment by continuous tracking; Fmj: Forceps major; Fmn: Forceps minor; FOV: Field of view; GLM: General linear model; IFOF: Inferior fronto-occipital fasciculus; ILF: Inferior longitudinal fasciculus; IQ: Intelligence quotient; MD: Mean diffusivity; MNI: Montreal Neurological Institute; rmANOVA: Repeated measure analysis of variance; ROI: Region of interest; RT: Repetition time; SLF: Superior longitudinal fasciculus; UNC: Uncinate fasciculus

Acknowledgement

This material is based on work of Cuban Project of Human Brain Mapping which comprise data base from a random sample of the population comprising medical, psychological and neuroimaging data.

Funding

None.

Authors' contributions

DG performed the protocols and wrote the article. MD participated in statistical analysis. MB participated in the design of the study. All authors read and approved the final manuscript.

Competing interest

The authors declare that they have no competing interests.

Author details

[1]Key Laboratory for NeuroInformation of Ministry of Education, Center for Information in Medicine, University of Electronic Science and Technology of China, 2006, Xiyuan Ave, West Hi-Tech Zone, Chengdu 61000, China. [2]Cuban Neuroscience Center, 190th Ave between 25th and 27th Ave, Havana 11300, Cuba. [3]IDIBELL Bellvitge Biomedical Research Institute, Barcelona, Spain.

References

1. Meyer JW, Makris N, Bates JF, Caviness VS, Kennedy DN. MRI-based topographic parcellation of human cerebral white matter: I. Technical foundations. Neuroimage. 1999;9(1):1–17.
2. Paus T, Zijdenbos A, Worsley K, Collins DL, Blumenthal J, Giedd JN, Rapoport JL, Evans AC. Structural maturation of neural pathways in children and adolescents: in vivo study. Science. 1999;283(5409):1908–11.
3. Xue R, van Zijl P, Crain BJ, Solaiyappan M, Mori S. In vivo three-dimensional reconstruction of rat brain axonal projections by diffusion tensor imaging. Magn Reson Med. 1999;42(6):1123–7.
4. Mori S, Crain BJ, Chacko V, Van Zijl P. Three-dimensional tracking of axonal projections in the brain by magnetic resonance imaging. Ann Neurol. 1999;45(2):265–9.
5. Le Bihan D, Mangin JF, Poupon C, Clark CA, Pappata S, Molko N, Chabriat H. Diffusion tensor imaging: concepts and applications. J Magn Reson Imaging. 2001;13(4):534–46.
6. Iturria Medina Y. Caracterización de la conectividad anatómica cerebral a partir de las neuroimágenes de la difusión y la teoría de grafos. Havana: Universidad de Ciencias Médicas de la Habana; 2013.
7. Wakana S, Jiang H, Nagae-Poetscher LM, Van Zijl PC, Mori S. Fiber tract-based atlas of human white matter anatomy 1. Radiology. 2004;230(1):77–87.
8. Mori S, Kaufmann WE, Davatzikos C, Stieltjes B, Amodei L, Fredericksen K, Pearlson GD, Melhem ER, Solaiyappan M, Raymond GV. Imaging cortical association tracts in the human brain using diffusion-tensor-based axonal tracking. Magn Reson Med. 2002;47(2):215–23.
9. Hua K, Zhang J, Wakana S, Jiang H, Li X, Reich DS, Calabresi PA, Pekar JJ, van Zijl PC, Mori S. Tract probability maps in stereotaxic spaces: analyses of white matter anatomy and tract-specific quantification. Neuroimage. 2008;39(1):336–47.
10. Huang H, Zhang J, van Zijl P, Mori S. Analysis of noise effects on DTI-based tractography using the brute-force and multi-ROI approach. Magn Reson Med. 2004;52(3):559–65.
11. Clark CA, Barrick TR, Murphy MM, Bell BA. White matter fiber tracking in patients with space-occupying lesions of the brain: a new technique for neurosurgical planning? Neuroimage. 2003;20(3):1601–8.
12. Field AS, Alexander AL, Wu YC, Hasan KM, Witwer B, Badie B. Diffusion tensor eigenvector directional color imaging patterns in the evaluation of cerebral white matter tracts altered by tumor. J Magn Reson Imaging. 2004;20(4):555–62.
13. Beals KL, Smith CL, Dodd SM, Angel JL, Armstrong E, Blumenberg B, Girgis FG, Turkel S, Gibson KR, Henneberg M. Brain size, cranial morphology, climate, and time machines [and comments and reply]. Curr Anthropol. 1984;25:301–30.
14. World Medical Organization. Declaration of Helsinki (1964). BMJ. 1996;313: 1448–1449.
15. Wechsler D, Sierra GP, Blanca L. WAIS-III: escala Weschler de inteligencia para adultos-III: El Manual Moderno. Mexico City; 2003.

16. Sheehan DV, Lecrubier Y, Sheehan KH, Amorim P, Janavs J, Weiller E, Hergueta T, Baker R, Dunbar GC. The Mini-International Neuropsychiatric Interview (MINI): the development and validation of a structured diagnostic psychiatric interview for DSM-IV and ICD-10. J Clin Psychiatry. 1998;59:22–33.

17. Anderson AW. Theoretical analysis of the effects of noise on diffusion tensor imaging. Magn Reson Med. 2001;46(6):1174–88.

18. Kreher B, Hennig J, Il'yasov K. DTI & FiberTools: a complete toolbox for DTI calculation, fiber tracking, and combined evaluation. In: Proceeding of ISMRM 14th International Scientific Meeting: 2006. 2006.

19. Basser PJ, Mattiello J, LeBihan D. Estimation of the effective self-diffusion tensor from the NMR spin echo. J Magn Reson B. 1994;103(3):247–54.

20. Wakana S, Jiang H, Hua K, Zhang J, Dubey P, Blite A, van Zijl P, Mori S. Reproducible protocol for human white matter fiber tracking and quantitative analysis of their status. In: International Society of Magnetic Resonance in Medicine: 2005. 2005.

21. Wakana S, Caprihan A, Panzenboeck MM, Fallon JH, Perry M, Gollub RL, Hua K, Zhang J, Jiang H, Dubey P. Reproducibility of quantitative tractography methods applied to cerebral white matter. Neuroimage. 2007;36(3):630–44.

22. Evans AC, Collins DL, Mills S, Brown E, Kelly R, Peters TM. 3D statistical neuroanatomical models from 305 MRI volumes. In: Nuclear Science Symposium and Medical Imaging Conference, IEEE Conference Record; 1993. p. 1813–1817.

23. Greenhouse SW, Geisser S. On methods in the analysis of profile data. Psychometrika. 1959;24(2):95–112.

24. Carpenter MB, Sutin J. Human neuroanatomy. Williams & Wilkins; 1983.

25. Nieuwenhuys R, Voogd J, Van Huijzen C. The human central nervous system: a synopsis and atlas. Springer Science & Business Media; 2007.

26. Mukherjee P, Chung S, Berman J, Hess C, Henry R. Diffusion tensor MR imaging and fiber tractography: technical considerations. Am J Neuroradiol. 2008;29(5):843–52.

27. Thomas B, Eyssen M, Peeters R, Molenaers G, Van Hecke P, De Cock P, Sunaert S. Quantitative diffusion tensor imaging in cerebral palsy due to periventricular white matter injury. Brain. 2005;128(11):2562–77.

28. Stadlbauer A, Nimsky C, Buslei R, Salomonowitz E, Hammen T, Buchfelder M, Moser E, Ernst-Stecken A, Ganslandt O. Diffusion tensor imaging and optimized fiber tracking in glioma patients: histopathologic evaluation of tumor-invaded white matter structures. Neuroimage. 2007;34(3):949–56.

29. Phillips OR, Nuechterlein KH, Clark KA, Hamilton LS, Asarnow RF, Hageman NS, Toga AW, Narr KL. Fiber tractography reveals disruption of temporal lobe white matter tracts in schizophrenia. Schizophr Res. 2009;107(1):30–8.

30. Jahanshad N, Lee AD, Barysheva M, McMahon KL, de Zubicaray GI, Martin NG, Wright MJ, Toga AW, Thompson PM. Genetic influences on brain asymmetry: a DTI study of 374 twins and siblings. Neuroimage. 2010;52(2):455–69.

31. Reich DS, Smith SA, Jones CK, Zackowski KM, van Zijl PC, Calabresi PA, Mori S. Quantitative characterization of the corticospinal tract at 3T. Am J Neuroradiol. 2006;27(10):2168–78.

32. Fabiano AJ, Horsfield MA, Bakshi R. Interhemispheric asymmetry of brain diffusivity in normal individuals: a diffusion-weighted MR imaging study. Am J Neuroradiol. 2005;26(5):1089–94.

33. Pierpaoli C, Basser PJ. Toward a quantitative assessment of diffusion anisotropy. Magn Reson Med. 1996;36(6):893–906.

34. Pierpaoli C, Jezzard P, Basser PJ, Barnett A, Di Chiro G. Diffusion tensor MR imaging of the human brain. Radiology. 1996;201(3):637–48.

35. Basser PJ, Jones DK. Diffusion-tensor MRI: theory, experimental design and data analysis–a technical review. NMR Biomed. 2002;15(7–8):456–67.

36. Alexander DC, Pierpaoli C, Basser PJ, Gee JC. Spatial transformations of diffusion tensor magnetic resonance images. IEEE Trans Med Imaging. 2001;20(11):1131–9.

37. Bizzi A. Presurgical mapping of verbal language in brain tumors with functional MR imaging and MR tractography. Neuroimaging Clin N Am. 2009;19(4):573–96.

38. Alexander AL, Hasan K, Kindlmann G, Parker DL, Tsuruda JS. A geometric analysis of diffusion tensor measurements of the human brain. Magn Reson Med. 2000;44(2):283–91.

39. Watkins K, Paus T, Lerch J, Zijdenbos A, Collins D, Neelin P, Taylor J, Worsley KJ, Evans AC. Structural asymmetries in the human brain: a voxel-based statistical analysis of 142 MRI scans. Cereb Cortex. 2001;11(9):868–77.

40. Büchel C, Raedler T, Sommer M, Sach M, Weiller C, Koch M. White matter asymmetry in the human brain: a diffusion tensor MRI study. Cereb Cortex. 2004;14(9):945 51.

41. Gur RC, Turetsky BI, Matsui M, Yan M, Bilker W, Hughett P, Gur RE. Sex differences in brain gray and white matter in healthy young adults: correlations with cognitive performance. J Neurosci. 1999;19(10):4065–72.

42. Mori S, Wakana S, Van Zijl PC, Nagae-Poetscher L. MRI atlas of human white matter. Am Soc Neuroradiology. 2005;16:276.

43. Filipek PA, Richelme C, Kennedy DN, Caviness VS. The young adult human brain: an MRI-based morphometric analysis. Cereb Cortex. 1994;4(4):344–60.

44. Passe TJ, Rajagopalan P, Tupler LA, Byrum CE, Macfall JR, Krishnan KRR. Age and sex effects on brain morphology. Progr Neuropsychopharmacol Biol Psychiatry. 1997;21(8):1231–7.

45. Luders E, Narr KL, Thompson PM, Rex DE, Woods RP, DeLuca H, Jancke L, Toga AW. Gender effects on cortical thickness and the influence of scaling. Hum Brain Mapp. 2006;27(4):314–24.

46. de Schotten MT, Bizzi A, Dell'Acqua F, Allin M, Walshe M, Murray R, Williams SC, Murphy DG, Catani M. Atlasing location, asymmetry and inter-subject variability of white matter tracts in the human brain with MR diffusion tractography. Neuroimage. 2011;54(1):49–59.

47. Ringo JL, Doty RW, Demeter S, Simard PY. Time is of the essence: a conjecture that hemispheric specialization arises from interhemispheric conduction delay. Cereb Cortex. 1994;4(4):331–43.

48. Kawashima R, Yamada K, Kinomura S, Yamaguchi T, Matsui H, Yoshioka S, Fukuda H. Regional cerebral blood flow changes of cortical motor areas and prefrontal areas in humans related to ipsilateral and contralateral hand movement. Brain Res. 1993;623(1):33–40.

49. Kim S-G, Ashe J, Hendrich K, Ellermann JM, Merkle H, Ugurbil K, Georgopoulos AP. Functional magnetic resonance imaging of motor cortex: hemispheric asymmetry and handedness. Science. 1993;261(5121):615–7.

50. Civardi C, Cavalli A, Naldi P, Varrasi C, Cantello R. Hemispheric asymmetries of cortico-cortical connections in human hand motor areas. Clin Neurophysiol. 2000;111(4):624–9.

51. Rodrigo S, Naggara O, Oppenheim C, Golestani N, Poupon C, Cointepas Y, Mangin J, Le Bihan D, Meder J. Human subinsular asymmetry studied by diffusion tensor imaging and fiber tracking. Am J Neuroradiol. 2007;28(8):1526–31.

52. Rademacher J, Bürgel U, Geyer S, Schormann T, Schleicher A, Freund H-J, Zilles K. Variability and asymmetry in the human precentral motor system. Brain. 2001;124(11):2232–58.

53. White L, Andrews T, Hulette C, Richards A, Groelle M, Paydarfar J, Purves D. Structure of the human sensorimotor system. II: Lateral symmetry. Cereb Cortex. 1997;7(1):31–47.

54. Glasser MF, Rilling JK. DTI tractography of the human brain's language pathways. Cereb Cortex. 2008;18(11):2471–82.

55. Iturria-Medina Y, Fernández AP, Morris DM, Canales-Rodríguez EJ, Haroon HA, Pentón LG, Augath M, García LG, Logothetis N, Parker GJ. Brain hemispheric structural efficiency and interconnectivity rightward asymmetry in human and nonhuman primates. Cereb Cortex. 2011;21(1):56–67.

56. Prasad KM, Patel AR, Muddasani S, Sweeney J, Keshavan MS. The entorhinal cortex in first-episode psychotic disorders: a structural magnetic resonance imaging study. Am J Psychiatry. 2004;161(9):1612–9.

57. Schmahmann JD, Pandya DN, Wang R, Dai G, D'Arceuil HE, de Crespigny AJ, Wedeen VJ. Association fibre pathways of the brain: parallel observations from diffusion spectrum imaging and autoradiography. Brain. 2007;130(3):630–53.

58. Highley JR, Walker MA, Esiri MM, Crow TJ, Harrison PJ. Asymmetry of the uncinate fasciculus: a post-mortem study of normal subjects and patients with schizophrenia. Cereb Cortex. 2002;12(11):1218–24.

59. Courchesne E, Chisum HJ, Townsend J, Cowles A, Covington J, Egaas B, Harwood M, Hinds S, Press GA. Normal brain development and aging: quantitative analysis at in vivo MR imaging in healthy volunteers 1. Radiology. 2000;216(3):672–82.

60. Lebel C, Beaulieu C. Longitudinal development of human brain wiring continues from childhood into adulthood. J Neurosci. 2011;31(30):10937–47.

61. Ge Y, Grossman RI, Babb JS, Rabin ML, Mannon LJ, Kolson DL. Age-related total gray matter and white matter changes in normal adult brain. Part I: volumetric MR imaging analysis. Am J Neuroradiol. 2002;23(8):1327–33.

62. Good CD, Johnsrude IS, Ashburner J, Henson RN, Fristen K, Frackowiak RS. A voxel-based morphometric study of ageing in 465 normal adult human brains. In: Biomedical Imaging, 5th IEEE EMBS International Summer School; 2002. p. 16.

63. Thomas C, Moya L, Avidan G, Humphreys K, Jung KJ, Peterson MA, Behrmann M. Reduction in white matter connectivity, revealed by diffusion tensor imaging, may account for age-related changes in face perception. J Cogn Neurosci. 2008;20(2):268–84.

64. Resnick SM, Pham DL, Kraut MA, Zonderman AB, Davatzikos C. Longitudinal magnetic resonance imaging studies of older adults: a shrinking brain. J Neurosci. 2003;23(8):3295–301.

65. Sullivan EV, Pfefferbaum A. Diffusion tensor imaging and aging. Neurosci Biobehav Rev. 2006;30(6):749–61.

66. Madden DJ, Spaniol J, Costello MC, Bucur B, White LE, Cabeza R, Davis SW, Dennis NA, Provenzale JM, Huettel SA. Cerebral white matter integrity mediates adult age differences in cognitive performance. J Cogn Neurosci. 2009;21(2):289–302.

67. De Bellis MD, Keshavan MS, Beers SR, Hall J, Frustaci K, Masalehdan A, Noll J, Boring AM. Sex differences in brain maturation during childhood and adolescence. Cereb Cortex. 2001;11(6):552–7.

68. Hsu J-L, Leemans A, Bai C-H, Lee C-H, Tsai Y-F, Chiu H-C, Chen W-H. Gender differences and age-related white matter changes of the human brain: a diffusion tensor imaging study. Neuroimage. 2008;39(2):566–77.

69. Bava S, Boucquey V, Goldenberg D, Thayer RE, Ward M, Jacobus J, Tapert SF. Sex differences in adolescent white matter architecture. Brain Res. 2011;1375:41–8.

70. Schmithorst VJ, Holland SK, Dardzinski BJ. Developmental differences in white matter architecture between boys and girls. Hum Brain Mapp. 2008;29(6):696–710.

71. Eluvathingal TJ, Hasan KM, Kramer L, Fletcher JM, Ewing-Cobbs L. Quantitative diffusion tensor tractography of association and projection fibers in normally developing children and adolescents. Cereb Cortex. 2007;17(12):2760–8.

72. Yu Q, Peng Y, Mishra V, Ouyang A, Li H, Zhang H, Chen M, Liu S, Huang H. Microstructure, length, and connection of limbic tracts in normal human brain development. Front Aging Neurosci. 2014;6:228.

73. Nir TM, Jahanshad N, Villalon-Reina JE, Toga AW, Jack CR, Weiner MW, Thompson PM, Initiative AsDN. Effectiveness of regional DTI measures in distinguishing Alzheimer's disease, MCI, and normal aging. Neuroimage Clin. 2013;3:180–95.

74. Park HJ, Westin CF, Kubicki M, Maier SE, Niznikiewicz M, Baer A, Frumin M, Kikinis R, Jolesz FA, McCarley RW: White matter hemisphere asymmetries in healthy subjects and in schizophrenia: a diffusion tensor MRI study. Neuroimage 2004:23(1):213–223.

75. Kitamura S, Morikawa M, Kiuchi K, Taoka T, Fukusumi M, Kichikawa K, Kishimoto T. Asymmetry, sex differences and age-related changes in the white matter in the healthy elderly: a tract-based study. BMC Res Notes. 2011;4(1):378.

76. Beaulieu C. The basis of anisotropic water diffusion in the nervous system–a technical review. NMR Biomed. 2002;15(7–8):435–55.

77. Mukherjee D, Nissen SE, Topol EJ. Risk of cardiovascular events associated with selective COX-2 inhibitors. JAMA. 2001;286(8):954–9.

78. Schmithorst VJ, Wilke M, Dardzinski BJ, Holland SK. Correlation of white matter diffusivity and anisotropy with age during childhood and adolescence: a cross-sectional diffusion-tensor MR imaging study 1. Radiology. 2002;222(1):212–8.

79. Lebel C, Walker L, Leemans A, Phillips L, Beaulieu C. Microstructural maturation of the human brain from childhood to adulthood. Neuroimage. 2008;40(3):1044–55.

80. Voineskos AN, Rajji TK, Lobaugh NJ, Miranda D, Shenton ME, Kennedy JL, Pollock BG, Mulsant BH. Age-related decline in white matter tract integrity and cognitive performance: a DTI tractography and structural equation modeling study. Neurobiol Aging. 2012;33(1):21–34.

81. Inano S, Takao H, Hayashi N, Abe O, Ohtomo K. Effects of age and gender on white matter integrity. Am J Neuroradiol. 2011;32(11):2103–9.

82. Ankney CD. Sex differences in relative brain size: The mismeasure of woman, too? Intelligence. 1992;16(3):329–36.

5

Prevalence and location of the secondary mesiobuccal canal in 1,100 maxillary molars using cone beam computed tomography

Pablo Betancourt[1,3]*, Pablo Navarro[1], Gonzalo Muñoz[2] and Ramón Fuentes[1]

Abstract

Background: Several articles have used cone beam computed tomography (CBCT) to study the morphology of the maxillary molars and to ascertain its ability to visualize the second mesiobuccal canal (MB2); however, its geometric location has not been examined in depth. The aim of this study was to describe in vivo the prevalence and location of the MB2 in the mesiobuccal root of the first maxillary molar (1MM) and the second maxillary molar (2MM) through CBCT imaging.

Methods: Five hundred fifty CBCT images of the 1MM and 550 of the 2MM were analyzed. To detect the MB2 canal, the observation and measurements were done 1 mm apically to the pulpal floor to standardize the methodology. The geometric location of the central point of the MB2 canal (PMB2) was measured in relation to the central point of the mesiobuccal canal (PMB1) and in relation to the line projected between the PMB1 and the central point of the palatal canals (PP). The data were analyzed using descriptive statistics, with a value of $P < 0.05$ being statistically significant.

Results: In the 1MM, the prevalence of the MB2 canal was 69.82% and was more frequent in women ($p = 0.005$). The distance between PMB1 and PP was 7.64 ± 1.04 mm. The average distance between PMB1 and PMB2 was 2.68 ± 0.49 mm, and for PMB2 and the line projected between the PMB1 and PP canals was 1.25 ± 0.34 mm. In the 2MM, the MB2 canal was identified in 46.91% and was more frequent in men ($p = 0.000$). The distance between PMB1 and PP was 7.02 ± 1.30. The average distance between PMB1 and PMB2 was 2.41 ± 0.64 mm, and for the PMB2 and the line projected between the PMB1 and PP canals was 0.98 ± 0.33 mm.

Conclusions: The MB2 canal was found in a high percentage of the sample. These results indicate that CBCT is an effective, high-precision diagnostic tool not only for detecting but also locating in vivo the MB2 canal in the mesiobuccal root of upper molars.

Keywords: Maxillary molars, Second mesiobuccal canal, Location, Cone-beam computed tomography

Background

The permanent first maxillary molar (1MM) and permanent second maxillary molar (2MM) are the teeth that present the greatest complexity and variation in the root canal system [1, 2], and this is reflected in them having the highest rates of endodontic failure and being a constant challenge for the clinician [3].

A high percentage of treatment failures is due to the impossibility of detecting the presence and location of the secondary mesiobuccal canal (MB2), located in the mesiobuccal root of the 1MM and the 2MM [4], which prevents the correct implementation of biomechanical instrumentation, irrigation and obturation (Fig. 1). Its location in clinical practice is highly complex due to the excessive dentin deposited in the opening of the canal and to the difficulty in visually accessing maxillary molars.

The percentage of visualization of the MB2 canal varies according to the technique used in each study,

---
* Correspondence: pablo.betancourt@ufrontera.cl
[1]Research Center in Dental Sciences (CICO), Endodontic Laboratory, Dental School, Universidad de La Frontera, Temuco, Chile
[3]Integral Adultos Department, Dental School, Universidad de La Frontera, Claro Solar 115, Temuco, Chile
Full list of author information is available at the end of the article

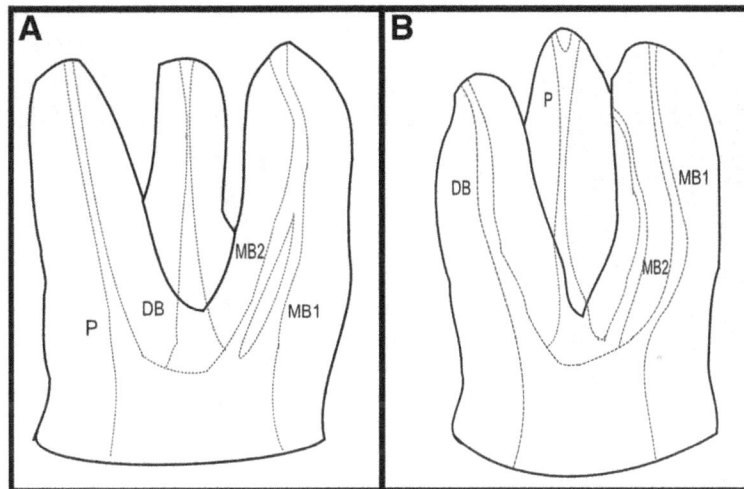

Fig. 1 Maxillary molar with 4 canals: first mesiobuccal canal (MB1), secondary mesiobuccal canal (MB2), distobuccal canal (DB) and palatal canal (P). **a** Maxillary molar with joining mesiobuccal canals. **b** Maxillary molar with two separate mesiobuccal canals

including histological sections [5], diaphanization [6], magnifying loupes [7], endodontic surgical microscope [8–10], scanning electron microscope [5], micro-computed tomographic analysis [11], and cone beam computed tomography (CBCT) [1, 3, 4, 12].

In recent years, CBCT has made it possible to visualize hard-to-reach anatomical structures in three dimensions, and it has become a valuable aid as a complementary examination for endodontic diagnosis and treatment with a lower dose of radiation than conventional computed tomography [13, 14]. Several articles [1, 3], [4, 12, 15], have used CBCT to study the morphology of the maxillary molars and to ascertain its ability to visualize the MB2 canal; however, its geometric location has not been examined in depth.

The aim of this study was to determine in vivo the prevalence of the MB2 canal in maxillary molars, and to describe a methodology to enable its geometric location through CBCT imaging.

Methods

This study was approved by the Ethics Committee of the Universidad de La Frontera, Temuco, Chile (Protocol n° 048/13). CBCT images that contained the 1MM and 2MM, from patients both men and women, were analyzed, The images were taken between January 2014 and March 2015, and belong to the radiology unit of the Universidad de La Frontera. The patient's identity was not revealed and only access to information regarding age and gender was provided.

The imaging examinations were taken as part of the diagnosis, examination and planning of surgical, endodontic, periodontal, orthodontic or rehabilitative treatment. The images were obtained on a Pax Zenith CBCT unit (Vatech, Hwaseong-si, Korea), using 120 kV and 9 mA; FOV 8 × 6 cm, voxel size 0.12 mm.

550 1MM (right and left) and 550 2MM (right and left) CBCT images were included where the presence of all maxillary molars could be observed. Inclusion criteria for the CBCT images were: aged between 15 and 75 years, and complete root formation. The exclusion criteria were: present metallic restoration, intra-radicular post or endodontic filling, rehabilitated using fixed prosthesis, canal calcification, evidence of radectomy or periapical surgery, and maxillary molars with developmental anomalies.

A learning process to reach a consensus in the identification of the MB2 based on the anatomical diagnosis of CBCT images took place prior to a data reliability assessment, because the MB2 is very fine, which reduces the contrast on the image, and its visualization also varies according to the area of the tooth in which the measurement is taken. Two endodontics specialists examined 20 previously selected CBCT images of maxillary molars. The observers analyzed the images on three occasions, at one-week intervals. When a consensus could not be reached, a radiologist with experience in endodontics helped to make the decision. The reliability data were analyzed using the Kappa concordance index, which determined that there was agreement between the observers ($p = 0.000$) and the strength of agreement was very good (0.886).

Observation methodology

The images were processed with the Ez 3D 2009 software (Vatech, Hwaseong-si, Korea) and projected onto a LED KDL-42W651A screen (Sony, Minato, Japan) to observe coronal (Fig. 2a), sagittal (Fig. 2b) and axial

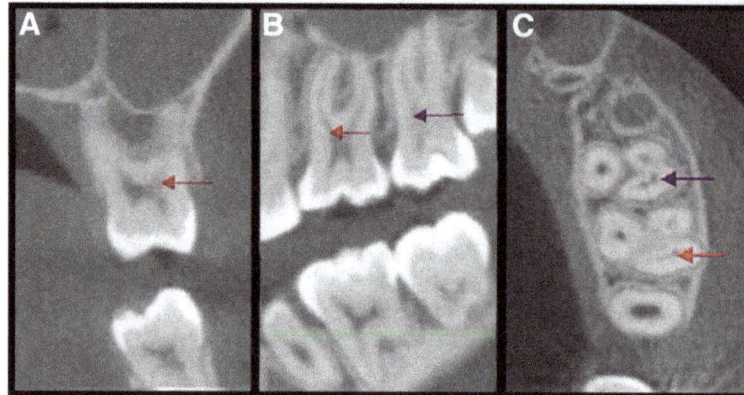

Fig. 2 CBCT images of a left maxillary first molar (red arrows) and left maxillary second molar (purple arrows). Mesiobuccal root with 2 canals as viewed in coronal, sagittal, and axial directions using Ez 3D 2009 software. **a** coronal view; **b** sagittal view; **c** axial view

sections (Fig. 2c). First, the sagittal and coronal sections was oriented parallel to the long axis of the root, and then sections were obtained on the axial plane at 0.5 mm intervals and a 1mm thickness for all the samples, using multiplanar reformatting (MPR). MPR constructs a three-dimensional model and shows all structures within the 1mm thickness overlapped on each other. A corono-apical exploration was made. To detect the MB2 canal, the observation and measurements were done 1 mm apically (2 sections of 0.5mm) to the pulpal floor to standardize the methodology (Fig. 3).

The geometric location of the MB2 canal was found in relation to the first mesiobuccal canal (MB1) and the palatal canal (P). The central points of each canal were located (PMB1, PMB2 and PP) and straight lines projected between them (PMB1–PP and PMB1–PMB2). A third line was drawn (PMB2–PT), perpendicular to the PMB1–PP line (PT point), according to the protocol described by Betancourt et al. [14]. The distances of the lines drawn between the points were measured in millimeters (Fig. 4).

The data were analyzed using descriptive statistics (mean ± SD). The association between the MB2 canal and gender and side were determined and evaluated using Pearson's chi-square test with the SPSS/PC v. 20.0 software (SPSS, Chicago, IL). The relation to age was also established using the t-test for independent samples, considering the normality of the data. 95% confidence intervals were used to calculate the average distances between the points PMB1-PMB2, PMB1-PP and PMB2-PT. A value of $p < 0.05$ was chosen as the threshold for statistical significance.

Results

550 1MM and 550 2MM were selected according to the established dates and inclusion criteria.

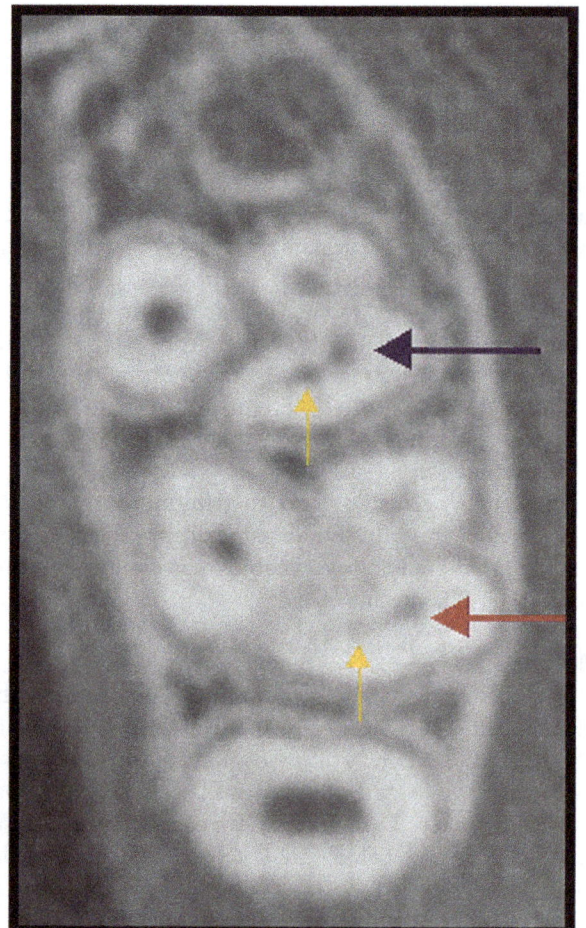

Fig. 3 Cross-sectional CBCT image of left maxillary first and second molar with a clearly distinguished MB2 canal (yellow arrows). The red arrows denote the mesiobuccal root in the maxillary first molar and the purple arrows denote the mesiobuccal root in the maxillary second molar

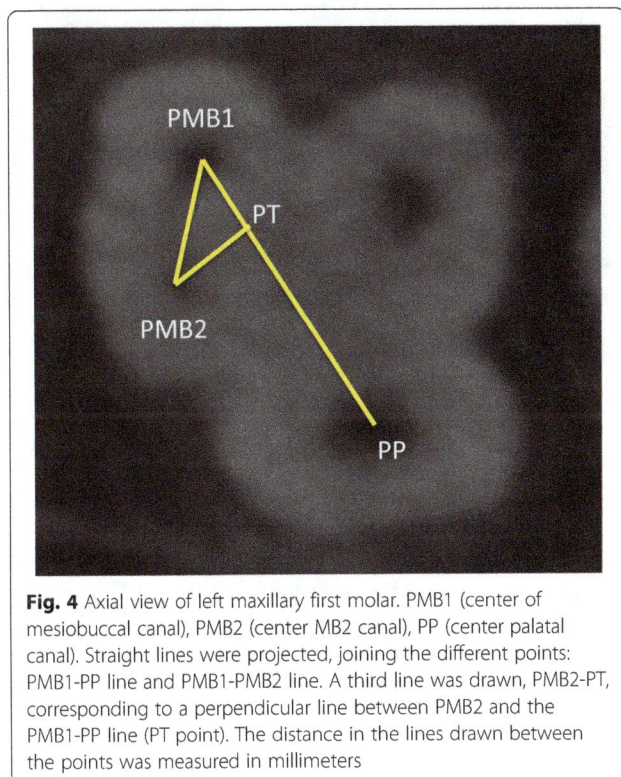

Fig. 4 Axial view of left maxillary first molar. PMB1 (center of mesiobuccal canal), PMB2 (center MB2 canal), PP (center palatal canal). Straight lines were projected, joining the different points: PMB1-PP line and PMB1-PMB2 line. A third line was drawn, PMB2-PT, corresponding to a perpendicular line between PMB2 and the PMB1-PP line (PT point). The distance in the lines drawn between the points was measured in millimeters

First maxillary molar

The MB2 canal was found in 69.82% of the analyzed cases (384/550). The percentage distribution of the MB2 canal according to side was homogenous: 50.5% on the right and 49.5% on the left (Fig. 5). With regard to the incidence of the MB2 canal according to gender, statistically significant differences were observed (p = 0.005), with 55.2% in men and 44.8% in woman (Fig. 6) (Table 1). The average age of the subjects where the MB2 canal was found was 27.40 ± 12.95 years. The distances between the points were analyzed with 95% confidence. The distance between PMB1-PP was 7.64 ± 1.04 mm. For PMB1-PMB2 the average of distance was 2.68 ± 0.49 mm, and for PMB2-PT it was 1.25 ± 0.34 mm.

Second maxillary molar

The MB2 canal was identified in 46.91% (258/550) of the cases. When the incidence of the MB2 canal was compared between the right side (49.2%) and left side (50.8%), there were no statistically significant differences (p = 0.560) (Fig. 5). Visualization of the MB2 canal was more frequent in men (59.3%) than in women (40.7%), with statistically significant differences between the two genders (p = 0.000) (Fig. 6) (Table 2). The average age of the subjects where the MB2 canal was found was 27.81 ± 12.66. The distances between the points were analyzed with 95% confidence. The distance between PMB1-PP was 7.02 ± 1.30. For PMB1-PMB2 the average distance was 2.41 ± 0.64 mm, and for PMB2-PT it was 0.98 ± 0.33 mm.

Discussion

Despite their usefulness in locating the MB2 canal, magnification systems pose a series of limitations, such as a limited view of the clinical field, showing only superficially the mean orifice of the MB2 canal and not the entire root canal system. However, if access is not gained correctly, then magnification cannot provide an image of the area where the MB2 canal is located. In cases of inclined or rotated molars, magnification becomes less effective, since a severe to moderate angulation of the tooth prevents a good view of the pulpal floor. Stopko [8] stated that these microsurgical devices alone are insufficient to locate and instrument the MB2 canal in every case. On the other hand, conventional periapical x-rays are essential for the endodontic preoperative diagnosis and they are the most frequently used method for detecting accessory canals in everyday practice; nevertheless, the periapical x-ray can only provide two-dimensional information, which limits its diagnostic effectiveness. Furthermore, interpretation becomes difficult in terms of such factors as the superposition of anatomical structures, excessive bone

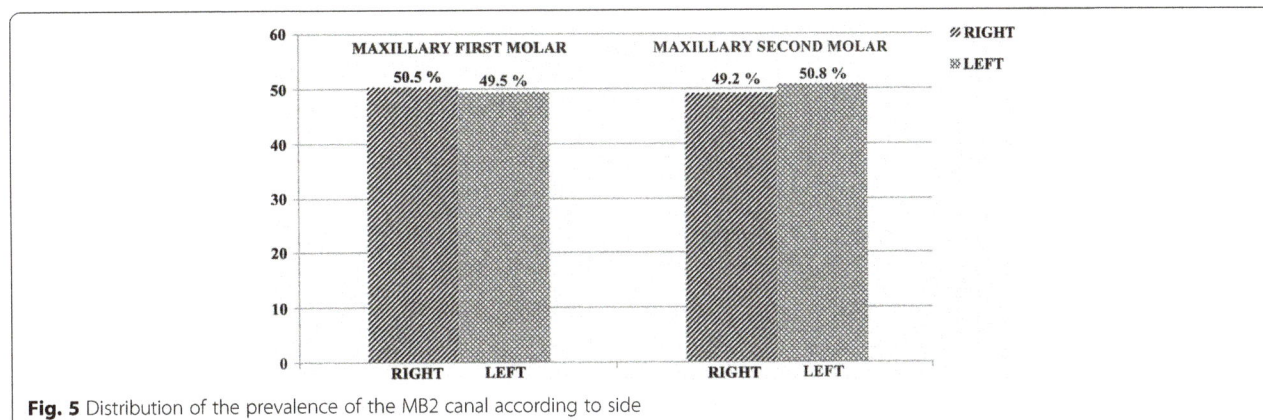

Fig. 5 Distribution of the prevalence of the MB2 canal according to side

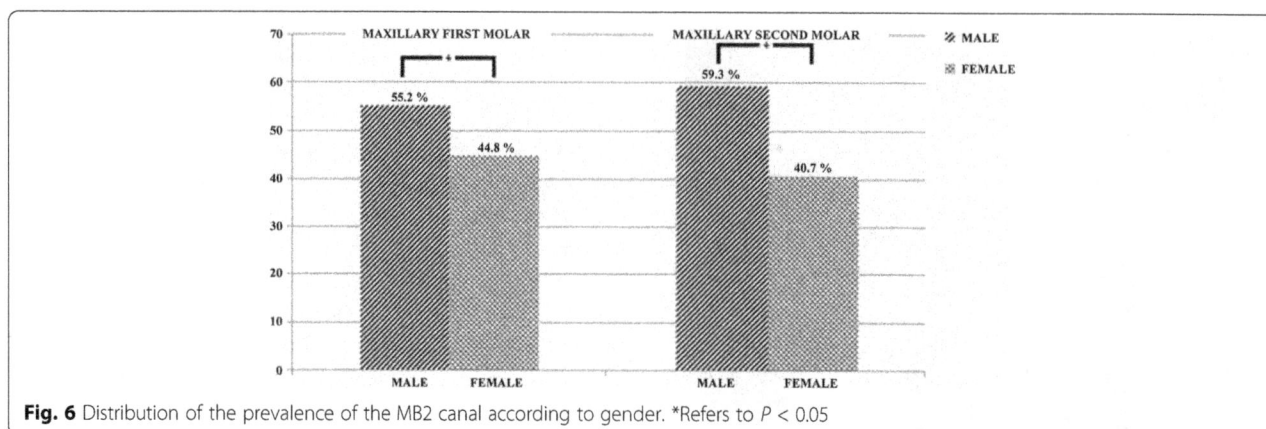

Fig. 6 Distribution of the prevalence of the MB2 canal according to gender. *Refers to $P < 0.05$

density of the zygomatic arch or impacted teeth [13]. Barton et al. [16] and Abuabuara et al. [17] detected the MB2 canal in maxillary molars in 39.2% and 8% respectively through conventional periapical x-rays, demonstrating the low effectiveness of the method. Nattress & Martin [18] concluded that x-ray images were not reliable for detecting multiple canals. Therefore, it is very important to know and use additional tools to aid in detecting the MB2 canal in the diagnostic phase.

Patel et al. [13] reported CBCT as a non-invasive high-precision three-dimensional technique that increases the percentage of therapeutic success. Matherne et al. [19], using an in vitro human model, showed the superiority of CBCT over conventional x-rays in detecting the presence of accessory channels, and Blattner et al. [4], in an in vitro study, found CBCT to be a reliable method for the detection of the MB2 canal compared to the gold standard of physically sectioning the specimen.

Various studies have suggested the use of CBCT as an in vivo diagnostic method to detect the MB2 canal in maxillary molars [1, 3, 12, 14, 15]. The results obtained in this study revealed a prevalence of the MB2 canal in 69.81% in the 1MM, similar to that reported with the same diagnostic method by Kim et al. (63.59%) [20], Lee et al. (70.5%) [15], Betancourt et al. (68.75%) [12] and higher than the 52% reported by Zhang et al. [3] and the 8.78% by Zheng et al. [1]. The MB2 canal in the 2MM was identified in 46.90% of the cases, a percentage similar to the results reported using CBCT by Betancourt et al. (48%) [14], Lee et al. (42.2%) [15], and higher than the 34.32% by Silva et al. [21] and the 22% observed by Zhang et al. [3]. If two separate orifices blended into a single canal it was not considered to be a separate canal. This morphology is classified as Vertucci type 1 canal configuration and is the most seen in the second maxillary molars. This criteria is probably one of the reasons

Table 1 Prevalence MB2 canal in the mesiobuccal root of the maxillary first molars by gender and tooth position

	MB2		
	Absent	Present	Total
Female	96	172	268
	57,8%	44,8%	48,7%
Male	70	212	282
	42,2%	55,2%*	51,3%
Total	166	384	550
	100%	100%	100%
Rigth Side	85	194	279
	51,2%	50,5%	50,7%
Left Side	81	190	271
	48,8%	49,5%	49,3%
Total	166	384	550
	100%	100%	100%

* refers to $p < 0.05$

Table 2 Prevalence MB2 canal in the mesiobuccal root of the maxillary second molars by gender and tooth position

	MB2		
	Absent	Present	Total
Female	167	105	272
	57,2%	40,7%	49,5%
Male	125	153	278
	42,8%	59,3%*	50,5%
Total	292	258	550
	100%	100%	100%
Rigth Side	151	127	278
	51,7%	49,2%	50,5%
Left Side	141	131	272
	48,3%	50,8%	49,5%
Total	292	258	550
	100%	100%	100%

* refers to $p < 0.05$

for the lower incidence of second mesiobuccal canals in this tooth.

The geometrical location of the MB2 canal has only been reported using in vitro studies [7, 22–24], however, a previous study by our group in second maxillary molars [14] demonstrated the efficiency of CBCT on MB2 canal location in vivo. This article is intended to expand the study sample used by Betancourt et al. [14], increasing the sample of 225 to 1,100 maxillary molars, also the study of the first maxillary molars were included. We observed that the MB2 canal was located in the 1MM 2.68 ± 0.49 mm palatally and 1.25 ± 0.34 mesially to the MB1 canal. In the 2MM it was located 2.41 ± 0.64 mm palatally and 0.98 ± 0.33 mm mesially, whereas Betancourt et al. [14], using the same technique, found it to be 2.2 ± 0.54 mm palatally and 0.98 ± 0.32 mesially to the MB1 canal. Gorduysus et al. [22] reported the MB2 location 1.65 ± 0.72 mm palatally and 0.69 ± 0.42 mesially to the MB1 canal in a combined study of first and second molars.

Our results regarding the location of the MB2 canal are lower than the results of Gilles & Reader [6], who located the MB2 canal mesially to the MB1 canal at a distance of 2.31 mm in the 1MM and 2.06 mm in the 2MM by scanning electronic microscopy, and Degerness & Bowles [24], who located it in the 1MM 1.2 ± 0.6 mm from the MB1 canal and in the 2MM 1.78 ± 0.6 mm through a stereomicroscope. Greater distances were reported by Kulid & Peter [25], who found no statistically significant differences between the 1MM and 2MM (1.82 ± 0.71mm), similarly to Görduysus et al. (1.81 ± 0.38 mm) [22]. This could be explained by the heightened sensitivity of in vitro studies or the use of microscopes with various magnifications that distort the images, whereas with CBCT the resolution of the resulting image is isotropic, i.e., the voxel, the minimum data unit, is equal in dimension on the 3 spatial axes, producing images without distortion or magnification (1:1).

We believe the variation in the geometric location of the MB2 canal mesially or palatally in relation to the MB1 canal depends on the type of study, because in vitro studies the anatomical relation and proportion on the arch is lost, where it is also not possible for all the axes and planes to be observed, which can be done with CBCT.

When relating the patient's gender to the incidence of the MB2 canal, we obtained a statistically significant association. The 1MM (p = 0.005) and the 2MM (p = 0.000) was more frequent in men. These results are consistent with those reported by Fogel et al. [26] and Betancourt et al. [14]. However, Zheng et al. [1] and Betancourt et al. [12] found no difference. The smaller detection percentage of the MB2 canal in women could be explained by the demineralization and loss of bone mass in adults being

three times greater in women [27], which would prevent the correct observation of the canal through computerized tomography due to lack of contrast.

The MB2 canal showed a high tendency to appear bilaterally, which is similar to that reported by Betancourt et al. [12], Betancourt et al. [14] and Lee et al. [15], all through in vivo CBCT images. This means that if a MB2 canal exists on one side, the clinician must consider searching in the contralateral mesiobuccal root.

Our results show that the observation of the MB2 canal is difficult at a higher age. This significant decrease in visibility through CBCT may be due to there being an increase in the porosity of the cortical bone and a reduction in bone mass after 50 years of age [28], which would cause an increase in the radiolucency of the bone and a subsequent lack of contrast with the MB2 canal, as this has a radiolucent structure. Another factor to consider is that with increasing age tertiary dentin dressing is being produced in certain places of the pulp-dentin interface due to the exposure of the tooth to external stressors, such as decay, dental trauma or restorative procedures. Finally, the elderly subjects presented greater canal calcification; therefore, the diameter of the additional canal is less than the diameter of the MB1 and palatal canals, a situation which is difficult to detect clearly on the CBCT images.

One significant problem which can affect the image quality and diagnostic accuracy of CBCT images is the scatter and beam hardening caused by high density neighboring structures, such as enamel, metal posts and restorations. If this scattering and beam hardening is associated close to or with the tooth being assessed the resulting CBCT images may be of minimal diagnostic value [29]. This difficulty did not arise in this study since the teeth with metallic restoration, intraradicular posts, root obturation or rehabilitated by means of a fixed prosthesis were excluded. Another point to consider is that the geometric location of the MB2 canal presents variations according to the height at which the measurements are taken; therefore, we recommend taking them at 1.0 mm (2 sections of 0.5mm) apically to the pulp chamber floor, because we regularly observed the MB2 at that level in every case where it was present.

These results indicate that CBCT is an effective, high-precision diagnostic tool for detecting and locating in vivo the MB2 canal in the mesiobuccal root of upper molars, thereby increasing the chances of endodontic success. This study demonstrates that the geometric location in vivo of the MB2 canal is possible through the methodology used in this article. Its tool helps to understand the root and canal morphology of maxillary molars in the diagnostic stage; as a result, it helps the clinician to perform the endodontic treatment safely, effectively, and predictively.

Conclusion

The MB2 canal is found in 69.82% of the 1MM and 46.91% of the 2MM. In order to obtain the geometric location of the MB2 canal in the mesiobuccal root, we suggest using the center of the main mesiobuccal canal as a reference parameter and from there exploring 2.68 ± 0.49 mm in a palatal direction and 1.25 ± 0.34 mm in a mesial direction in the 1MM, while exploring 2.41 ± 0.64 mm in a palatal direction and 0.98 ± 0.33 mm in a mesial direction in the 2MM. Given our study results, we recommend that CBCT be considered a complementary diagnostic method before establishing an endodontic treatment in maxillary molars so as to obtain an optimal result.

Abbreviations

1MM: First maxillary molar; 2MM: Second maxillary molar; CBCT: Cone beam computed tomography; MB1: Mesiobuccal canal; MB2: Second mesiobuccal canal; MPR: Multiplanar reformatting; P: Palatal canal; PMB1: Central point of the mesiobuccal canal; PMB2: Central point of the MB2 canal; PP: Central point of the palatal canal

Acknowledgements

The authors are grateful for project DIUFRO # DI14-0034 and Endodontic Laboratory, Research Center in Dental Sciences (CICO), Universidad de La Frontera.

Funding

The DIUFRO project # DI14-0034 provided funds to purchase a PC to analyze the images and data of the study. This project was sponsored by the Universidad de La Frontera, Temuco, Chile.

Authors' contributions

PB Devised the study concept, designed the study, supervised the intervention, data collection and analysis, participated in the coordination of the study, critically revised and drafted the manuscript, manuscript preparation, edited the manuscript before submission. PN Contributed to the design and analysis of the study data, statistical analysis, statistical plots and revised the manuscript, edited the manuscript before submission. GM Image analysis, Image processing, data collection, revised the manuscript and manuscript preparation. RF Participated in the study concept, designed the study, ran the study intervention, collected data, performed the analyses, critically revised and drafted the manuscript, edited the manuscript before submission. All authors read and approved the final manuscript.

Competing interests

The authors declare that they have no competing interests.

Author details

[1]Research Center in Dental Sciences (CICO), Endodontic Laboratory, Dental School, Universidad de La Frontera, Temuco, Chile. [2]Dental School, Universidad de La Frontera, Temuco, Chile. [3]Integral Adultos Department, Dental School, Universidad de La Frontera, Claro Solar 115, Temuco, Chile.

References

1. Zheng Q, Wang Y, Zhou X, Wang Q, Zheng G, Huang D. A Cone-Beam Computed Tomography Study of Maxillary First Permanent Molar Root and Canal Morphology in a Chinese Population. J Endod. 2010;36:1480–4.
2. Badole GP, Bahadure RN, Warhadpande MM, Kubde R. A rare root canal configuration of maxillary second molar: a case report. Case Rep Dent. 2012;2012:767582.
3. Zhang R, Yang H, Yu X, Wang H, Hu T, Dummer PMH. Use of CBCT to identify the morphology of maxillary permanent molar teeth in a Chinese subpopulation. Int Endod J. 2011;44:162–9.
4. Blattner T, George N, Lee C, Kumar V, Yelton C. Efficacy of Cone-Beam Computed Tomography as a Modality to Accurately Identify the Presence of Second Mesiobuccal Canals in Maxillary First and Second Molars: A Pilot Study. J Endod. 2010;36:867–70.
5. Schwarze T, Baethge C, Stecher T, Geurtsen W. Identification Of Second Canals In The Mesiobuccal Root Of Maxillary First And Second Molars Using Magnifying Loupes Or An Operating Microscope. Aust Endod J. 2002;28:57–60.
6. Gilles J, Reader A. An SEM investigation of the mesiolingual canal in human maxillary first and second molars. Oral Surg Oral Med Oral Pathol. 1990;70:638–43.
7. Peeters H, Suardita K, Setijanto D. Prevalence of a second canal in the mesiobuccal root of permanent maxillary first molars from an Indonesian population. J Oral Sci. 2011;53:489–94.
8. Stropko JJ. Canal morphology of maxillary molars: clinical observations of canal configurations. J Endod. 1999;25:446–50.
9. Karaman GT, Onay EO, Ungor M. Colak M Evaluating the potential key factors in assessing the morphology of mesiobuccal canal in maxillary first and second molars. Aust Endod J. 2011;37:134–40.
10. Das S, Warhadpande MM, Redij SA, Jibhkate NG, Sabir H. Frequency of second mesiobuccal canal in permanent maxillary first molars using the operating microscope and selective dentin removal: A clinical study. Contemp Clin Dent. 2015;6:74–8.
11. Verma P, Love RM. A Micro CT study of the mesio- buccal root canal morphology of the maxillary first molar tooth. Int Endod J. 2011;44:210–7.
12. Betancourt P, Fuentes R, Aracena Rojas S, Cantín M, Navarro CP. Prevalencia del segundo canal en la raíz mesiovestibular de los primeros molares maxilares mediante tomografía computarizada de haz de cono. Av Odontoestomatol. 2013;29:31–6.
13. Patel S, Dawood A, Whaites E, Pitt FT. New dimensions in endodontic imaging: part 1. Conventional and alternative radiographic systems. Int Endod J. 2009;42:447–62.
14. Betancourt P, Navarro P, Cantín M, Fuentes R. Cone-beam computed tomography study of prevalence and location of MB2 canal in the mesiobuccal root of the maxillary second molar. Int J Clin Exp Med. 2015;8:9128–34.
15. Lee J, Kim K, Lee J, Park W, Jeong J, Lee Y, Gu Y, Chang S, Son W, Lee W, Baek S, Bae K, Kum K. Mesiobuccal root canal anatomy of Korean maxillary first and second molars by cone-beam computed tomography. Oral Surg Oral Med Oral Pathol Oral Radiol Endod. 2011;111:785–91.
16. Barton DJ, Clark SJ, Eleazer PD, Scheetz JP, Farman AG. Tuned-aperture computed tomography versus parallax analog and digital radiographic images in detecting second mesiobuccal canals in maxillary first molars. Oral Surg Oral Med Oral Pathol Oral Radiol Endod. 2003;96:223–8.
17. Abuabara A, Baratto-Filho F, Aguiar Anele J, Leonardi DP, Sousa-Neto MD. Efficacyofclinical and radiological methods to identify second mesiobuccal canals in maxillary first molars. Acta Odontol Scand. 2013;71:205–9.
18. Nattress BR, Martin DM. Predictability of radiographic diagnosis of variations in root canal anatomy in mandibular incisors and premolar teeth. Int Endod J. 1991;24:58–62.
19. Matherne RP, Angelopoulos C, Kulild JC, Tira D. Use of cone-beam computed tomography to identify root canal systems in vitro. J Endod. 2008;34:87–9.
20. Kim Y, Lee SJ, Woo J. Morphology of maxillary fisrt and second molars analyzed by cone beam computed tomography in a korean population: Varitations in the number of roots and Canals and the incidence of fusion. J Endod. 2012;38:1063–8.
21. Silva EJ, Nejaim Y, Silva AI, Haiter-Neto F, Zaia AA, Cohenca N. Evaluation of root canal configuration of maxillary molars in a Brazilian population using cone-beam computed tomo- graphic imaging: An in vivo study. J Endod. 2014;40:173–6.

22. Görduysus MO, Görduysus M, Friedman S. Operating microscope improves negotiation of second mesiobuccal canals in maxillary molars. J Endod. 2001;27:683–6.

23. Tuncer A, Haznedaroglu F, Sert S. The Location and Accessibility of the Second Mesiobuccal Canal in Maxillary First Molar. Eur J Dent. 2010;4:12–6.

24. Degerness R, Bowles W. Anatomic Determination of the Mesiobuccal Root Resection Level in Maxillary Molars. J Endod. 2008;34:1182–6.

25. Kulild J, Peters D. Incidence and configuration of canal systems in the mesiobuccal root of maxillary first and second molars. J Endod. 1990;16:311–7.

26. Fogel HM, Peikoff MD, Christie WH. Canal configuration in the mesiobuccal root of the maxillary first molar: A clinical study. J Endod. 1994;20:135–7.

27. Benson BW, Prihoda TJ, Glass BJ. Variations in adult cortical bone mass as measured by a panoramic mandibular index. Oral Surg Oral Med Oral Pathol. 1991;71(3):349–56.

28. Hildebolt CF. Osteoporosis and oral bone loss. Dentomaxillofac Radiol. 1997;26:3–15.

29. Estrela C, Bueno MR, Leles CR, Azevedo B, Azevedo JR. Accuracy of cone beam computed tomography and panoramic radiography for the detection of apical periodontitis. J Endod. 2008;34:273–9.

6

The correlation between radiographic and pathologic grading of lumbar facet joint degeneration

Xin Zhou[1,2†], Yuan Liu[1,2†], Song Zhou[1,2†], Xiao-Xing Fu[1,2], Xiao-Long Yu[1,2], Chang-Lin Fu[1,2], Bin Zhang[1,2*] and Min Dai[1,2*]

Abstract

Background: Before performing spine non-fusion surgery that retains the facet joints, choosing an accurate radiographic method to evaluate the degree of facet joint degeneration is extremely important. Therefore, the objective of this study was to determine the accuracy and reliability of different radiographic classifications by analyzing the correlation between radiographic and pathologic grading of lumbar facet joint degeneration. Taking the pathologic examination as standard, the consistency of computed tomography (CT) and magnetic resonance imaging (MRI) assessment of lumbar facet joint degeneration was compared.

Methods: A total of 74 facet joints obtained from 42 patients who underwent posterior lumbar surgery were evaluated. All patients underwent CT and MRI before surgery. The pathologic grade was evaluated with a method based on hematoxylin-eosin and toluidine blue staining. The radiographic grade was evaluated using the methods proposed by different authors.

Results: There was a moderate consistency between pathologic and radiographic grading for facet joint degeneration. The weighted kappa coefficients comparing pathologic with radiographic grading were 0.506 for CT, 0.561 for MRI, and 0.592 for CT combined with MRI, respectively. Taking the pathologic examination as standard, the consistency of CT and MRI examination was also moderate, and the weighted kappa coefficient was 0.459.

Conclusion: The radiographic examination has moderate accuracy and reliability for evaluating degeneration of facet joints. Therefore, a more accurate method for evaluating the degeneration of facet joints is necessary before performing spine non-fusion surgery that retains the facet joints.

Keywords: Lumbar facet joint, Degeneration, Radiography, Pathology, Spine non-fusion technique

Background

In patients with low back pain, the proportion of lumbar facet joint osteoarthritis (FJOA) is as high as 40–85 % [1]. It has been reported that 15–40 % of low back pain may be caused by FJOA [2, 3]. The facet joint is a synovial joint composed of cartilage, synovium, and an articular capsule [4, 5]. The characteristics of FJOA are similar to other synovial joints such as the knee [4, 6].

The degeneration of the lumbar facet joint will not only cause low back pain but also lead to instability of the spine, resulting in degenerative spondylolisthesis and scoliosis [7].

Spinal fusion is currently the most common operation for treatment of lumbar degenerative disease, but postoperative complications such as loss of motion and adjacent segment degeneration may occur [8]. Motion preservation devices and intervertebral disc replacement may help to reduce these disadvantages. Moreover, interspinous devices have been used to treat low back pain originating from facet joints, but were not suitable for severe facet joint pain [9]. Patients with severe degeneration of the facet joint could still have low back pain after successful

* Correspondence: 609901889@qq.com; 764932881@qq.com
Xin Zhou, Yuan Liu and Song Zhou are co-first authors.
†Equal contributors
[1]Department of Orthopedics, The First Affiliated Hospital of Nanchang University, Nanchang 330006, China
Full list of author information is available at the end of the article

intervertebral disc replacement [10]. Therefore, preoperative accurate assessment of facet joint degeneration will contribute to the choice of the appropriate surgical treatment of lumbar degenerative disease.

Recently, the pathologic grading of facet joint degeneration described by Gries [11] has been widely accepted. Radiographic grading was evaluated with methods reported by Pathria, Grogan, and Weishaupt, respectively [12–14]. Determination of the correlation between facet joint pathologic and radiographic grading to facilitate the choice of an appropriate radiographic examination for evaluation of facet joint degeneration is necessary. Our study evaluated the correlation between pathologic and radiographic grading to determine the accuracy and reliability of radiographic grading of facet joint degeneration to facilitate accurate evaluation of facet joint degeneration before lumbar spine surgery, and to aid in selection of the appropriate operation.

Methods

Subjects

We recruited 42 patients (19 women and 23 men), 21 to 68 years old (mean: 52 years), who underwent posterior lumbar surgery after being symptomatic for 3 to 240 months (mean: 48 months). All patients underwent CT and MRI before surgery, and 74 inferior articular processes (2 facets at L1/2, 3 at L2/3, 17 at L3/4, 35 at L4/5, and 17 at L5/S1) were obtained at surgery.

We included patients with lumbar spinal stenosis, lumbar disc herniation, and spondylolisthesis. All patients underwent routine CT (64-layer, high-speed helical CT, Siemens) and MRI (1.5 T, Siemens) preoperatively, and the inferior articular processes were resected intraoperatively. Exclusion criteria were patients with lumbar spinal tumor, infectious disease, fracture, or prior surgical treatment.

Image evaluation

Criteria proposed by Pathria to estimate the degeneration of the facet joint on CT were used [12]. Grade 1, normal; Grade 2, narrowing of facet joint; Grade 3, narrowing plus sclerosis or hypertrophy; and Grade 4, severe osteoarthritis with narrowing, sclerosis, and osteophytes (Figs. 1, 2 and 3).

Degeneration of the facet joint on MRI was evaluated according to the criteria used by Grogan [13]. Grade 1,

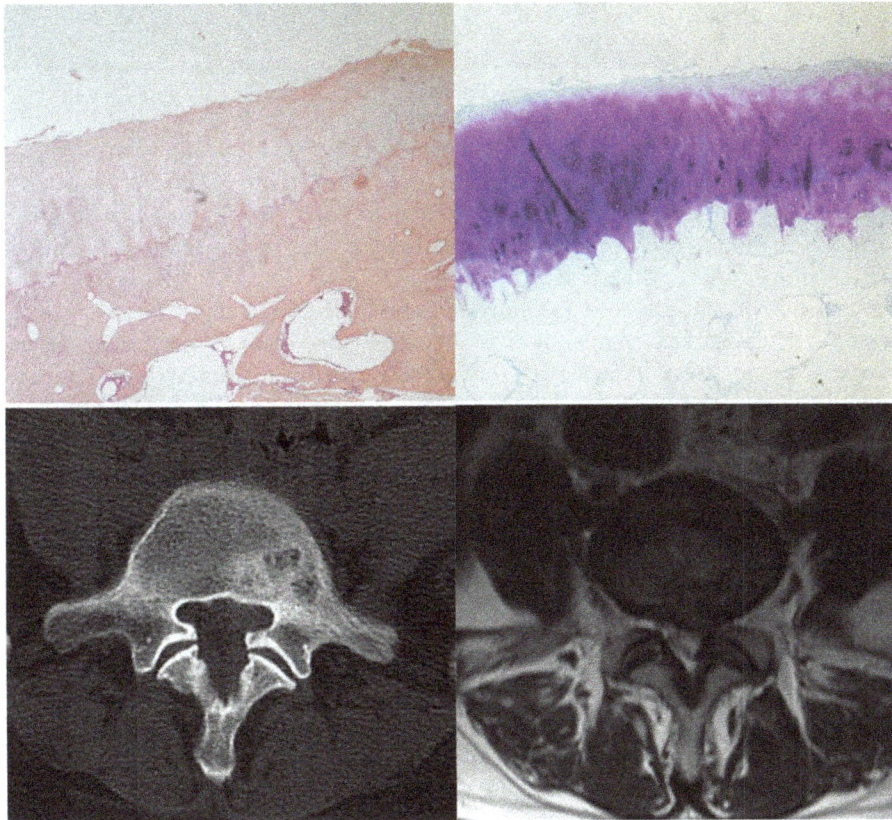

Fig. 1 A 43 years old woman with L5-S1 lumbar disc herniation suffered posterior lumbar surgery. The left inferior articular process of L5 was examined by hematoxylin and eosin (40×) (left) and toluidine blue (40×) (right) stain. The pathologic grading was 2. The CT grading, the MR grading and the CT combined MR grading were also 2

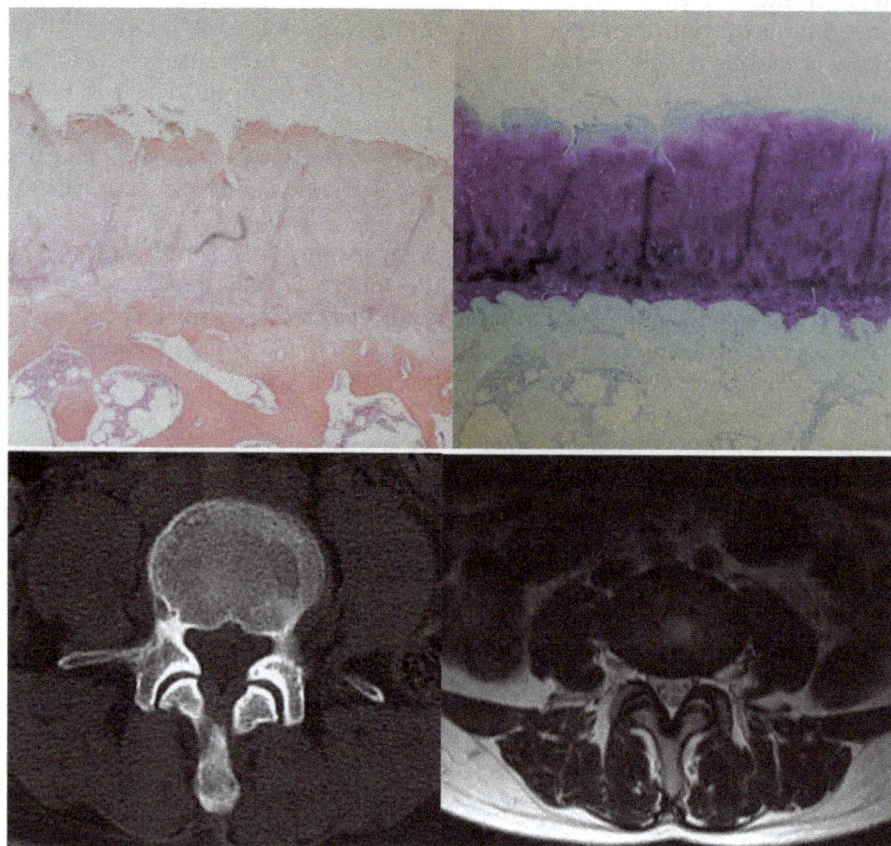

Fig. 2 The pathologic grading of the left L4/5 facet joint was 3. While the CT and MR grading was 2, the CT combined MR grading was 3. Both the CT and the MR grading underestimated the degree of facet joints degeneration

uniformly thick cartilage covering both articular surfaces completely; a uniform thin band of cortical bone. Grade 2, cartilage covering the entire surface with eroded or irregular regions; a thin band of cortical bone extended into the space from the articular surface. Grade 3, cartilage incompletely covering the articular surface, with the underlying bone exposed to the joint space; dense bone extended into the joint space but covering less than half the facet. Grade 4, complete absence of cartilage except for traces evident on the articular surface; presence of osteophytes or dense cortical bone covered greater than half the facet joint (Figs. 1, 2 and 3).

We also used Weishaupt proposed criteria adapted from those by Pathria to define the degree of facet degeneration using CT combined with MRI [14]. Grade 1, normal facet joint space (2–4 mm width); Grade 2, narrowing of the facet joint space (<2 mm) and/or small osteophytes, and/or mild hypertrophy of the articular process; Grade 3, narrowing of the facet joint space and/or moderate osteophytes, and/or moderate hypertrophy of the articular process, and/or mild subarticular bone erosions; and Grade 4, narrowing of the facet joint space and/or large osteophytes, and/or severe hypertrophy of

the articular process, and/or severe subarticular bone erosions, and/or subchondral cysts (Figs. 1, 2 and 3).

Pathologic evaluation

The inferior articular processes were resected during the posterior lumbar surgery, and were fixed in 10 % neutral buffered formalin. The specimens were immersed in a solution containing 10 % nitric acid and 1 % ethylenediaminetetraacetic acid (EDTA) for decalcification. After dehydration the specimens were embedded in paraffin, and a microtome was used to section the specimens into 5-um thickness, followed by dewaxing and washing. Finally the sections were stained by hematoxylin-eosin and toluidine blue, respectively.

The pathologic grade was evaluated with a method proposed by Gries [11]. Grade 1, smooth intact surface, orderly chondrocyte distribution, orderly collagen framework; uniform lamellar subchondral bone plate, uniform vascular budding into cartilage. Grade 2, tangential surface flaking, minimal chondrocyte death, few chondrones; minor thickening of trabeculae, small fissures at bone-cartilage junction, occasional fibrous tissue formation. Grade 3, fissures < 1/2 total depth,

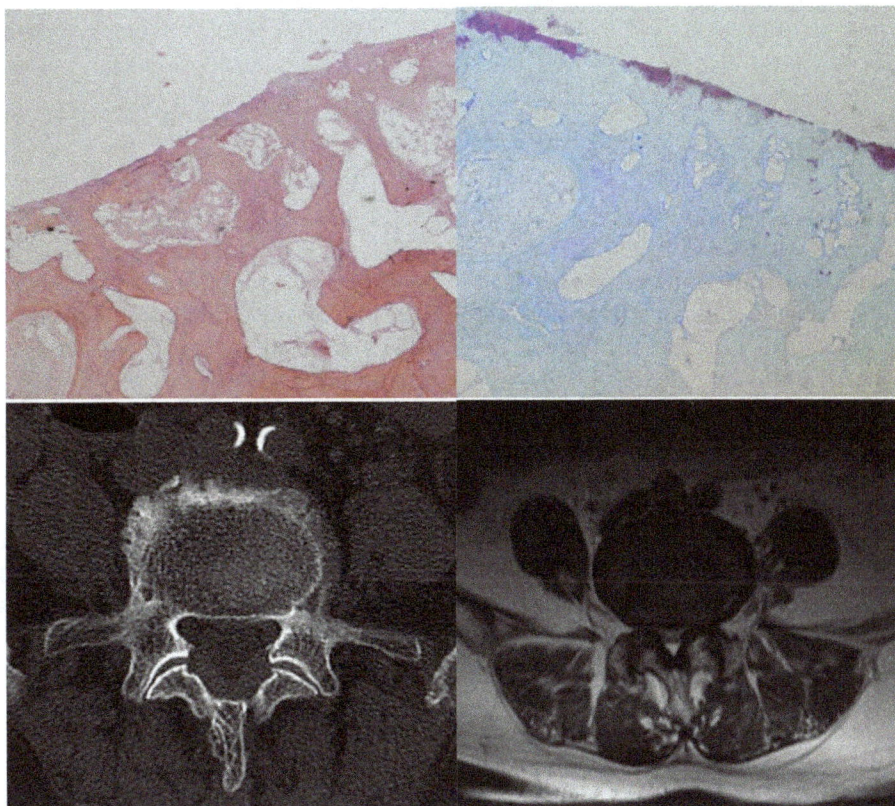

Fig. 3 The pathologic grading of the right L4/5 facet joint was 4. While the CT grading was 3, the MR and CT combined MR grading was 4. The CT grading underestimated the degree of facet joints degeneration

loss of cartilage < 1/2 depth, moderate chondrocyte death, many chondrones; moderate trabecular thickening, woven bone formation, moderate fibrous tissue formation. Grade 4, deep fissures, areas of total cartilage loss, extensive chondrocyte death; eburnation of exposed bone, bone sclerosis, cysts, extensive fibrosis (Figs. 1, 2 and 3).

Statistical analysis

The consistency of radiographic and pathologic grading as well as the consistency of CT and MRI grading based on the histologic examination were evaluated by consistent percentage and weighted kappa statistics. The kappa scores were classified into six categories: less than 0.00 (poor), 0.00 to 0.20 (slight), 0.21 to 0.40 (fair), 0.41 to 0.60 (moderate), 0.61 to 0.80 (substantial), and 0.81 to 1.00 (almost perfect) [15].

All radiographic and pathologic grading was assessed by two independent professionals. Grading was reevaluated up to 4 weeks after the first assessment. The interobserver and intraobserver agreement was estimated. The sensitivity, specificity, false negative rates (FNR).and false positive rate (FPR) were also calculated. SPSS (SPSS Statistics 13) was used for the statistical analyses.

Results

Consistency of radiographic and pathologic grading

The results showed moderate consistency between the CT and pathologic grading. Results for readers 1 and 2 and the consensus evaluation were the same for image and histologic grading in 39 (52.70 %), 41 (55.41 %), and 51 (68.92 %) of 74 facets, respectively. The agreement of CT and pathologic grading showed weighted kappa coefficients of 0.291, 0.297, and 0.506 for readers 1 and 2 and the consensus evaluation, respectively. Readers 1 and 2 and the consensus evaluation underestimated 26 (35.14 %), 23 (31.08 %), and 16 (21.62 %) facets (rate), and overestimated 9 (12.16 %), 10 (13.51 %), and 7 (9.46 %) facets (rate), respectively (Table 1). With the pathologic grade set as a standard, and with pathologic grades 1 and 2 defined as not degeneration, and grades 3 and 4 defined as degeneration, the facets were graded as not degeneration by CT, but as degeneration by pathologic grading in 19 (25.68 %), 14 (18.92 %), and 8 (10.81 %) facets by readers 1 and 2 and the consensus evaluation, respectively. The false negative rate (FNR) was 31.67, 23.33, and 13.33 %, and the false positive rate (FPR) was 28.57, 42.86, and 21.43 % for readers 1 and 2 and the consensus evaluation. The sensitivity and specificity of CT were 68.33, 76.67, and 86.67 %, and 71.43,

Table 1 Consistency of CT grading and pathologic grading for facet joint degeneration

Reader	Underestimate	Exact estimate	Overestimate	Weighted kappa coefficient
Reader 1	26(35.14 %)	39(52.70 %)	9(12.16 %)	0.291
Reader 2	23(31.08 %)	41(55.41 %)	10(13.51 %)	0.297
Consensus	16(21.62 %)	51(68.92 %)	7(9.46 %)	0.506

57.14, and 78.57 % for readers 1 and 2 and the consensus evaluation, respectively (Table 4).

The results showed moderate consistency between MRI and pathologic grading. Results for readers 1 and 2 and the consensus evaluation were the same grade for images and histologic grade in 49 (66.22 %), 49 (66.22 %), and 54 (72.97 %) of 74 facets, respectively. The agreement of MRI and pathologic grading showed weighted kappa coefficients of 0.458, 0.445, and 0.561 for readers 1 and 2 and the consensus evaluation, respectively. Readers 1 and 2 and the consensus evaluation underestimated 13 (17.57 %), 16 (21.62 %), and 12 (16.22 %) facets (rate), and overestimated 12 (16.22 %), 9 (12.16 %), and 8 (10.81 %) facets (rate), respectively (Table 2). The facets were graded as not degeneration by MRI but as degeneration by pathologic grading in 9 (15 %), 7 (11.67 %), and 6 (10 %) facets by readers 1 and 2 and the consensus evaluation, respectively. The false negative rate was 15, 11.67, and 10 %, and the false positive rate was 50, 42.86, and 35.71 % for readers 1 and 2 and the consensus evaluation, respectively. The sensitivity and specificity of MRI were 85, 88.33, and 90 %, and 50, 57.14, and 64.29 % for readers 1 and 2 and the consensus evaluation, respectively (Table 4).

The results showed moderate consistency between CT combined with MRI grading and pathologic grading. Results for readers 1 and 2 and the consensus evaluation were the same for images and histologic grade in 45 (60.81 %), 48 (64.86 %), and 55 (74.32 %) of 74 facets, respectively. The agreement of CT combined with MRI and pathologic grading showed weighted kappa coefficients of 0.394, 0.426, and 0.592 for readers 1 and 2 and the consensus evaluation, respectively. Readers 1 and 2 and the consensus evaluation underestimated 23 (31.08 %), 20 (27.03 %), and 14 (18.92 %) facets (rate), and overestimated 6 (8.11 %), 6 (8.11 %), and 5 (6.76 %) facets (rate), respectively (Table 3). The facets were graded as not degeneration by CT combined with MRI but as degeneration by pathologic grading in 15 (25 %), 9 (15 %), and 9 (15 %) facets by readers 1 and 2 and the consensus evaluation. The false negative rate was

25, 15, and 15 %, and the false positive rate was 28.57, 35.71, and 28.57 % for readers 1 and 2 and the consensus evaluation. The sensitivity and specificity of CT combined with MRI were 75, 85, and 85 %, and 71.43, 64.29, and 71.43 % for readers 1 and 2 and the consensus evaluation, respectively (Table 4).

Consistency of CT and MRI classification based on pathologic grading

With the pathologic grade set as a standard, results for readers 1 and 2 and the consensus evaluation were the same for at least one of the two image grades as for histologic grade in 55, 56, and 63 of 74 facets, respectively. The numbers of CT and MRI classifications which were the same as for the pathologic grade were 38, 41, and 51, and 43, 45, and 54 for readers 1 and 2 and the consensus evaluation, respectively. Results for readers 1 and 2 and the consensus evaluation yielded the same grade for CT and MRI in 26 (47.27 %), 30 (53.57 %), and 42 (66.67 %) facets, and the weighted kappa coefficients were 0.212, 0.235, and 0.459 respectively.

Intraobserver and interobserver agreement
Intraobserver agreement
Two observers evaluated the histologic and radiographic grading twice to determine the intraobserver agreement. The weighted kappa coefficients of the two histology observers were 0.852 and 0.833, respectively (almost perfect).

The weighted kappa coefficients of reader 1 for CT, MRI, and CT combined with MRI grading were 0.655, 0.646, and 0.653, respectively. The weighted kappa coefficients of reader 2 were 0.654, 0.656, and 0.669, respectively; all they corresponded to substantial agreement (Table 5).

Interobserver agreement
The weighted kappa coefficients of the two histology observers were 0.810 and 0.812, respectively (almost perfect agreement).

Table 2 Consistency of MR grading and pathologic grading for facet joint degeneration

Reader	Underestimate	Exact estimate	Overestimate	Weighted kappa coefficient
Reader 1	13(17.57 %)	49(66.22 %)	12(16.22 %)	0.458
Reader 2	16(21.62 %)	49(66.22 %)	9(12.16 %)	0.445
Consensus	12(16.22 %)	54(72.97 %)	8(10.81 %)	0.561

Table 3 Consistency of CT combined with MR grading and pathologic grading for facet joint degeneration

Reader	Underestimate	Exact estimate	Overestimate	Weighted kappa coefficient
Reader 1	13(17.57 %)	45(60.81 %)	12(16.22 %)	0.394
Reader 2	16(21.62 %)	48(64.86 %)	9(12.16 %)	0.426
Consensus	12(16.22 %)	55(74.32 %)	8(10.81 %)	0.592

For the first time, the weighted kappa coefficients of readers 1 and 2 for CT, MRI, and CT combined with MRI grading were 0.653, 0.645, and 0.553, respectively. The second time, the weighted kappa coefficients were 0.630, 0.615, and 0.572. The interobserver agreement of the two readers was substantial evaluating facets with CT or MRI, but only moderate combining CT and MRI (Table 6).

Discussion

Consistency between radiographic and pathologic grading

This study showed that radiographic grading of facet joint degeneration demonstrated moderate consistency with pathologic grading; CT combined with MRI grading exhibited the best agreement, followed by MRI grading and CT grading. The sensitivity of evaluation of facet joint degeneration was better than the specificity, indicating that imaging examination could efficiently detect degeneration of the facet joint, but that accuracy needed improvement. Moreover, imaging classification had a tendency to underestimate degeneration compared to pathologic classification; this finding suggests that clinicians should expect more severe facet degeneration than the degeneration estimated through CT or MRI.

In this study, we adopted the grading system proposed by Grogan, and first evaluated both cartilage and subchondral bone degeneration. Studies had shown that

Table 4 Sensitivity, specificity, false negative rate, false positive rate of radiographic examination for facet joint degeneration by the pathologic grading

Radiography	Sensitivity	Specificity	FNR	FPR
CT				
Reader 1	68.33 %	71.43 %	31.67 %	28.57 %
Reader 2	76.67 %	57.14 %	23.33 %	42.86 %
Consensus	86.67 %	78.57 %	13.33 %	21.43 %
MR				
Reader 1	85.00 %	50.00 %	15.00 %	50.00 %
Reader 2	88.33 %	57.14 %	11.67 %	42.86 %
Consensus	90.00 %	64.29 %	10.00 %	35.71 %
CT combined with MR				
Reader 1	75.00 %	71.43 %	25.00 %	28.57 %
Reader 2	85.00 %	64.29 %	15.00 %	35.71 %
Consensus	85.00 %	71.43 %	15.00 % ·	28.57 %

subchondral bone plays an important role in the development of osteoarthritis [16–19]. In the early period of osteoarthritis, transformation enhancement of subchondral bone, change of trabecular bone structure, and sclerosis of subchondral bone appear [20]. Because articular cartilage derives nutrition from the terminal vessels in the subchondral bone plate and calcified cartilage layer [21], subchondral bone sclerosis can not only accelerate the disease process, but also is likely to be an originating factor in the onset of osteoarthritis [22]. Considering the role of the subchondral bone in osteoarthritis, this study introduced the grade of facet joint subchondral bone degeneration to obtain more accurate radiographic and pathologic classification.

Since CT examination could better display osteophyte formation, hypertrophy of articular processes, sclerosis, calcification of the joint capsule, and the vacuum joint phenomenon [23], previous research reported that CT was the best radiographic examination for evaluating facet joint degeneration [4, 24–26]. However, our study found that MRI examination was slightly superior to CT in assessing facet joint degeneration. The different results may be explained because the studies that reported CT facet evaluation being better than MRI assessment were published years ago, when MRI technique was limited, thus leading to low accuracy on MRI examination.

Our study used a 1.5 T MRI, which not only better displayed the articular cartilage, joint fluid, and joint capsule, but also showed osteophytes, subchondral bone, and other osseous structures. Use of a 3 T MRI device may be able to identify minimal and early phase degeneration of facet joints, and improve the accuracy of MRI examination. The intraobserver and interobserver agreements of MRI classification were inferior to CT, indicating that MRI grading was more prone to produce divergence between the observers. Therefore, trained and experienced observers are needed to evaluate MRI grading to obtain adequate accuracy.

In this study, the consistency between CT combined with MRI grading and pathology grading was better, the sensitivity was highest, and the false negative rate was lowest than other method alone. However, both CT and MRI examination underestimated facet joint degeneration; thus, advanced imaging technology and more accurate grading methods for facet joint degeneration are necessary to improve the accuracy and reliability of evaluation of the degenerative facet joint.

Table 5 Intraobserver agreement

Reader	Histology		CT		MR		CT combined with MR	
	1	2	1	2	1	2	1	2
Exact estimate	67	66	57	58	57	58	58	60
	90.54 %	89.19 %	77.03 %	78.38 %	77.03 %	78.38 %	78.38 %	81.08 %
Wĸ	0.852	0.833	0.655	0.654	0.646	0.656	0.653	0.669

Wĸ weighted kappa coefficient

Consistency of CT grading and MRI grading based on pathologic grading

With the pathologic examination set as a standard, the CT and MRI grading showed moderate consistency. This result may be related to the features of CT and MRI examination, in which CT mainly observed the degeneration of bony structures, whereas MRI detected articular cartilage degeneration. Therefore, we do not think that CT examination can replace MRI for evaluation of facet joint degeneration.

Clinical implications of radiographic grading for facet joint degeneration

Facet joint degeneration is an important cause of low back pain [2–4], and the amount of low back pain is associated with the degree of facet joint degeneration in some patients [27]. In the spine arthrodesis, facet joints are usually fused along with intervertebral fusion. As a result, the possible facet pain may be cured, in other words, the facet pain may be eliminated through the fusion procedure. Nevertheless, in non-fusion surgeries that retain the facet joints, such as artificial disc replacement or discectomy, patients with low back pain may still have symptoms secondary to facet joint degeneration. Therefore, an accurate evaluation of facet joint degeneration is particularly important before surgery. This study found that CT and MRI examination in the evaluation of facet joint degeneration had moderate accuracy and reliability, and CT combined with MRI was the best choice for assessment of facet joint degeneration. Clinically, use of CT and MRI examination to evaluate facet joint degeneration before spinal non-fusion surgery is presently the best option to detect FJOA.

There were some limitations in this study. First, patients with lumbar spinal stenosis, lumbar disc herniation, or spondylolisthesis were chosen in this study, and

were not clearly diagnosed with FJOA. Therefore, this study did not evaluate the correlation between symptoms and facet joint degeneration. Second, the majority of patients had a long course of disease and severe degeneration of the facet joints, and normal facet joint specimens were not obtained. Increasing the sample size or collecting facets from patients with lumbar fractures could be implemented in further research. Third, the facet samples were excised from living patients, so only the inferior articular specimens which were resected during fusion surgery were used. However, previous studies proved that the degeneration of superior and inferior articular facets made no obvious difference [28, 29]. Thus, we surmise that the inferior articular processes represent degeneration of the entire facet joint.

Facet joints play an important role in non-fusion surgery, but our study showed that the accuracy and reliability of the radiographic examination to evaluate facet joint degeneration was still limited. Therefore, using more advanced radiographic technology and thin-layer scanning, and developing more accurate and effective radiographic grading for facet joint degeneration will be the direction of our further research.

Conclusion

This study found that current radiographic techniques had moderate accuracy and reliability for assessing facet joint degeneration. CT combined with MRI was better for assessing facet joint degeneration than CT or MRI alone. However, more accurate radiographic grading for evaluating facet joint degeneration is still needed.

Ethics and consent statements

This study conformed to human experimentation standards of the ethics committee of the First Affiliated

Table 6 Interobserver agreement

Time	Histology		CT		MR		CT combined with MR	
	1st	2nd	1st	2nd	1st	2nd	1st	2nd
Exact estimate	65	65	57	56	57	56	55	54
	87.84 %	87.84 %	77.03 %	75.68 %	77.03 %	75.68 %	74.32 %	72.97 %
Wĸ	0.810	0.812	0.653	0.630	0.645	0.615	0.553	0.572

Wĸ weighted kappa coefficient

Hospital of Nanchang University, and informed consents were obtained from the subjects.

Abbreviations
CT: computed tomography; FJOA: facet joint osteoarthritis; FNR: false negative rate; FPR: false positive rate; MRI: magnetic resonance imaging.

Competing interests
The authors declare that they have no competing interests.

Authors' contributions
BZ carried out the conception and design, revised the manuscript, and approved the final version to be published. MD carried out conception and design and approved the final version to be published. XZ participated in the conception and design, drafted and revised the manuscript, and analyzed and interpreted the data. YL participated in the design of the study and performed the statistical analysis. SZ conceived of the study, participated in its design and coordination, and helped to revise the manuscript. XXF: acquisition of data, analysis and interpretation of data. XLY: acquisition of data. CLF: acquisition of data. All authors read and approved the final manuscript.

Acknowledgements
We would like to thank radiologist Yu-Ling He of the Department of Radiology, the First Affiliated Hospital of Nanchang University, for his advice in the evaluation of radiographic grading. We thank pathologist San-San Wang of the Department of Pathology, the First Affiliated Hospital of Nanchang University, for her direction in the evaluation of pathologic grading.

Foundation item
1. Science and technology support project of Jiangxi Province (20151122070282);
2. Science and technology project of Health and Family Planning Commission of Jiangxi Province (20155195).

Author details
[1]Department of Orthopedics, The First Affiliated Hospital of Nanchang University, Nanchang 330006, China. [2]Artificial Joint Engineering and Technology Research Center of Jiangxi Province, Nanchang 330006, China.

References
1. Goode AP, Carey TS, Jordan JM. Low back pain and lumbar spine osteoarthritis: how are they related? Curr Rheumatol Rep. 2013;15:305–17.
2. Schwarzer AC, Aprill C, Derby R, et al. Clinical features of patients with pain stemming from the lumbar zygapophyseal joints. Is the lumbar facet syndrome a clinical entity? Spine. 1994;10:1132–7.
3. Manchkanti L, Pampati V, Fellows B, et al. Prevalence of facet joint pain in chronic low back pain. Pain Physician. 1999;2:59–64.
4. Kalichman L, Hunter DJ. Lumbar facet joint osteoarthritis: a review. Semin Arthritis Rheum. 2007;37:69–80.
5. Fujiwara A, Lim TH, An HS, et al. The effect of disc degeneration and facet joint osteoarthritis on the segmental flexibility of the lumbar spine. Spine. 2000;25:3036–44.
6. Gellhorn AC, Katz JN, Suri P. Osteoarthritis of the spine: the facet joints. Nat Rev Rheumatol. 2013;9:216–24.
7. Louis R. Spinal stability as defined by the three-column spine concept. Anat Clin. 1985;7:33–42.
8. Kumar MN, Jacquot F, Hall H. Long-term follow-up of functional outcomes and radiographic changes at adjacent levels following lumbar spine fusion for degenerative disc disease. Eur Spine J. 2001;10:309–13.
9. Mario C, Alexander A, Christian W, et al. The short- and mid-term effect of dynamic interspinous distraction in the treatment of recurrent lumbar facet joint pain. Eur Spine J. 2009;18:1686–94.
10. Trouillier H, Kern P, Refior HJ, et al. A prospective morphological study of facet joint integrity following intervertebral disc replacement with the CHARITE Artificial Disc. Eur Spine J. 2006;15:174–82.
11. Gries NC, Berlemann U, Moore RJ, et al. Early histologic changes in lower lumbar discs and facet joints and their correlation. Eur Spine J. 2000;9:23–9.
12. Pathria M, Sartoris DJ. Osteoarthritis of the lumbar facet joints: accuracy of oblique radiographic assessment. Radiology. 1987;164:227–30.
13. Grogan J, Nowicki BH, Schmidt TA, et al. Lumbar facet joint tropism does not accelerate degeneration of the facet joints. Am J Neuroradiol. 1997;18:1325–9.
14. Weishaupt D, Zanetti M, Boos N, et al. MR imaging and CT in osteoarthritis of the lumbar facet joints. Skeletal Radiol. 1999;28:215–9.
15. Landis JR, Koch GG. The measurement of observer agreement for categorical data. Biometrics. 1977;33:159–74.
16. Sniekers YH, Intema F, Lafeber FP, et al. A role for subchondral bone changes in the process of osteoarthritis: a micro-CT study of two canine models. BMC Musculoskelet Disord. 2008;9:20.
17. Botter SM, Van Osch GJ, Waarsing JH, et al. Cartilage damage pattern in relation to subchondral plate thickness in a collagenase-induced model of osteoarthritis. Osteoarthritis Cartilage. 2008;16:506–14.
18. Botter SM, Van Osch GJ, Clockaerts S, et al. Osteoarthritis induction leads to early and temporal subchondral plate porosity in the tibial plateau of mice: an in vivo microfocal computer tomography study. Arthritis Rheum. 2011;63:2690–9.
19. Hayami T, Pickarski M, Zhuo Y, et al. Characterization of articular cartilage and subchondral bone changes in the rat anterior cruciate ligament transaction and meniscectomized models of osteoarthritis. Bone. 2006;38:234–43.
20. Tomoya M, Hiroshi H, Toru O, et al. Role of subchondral bone in osteoarthritis development: a comparative study of two strains of guinea pigs with and without spontaneously occurring osteoarthritis. Arthritis Rheum. 2007;56:3366–74.
21. Lyons TJ, McClure SF, Stoddart RW, et al. The normal human chondro-osseous junctional region: evidence for contact of uncalcified cartilage with subchondral bone and marrow spaces. BMC Musculoskelet Disord. 2006;7:52.
22. Burr DB. Anatomy and physiology of the mineralized tissues: role in the pathogenesis of osteoarthrosis. Osteoarthritis Cartilage. 2004;12:20–30.
23. Carrera GF, Haughton VM, Syvertsen A, et al. Computed tomography of the facet joints. Radiology. 1980;134:145–8.
24. Raskin SP. Degenerative changes of the lumbar spine: assessment by computed tomography. Orthopedics. 1981;4:186–95.
25. Grenier N, Kressel HY, Schiebler ML, et al. Normal and degenerative posterior spinal structures: MR imaging. Radiology. 1987;165:517–25.
26. Modic MT, Ross JS. Magnetic resonance imaging in the evaluation of low back pain. Orthop Clin North Am. 1991;22:283–301.
27. Suri P, Hunter DJ, Rainville J. Presence and extent of severe facet joint osteoarthritis are associated with back pain in older adults. Osteoarthritis Cartilage. 2013;21:1199–206.
28. Tanno I, Murakami G, Oguma H, et al. Morphometry of the lumbar zygapophyseal facet capsule and cartilage with special reference to degenerative osteoarthritic changes: an anatomical study using fresh cadavers of elderly Japanese and Korean subjects. J Orthop Sci. 2004;9:468–77.
29. Tischer T, Aktas T, Milz S, et al. Detailed pathological changes of human lumbar facet joints L1-L5 in elderly individuals. Eur Spine J. 2006;15:308–15.

7

A comparison of pediatric and adult CT organ dose estimation methods

Yiming Gao[1] ⓘ, Brian Quinn[1], Usman Mahmood[1], Daniel Long[1], Yusuf Erdi[1], Jean St. Germain[1], Neeta Pandit-Taskar[2], X. George Xu[3], Wesley E. Bolch[4] and Lawrence T. Dauer[1,2]*

Abstract

Background: Computed Tomography (CT) contributes up to 50% of the medical exposure to the United States population. Children are considered to be at higher risk of developing radiation-induced tumors due to the young age of exposure and increased tissue radiosensitivity. Organ dose estimation is essential for pediatric and adult patient cancer risk assessment. The objective of this study is to validate the VirtualDose software in comparison to currently available software and methods for pediatric and adult CT organ dose estimation.

Methods: Five age groups of pediatric patients and adult patients were simulated by three organ dose estimators. Head, chest, abdomen-pelvis, and chest-abdomen-pelvis CT scans were simulated, and doses to organs both inside and outside the scan range were compared. For adults, VirtualDose was compared against ImPACT and CT-Expo. For pediatric patients, VirtualDose was compared to CT-Expo and compared to size-based methods from literature. Pediatric to adult effective dose ratios were also calculated with VirtualDose, and were compared with the ranges of effective dose ratios provided in ImPACT.

Results: In-field organs see less than 60% difference in dose between dose estimators. For organs outside scan range or distributed organs, a five times' difference can occur. VirtualDose agrees with the size-based methods within 20% difference for the organs investigated. Between VirtualDose and ImPACT, the pediatric to adult ratios for effective dose are compared, and less than 21% difference is observed for chest scan while more than 40% difference is observed for head-neck scan and abdomen-pelvis scan. For pediatric patients, 2 cm scan range change can lead to a five times dose difference in partially scanned organs.

Conclusions: VirtualDose is validated against CT-Expo and ImPACT with relatively small discrepancies in dose for organs inside scan range, while large discrepancies in dose are observed for organs outside scan range. Patient-specific organ dose estimation is possible using the size-based methods, and VirtualDose agrees with size-based method for the organs investigated. Careful range selection for CT protocols is necessary for organ dose optimization for pediatric and adult patients.

Keywords: CT dosimetry, Organ dose, Effective dose, Pediatric, Adult, Monte Carlo

Background

Besides the natural background, medical exposure is the largest source of ionizing radiation exposure to the human population [1, 2]. Computed Tomography (CT) is one of the most widely adopted medical imaging modalities in clinical use, and is increasingly used because of the technology advancements and the improvements in medical infrastructure [1, 3–5]. CT scans contribute up to 50% of the medical exposure to the United States (US) populations in 2006 [1, 2]. The annual number of CT examinations in the US has increased by 10% each year from 1993 through 2011, up to 85 million in 2011, and stabilized around 80 million with 0.6 million annual change at most since 2011 [6]. With a population of 325 million in the US in 2016 where 24% of the population is pediatrics and adolescents under age of 18, one in four Americans has a CT scan each year [7]. The high number of CT scans and high contribution of CT scans to medical exposure raised concerns in the radiation protection and radiology

* Correspondence: dauerl@mskcc.org
[1]Department of Medical Physics, Memorial Sloan Kettering Cancer Center, 1275 York Avenue, Box 84, New York, NY 10065, USA
[2]Department of Radiology, Memorial Sloan Kettering Cancer Center, 1275 York Avenue, New York, NY 10065, USA
Full list of author information is available at the end of the article

community. The International Commission on Radiological Protection (ICRP) addressed the importance of multi-detector CT patient dose management in 2007 [4]. The principles of optimization and 'as low as reasonably achievable' (ALARA) have been major principles and have been adopted in the radiation protection of patients, the public, and radiological workers for decades [8–11]. The American College of Radiology (ACR) introduced the Dose Index Registry in 2011 to facilitate the collection and comparison of the CT dose indices for all participating medical entities [12]. A group of radiologists formed the Alliance for Radiation Safety in Pediatric Imaging & the Image Gently Alliance, and started the Image Gently campaign in 2007 to send a message of reducing the amount of radiation when performing pediatric CT scans [13]. For adults, ACR introduced the Image Wisely campaign in 2010 to raise awareness of eliminating unnecessary exams as well as using only the amount of radiation necessary for required image quality [14].

Children are generally considered to be at higher risks of developing radiation-induced tumors because of the young age of exposure and increased tissue radiosensitivity in some of the organs [15–17]. For the 23 types of cancers reviewed recently by the United Nations Scientific Committee on the Effects of Atomic Radiation (UNSCEAR) committee, children are clearly more likely to develop one of a quarter of these types, including leukemia, brain, breast, skin, and thyroid cancer [15]. However, for the other three quarters of the cancer types, children are no more sensitive (such as colon cancer or lung cancer) than adults, or there is either not enough data or no clear relationship between radiation exposure and cancer risks [15]. The UNSCEAR committee recommends avoiding the use of generalized radiation risks for children and emphasizes the evaluating of and using specific organ dose, the importance of which has been recognized by the radiology community with respect to radiation induced cancer risk estimations [15, 18–24].

Organ dose is the absorbed dose to a specific organ in the body, and is generally estimated as the ratio of the amount of ionizing radiation energy deposited in the organ to the mass of the organ, representing an estimate of the average damage to the organ per unit mass. Organ dose is not a dose estimate that is readily available to radiologists or physicians in clinical CT scans. Rather, the CT scanners commonly report volumetric CT dose index ($CTDI_{vol}$) and dose length product (DLP) at the end of examinations [25]. $CTDI_{vol}$ represents the average radiation dose for a standardized CTDI phantom over the entire field of view and through a scan length of 100 mm along the longitudinal axis after taking the pitch of the scan into consideration [25]. DLP is the integrated dose for the entire CT scan length, and is equal to the product of $CTDI_{vol}$ and scan length [25]. It is clear that either $CTDI_{vol}$ or DLP, when $CTDI_{vol}$ is an average radiation dose estimate and DLP is an overall radiation dose estimate to standardized phantoms, is not a good estimate of patient organ dose. Size-specific dose estimates (SSDE) were introduced in 2011 to adjust the $CTDI_{vol}$ to address the effect of the patient sizes on the average radiation dose, especially for small-size pediatric patients and large-size overweight patients [26]. Methods and recommendations of the calculations and usage of SSDE were updated in a later publication [27], but the quantity itself remained a poor estimate for individual organ dose that did not account for the tissue differences or the geometric location of the organ [22, 23, 28].

Although organ dose cannot be directly measured on living tissues or organs, measurements in physical anthropomorphic phantoms are possible. However, they require great amounts of time, equipment, and skilled staff to perform [19, 29–35]. A practical method of accurate organ dose estimation is to use Monte Carlo (MC) methods and anatomically realistic computational anthropomorphic phantoms to simulate the CT scans and to calculate the organ doses [18, 20, 21, 23, 36, 37]. Sophisticated computation codes such as MCNPX incorporate the Monte Carlo method and can be used to model the CT scanner and simulate the transport of ionizing radiation in anthropomorphic phantoms [38–40]. Unlike stylized phantoms which are composed of three dimensional geometric objects such as spheres and cylinders, computational anthropomorphic phantoms resemble the realistic anatomical features of patient morphologies and faithfully apply the compositions of the body tissues according to standards or reference sets [41–43]. Thus, the use of realistic phantoms generates more accurate dose results than using stylized phantoms [20, 42, 44–46]. Pediatric patient phantoms, pregnant patient phantoms, and adult patient phantoms with various body sizes were developed to address the age, pregnancy, or body size variations among patient populations [47–51].

Various MC-based organ dose calculators can be currently acquired, allowing quick dose calculations for medical physicists and physicians. Most of the widely used calculators are based on the unrealistic stylized phantoms, such as ImPACT and CT-Expo [52, 53]. CT-Expo integrated two adult phantoms and two pediatric phantoms, allowing for some representative pediatric organ dose estimations [53]. However, ImPACT provides no intrinsic calculation method for pediatric organ dose estimation, while supplying a set of ranges of adjustment factors for roughly estimating effective dose to pediatric patients [52]. A few newly developed dose calculators utilize anatomically realistic phantoms and provide better patient-matching options for organ dose calculation. VirtualDose is the first online organ dose and effective dose calculator that incorporates anatomically realistic phantoms for patients of various ages (including pediatric ages 0 through 15), gender, pregnancy stages, or body sizes [23].

The objective of this study is to validate the Virtual-Dose software in comparison to currently available software and methods for pediatric and adult CT organ dose estimation. First, CT-Expo and VirtualDose are used to generate the major portion of the organ dose data. Then, ImPACT is used to calculate and compare adult organ doses as it lacks specific pediatric phantoms [52]. Thirdly, body-size based MC methods for organ doses of patients of various sizes are also investigated, and compared with the doses by VirtualDose [18, 22, 24, 28]. Finally, pediatric-to-adult effective dose ratios are also calculated with VirtualDose and compared to the ranges of the effective dose ratios provided by ImPACT. Additionally, the effect of the scan range change on organ dose is discussed to show the importance of scan range selection on dose optimization.

Methods

Organ dose and effective dose for pediatric patients who received CT scans were calculated with three dose calculators: VirtualDose, CT-Expo, and ImPACT. Four CT protocols were investigated: head, chest, abdomen-pelvis (AP), and chest-abdomen-pelvis (CAP). With Virtual-Dose, pediatric patients at 5 different age groups were covered: 0-year-old, 1-year-old, 5-year-old, 10-year-old, and 15-year-old. Adult patients of normal sizes were also included in the calculations. Organ doses by VirtualDose were also compared to the organ doses based on size-dependent functions from literature [18, 22, 24, 28]. The ratios of the effective doses of the 5 pediatric groups to the normal size adults were calculated and compared to the ranges of pediatric-to-adult effective dose ratios by ImPACT.

CT protocols

Four CT protocols were simulated in the study to cover the head and the trunk of patients: head, chest, AP, and CAP. Since the dose calculator VirtualDose provided the largest collection of pediatric phantoms, the scan range defined in VirtualDose for the four protocols was also applied to CT-Expo and ImPACT as best as possible. For head protocol, the scan range was from the top of head through C1 lamina. For chest protocol, the scan range was from the clavicles through the diaphragm. For AP protocol, the scan range was from the top of liver through the pubic symphysis. For CAP protocol, the scan range was from the clavicles through the pubic symphysis. No over-scan was taken into account, as a

pitch of 1 was used. A Siemens Somatom Sensation 16 CT model, which was the scanner model employed in the Monte Carlo simulations of the pediatric phantoms [23], was used in the calculation of dose data for the three dose calculators. In VirtualDose, for 0-year-old, 1-year-old, 5-year-old, and 10-year-old patients, head bowtie filters were used in all four protocols. For 15-year-old and adult patients, head bowtie filters were used for head protocols, and body bowtie filters were used for other protocols. The rest of CT scan parameters were kept the same for all protocols and all phantoms to enable more direct comparisons: 120 kVp tube voltage, 100 mAs tube current time product, a pitch of 1, and 10 mm beam collimation. The effective dose was calculated using tissue weighting factors from ICRP No. 103 publication employing the gender-average methodology [10].

Organ dose calculators

VirtualDose was a web-based CT organ dose and effective dose calculator that incorporated 25 "virtual patient" phantoms covering pediatric patients, pregnant patients, normal size adult patients, and overweight adult patients [23]. The 5 pairs of male and female pediatric phantoms covering 0-year-old, 1-year-old, 5-year-old, 10-year-old and 15-year-old patients were used in this study, in addition to a pair of normal size male and female adults. The doses to 15 organs to which tissue weighting factors were assigned in the ICRP No. 103 Publication, as well as doses to the 13 organs defined as remainder in the report and the effective dose, were estimated [10]. The $CTDI_{vol}$ was 16.6 mGy for the protocols using head bowtie filters, and it was 6.8 mGy for the protocols using body bowtie filters. Organ dose and effective dose were normalized with these $CTDI_{vol}$ values accordingly, to reduce the scanner dependency [54]. The scan range of the four protocols simulated by VirtualDose was listed in Table 1. For 0-year-old, 1-year-old, 5-year-old, and 10-year-old patients, the scan range were the same between males and females.

CT-Expo was a Microsoft Excel based application for patient CT dose calculation, and used the dose evaluation methods mentioned in CT exposure surveys in Germany [53, 55]. The application was capable of reporting organ doses and effective doses using the tissue weighting factors of the ICRP No. 103 Publication [10]. However, the application only included 4 stylized patient phantoms: one for adult male (ADAM), one for adult female (EVA), one for children at age of seven (CHILD), and one for infants (BABY) [53, 56]. The doses for 31 organs and tissues were available, but for comparison purposes the 28 organ doses available in VirtualDose were also collected in CT-Expo. The average of the lower large intestine dose and the upper large intestine dose was considered as the colon dose for

Table 1 Scan range for VirtualDose in this study

Patient	Height	Head		Chest		AP[a]		CAP[b]	
		Start	End	Start	End	Start	End	Start	End
0YM	47.5	39.8	47.1	28.0	35.8	13.5	29.6	13.5	35.8
0YF	47.5	39.8	47.1	28.0	35.8	13.5	29.6	13.5	35.8
1YM	76.5	64.4	75.6	47.8	58.4	28.7	49.0	28.7	58.4
1YF	76.5	64.4	75.6	47.8	58.4	28.7	49.0	28.7	58.4
5YM	110.5	96.0	108.8	75.9	89.4	50.0	76.9	50.0	89.4
5YF	110.5	96.0	108.8	75.9	89.4	50.0	76.9	50.0	89.4
10YM	140.5	125.2	138.6	100.0	117.8	66.7	102.0	66.7	117.8
10YF	140.5	125.2	138.6	100.0	117.8	66.7	102.0	66.7	117.8
15YM	166.5	152.0	165.0	117.4	140.4	81.8	120.6	81.8	140.4
15YF	161.7	147.8	159.8	114.8	136.2	80.2	118.1	80.2	136.2
RPIM	176.0	164.0	176.0	124.0	151.0	86.8	124.8	86.8	151.0
RPIF	163.5	152.5	163.0	115.0	140.0	82.0	115.1	82.0	140.0

[a] AP abdomen-pelvis, [b] CAP, chest-abdomen-pelvis
Note: both scan range and phantom height are in unit of cm. The simulated CT scans start from inferior location (Start) through superior location (End). The bottom of the feet of phantoms is defined as 0 cm

calculations with CT-Expo. Due to lacking anatomical details in organs and tissues of the stylized phantoms, the scan range was matched on these phantoms as best as possible, and the start and end locations were listed in Table 2. The location of pubic symphysis was surrogated by the location of the bottom of the trunk, and the location of C1 vertebrae was approximated by the location where the cylindrical spine intercepts the oval head.

Several comparisons of the estimated organ dose by VirtualDose to the estimated organ dose by CT-Expo were made. The 0-year-old and 1-year-old doses of VirtualDose were compared to the BABY doses of CT-Expo. The 5-year-old and 10-year-old doses of VirtualDose were compared to the CHILD doses of CT-Expo. The 15-year-old and adult doses of VirtualDose were compared to the adult doses of CT-Expo. The comparisons were performed for both males and females, although for patients younger than 10-year-old there were no differences in doses to most organs between males and females except for doses to gonads. Organs that were outside the scan range and with doses

Table 2 Scan range for CT-Expo in this study

Patient	Head		Chest		AP		CAP	
	Start	End	Start	End	Start	End	Start	End
BABY	29	38	14	25	0	18	0	25
CHILD	47	63	28	42	0	32	0	42
ADAM	81	94	41	71	-2	43	-2	71
EVA	75	89	38	67	0	40	0	67

Note: both scan range and phantom height are in unit of cm. The simulated CT scans start from inferior location (Start) through superior location (End). The trunk base of the phantoms is defined as 0 cm

smaller than 0.5 mGy were not included in dose comparisons as the inherent errors of the doses might be comparable to the doses themselves. Effective doses calculated with tissue weighting factors from ICRP No.103 publication were also included in the comparisons, and were noted as ED103 in figures [10]. Two-sample t-test was performed for a list of in-field organs in each scanned region between VirtualDose and CT-Expo for 0-year-old (or BABY), 5-year-old (or CHILD), and adult. For head scan, the organ list included the brain and the lens of eye. For chest scan, the organ list included the breast, the esophagus, the lungs, and the thymus. For AP scan, the organ list includes the colon, the liver, the stomach, the urinary bladder, the adrenals, the gall bladder, the kidneys, the pancreas, the small intestine, the spleen, and the uterus (female)/prostate (male). For CAP scan, the organ list was the combination of the lists of chest scan and AP scan. For each of the aforementioned scan region, the null hypothesis was the VirtualDose doses and the CT-Expo doses were from distributions of equal means and equal variances. In each t-test, the dose lists of 0-year-old, 5-year-old, and adult for both male and female were concatenated into one list for VirtualDose, and the dose lists of BABY, CHILD, and adult were concatenated into one list for CT-Expo before the test was performed on the resultant lists of the two software. Similar t-test was also performed for effective dose of the two by concatenating the effective dose results across patients and scan regions into one list for each tool and using the resultant lists in the test. Statistical significance was defined as $p < 0.05$.

ImPACT was also a Microsoft Excel based spreadsheet application for patient CT dose calculation, and used the Monte Carlo data by the National Radiological Protection Board (NRPB) in the United Kingdom [52]. The application only included the MIRD hermaphrodite adult phantom, and employed adjustment factors for the effective dose of pediatric patients [57, 58]. For adults, organ doses were calculated using the ImPACT spreadsheet and the scan range for ImPACT calculations was listed in Table 3. The adult organ doses were compared between VirtualDose, CT-Expo, and ImPACT. Ratios of VirtualDose to CT-Expo, and ratios of VirtualDose to ImPACT were calculated and demonstrated for the simulated head CT scan and the simulated CAP CT scan.

Table 3 Scan range for ImPACT in this study

Patient	Head		CAP	
	Start	End	Start	End
MIRD	80	94	-1	71

Note: both scan range and phantom height are in unit of cm. The simulated CT scans start from inferior location (Start) through superior location (End). The trunk base of the phantoms is defined as 0 cm

Effective doses with tissue weighting factors from ICRP No.103 publication were also compared between the three codes [10]. Two-sample t-test was performed between VirtualDose and ImPACT, VirtualDose and CT-Expo, and ImPACT and CT-Expo for adult. The included in-field organs were the same as the ones defined previously for head scan and CAP scan. The organ doses of the two scan regions and both genders were concatenated into one list for each tool before the test was performed on the resultant lists. The null hypothesis was the doses of the two compared tools were from distributions of equal means and equal variances. Statistical significance was defined as $p < 0.05$.

In addition, the ratios of pediatrics effective dose to adult effective dose were provided in the form of ranges in ImPACT spread sheet, allowing rough estimation of pediatric effective dose from adult effective dose for head and neck (HN), chest, and AP CT scans [52]. Similar pediatric-to-adult effective dose ratios were calculated with VirtualDose using the tissue weighting factors of the ICRP No. 103 Publication [10]. The ratios calculated by VirtualDose were compared to the ranges of ratios by ImPACT.

Body-size based methods

The organ doses of patients were affected by the size of the body region being scanned. Besides the SSDE metric introduced by AAPM, several groups investigated the effects of the body sizes on organ doses, and developed empirical functions [18, 21, 22, 24, 28]. Turner et al. found a strong exponential relationship between body-$CTDI_{vol}$–normalized organ doses and patient perimeter of the abdominal region [18]. Care must be taken in utilizing the exponential function proposed by Turner et al., because typically one would apply head bowtie filter for pediatric CT exams and calculate head-$CTDI_{vol}$-normalized organ doses as in the following studies by three other groups [18]. Tian et al. found the head-$CTDI_{vol}$-normalized organ doses decreased exponentially with the patient diameter increasing [21, 28]. Kost et al. calculated the diameters of patients by assuming a cylindrical volume of the scanned region and performed exponential regression for head-$CTDI_{vol}$-normalized organ doses as a function of these diameters [22]. Papadakis et al. developed exponential equations for head-$CTDI_{vol}$-normalized organ doses as a function of the water equivalent diameters of the scanned regions of patients [24]. In this study, we applied size parameters of the pediatric phantoms in VirtualDose to the methods proposed by the aforementioned four groups and calculated the doses for a limited number of organs. The reasons for the limited number of organs are: Turner et al. only reported doses to several organs of abdominal region [18]; only the effective diameters of abdominal

regions of the pediatric phantoms in VirtualDose were available; the effective diameters could be assumed to be the same as the water equivalent diameters for abdominal region [27]. We calculated the absolute absorbed doses to six organs (adrenals, kidneys, liver, pancreas, spleen and stomach) using the methods by the four groups with either effective diameters or the derived perimeters for abdomen-pelvis scans of pediatric patients [18, 22, 24, 28]. To obtain absolute absorbed doses, the head $CTDI_{vol}$ of the Siemens Sensation 16 scanner was applied to the normalized organ doses calculated with three of the four methods, and the body $CTDI_{vol}$ was applied to the normalized organ doses calculated with the method by Turner et al [18]. Organ doses calculated with VirtualDose were compared to the doses calculated with the four methods. Two-sample t-test was performed for dose to each organ across patients of various ages with a null hypothesis that VirtualDose results and results of a size-based method were from distributions of equal means and equal variances. Statistical significance was defined as $p < 0.05$. The tests were carried out for four times for each comparison of VirtualDose and one of the four size-based methods.

Effective dose estimation for pediatrics based on adult doses

Effective dose was the sum of the gender-averaged weighted organ dose equivalents using recommended tissue weighting factors from ICRP for the purpose of estimating the dose and risk to the population being irradiated [8–10]. In this study we used the tissue weighting factors from the ICRP No. 103 publication [10]. Khursheed et al. calculated the ratios of the effective dose for pediatrics to the effective dose of adults by Monte Carlo simulations of a family of six stylized phantoms representing pediatrics and adults [58]. The range of the ratios was adopted by ImPACT for users to estimate pediatric effective doses [52]. However, ranges of ratios were difficult to use in practice. In addition, these ratios were derived based on unrealistic stylized phantoms that lack anatomical details in geometrically simplified organs, while the phantoms in VirtualDose were created based on patient CT images [23, 47, 59]. Considering such ratios as quick adjustment factors of effective doses for clinic applications, these ratios were calculated in this study with VirtualDose using the anthropomorphic pediatric phantoms and were compared with the ratio range in ImPACT [52].

Results
Comparison of VirtualDose and CT-Expo

For head CT scan, the doses to eleven organs as well as the effective dose are compared between VirtualDose and CT-Expo, as demonstrated in Fig. 1. For distributed organs such as bone surface, red marrow, skin, lymph nodes, and muscle, VirtualDose results are within 0.3 and 2.7 times of CT-Expo results, where consistently significant differences are found for bone surface dose and red marrow dose among various patients. The skin doses are within 30% difference between the two codes. The lymph nodes dose is approximated with the muscle dose in CT-Expo, so it shares similar trend with the muscle dose. For organs inside the scan range such as brain and eye lens, VirtualDose results are within 0.9 and 1.2 times of CT-Expo results. However, the t-test shows the VirtualDose results are different from the CT-Expo results with a p-value of 0.0011 ($p < 0.05$). For organs partially in the scan range or outside the scan range such as salivary glands, thyroid, ET (extrathoracic) region, and oral mucosa, VirtualDose results are within 0.2 and 2.0 times of CT-Expo results. The effective doses calculated by VirtualDose are within 0.8 and 1.7 times of the effective doses calculated by CT-Expo across various patients.

For chest CT scan, the doses to twenty-one organs as well as the effective doses are compared between VirtualDose and CT-Expo, as demonstrated in Fig. 2. For distributed organs such as bone surface, red marrow, skin, lymph nodes, and muscle, VirtualDose results are within 0.2 and 2.0 times of CT-Expo results. Again, large differences are found in bone surface doses and red marrow doses among various patients. For organs within scan range such as breasts, esophagus, lungs, heart, and thymus, VirtualDose results are within 0.7 and 1.3 times of CT-Expo results. The t-test of this scan region shows that there are no statistically significant differences between VirtualDose and CT-Expo in-field organ doses with a p-value of 0.26 ($p > 0.05$). One should note that CT-Expo does not provide breast doses for males and in this study the male breast dose is assumed to be the same as female breast dose, and it does not provide heart doses for pediatrics either. Thus, only the female breast doses and the adult heart doses are obtained from CT-Expo and used for comparison. For organs partially in the scan range or outside the range such as liver, salivary glands, stomach, thyroid, adrenals, ET region, gall bladder, kidneys, oral mucosa, pancreas, and spleen, VirtualDose results are within 0.2 and 1.8 times of CT-Expo results. For effective doses, VirtualDose results are within 0.9 and 1.2 times of CT-Expo results.

For abdomen-pelvis scan, the doses to eighteen organs as well as the effective doses are compared between VirtualDose and CT-Expo, as demonstrated in Fig. 3. For distributed organs such as bone surface, red marrow, skin, lymph nodes, and muscle, VirtualDose results are within 0.2 and 1.6 times of CT-Expo results, where large discrepancies occur for bone surface doses across

various patients. For organs within the scan range such as colon, liver, stomach, urinary bladder, adrenals, gall bladder, kidneys, pancreas, small intestine, spleen, and uterus (female)/prostate (male), VirtualDose results are within 0.7 and 1.6 times of CT-Expo results. The t-test of this scan region shows that there are no statistically significant differences between VirtualDose and CT-Expo in-field organ doses with a p-value of 0.92 ($p > 0.05$). For the organs partially in the scan range or outside the scan range such as gonads and lungs, VirtualDose results are within 0.4 and 1.7 times of CT-Expo results. For effective doses, VirtualDose results are within 0.8 and 1.3 times of CT-Expo results.

For chest-abdomen-pelvis scan, the doses to twenty-six organs as well as the effective doses are compared between VirtualDose and CT-Expo, as demonstrated in Fig. 4. For distributed organs such as bone surface, red marrow, skin, lymph nodes, and muscle, VirtualDose results are within 0.3 and 1.5 times of CT-Expo results, where large discrepancies exist for bone surface dose and red marrow dose across patients of various ages. For organs partially in the scan range or outside the range such as male gonads, salivary glands, thyroid, ET region, and oral mucosa, VirtualDose results are within 0.2 and 1.9 times of CT-Expo results. The rest of the twenty-six organs are within the scan range, where VirtualDose results are within 0.7 and 1.6 times of CT-Expo results. The t-test of this scan region shows that there are no statistically significant differences between VirtualDose and CT-Expo in-field organ doses with a p-value of 0.30 ($p > 0.05$). For effective doses, VirtualDose results are within 0.98 and 1.22 times of CT-Expo results. The t-test of the effective doses from all scans shows that there is no statistically significant difference between VirtualDose and CT-Expo with a p-value of 0.83 ($p > 0.05$).

Comparison of VirtualDose, CT-Expo, and ImPACT for adults

For head scan, the doses to ten organs as well as effective dose are compared. In general the dose ratios of VirtualDose to ImPACT are similar to the ratios of VirtualDose to CT-Expo, except for red marrow, salivary glands and oral mucosa, as shown in Fig. 5. For distributed organs and between VirtualDose and ImPACT, VirtualDose results are within 0.4 and 1.7 times of ImPACT results. For brain in the scan range, VirtualDose results are within 1.08 and 1.13 times of ImPACT results. For organs partially in the range or outside the range, VirtualDose results are within 0.2 and 1.7 times of ImPACT results. For the effective doses, the difference between VirtualDose result and ImPACT result is 32%.

For CAP scan, the doses to twenty-four organs as well as the effective doses are compared as shown in Fig. 6. For distributed organs and between VirtualDose and

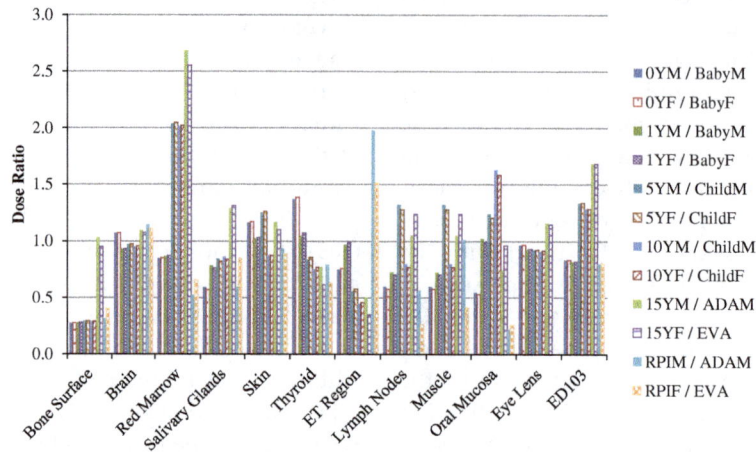

Fig. 1 Comparisons of organ doses* and effective doses between VirtualDose and CT-Expo: Head CT scan with 120 kVp tube voltage; ET region stands for extrathoracic region (nose, mouth, pharynx, larynx), and ED103 stands for effective dose with ICRP 103 tissue weighting factors [10]. *Note: Organs outside scan range and with dose smaller than 0.5 mGy are not included in Figs. 1, 2, 3, 4, 5 and 6, since the statistical error in the Monte Carlo results for these organs are high and can be as high as the dose itself

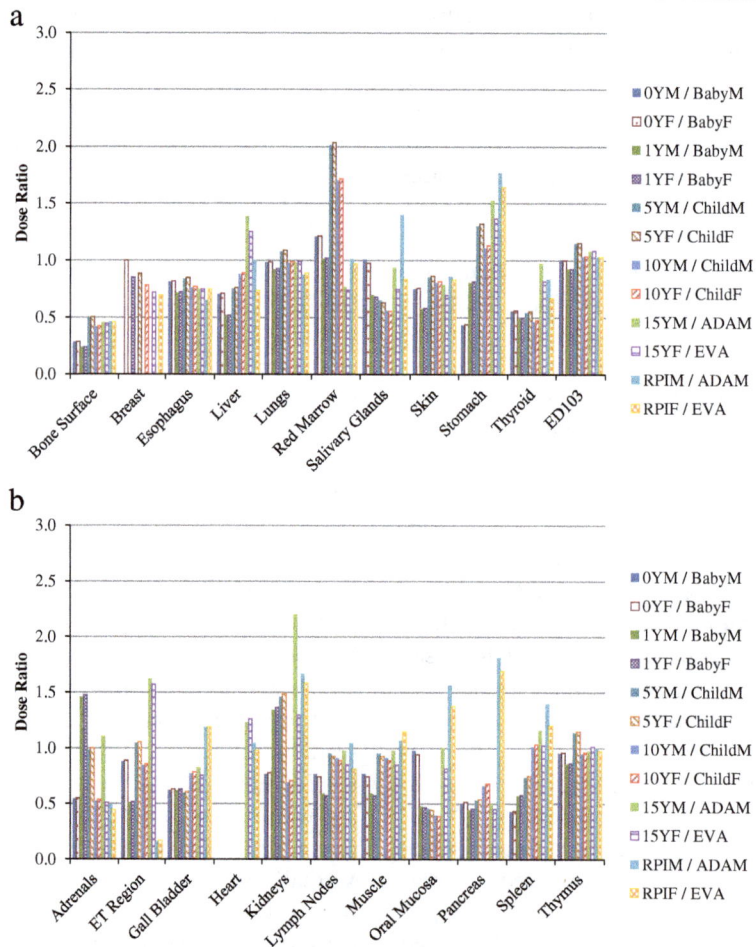

Fig. 2 Comparisons of organ doses and effective doses between VirtualDose and CT-Expo: Chest CT scan with 120 kVp tube voltage; the results are broken into subfigure **a)** and **b)** for ease of display; ET region stands for extrathoracic region (nose, mouth, pharynx, larynx), and ED103 stands for effective dose with ICRP 103 tissue weighting factors [10]

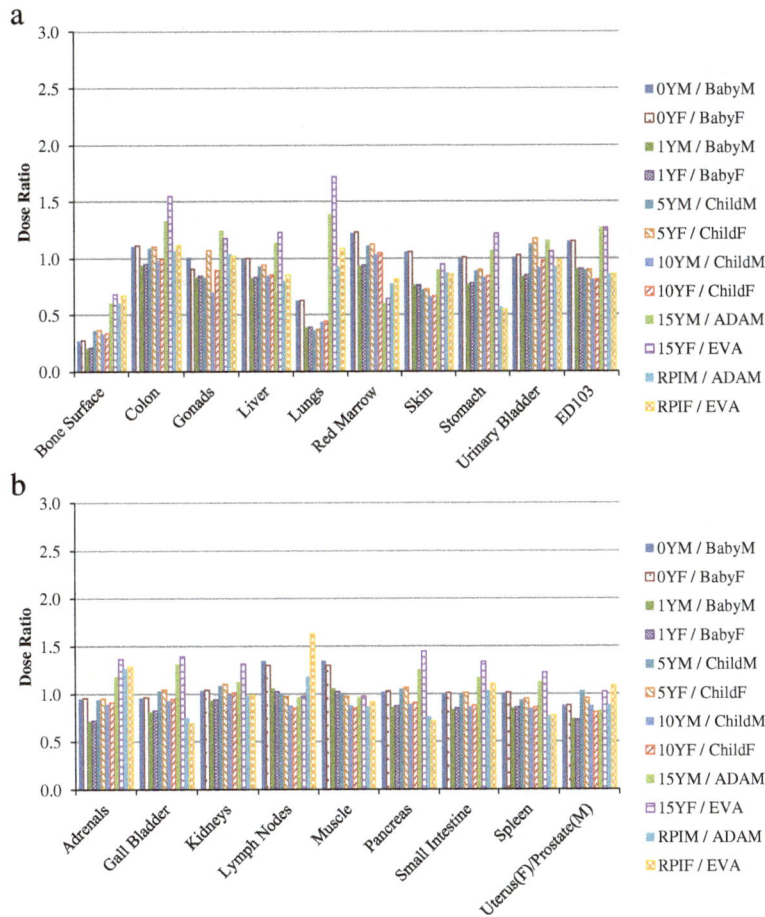

Fig. 3 Comparisons of organ doses and effective doses between VirtualDose and CT-Expo: Abdomen-Pelvis (AP) CT scan with 120 kVp tube voltage; the results are broken into subfigure **a**) and **b**) for ease of display; ED103 stands for effective dose with ICRP 103 tissue weighting factors [10]

ImPACT, VirtualDose results are within 0.7 and 1.5 times of ImPACT results. For organs within the scan range, VirtualDose results are within 0.7 and 1.2 times of ImPACT results. For organs partially in the range or outside the range, VirtualDose results are within 0.3 and 1.3 times of ImPACT results. For effective dose, the difference between VirtualDose result and ImPACT result is 3%.

The breast dose ratio of VirtualDose to ImPACT is different from the ratio of VirtualDose to CT-Expo, where the VirtualDose breast dose is very close to the ImPACT breast dose while the VirtualDose breast dose is 49% higher than the CT-Expo breast dose. Besides breast dose, the ImPACT doses of several organs (gonads, skin, thyroid, and lymph nodes) are different from the CT-Expo doses by more than 15%, even though both codes use stylized phantoms for dose calculations. Between VirtualDose and ImPACT, the t-test shows there are no statistically significant differences with a p-value of 0.96 ($p > 0.05$). Between VirtualDose and CT-Expo, the t-test shows the tools are statistically different

for adult head scan and CAP scan with a p-value of 0.0054 ($p < 0.05$). Between CT-Expo and ImPACT, the t-test also shows the tools are statistically different with a p-value of 0.0009 ($p < 0.05$).

Comparison of VirtualDose and body-size based methods
The organ doses by the four different empirical functions are compared to the VirtualDose results for abdomen-pelvis scan of pediatric patients at ages of 0-year-old, 1-year-old, 5-year-old, 10-year-old, and 15-year-old, as shown in Fig. 7. As patient age decreases, the organ doses show consistent increasing trends for all methods. The organ doses for 0-year-old patients are 1.4 to 2.1 times of the doses for 15-year-old patients, given the same scan parameters. Across the five methods, the variations of organ doses are smaller than 16% for adrenals, 17% for liver, 18% for pancreas, 16% for spleen, and 16% for stomach. Across the five patient ages, the largest variations are observed for 15-year-old patients (18%), and the smallest variations are for 0-year-old patients (5%). The doses by VirtualDose are within the dose

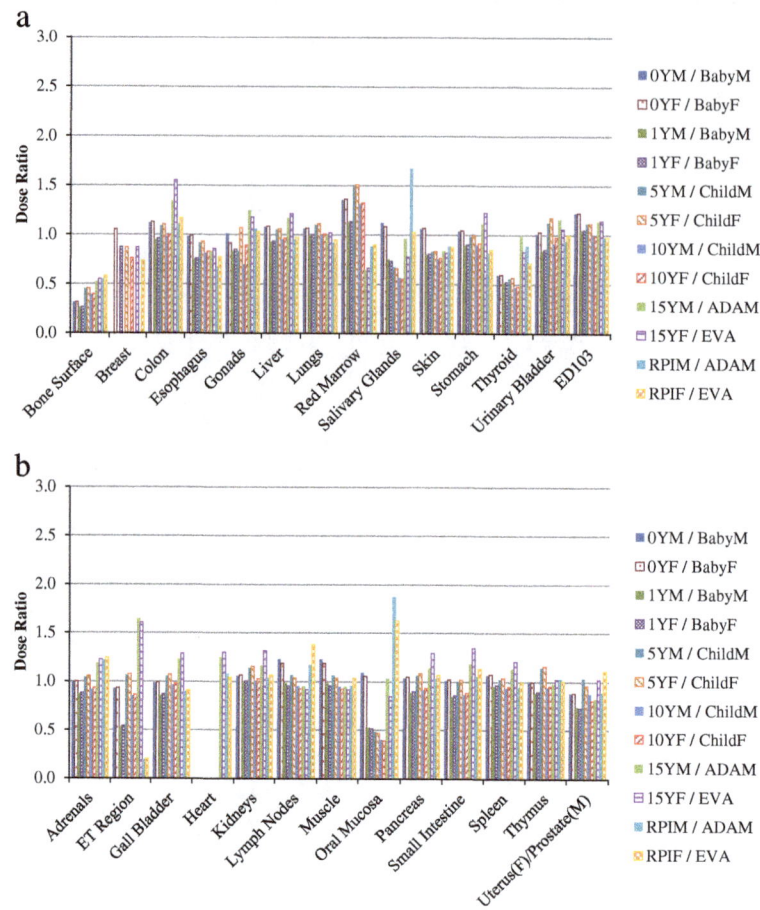

Fig. 4 Comparisons of organ doses and effective doses between VirtualDose and CT-Expo: Chest-Abdomen-Pelvis (CAP) CT scan with 120 kVp tube voltage; the results are broken into subfigure **a**) and **b**) for ease of display; ET region stands for extrathoracic region (nose, mouth, pharynx, larynx), and ED103 stands for effective dose with ICRP 103 tissue weighting factors [10]

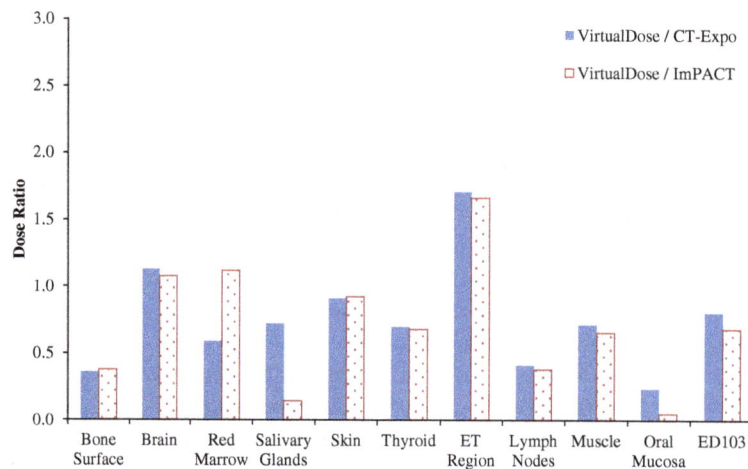

Fig. 5 Comparisons of adult gender-averaged organ doses and effective doses among VirtualDose, CT-Expo, and ImPACT: Head CT scan with 120 kVp tube voltage; ET region stands for extrathoracic region (nose, mouth, pharynx, larynx), and ED103 stands for effective dose with ICRP 103 tissue weighting factors [10]

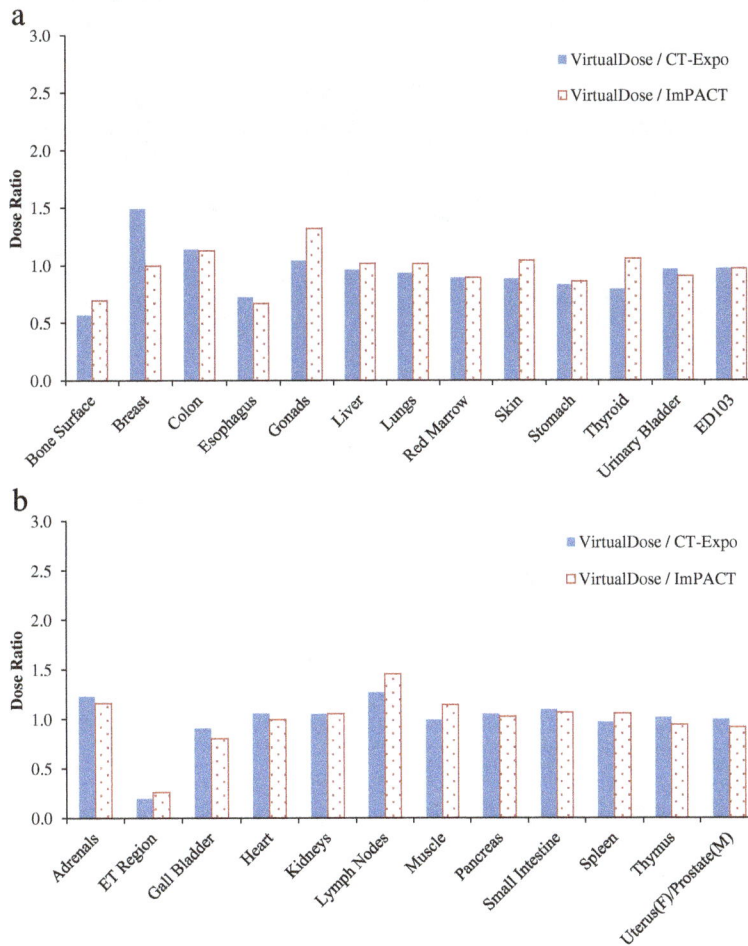

Fig. 6 Comparisons of adult gender-averaged organ doses and effective doses among VirtualDose, CT-Expo, and ImPACT: CAP CT scan with 120 kVp tube voltage; the results are broken into subfigure **a**) and **b**) for ease of display; ET region stands for extrathoracic region (nose, mouth, pharynx, larynx), and ED103 stands for effective dose with ICRP 103 tissue weighting factors [10]

range of the four size-based methods, except for kidneys where VirtualDose results are higher than other methods for patients under 10 years old. The doses estimated with Tian et al. method and Turner et al. method are generally relatively low for the six organs studied and the five age groups of patients, while the doses with Papadakis et al. method, with Kost et al. method, and with VirtualDose are generally relatively high [18, 21, 22, 24, 28]. Table 4 shows that VirtualDose was not statistically different ($p > 0.05$) for all the six organs from any of the four size-based methods.

Effective dose adjustment factors for pediatrics based on adult doses

The ratios of the pediatric effective doses to the adult effective doses are calculated for the five age groups of phantoms in VirtualDose and for three types of scans: HN, chest, and AP, as shown in Table 5. HN scans are assumed to start at the top of skull through the level of clavicles. The ratios increase as the patients become

younger, and range from 1.0 to 1.5 for HN scan, from 1.1 to 2.0 for chest scan, and from 1.5 to 2.9 for AP scan. For HN scan, the ratio changes by no more than 10% until patient is younger than 1 year old.

Compared to the ranges of pediatric to adult effective dose ratios provided in the ImPACT spreadsheet, the factors by VirtualDose ratios are lower than the range for HN scans, within the range for chest scans, and above the range for AP scans, as shown in Fig. 8. For 0-year-old patients and HN scans, the VirtualDose ratio is below 0.65 times of effective dose ratios derived from the ranges provided in the ImPACT spreadsheet. For 5-year-old patients and AP scans, the VirtualDose ratio is above 1.38 times of effective dose ratios derived from the range of ImPACT sheet.

Discussion

Fast and accurate estimation of organ doses for patients, especially for pediatric patients, are essential for radiologists and radiation protection professionals in clinical practice.

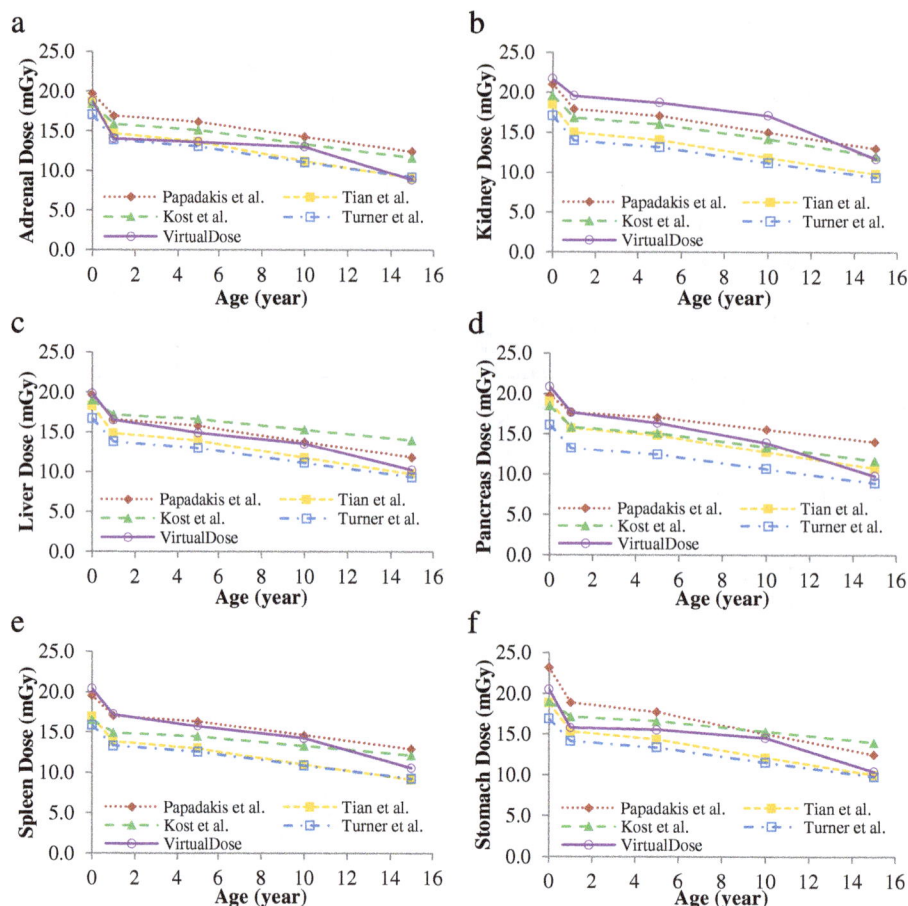

Fig. 7 Comparison of VirtualDose with the size-based empirical functions: Organ doses for **a**) Adrenals, **b**) Kidneys, **c**) Liver, **d**) Pancreas, **e**) Spleen, and **f**) Stomach in AP CT scans [18, 22, 24, 28]

In this study we compared existing methods of CT dose calculations for pediatric and adult patients by various groups.

Two sets of software that enable fast organ dose estimations in a few clicks of the computer mouse are compared in the beginning: VirtualDose and CT-Expo. VirtualDose is inherently more preferable to CT-Expo in that it includes more pediatric phantoms that can represent wider patient ages, and that it utilizes anatomically realistic phantoms for dose calculations. In addition, CT-Expo does not provide male breast dose at all, or heart dose to pediatric patients [53]. Four CT protocols are simulated to cover most of the radiosensitive organs

in patient body. The comparisons of the results by the two pieces of software show large discrepancies as expected; with the results between each software deviating up to five times from each other. Across the four protocols, the bone surface doses by VirtualDose are consistently smaller than the doses for CT-Expo by about 70%. The mathematical phantoms used in CT-Expo do not have specific representations of the bone surface, so calculations based on such phantoms approximate the bone surface dose with the dose to the entire skeleton [60]. Such approximation explains the over-estimated bone surface doses by CT-Expo. The mathematical phantoms do not possess explicit red bone

Table 4 Two-sample t-test p-values from comparisons of VirtualDose (VD) to size-based methods for six organs of pediatric patients underwent simulated abdomen-pelvis CT scan

Compared methods	Adrenal	Kidney	Liver	Pancreas	Spleen	Stomach
VD and Papadakis et al. [24]	0.30	0.67	0.82	0.63	0.82	0.41
VD and Tian et al. [28]	0.93	0.12	0.56	0.64	0.21	0.60
VD and Kost et al. [22]	0.55	0.36	0.46	0.71	0.47	0.58
VD and Turner et al. [18]	0.71	0.054	0.31	0.16	0.14	0.30

Table 5 Relative effective doses for pediatric patients

Patients	Head & neck	Chest	AP
Adult	1.0	1.0	1.0
15 y	1.0	1.1	1.5
10 y	1.1	1.5	2.0
5 y	1.3	1.6	2.2
1 y	1.4	1.8	2.3
Newborn (0 y)	1.5	2.0	2.9

Note: The relative effective doses are calculated against the effective doses for adults

marrow models and approximate the red marrow dose by applying correction factors to dose to the whole bones, while the anthropomorphic phantoms explicitly model the spongiosa of bones for red bone marrow dose calculations [47, 59, 60]. Due to the anatomical differences between anthropomorphic phantoms and mathematical phantoms, large differences exist for red marrow dose between VirtualDose and CT-Expo, where VirtualDose results can be two times higher than the CT-Expo results.

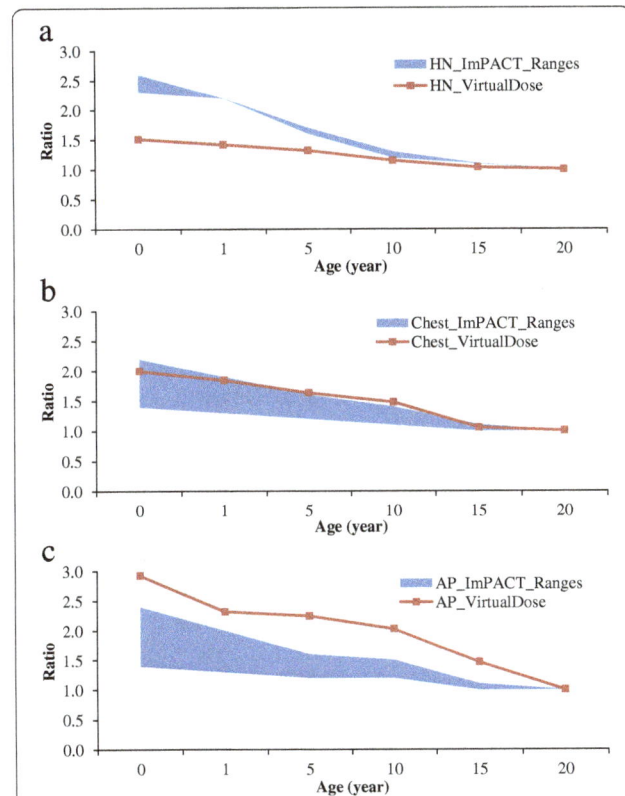

Fig. 8 Ratios of pediatric effective doses to adult effective doses: VirtualDose ratios compared to ratio ranges provided in ImPACT for **a)** Head and Neck (HN) scans, **b)** Chest scans, and **c)** AP scans, where adults are assumed to be 20 years old, and ratio equals to pediatric effective dose (mSv) divided by adult effective dose (mSv)

Dose estimates to organs inside the scan range vary less between various methods than dose estimates to organs at the edge of the scan range or outside the scan range. Even between two generations of phantoms, the mathematical phantoms and the anthropomorphic phantoms, at various patient ages our study show dose differences within 60% for organs inside scan range. Between VirtualDose and CT-Expo, differences up to 5 times can occur for organs outside scan range, such as the ET region dose in CAP scans. The doses to these outside organs are contributed by scattered photons, and are typically one or two magnitudes smaller than doses to organs inside the scan range [18, 61]. In addition, large statistical errors exist in doses to outside organs from Monte Carlo simulations without high enough number of photons simulated [61].

Doses to the organs at the edge of the scan range are subject to the definitions of scan range, and are sensitive to changes of scan range by centimeters or even by millimeters. Additional calculations were performed using VirtualDose to determine the magnitudes of dose sensitivity of organs at the edges of scan range. The inferior edges of head protocols, the superior and inferior edges of chest protocols, and the superior and inferior edges of AP protocols are moved by 0.5 cm steps for 3cm superiorly and then 3cm inferiorly. The dose sensitivity to changes in scan range are investigated for five representative organs in male patients: the salivary gland for head scans, the thyroid at superior edges of chest scans, the stomach at inferior edges of chest scans, the lungs at superior edges of AP scans, and the testes at inferior edges of AP scans, as shown in Fig. 9. In addition, for relatively small organs such as the salivary gland, the thyroid, and the testes, the scan range is further extended such that the inflection points (beyond which the organs are less sensitive to scan range changes) of the curves are shown in the figure. Further range extension beyond inflection points impact less on the doses of the partially scanned organs, where plateau of slowly increasing dose ratios are observed.

Salivary glands are located in the jaws of the lower part of the head, and are at the edges of the head (Brain) CT scans simulated in this study. Extension of the scan range inferiorly includes more or even the entire glands into the head scans. The dose to the glands can be 7.5 times of the default dose after an inferior extension of 3 cm for new-born (0-year-old) patients. For older patients, a 3-cm extension can still increase the dose to the glands by more than 2 times. With a 1-cm inferior extension or a 1-cm superior retraction, the dose to the glands can be doubled or halved, indicating the salivary gland dose is very sensitive to the location of the inferior edge of the head scan. Comparing the doses with 3cm superior retraction and the doses with 3cm inferior

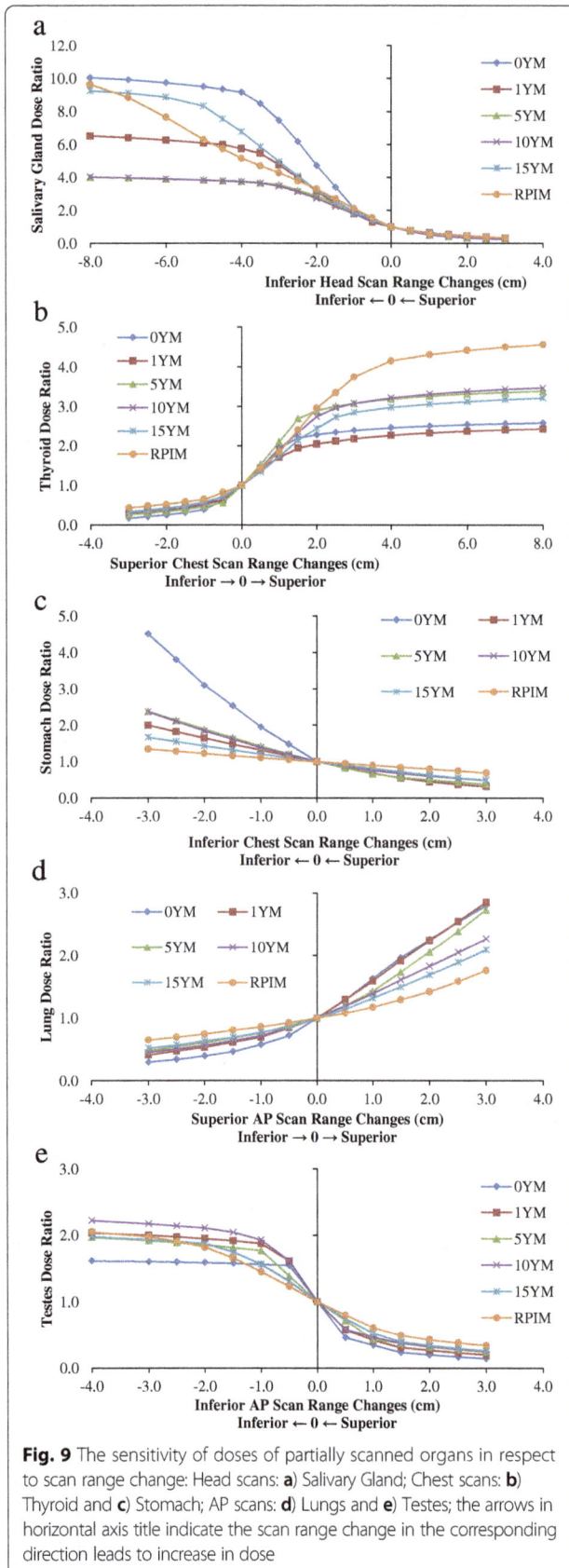

Fig. 9 The sensitivity of doses of partially scanned organs in respect to scan range change: Head scans: **a**) Salivary Gland; Chest scans: **b**) Thyroid and **c**) Stomach; AP scans: **d**) Lungs and **e**) Testes; the arrows in horizontal axis title indicate the scan range change in the corresponding direction leads to increase in dose

extension of the inferior range, the changes in salivary gland dose can be 27 times for newborn patients and 13 times for adults. The inferior extension of head scan range increases the salivary dose, and the extension is up to 8cm to show the inflection points on the dose ratio curves. For patients under 10 years old, a 4cm inferior range extension is enough to show the inflection points. For 15-year old patients and adult patients, because of the relative large size of the gland, the organ remains sensitive to scan range change until relative large extension is made (a 5cm extension for 15-year-old, and an 8cm extension for adults).

The thyroid gland lies at the levels of the fifth cervical vertebrae through the first thoracic vertebrae of patient body, and can be partially covered in the chest CT scan. In our calculations the chest scans ended at the level of clavicles, which position at levels of the first and the second vertebrae of the body. As expected, the 3cm superior extension of the chest scan range increases the thyroid dose by up to 2.7 times for adult patients. For pediatric patients less than 5 years old the thyroid is completely covered after a 2-cm increase in scan range superiorly, and the increase in thyroid dose is small for any further range extensions. The thyroid dose is sensitive to the location of the superior edge of the chest scan, as the dose can be doubled or halved for a 1-cm change in the location. Comparing the doses with 3cm superior extension and the doses with 3cm inferior retraction of the superior range, the changes in thyroid dose can be 14 times for newborn patients and 8.5 times for adults. The superior extension of chest scan range increases the thyroid dose, and the extension is up to 8cm to show the inflection points as well as the plateau on the dose ratio curves. For all patients, a 4cm inferior range extension is enough to show the inflection points. For patients under 10 years old, the thyroid is less sensitive to scan range change after a 2cm inferior range extension.

The stomach sits inferiorly to esophagus, diaphragm and lungs, and it can be partially included in the chest CT scans at the inferior ends of the scan range. The stomach dose increases as the chest scan range are extended inferiorly, and for new-born patients the stomach doses can be 3.5 times higher with a 3 cm inferior range extension. For adult patients, however, the changes in scan range by 3cm do not have great impact on the stomach dose, where the dose changes are smaller than 34%. With 1cm change in range, the stomach dose can change by 90% for newborn patients but only 21% for adult patients. Comparing the doses with 3cm superior retraction and the doses with 3cm inferior extension of the inferior range, the changes in stomach dose can be 14 times for newborn patients but only 2 times for adults.

For AP scans, the lung doses and the testes doses are analyzed regarding to changes in scan range. The lungs are large organs in the chest cavity and can be partially included in the superior ends of the AP scans. The lungs receive more scattered photons than small organs such as salivary glands, and the lung doses are not as sensitive as salivary gland doses in regarding to the scan range changes. A 3cm increase in superior ends of range lead to 180% increase in dose for new-born patients and 76% increase in dose for adult patients. A 1cm change in scan range can lead to 60% change in dose for new-born patients, but the change can only lead to less than 17% change in dose for adult patients. Comparing the doses with 3cm superior extension and the doses with 3cm inferior retraction of the superior range, the changes in lung dose can be 9.5 times for new-born patients and 2.5 times for adults.

The testes are male gonads inferior to the pubic symphysis, and they can be potentially partially covered in the inferior end of the AP scans. In our default simulations we included part of the testes inside the scan range. As a result, the scan range changes seem to have relatively low effects on the testes doses, where a 3cm inferior extension of the scan range only increases the dose by 120% across patients of various ages. However, one should note that by comparing the doses with 3cm inferior extension and the doses with 3cm superior retraction, the changes in the testes doses can be 11 times for new-born patients and 6 times for adult patients. The inferior extension of AP scan increases the testes dose, and the extension is up to 4cm to show the inflection points on the dose ratio curves. For patients under 10 years old, the testes are less sensitive to scan range change after just a 1cm inferior range extension.

Overall the doses to organs partially included in the scan range are subject to specific scan range in practices, where 1cm change in range can lead to 60% change in dose to large organs such as stomach and lungs for new-born patients and 100% change in dose to small organs such as thyroid and salivary glands. The organs in adults are in most times less sensitive to scan range changes, and the organs in other pediatric patients are more sensitive than adults but less sensitive than newborn patients. One should note that for small organs such as thyroid and testes, dose changes of 5 times or more can occur in only a 2 cm scan range extension or retraction, especially for pediatric patients. For adults the effect of scan range changes on organ doses may not fully manifest itself until more than 3 cm changes have occurred. For example, the 3cm superior extensions of chest scan range lead to greater changes for the thyroid doses of adults than these of pediatrics. In addition, one should note that the dose ratios are calculated against the default scan range, where the five discussed organs are already partially covered in the scan range. If the organs are not included in the scan range and scan range extension is made to begin to cover such organs, more drastic dose increases should be expected. Moreover, the high sensitivity of doses of small organs to scan range implies high impact of overscan on doses to these organs when volumetric helical CT scans are performed with large beam collimations.

The comparisons between VirtualDose and CT-Expo, and the comparisons between VirtualDose and ImPACT illustrate that anatomical differences between anthropomorphic phantoms and mathematical/stylized phantoms as well as calculation methodology differences lead to large discrepancies between organ doses calculated by these tools. Across patients of various ages the statistical tests show that VirtualDose does not differ from CT-Expo significantly except for head scans. However, when comparing results for adults the t-test shows that VirtualDose is different from CT-Expo. Between VirtualDose and ImPACT, the t-test shows that the two are not different for adult head and CAP CT scan in-field organ dose estimation. Even between CT-Expo and ImPACT doses to several organs such as salivary glands and breasts are different as the scan range cannot be exactly the same due to the modifications made to the stylized phantoms [62, 63]. The t-test shows that CT-Expo is statistically different from ImPACT for adult head and CAP CT scan in-field organ dose estimation. The methods based on realistic anthropomorphic phantoms should be considered more preferable, as the software with stylized phantoms either do not provide direct pediatric dose calculations, or are lack of a variety of pediatric phantoms that can represent newborn, child, and adolescent pediatric patients [52, 53]. Besides the unrealistic geometries of stylized phantoms, crude approximations are made for bone surface and red bone marrow dose calculations, and doses to a few organs such as male breasts and pediatric heart are not available [52, 53].

VirtualDose provides 5 age groups of pediatric phantoms for organ doses calculations for pediatric patients. Four different research groups proposed size-based organ dose functions that were based on Monte Carlo calculations of simulated CT scans on several anthropomorphic phantoms or even tens of phantoms. The comparisons of the doses to several organs inside abdominal regions show that VirtualDose is within relatively small variations (less than 20%) of the four comparison methods. If the size parameters such as perimeters, effective diameters, or water equivalent diameters are available for specific patients, it is reasonable to use the size-based methods to estimate patient specific organ doses. However, one has to decide among the different methods, which do not match each other exactly and have variations of about 20%. More importantly, the size parameters are normally not readily available and currently require trained staff to measure them on patient CT images. Statistical analysis shows that VirtualDose is not different from the size-based methods for the organs investigated. In the cases when such parameters are not available and fast organ dose calculations are required to response to patients' questions, VirtualDose can be the tool that conveys the dose estimates in seconds.

The effective dose ratios of pediatrics to adults by VirtualDose share similar trends with the range of ratios provided by ImPACT, although the magnitudes of the ratios are different between the two codes. For HN scans, the VirtualDose ratios are lower than the ImPACT ratios, especially for small pediatric patients. For chest scans, the VirtualDose ratios are within 10% of the ratios of ImPACT. For AP scans, the VirtualDose ratios are higher than the ImPACT ratios. The anatomical differences between the anthropomorphic phantoms used in VirtualDose and the stylized phantoms used in ImPACT have likely caused the differences. In addition, the ImPACT effective doses are normalized by air kerma before the ratios of effective doses are calculated, while no such normalizations are performed when calculating the effective dose ratios with VirtualDose.

A limitation of this study was that no physical measurement was involved and it was not practical to determine if one method was more accurate than another. In addition, the calculations in this study were performed on only a few virtual patients and it was hard to obtain enough data for statistical testings. Measurements on physical human phantoms are planned to validate the computational methods based on experiment design in literature [34, 35, 64–66]. Future work involves the application of the methods discussed in this study to a number of adult and pediatric patients for organ doses and effective dose estimation.

Conclusion

VirtualDose has been validated in comparison to two different organ dose estimation tools and four size-based methods for pediatric and adult patients. Up to five times discrepancies in doses to organs outside the scan range or distributed organs are found between Virtual-Dose and the other two tools (CT-Expo and ImPACT). For organs inside scan range, the differences are smaller than 60% and may not be statistically significant. The size-based methods require patient size information such as patient diameters, and can provide estimations of organ doses for specific patients. The organ doses generated using VirtualDose are within 20% of such size-based methods and show no significant difference.

ImPACT spread sheet and CT-Expo can provide organ dose estimation for average-size adult patients, and CT-Expo can provide organ dose estimations for 7-year-old and new born pediatric patients. VirtualDose can provide organ dose estimation for pediatric patients from new-born to 15 years old and for adults. Patient-specific organ dose can be estimated with the size-based methods and the patient-specific size information, but one has to acquire the size information. Finally, one should be careful about the calculations of doses to organs partially involved in the scan range, as even change in scan range of just 2 cm can lead to a 5 times difference in doses to such organs for pediatric patients. Careful range selection for CT protocols is necessary for organ dose optimization for pediatric and adult patients.

Abbreviations

0YF: 0 year old female; 0YM: 0 year old male; 10YF: 10 years old female; 10YM: 10 years old male; 15YF: 15 years old female; 15YM: 15 years old male; 1YF: 1 year old female; 1YM: 1 year old male; 5YF: 5 years old female; 5YM: 5 years old male; AAPM: American Association of Physicists in Medicine; ACR: American College of Radiology; ALARA: As low as reasonably achievable; AP: Abdomen and pelvis; CAP: Chest, abdomen and pelvis; CT: Computed tomography; CTDI: Computed tomography dose index; DIR: Dose Index Registry; DLP: Dose length product; ED103: Effective Dose calculated with tissue weighting factors from ICRP Publication 103; ET: Extrathoracic; HN: Head and neck; ICRP: International Commission on Radiological Protection; MC: Monte Carlo; NCRP: National Council on Radiation Protection and Measurements; NRPB: National Radiological Protection Board; OECD: Organisation for economic co-operation and development; RPIF: Rensselaer Polytechnic Institute Adult Female; RPIM: Rensselaer Polytechnic Institute Adult Male; SSDE: Size-specific dose estimates; UNSCEAR: United Nations Scientific Committee on the Effects of Atomic Radiation; US: United States; VD: VirtualDose

Acknowledgements

The authors wish to acknowledge the support from National Institute of Biomedical Imaging and Bioengieering Grant (R01EB015478) to the development of VirtualDose.

Funding

This research was funded in part through the NIH/NCI Cancer Center Support Grant P30 CA008748.

Authors' contributions

YG collected and analyzed the data, drafted the manuscript, and participated in designing the study. BQ participated in designing the study and provided technical insights. UM, DL, YE, JSG, and NPT provided practical and clinical input and helped draft the manuscript. XGX and WEB provided the VirtualDose estimator and helped draft the manuscript. LTD conceived of and designed the study, provided technical oversight for dose calculation methods and results. All authors read and approved the manuscript.

Competing interests

Dr. George X. Xu is the CEO of Virtual Phantoms, Inc., which is in charge of the business related to VirtualDose.

Author details

¹Department of Medical Physics, Memorial Sloan Kettering Cancer Center, 1275 York Avenue, Box 84, New York, NY 10065, USA. ²Department of Radiology, Memorial Sloan Kettering Cancer Center, 1275 York Avenue, New York, NY 10065, USA. ³Department of Mechanical, Aerospace, and Nuclear Engineering, Rensselaer Polytechnic Institute, Troy, NY 12180, USA. ⁴J. Crayton Pruitt Family Department of Biomedical Engineering, University of Florida, Gainesville, FL 32611, USA.

References

1. UNSCEAR. Sources And Effects Of Ionizing Radiation, UNSCEAR Publications. vol. I. New York: United Nations Scientific Committee on the Effects of Atomic Radiation; 2008.
2. NCRP. Ionizing Radiation Exposure of the Population of the United States. In: NCRP Publications. Bethesda, MD; 2009.
3. ICRP. Managing patient dose in computed tomography. ICRP Publication 87. Ann ICRP. 2000;30(4):1–86.
4. Valentin J, ICRP. Managing patient dose in multi-detector computed tomography(MDCT). ICRP Publication 102. Ann ICRP. 2007;37(1):1–79.
5. Dauer LT, Hricak H. Addressing the Challenge of Managing Radiation Use in Medical Imaging: Paradigm Shifts and Strategic Priorities. Oncology-Ny. 2014;28(3):243–+.
6. (OECD) TOfEC-oaD. Computed tomography (CT) exams (indicator) [https://data.oecd.org/healthcare/computed-tomography-ct-exams.htm] Accessed 29 Sept 2016.
7. USCB. United States Population by Age and Sex. U.S. Census Bureau [https://www.census.gov/popclock/]. Accessed 29 Sept 2016.
8. ICRP. Recommendations of the International Commission on Radiological Protection. ICRP Publication 26. Annals ICRP. 1977;1(3):1–80.
9. ICRP. 1990 Recommendations of the International Commission on Radiological Protection. ICRP Publication 60. Ann ICRP. 1991;21(1-3):1–201.
10. ICRP. The 2007 Recommendations of the International Commission on Radiological Protection. ICRP Publication 103. Ann ICRP. 2007;37(2-4):1–332.
11. ICRP. Radiation Protection in Medicine. ICRP Publication 105. Ann ICRP. 2007;37(6):1–63.
12. ACR. DIR User Guide. American College of Radiology [http://www.acr.org/Quality-Safety/National-Radiology-Data-Registry/Dose-Index-Registry] Accessed 29 Sept 2016.
13. Goske MJ, Applegate KE, Boylan J, Butler PF, Callahan MJ, Coley BD, Farley S, Frush DP, Hernanz-Schulman M, Jaramillo D, et al. The Image Gently campaign: working together to change practice. AJR Am J Roentgenol. 2008;190(2):273–4.
14. Brink JA, Amis ES. Image Wisely: A Campaign to Increase Awareness about Adult Radiation Protection. Radiology. 2010;257(3):601–2.
15. UNSCEAR. Sources, Effects And Risks Of Ionizing Radiation, UNSCEAR Publications. vol. II. New York: United Nations Scientific Committee on the Effects of Atomic Radiation; 2013.
16. Brenner D, Elliston C, Hall E, Berdon W. Estimated risks of radiation-induced fatal cancer from pediatric CT. AJR Am J Roentgenol. 2001;176(2):289–96.
17. Brenner DJ. Estimating cancer risks from pediatric CT: going from the qualitative to the quantitative. Pediatr Radiol. 2002;32(4):228–1. discussion 242-224.
18. Turner AC, Zhang D, Khatonabadi M, Zankl M, DeMarco JJ, Cagnon CH, Cody DD, Stevens DM, McCollough CH, McNitt-Gray MF. The feasibility of patient size-corrected, scanner-independent organ dose estimates for abdominal CT exams. Med Phys. 2011;38(2):820–9.
19. Brady Z, Cain TM, Johnston PN. Comparison of organ dosimetry methods and effective dose calculation methods for paediatric CT. Australas Phys Eng Sci Med. 2012;35(2):117–34.
20. Lee C, Kim KP, Long DJ, Bolch WE. Organ doses for reference pediatric and adolescent patients undergoing computed tomography estimated by Monte Carlo simulation. Med Phys. 2012;39(4):2129–46.
21. Tian X, Li X, Segars WP, Frush DP, Paulson EK, Samei E. Dose coefficients in pediatric and adult abdominopelvic CT based on 100 patient models. Phys Med Biol. 2013;58(24):8755–68.
22. Kost SD, Fraser ND, Carver DE, Pickens DR, Price RR, Hernanz-Schulman M, Stabin MG. Patient-specific dose calculations for pediatric CT of the chest, abdomen and pelvis. Pediatr Radiol. 2015;45(12):1771–80.
23. Ding A, Gao Y, Liu H, Caracappa PF, Long DJ, Bolch WE, Liu B, Xu XG. VirtualDose: a software for reporting organ doses from CT for adult and pediatric patients. Phys Med Biol. 2015;60(14):5601–25.
24. Papadakis AE, Perisinakis K, Damilakis J. Development of a method to estimate organ doses for pediatric CT examinations. Med Phys. 2016;43(5):2108.
25. AAPM. The Measurement, Reporting, and Management of Radiation Dose in CT. AAPM Report No. 96. College Park: AAPM Publications; 2008. Online.
26. AAPM. Size-Specific Dose Estimates (SSDE) in Pediatric and Adult Body CT Examinations. AAPM Report No. 204. College Park: AAPM Publications; 2011. Online.
27. AAPM. Use of Water Equivalent Diameter for Calculating Patient Size and Size-Specific Dose Estimates (SSDE) in CT. AAPM Report No. 220. College Park: AAPM Publications; 2014. Online.
28. Tian X, Li X, Segars WP, Paulson EK, Frush DP, Samei E. Pediatric chest and abdominopelvic CT: organ dose estimation based on 42 patient models. Radiology. 2014;270(2):535–47.
29. Fahey FH, Palmer MR, Strauss KJ, Zimmerman RE, Badawi RD, Treves ST. Dosimetry and adequacy of CT-based attenuation correction for pediatric PET: phantom study. Radiology. 2007;243(1):96–104.
30. Fujii K, Aoyama T, Koyama S, Kawaura C. Comparative evaluation of organ and effective doses for paediatric patients with those for adults in chest and abdominal CT examinations. Br J Radiol. 2007;80(956):657–67.
31. Hollingsworth CL, Yoshizumi TT, Frush DP, Chan FP, Toncheva G, Nguyen G, Lowry CR, Hurwitz LM. Pediatric cardiac-gated CT angiography: assessment of radiation dose. AJR Am J Roentgenol. 2007;189(1):12–8.
32. Nishizawa K, Mori S, Ohno M, Yanagawa N, Yoshida T, Akahane K, Iwai K, Wada S. Patient dose estimation for multi-detector-row CT examinations. Radiat Prot Dosim. 2008;128(1):98–105.
33. Brisse HJ, Robilliard M, Savignoni A, Pierrat N, Gaboriaud G, De Rycke Y, Neuenschwander S, Aubert B, Rosenwald JC. Assessment of organ absorbed doses and estimation of effective doses from pediatric anthropomorphic phantom measurements for multi-detector row CT with and without automatic exposure control. Health Phys. 2009;97(4):303–14.
34. Huang B, Law MW, Khong PL. Whole-body PET/CT scanning: estimation of radiation dose and cancer risk. Radiology. 2009;251(1):166–74.
35. Zhang D, Li X, Gao Y, Xu XG, Liu B. A method to acquire CT organ dose map using OSL dosimeters and ATOM anthropomorphic phantoms. Med Phys. 2013;40(8):081918.
36. Pearce MS, Salotti JA, Little MP, McHugh K, Lee C, Kim KP, Howe NL, Ronckers CM, Rajaraman P, Craft AW, et al. Radiation exposure from CT scans in childhood and subsequent risk of leukaemia and brain tumours: a retrospective cohort study. Lancet. 2012;380(9840):499–505.
37. Miglioretti DL, Johnson E, Williams A, Greenlee RT, Weinmann S, Solberg LI, Feigelson HS, Roblin D, Flynn MJ, Vanneman N, et al. The use of computed tomography in pediatrics and the associated radiation exposure and estimated cancer risk. JAMA Pediatr. 2013;167(8):700–7.
38. Pelowitz DB. MCNPX user's manual, version 2.6.0. Los Alamos: Los Alamos National Laboratory; 2008.
39. Gu J, Bednarz B, Caracappa PF, Xu XG. The development, validation and application of a multi-detector CT (MDCT) scanner model for assessing organ doses to the pregnant patient and the fetus using Monte Carlo simulations. Phys Med Biol. 2009;54(9):2699–717.
40. Turner AC, Zhang D, Kim HJ, DeMarco JJ, Cagnon CH, Angel E, Cody DD, Stevens DM, Primak AN, McCollough CH, et al. A method to generate equivalent energy spectra and filtration models based on measurement for multidetector CT Monte Carlo dosimetry simulations. Med Phys. 2009;36(6):2154–64.
41. Eckerman KF, Poston JWS, Bolch WE, Xu XG. The stylized computational phantoms developed at ORNL and elsewhere, Handbook of Anatomical Models for Radiation Dosimetry. New York: Taylor & Francis; 2010. p. 43–64.
42. Xu XG. An exponential growth of computational phantom research in radiation protection, imaging, and radiotherapy: a review of the fifty-year history. Phys Med Biol. 2014;59(18):R233–302.
43. Valentin J, Streffer C. Basic anatomical and physiological data for use in radiological protection: Reference values. ICRP Publication 89. Ann ICRP. 2002;32(3-4):1–265.
44. Zankl M, Fill U, Petoussi-Henss N, Regulla D. Organ dose conversion coefficients for external photon irradiation of male and female voxel models. Phys Med Biol. 2002;47(14):2367–85.
45. Liu H, Gu J, Caracappa PF, Xu XG. Comparison of two types of adult phantoms in terms of organ doses from diagnostic CT procedures. Phys Med Biol. 2010;55(5):1441–51.

46. Lee C, Kim KP, Long D, Fisher R, Tien C, Simon SL, Bouville A, Bolch WE. Organ doses for reference adult male and female undergoing computed tomography estimated by Monte Carlo simulations. Med Phys. 2011;38(3): 1196–206.

47. Lee C, Lodwick D, Hurtado J, Pafundi D, Williams JL, Bolch WE. The UF family of reference hybrid phantoms for computational radiation dosimetry. Phys Med Biol. 2010;55(2):339–63.

48. Xu XG, Taranenko V, Zhang J, Shi C. A boundary-representation method for designing whole-body radiation dosimetry models: pregnant females at the ends of three gestational periods–RPI-P3, -P6 and -P9. Phys Med Biol. 2007;52(23):7023–44.

49. Ding A, Mille MM, Liu T, Caracappa PF, Xu XG. Extension of RPI-adult male and female computational phantoms to obese patients and a Monte Carlo study of the effect on CT imaging dose. Phys Med Biol. 2012;57(9):2441–59.

50. Segars WP, Bond J, Frush J, Hon S, Eckersley C, Williams CH, Feng J, Tward DJ, Ratnanather JT, Miller MI, et al. Population of anatomically variable 4D XCAT adult phantoms for imaging research and optimization. Med Phys. 2013;40(4):043701.

51. Geyer AM, O'Reilly S, Lee C, Long DJ, Bolch WE. The UF/NCI family of hybrid computational phantoms representing the current US population of male and female children, adolescents, and adults–application to CT dosimetry. Phys Med Biol. 2014;59(18):5225–42.

52. ImPACT. ImPACT CT dosimetry calculator, version 1.0.4. London: St. George's Healthcare NHS Trust; 2011.

53. Stamm G, Nagel HD. CT-Expo V2.4: a tool for dose evaluation in computed tomography. Hannover; 2014.

54. Turner AC, Zankl M, DeMarco JJ, Cagnon CH, Zhang D, Angel E, Cody DD, Stevens DM, McCollough CH, McNitt-Gray MF. The feasibility of a scanner-independent technique to estimate organ dose from MDCT scans: using CTDIvol to account for differences between scanners. Med Phys. 2010;37(4):1816–25.

55. Brix G, Nagel HD, Stamm G, Veit R, Lechel U, Griebel J, Galanski M. Radiation exposure in multi-slice versus single-slice spiral CT: results of a nationwide survey. Eur Radiol. 2003;13(8):1979–91.

56. Zankl M, Panzer W, Petoussihenss N, Drexler G. Organ Doses for Children from Computed Tomographic Examinations. Radiat Prot Dosim. 1995;57(1-4):393–6.

57. Cristy M, Eckerman KF. Specific absorbed fractions of energy at various ages from internal photon sources (I. Methods). Oak Ridge National Laboratory: Oak Ridge; 1987.

58. Khursheed A, Hillier MC, Shrimpton PC, Wall BF. Influence of patient age on normalized effective doses calculated for CT examinations. Br J Radiol. 2002;75(898):819–30.

59. Zhang J, Na YH, Caracappa PF, Xu XG. RPI-AM and RPI-AF, a pair of mesh-based, size-adjustable adult male and female computational phantoms using ICRP-89 parameters and their calculations for organ doses from monoenergetic photon beams. Phys Med Biol. 2009;54(19):5885–908.

60. Zankl M, Drexler G, Petoussi-Henss N, Saito K. The calculation of dose from external photon exposures using reference human phantoms and Monte Carlo methods: Part VII. Organ doses due to parallel and environmental exposure geometries. 1997.

61. Li X, Samei E, Segars WP, Sturgeon GM, Colsher JG, Toncheva G, Yoshizumi TT, Frush DP. Patient-specific radiation dose and cancer risk estimation in CT: part II. Application to patients. Med Phys. 2011;38(1):408–19.

62. Kramer R, Khoury HJ, Vieira JW, Loureiro EC, Lima VJ, Lima FR, Hoff G. All about FAX: a Female Adult voXel phantom for Monte Carlo calculation in radiation protection dosimetry. Phys Med Biol. 2004;49(23):5203–16.

63. Kramer R, Vieira JW, Khoury HJ, de Andrade Lima F. MAX meets ADAM: a dosimetric comparison between a voxel-based and a mathematical model for external exposure to photons. Phys Med Biol. 2004;49(6):887–910.

64. Groves AM, Owen KE, Courtney HM, Yates SJ, Goldstone KE, Blake GM, Dixon AK. 16-detector multislice CT: dosimetry estimation by TLD measurement compared with Monte Carlo simulation. Br J Radiol. 2004;77(920):662–5.

65. Feng ST, Law MWM, Huang BS, Ng S, Li ZP, Meng QF, Khong PL. Radiation dose and cancer risk from pediatric CT examinations on 64-slice CT: A phantom study. Eur J Radiol. 2010;76(2):E19–23.

66. Moore BM, Brady SL, Mirro AE, Kaufman RA. Size-specific dose estimate (SSDE) provides a simple method to calculate organ dose for pediatric CT examinations. Med Phys. 2014;41(7):071917.

8

Qualitative analysis of small (≤2 cm) regenerative nodules, dysplastic nodules and well-differentiated HCCs with gadoxetic acid MRI

Michele Di Martino*[iD], Michele Anzidei, Fulvio Zaccagna, Luca Saba, Sandro Bosco, Massimo Rossi, Stefano Ginanni Corradini and Carlo Catalano

Abstract

Background: The characterization of small lesions in cirrhotic patients is extremely difficult due to the overlap of imaging features among different entities in the step-way of the hepatocarcinogenesis. The aim of our study was to evaluate the role of gadoxetic-acid MRI in the differentiation of small (≤2 cm) well-differentiated hepatocellular carcinomas from regenerative and dysplastic nodules.

Methods: Seventy-three cirrhotic patients, with 118 focal liver lesions (≤2 cm) were prospectively recruited. MRI examination was performed with a 3T magnet and the study protocol included T1 - and T2-weighted pre-contrast sequences and T1 -weighted gadoxetic-acid enhanced post-contrast sequences obtained during the arterial, venous, late dynamic and hepatobiliary phases. All lesions were pathologically confirmed. Two radiologists blinded to clinical and pathological information evaluated two imaging datasets; another radiologist analysed the signal intensity characteristics of each lesion. Sensitivity, specificity and diagnostic accuracy were considered for statistical analysis.

Results: Good agreement was reported between the two readers (κ 0.70). Both readers reported a significantly improved sensitivity (57.7 and 66.2 vs 74.6 and 83.1) and diagnostic accuracy (0.717 and 0.778 vs 0.843 and 0. 901) with the adjunction of the hepatobiliary phase 57.7 vs 74.6 and 66.2 vs 83.1 ($p \leq 0.04$).

Conclusions: Gadoxetic-acid MRI is a reliable tool for the characterization of HCC and lesions at high risk to further develop.

Keywords: Regenerative nodule, Dysplastic nodule, Well-differentiated HCC, Magnetic resonance, Liver specific contrast agent

Background

Hepatocellular carcinoma (HCC) occurs primarily in subjects with chronic liver disease or liver cirrhosis and is the cause of death in this population. The development of HCC may arise from de novo hepatocarcinogenesis or by means of a multistep progression from regenerative nodule, through dysplastic nodule to HCC [1, 2]. Especially for small nodules, it is sometimes very difficult to characterize a liver lesion due to the overlap of imaging features among different entities especially between dysplastic nodules and well-differentiated HCCs. Magnetic resonance imaging (MRI)

has shown a poor diagnostic performance in this setting with a sensitivity ranging from 55 to 72 % [3, 4]. With the introduction of hepatobiliary system–specific contrast media in clinical practice, MRI can improve the detection and characterization of liver tumours with a sensitivity value ranging from 72 to 92 % [4–6]. Gadoxetic acid is a paramagnetic, gadolinium-based contrast medium that combines perfusion and hepatocyte-selective properties. In a single examination, gadoxetic acid enables the standard dynamic MRI study of the liver and the evaluation of the functional liver tissue, due to the uptake of approximately 50 % of the contrast agent by the hepatocytes [7]. The role of a liver specific contrast agent in the detection of HCC in cirrhotic liver

* Correspondence: micdimartino@hotmail.it
Sapienza, University of Rome, Rome, Italy

has been well established in the literature, but definitive data on the role of MRI in the "grey zone" of the hepatocarcinogenesis (regenerative nodule, dysplastic nodule and well-differentiated HCC) are still partially lacking [8, 9]. The purpose of the present study is to distinguish well-differentiated HCCs from regenerative nodules and dysplastic nodules using gadoxetic acid MRI, mainly focused at the hepatobiliary phase.

Methods

Patient population

This prospective study was approved by the Institutional Review Board of "Sapienza" University of Rome, Department Radiological Sciences, Oncology and Anatomical Pathology and followed the principles of the 1964 Declaration of Helsinki and subsequent amendments. Informed consent was obtained from all individual participants included in the study. Between January 2014 and July 2015, 230 consecutive patients with chronic liver disease were evaluated prospectively within the Liver Unit of the Department of Gastroenterology for the examination of their pathology and the evaluation of suspected lesion at Ultrasound. Among these, 157 patients were excluded from data analysis for the following reasons: 1) absence of focal lesion at MR exam $n° = 35$; 2) focal lesion greater than 2 cm $n° = 37$; 3) lack of histologically proven lesion $n° = 57$; 4) inadequate specimen for pathological analysis at liver biopsy $n° = 15$; and 5) moderate/high grade of HCC n $° = 13$. The inclusion criteria were focal liver lesions ≤ 2 cm in diameter and their histological confirmation. The final study population was composed of seventy-three patients (47 males – 26 females; mean age 64 years; range 23–82 years), with 118 focal liver lesions (Fig. 1). Histological information had been obtained by liver transplantation, surgery and liver biopsy according to the best clinical care for the patient. Liver biopsy was mainly performed for the characterization of nodules with MRI patterns that were not suggestive of HCC (wash-in and wash-out), and in a few cases of HCC with typical aspects, a liver biopsy was performed before radiofrequency ablation. Patients who had undergone surgery or biopsy were followed by CT or MR examinations with a surveillance interval of 6 months [10]. Chronic hepatitis or cirrhosis were related to viral infection (hepatitis C $[n° = 31]$, hepatitis B $[n° = 13]$, both $[n° = 2]$), alcohol abuse ($n° = 7$), alcohol + HCV infection ($n° = 11$) or cryptogenic ($n° = 9$). Forty patients were Child-Pugh A classified, 22 were class B, and 11 were class C.

MRI technique

MRI was performed using a 3 Tesla scanner (Discovery MR750; General Electric Systems, Milwaukee, Wisconsin, US) equipped with a high-performance gradient system (50 mT/m). Signal reception was achieved using a combined antero-posterior phased-array surface coil and a spine array coil. MRI sequences and parameters are detailed in Table 1.

Timing for the initial post-contrast arterial phase acquisition was determined using an automated bolus detection technique (SmartPrep, General Electric) [11]. The full 0.025 mmol/kg body weight dose of gadoxetic-acid (Primovist Bayer Schering Pharma, Berlin, Germany: 0.1 mL/kg body weight) was administered at the flow rate of 2 mL/sec through an 18–22-gauge intravenous catheter by means of a power injector (Spectris; Medrad, Indianola, Pa), followed by a 20-mL saline flush at the same injection rate. Post contrast images were obtained ≈ 25, 70, and 180 s after contrast medium injection, during the hepatic arterial, hepatic venous, and late dynamic phases, respectively, as well as during the hepatobiliary phase

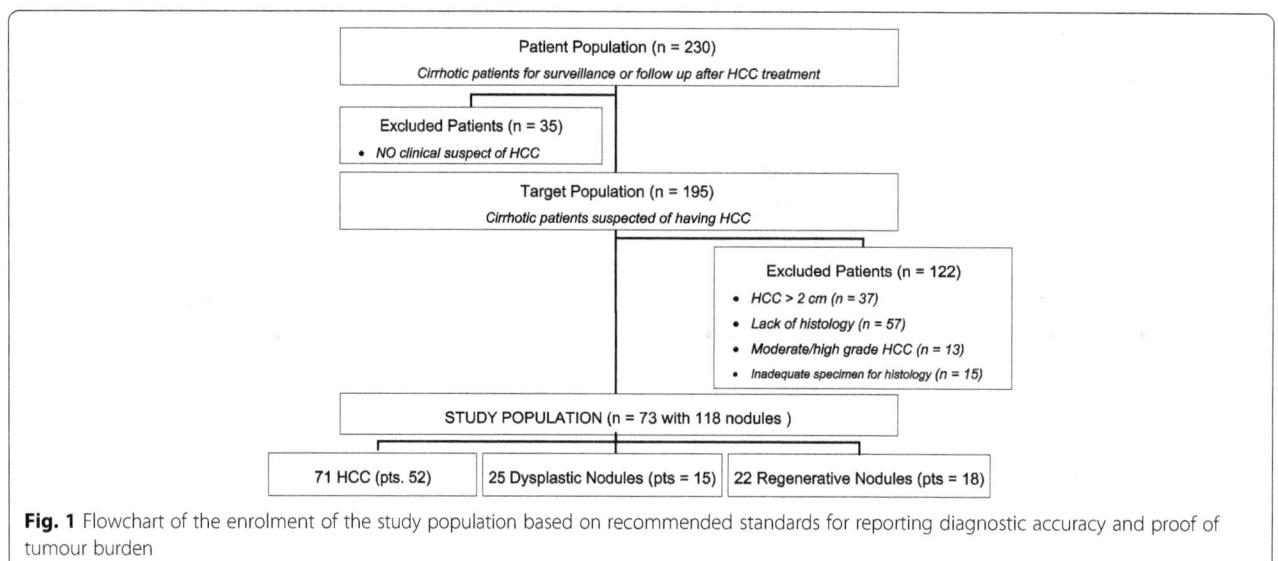

Fig. 1 Flowchart of the enrolment of the study population based on recommended standards for reporting diagnostic accuracy and proof of tumour burden

Table 1 MR imaging sequences and parameters

MR Sequence	Fat suppression	TR/TE (OP/IP) (ms)	Flip angle (degrees)	Section thickness (mm)	Matrix size	Bandwidth (Hz/pixel)	Field of view (cm)	Time (s)
T2-weighted 2D SSFSE	w/ and w/out	3000/110	90	5	320 × 324	260	30–40	32
T1-weighted 2D dual GRE	Not used	4/1.2–2.4	12	5	320 × 324	260	30–40	32
SS-EPI-DWI	Used	5455/77	90	6	100 × 192	250	30–40	30
T1-weighted 3D GRE LAVA[a]	Used	4.2/1.3	12	5 (interpolated 2.5)	320 × 224	250	30–40	23

[a]Acquired before and after contrast medium administration during the arterial (≈25 s), venous (70 s.), late dynamic (180 s.) and hepatobiliary phases (20 min)

(20 min after contrast medium administration). Before the administration of gadoxetic-acid, a respiratory-triggered single-shot echo-planar imaging DWI MR sequence was also acquired with b values of 0, 50, 400 and 800 s/mm2. A spectral attenuated inversion-recovery technique was used for fat suppression of DW images.

Image analysis

One radiologist (with 3 years of experience in liver imaging), who was not involved in the data set analysis, evaluated the signal intensity of each lesion at all acquired sequences (precontrast, dynamic and hepatobiliary phases) as hyperintense, isointense, or hypointense relative to liver parenchyma. Two data sets of images were generated: a) pre-contrast sequences + dynamic phase sequences and b) pre-contrast sequences + dynamic phase sequences + hepatobiliary phase sequences.

All data sets of images were independently reviewed by two radiologist experts in abdominal MRI (C.C. 18 years, M.D.M. 10 years), in two reading sessions with a time interval of four weeks to avoid any recall bias, by using a commercially available workstation (Leonardo; Siemens Medical Systems) with standard interpretation tools (window width, pan, level). The readers were blinded to the results of histopathologic analysis. HCC was unequivocally diagnosed if it was hypervascular during the hepatic arterial phase and fulfilled any one of the following five criteria: (a) hypointensity compared with the surrounding liver during portal venous or late dynamic phases (wash-out sign), (b) peripheral rim enhancement during the late dynamic phase (capsular appearance), (c) invasion line of adjacent vessels, and (d) hypointensity during the hepatobiliary phase. In addition, suggestive but non-conclusive criterion of HCC included (a) mild hyperintensity on T2-weighted MR images or (b) nodular early enhancement without washout.

Pathologic analysis

All resected and explanted livers were analysed by the same experienced (30 years of experience) pathologist. They were sectioned in the axial plane with a slice thickness of 5–10 mm. The MRI images had been directly correlated with histological findings by an expert radiologist (10 years of experience in abdominal imaging) who was present when the specimens were prepared for evaluation. Percutaneous needle nodule biopsy was performed with an 18-gauge needle, under local anaesthesia and ultrasound guidance. Each biopsy specimen was approximately 1.5 cm in length. No complications, such as bleeding and/or seeding, were reported after liver biopsy. The diagnosis of hepatocellular nodules was performed according to criteria of the International Working Party on haematoxylin and eosin (H&E)-stained sections supplemented by CD34 immunostaining for nodule vascularization. Criteria for the differentiation of HCC from dysplastic nodule were tumour invasion into portal tracts (stromal invasion) and presence of multi-foci of neo-angiogenesis [12, 13].

Statistical analysis

Inter-reader variability between the readers for lesion detection was assessed by using the weighted κ statistic. K values of 0.4 or less were considered positive but fair agreement, those of 0.41–0.60 moderate agreement, those of 0.61–0.80 a good agreement and greater than 0.80 indicated an excellent agreement [14]. The accuracy of each imaging method was determined using a jackknife alternative, free-response receiver operating characteristic (JAFROC_v3b_BETA), considering fixed readers and random cases [15]. The area under each curve (AUC) was used to indicate the overall diagnostic performance of each reader on each image set. Determinations of the sensitivity, specificity, and positive and negative predictive values (PPV and NPV, respectively) for lesion detection on each image set for each reader were calculated against reference standard findings. The 95 % confidence interval (CI) was also calculated for each evaluation. To consider the possible presence of multiple lesions within the same patient, the significance of differences in sensitivity and PPV among the different image sets was assessed using a generalized linear mixed model with P values calculated using an adjustment of the McNemar test [16]. Statistical analyses were conducted using dedicated software (SPSS version 13.0, SPSS, Chicago, Ill, US).

Results

Qualitative analysis

Among the 118 identified lesions (1 to 4 per patient), 71 in 52 patients were well-differentiated HCC (range 5–20 mm; median 15 mm) of which 32 were confirmed at liver transplantation, 15 at surgery and 24 at biopsy; 25 lesions in 15 patients were dysplastic nodules (range 5–20 mm, median 15 mm), of which 14 were confirmed at liver transplantation, 6 at surgery and 5 at biopsy. Additionally, 22 in 18 patients were regenerative nodules (range 6–20 mm; median 15 mm) of which 16 were confirmed at liver transplantation and 6 at biopsy. MRI appearance of regenerative, dysplastic nodules and well-differentiated HCC at different MRI sequences are summarized in Table 2. Well-differentiated HCC showed the typical imaging pattern (wash-in and wash-out) in 43/71 lesions (60.5 %), 16/71 (21.1 %) were hypervascular without wash-out and 12/71 (16.9 %) were hypointense during the arterial phase with loss of signal intensity during the late dynamic phase (Fig. 1). During the hepatobiliary phase, six typical HCCs showed uptake of the contrast medium (13.9 %); by contrast among hypervascular lesions without wash out, 7 nodules out of 16 (43.7 %) showed loss of signal intensity during the hepatobiliary phase, which means that there is an absence of functional hepatocytes and that it should be considered a sign of malignancy. All hypovascular HCCs reported a loss of signal intensity during the late dynamic phase, and four of these were isointense during the hepatobiliary phase. Additionally, 35 out of 71 (50.7 %) of the well-differentiated HCCs, mostly HCCs with the typical imaging pattern, were hyperintense on T2-weighted images. Data of Low Grade Dysplastic Nodules (LGDN) and High Grade Dysplastic Nodules (HGDN) were pooled because only 7 cases of LGDN out of 29 were identified. Dysplastic nodules, in most cases, appeared as a nodule without enhancement (hypo- or isointense) during the arterial phase and were relatively hypointense during the late dynamic phase 20/25 (80 %). Among these, 7 (40 %) were hypointense during the hepatobiliary phase (Fig. 2). Eight dysplastic nodules,

confirmed at liver biopsy and showing a loss of signal intensity on both late dynamic and hepatobiliary phases, subsequently developed the typical imaging pattern of HCC (wash-in and wash-out) within 6–12 months. In four cases (16 %) confirmed at liver transplantation, dysplastic nodules demonstrated the typical pattern of HCC and represented the main cause of false positive calls. None of the dysplastic nodules were hyperintense on T2-weighted images and most of them (20/25, 80 %) were hypointense to the surrounding liver parenchyma: in effect at histological examination some iron particles were found within the nodules. Regenerative nodules tend to be isointense to liver parenchyma in all pre-contrast and post-contrast dynamic phases. Only 4 out of 22 nodules (18.8 %) were hypervascular during the arterial phase (Fig. 3) and 2 lesions were slightly hypointense during the delayed phase. One lesion out of two showed high signal intensity on hepatobiliary phase and none of the regenerative nodules reported low signal intensity during the hepatobiliary phase. The other regenerative nodules were localized because they were hyperintense on T1-weighted images 6/22 (27.3 %) and/or slightly hypointense on T2-weighted images 10/22 (45.5 %) and/or 10/22 (45.5 %) hyperintense on hepatobiliary phase. Diagnostic performance regarding the detection of HCC showed a good inter-reader agreement (κ .70) between the two observers. Both readers detected significantly more malignant lesions on MRI datasets that included pre-contrast, dynamic and hepatobiliary phases than on MRI datasets that included only pre-contrast and dynamic phases (57.7 and 66.2 vs 74.6 and 83.1 : $p = 0.049$ and $p = 0.03$) (Table 3). The overall accuracy for the detection of HCC was higher on dynamic + hepatobiliary phase MRI for both readers compared to dynamic MRI alone, and both radiologists reported a significant difference (0.717 and 0.778 vs 0.843 and 0.901: $p = 0.03$) (Table 3). The hepatobiliary phase was useful for a definitive diagnosis of malignancy in 7 of 16 cases (43.7 %): these nodules showed enhancement during the arterial phase and no wash-out sign during the venous and late dynamic phase.

Both the PPV and NPV for HCC identification were higher on dynamic + hepatobiliary phases MRI compared to dynamic phases MRI alone (Table 3).

Table 2 Signal intensities of different lesions at each MR sequence

	T1-w	T2-w	T1-Art	T1-Ven	T1-LD	T1-Hepatobiliary
Well diff. HCC -	57,7 hyper (27/45)	53.3 hyper (24/45)	82.2 hyper (37/45)	64.4 iso (29/45)	66.6 hypo (30/45)	84.2 hypo (38/45)
D.N. -	55,1 hyper (16 /29)	58.6 hypo (17/29)	58.6 iso/hypo (25/29)	68 hypo (17/29)	89.6 hypo (26 /29)	58.6 iso/hyper (17/29)
R.N. -	51 iso / hyper (17/33)	75.7 iso (25/33)	57.7 iso (19/33)	87.8 iso (29/33)	84.8 iso (28/33)	100 iso / hyper (33/33)

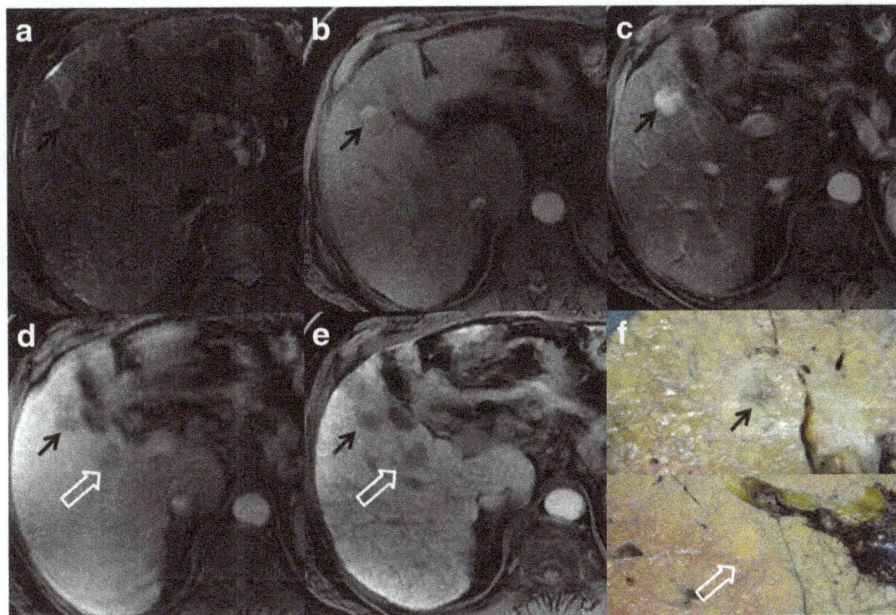

Fig. 2 MR scans in a patient with chronic hepatitis, HCV related, and HCC and dysplastic nodule in liver segment V. **a-b** T2- and T1-weighted fast images show a heterogeneous nodule in liver segment V (*arrow*). The lesion shows the typical pattern of HCC with enhancement during the arterial phase **c**) and a wash-out sign on late dynamic phase **d**). On the late dynamic phase, a lesion near the "hilum-hepatis" is also detectable with loss of signal intensity to the surrounding liver parenchyma (open arrow). **e** On the fat-suppressed T1-weighted 3D GRE image obtained during the hepatobiliary phase at 20 min after contrast injection, both lesions are hypointense to the surrounding liver parenchyma. **f** Histological analysis shows a hepatocellular carcinoma (*upper image*) and dysplastic nodule (*lower image*)

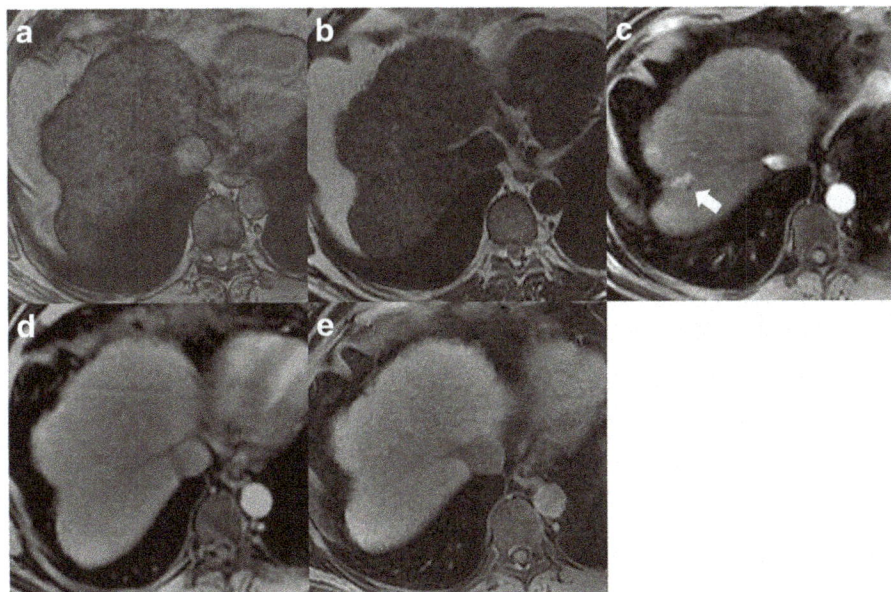

Fig. 3 MR scans in a patient with chronic hepatitis, HCV related, and a regenerative nodule in liver segment VIII. **a-b** T1- and T2-weighted images do not reveal any focal liver lesion. **c** T1-weighted gradient-echo shows a hypervascular lesion without wash-out during the late dynamic phase **d**). On the corresponding MR image obtained during the liver-specific hepatobiliary phase (**e**), the lesion is isointense to adjacent hepatic parenchyma. At pathologic examination of the explanted liver, this lesion corresponded to a multiacinar cirrhotic nodule

Table 3 Diagnostic performance for HCC detection

		Sensitivity	Specificity	Positive predictive value	Negative predictive value	Accuracy
Observer 1	Dynamic phases	57.7 %(41/71) [.45–.69]	91.5 %(43/47) [.80–.97]	91.1 %(41/45) [.78–.97]	58.9 %(43/73) [.49–.71]	0.717 [.60–.83]
	Dynamic + hept phases	*74.6 %(53/71) [.61–.83]	91.5 %(43/47) [.80–.97]	92.9 %(53/57) [.79–.97]	70.5 %(43/61) [.53–.75]	§0.843 [.73–.95]
Observer 2	Dynamic phases	66.2 %(47/71) [.54–.77]	91.5 %(43/47) [.80–.97]	92.2 %(47/51) [.85–.98]	62.7 %(42/67) (54/85)	0.778 [.64–.88]
	Dynamic + hept phases	*83.1 %(59/71) [.72–.91]	95.7 %(45/47) [.85–.99]	96.7 %(59/61) [.87–.98]	78.9 %(45/57) [.52–.73]	§0.901 [.78–.99]

Numbers in brackets are the 95 % CIs
*Significantly higher sensitivity for both readers $p = 0.04$ and $p = 0.03$
§Significantly higher sensitivity for both readers $p = 0.03$

Discussion

Our experience confirmed that Gadoxetic acid MRI is a reliable tool for the identification of HCC or lesions at high risk of developing into HCC. Loss of signal intensity during the hepatobiliary phase helps to improve the detection of small (≤20 mm) hypervascular well-differentiated HCCs without washout during the dynamic phases. With the development of fast sequences and the acquisition of images at different vascular phases, MRI has demonstrated a trend to a better sensitivity and accuracy over CT, and with the introduction in clinical practice of liver specific contrast agent, this difference has become more significant [17, 18]. At present, indeed, MRI is considered the best imaging approach in the evaluation of nodules in cirrhotic patients. However, the detection and characterization of small HCC in cirrhotic patients is still challenging because it is difficult to distinguish HCC from other entities that could develop in cirrhotic liver. Considering imaging patterns of the three groups of lesions that were mentioned in the study (well-differentiated HCC, dysplastic nodule and regenerative nodule) at dynamic phases, HCCs tend to have a typical imaging pattern in 60.5 % of cases. In 14 out of 71 cases (19 %), HCC appears as isointense lesions with wash-out signs. This imaging pattern suggests that tumour neo-angiogenesis starts after the disruption of peri-portal space [19, 20]. The main feature of dysplastic nodules was hypovascular lesion (iso/hypointense) with a loss of signal intensity during the late dynamic phase. This is probably because in the dysplastic nodules there are only a few foci of neo-angiogenesis and the blood is drained to the sinusoid by the surrounding liver parenchyma, but it could also be explained by the early uptake of the gadoxetic acid from the liver parenchyma near the lesion. Ten dysplastic nodules showed a loss of signal intensity on both late dynamic and hepatobiliary phases. These image findings overlapped in our study population with some hypovascular HCCs. Eight of those dysplastic nodules changed their imaging patterns to that of HCC at follow-up imaging. Loss of signal intensity on both the late dynamic and hepatobiliary phase should then be considered a high feature of malignancy and could predict malignant transformation, and a more intensive management would be required (strict follow-up or biopsy) [21–23]. As suggested by previously published papers, in our experience, gadoxetic-acid MRI significantly increases sensitivity and diagnostic accuracy in the detection of small hepatocellular carcinoma. [24–27]. In our experience, a high signal intensity on T2 should be certainly considered a sign of malignant transformation because it was encountered only in HCCs, although with a poor detection rate (53.3 %) [28]. Our study certainly has some limits. Firstly, in our study we considered low grade and high grade dysplastic nodules in the same group due to the small number of low grade dysplastic nodules. We are aware that there is a significant difference between these two entities in developing HCC. Secondly, some histological confirmations were obtained with liver biopsy, which in small nodules may lead to a small amount of sampling tissue and difficult nodule characterization. Finally, although DWI MRI sequence is a part of the MRI protocol at our institution, data were not reported in this paper because the preliminary results showed no significant differences of adding DW images for the detection of HCC. The role of DW images in cirrhotic liver is still a matter of debate. Some authors emphasize that it is useful for the detection and characterization of nodules in cirrhotic liver [29], while others affirm that it only slightly increases MRI sensitivity [30, 31].

Conclusion

In our experience, loss of signal intensity at gadoxetic acid MRI hepatobiliary phase is a reliable tool in the identification of HCC and lesions at high risk to develop into HCC. Cirrhosis-associated hepatocellular nodules with non specific findings at MR imaging, that show loss of signal intensity during the hepatobiliary phase should undergone more intensive management.

Abbreviation

DN: Dysplastic nodule; DWI: Diffusion weighted imaging; HCC: Hepatocellular carcinoma; HGDN: High grade dysplastic nodules; LGDN: Low grade dysplastic nodules; MRI: Magnetic resonance imaging; RN: Regenerative nodule

Acknowledgements
Not applicable.

Funding
No Finding were used.

Authors' contributions
MDM and MA contributed to study conception, design and writing of the article; MR, SB and SGC S contributed to data acquisition; LS and FZ contributed to data analysis and interpretation, and writing of article; MR, MDM and CC contributed to editing, reviewing and final approval of article.

Authors' information
Authors information are available on the full-title page.

Competing interests
The authors declare that they have nocompeting interests.

References

1. Coleman WB. Mechanisms of human hepatocarcinogenesis. Curr Mol Med. 2003;3:573–88.
2. Efremidis SC, Hytiroglou P. The multistep process of hepatocarcinogenesis in cirrhosis with imaging correlation. Eur Radiol. 2002;12:753–64.
3. Krinsky GA, Lee VS, Theise ND, et al. Hepatocellular carcinoma and dysplastic nodules in patients with cirrhosis: prospective diagnosis with MR imaging and explantation correlation. Radiology. 2001;219:445–54.
4. Bartolozzi C, Battaglia V, Bargellini I, et al. Contrast-enhanced magnetic resonance imaging of 102 nodules in cirrhosis: correlation with histological findings on explanted livers. Abdom Imaging. 2013;38:290–6.
5. Grazioli L, Morana G, Caudana R, et al. Hepatocellular carcinoma: correlation between gadobenate dimeglumine-enhanced MRI and pathologic findings. Invest Radiol. 2000;35:25–34.
6. Semelka RC, Helmberger TK. Contrast agents for MR imaging of the liver. Radiology. 2001;218:27–38.
7. Huppertz A, Haraida S, Kraus A, et al. Enhancement of focal liver lesions at gadoxetic acid-enhanced MR imaging: correlation with histopathologic findings and spiral CT–initial observations. Radiology. 2005;234:468–78.
8. Kim SH, Kim SH, Lee J, et al. Gadoxetic acid–enhanced MRI versus triple-phase MDCT for the preoperative detection of hepatocellularcarcinoma. Am J Roentgenol. 2009;192:1675–81.
9. Kim JI, Lee MJ, Choi JY, et al. The value of gadobenate dimeglumine-enhanced delayed phase MR imaging for characterization of hepatocellular carcinoma nodules in the cirrhotic liver. Invest Radiol. 2008;43:202–10.
10. Bruix J, Sherman M. Management of hepatocellular carcinoma: an update. Hepatology. 2011;53:1020–2.
11. HO VB, Foo TK. Optimization of gadolinium-enhanced magnetic resonance angiography using an automated bolus-detection algorithm (MR SmartPrep). Original investigation. Invest Radiol. 1998;33:515–23.
12. Llovet JM, Chen Y, Wurmbach E, et al. A molecular signature to discriminate dysplastic nodules from early hepatocellular carcinoma in HCV cirrhosis. Gastroenterology. 2006;131:1758–67.
13. Kojiro M. Histopathology of liver cancer. Best Pract Res CLin Gastroenterol. 2005;19:39–62.
14. Viera AJ, Garret JA. Understanding interobserver agreement: the kappa statistic. Fam Med. 2005;37:360–3.
15. Chakraborty DP. Analysis of location specific observer performance data: validated extensions of the jackknife free-response (JAFROC) method. Acad Radiol. 2006;13:1187–93.
16. Eliassziw M, Donner A. Application of the McNemar test to non-independent matched pair data. Statist Med. 1991;10:1981–91.
17. Burrel M, Llovet JM, Ayuso C, et al. MRI angiography is superior to helical CT for detection of HCC prior to liver transplantation: an explant correlation. Hepatology. 2003;38:1034–42.
18. Di Martino M, De Filippis G, De Santis A, et al. Hepatocellular carcinoma in cirrhotic patients: prospective comparison of US, CT and MR imaging. Eur Radiol. 2013;23:887–96.
19. Gatto A, De Geetano AM, Giuga M, et al. Differentiating hepatocellular carcinoma from dysplastic nodules at gadobenate dimeglumine-enhanced hepatobiliary-phase magnetic resonance imaging. Abdom Imaging. 2013;38:736–44.
20. Matsui O. Imaging of multistep human hepatocarcinogenesis by CT during intraarterial contrast injection. Intervirology. 2004;47:271–6.
21. Kogita S, Imai Y, Okada M, Kim T, Onishi H, Takamura M, et al. Gd-EOB-DTPAenhanced magnetic resonance images of hepatocellular carcinoma: correlation with histological grading and portal blood flow. Eur Radiol. 2010;20:2405–13.
22. Park MJ, Kim JK, Lee MW, et al. Small hepatocellular carcinomas: improved sensitivity by combining Gadoxetic-acid-enhanced and diffusion-weighted imaging patterns. Radiology. 2012;264:761–70.
23. Golfieri R, Renzulli M, Lucidi V, et al. Contribution of the hepatobiliary phase of Gd-EOB-DTPA-enhanced MRI to Dynamic MRI in the detection of hypovascular small (≤2 cm) HCC in cirrhosis. Eur Radiol. 2011;21:1233–42.
24. Takayama Y, Nishie A, Nakayama T, et al. Hypovascular hepatic nodule showing hypointensity in the hepatobiliary phase of gadoxetic acid-enhanced MRI in patients with chronic liver disease: Prediction of malignant transformation. Eur J Radiol. 2012;81:3072–8.
25. Golfieri R, Grazioli L, Orlando E, et al. Which is the best MRI marker of malignancy for atypical cirrhotic nodules: hypointensity in hepatobiliary phase alone or combined with other features? Classification after Gd-EOB-DTPA administration. J Magn Reson Imaging. 2012;36:648–57.
26. Granito A, Galassi M, Piscaglia F, et al. Impact of gadoxetic acid (Gd-EOB-DTPA)-enhanced magnetic resonance on the non-invasive diagnosis of small hepatocellular carcinoma: a prospective study. Aliment Pharmacol Ther. 2013;37:355–63.
27. Doo KW, Lee CH, Choi JW, Lee J, Kim HA, Park CM. Pseudo washout" sign in high-flow hepatic hemangioma on gadoxetic acid contrast-enhanced MRI mimicking hypervascular tumor. Am J Roentgenol. 2009;193:W490–6.
28. Chou CT, Chou JM, Chang TA, et al. Differentiation between dysplastic nodule and early-stage hepatocellular carcinoma: the utility of conventional MR imaging. World J Gastroenterol. 2013;19:7433–9.
29. Vandecaveye V, De Keyzer F, Verslype C, et al. Diffusion weighted MRI provides additional value to conventional dynamic contrast-enhanced MRI for detection of hepatocellular carcinoma. Eur Radiol. 2009;19:2456–66.
30. Park MS, Kim S, Patel J, et al. Hepatocellular carcinoma: detection with diffusionweighted versus contrast-enhanced magnetic resonance imaging in pretransplant patients. Hepatology. 2012;56:140–8.
31. Di Martino M, Di Miscio R, De F, et al. Detection of small (≤2 cm) HCC in cirrhotic patients: added value of diffusion MR-imaging. Abdom Imaging. 2013;38:1254–62.

9

Detection of articular perforations of the proximal humerus fracture using a mobile 3D image intensifier – a cadaver study

Jan Theopold[1*], Kevin Weihs[1], Christine Feja[2], Bastian Marquaß[1], Christoph Josten[1] and Pierre Hepp[1]

Abstract

Background: The purpose of this study was to investigate the accuracy of perforation detection with multiplanar reconstructions using a mobile 3D image intensifier.

Methods: In 12 paired human humeri, K-wires perforating the subchondral bone and placed just below the cartilage level were directed toward five specific regions in the humeral head. Image acquisition was initiated by a fluoroscopy scan. Within a range of 90°, 45° external rotation (ER) and 45° internal rotation (IR). The number and percentage of detected perforating screws were grouped and analyzed. Furthermore, the fluoroscopic images were converted into multiplanar CT-like reconstructions. Each K-wire perforation was characterized as "detected" or "not detected".

Results: In the series of fluoroscopy images in the standard neutral position at 30° internal rotation, and 30° external rotation, the perforations of all K-wires ($n = 56$) were detected. Twenty-nine (51.8%) of them were detected in one AP view, 22 (39.3%) in two AP views, and five (8.9%) in three AP views. All K-wire perforations (100%, $n = 56$) were detected in multiplanar reconstructions.

Conclusion: In order to reveal all of the intraoperative and postoperative screw perforations in a "five screw configuration", conventional AP images should be established in both the neutral positions (0°), at 30° internal rotation and 30° external rotation. Alternatively, the intraoperative 3D scan with multiplanar reconstructions enables a 100% rate of detection of the screw perforations.

Keywords: Proximal humerus fracture, Screw perforation, 3D imaging, Patient safety, Shoulder

Background

Correct fracture classification, anatomical reduction, and stable fixation, along with avoidance of iatrogenic and material-related complications, may provide the basis for a good functional outcome following proximal humerus fracture surgery. In recent years, locking plates have been widely used for the treatment of proximal humerus fractures [1–4]. Nevertheless, high complication rates, comprising primary and secondary screw perforation, malreduction, malunion, nonunion, avascular necrosis, and infection, have been observed [5]. One area of particular concern involves the reportedly high rates of intraoperative humeral head screw perforation or screw

cutout in the follow-up period [6–10]. This is likely the result of several factors, including diverging and converging locking screw vectors, the convex morphology of the humeral head, and poor bone quality limiting the tactile feedback of the drill bit, among other things. Iatrogenic articular screw penetration can lead to the destruction of the glenoid, which has been found to be unsatisfactorily treatable [7, 11]. The reduction is usually assessed intraoperatively while utilizing fluoroscopy in the anterior-posterior radiographic (AP) and Velpeau axillary views [12, 13]. The standard postoperative radiological control involves anteroposterior scapular, lateral scapular, and axillary radiographs.

The introduction of mobile 3D fluoroscopy has made intraoperative multiplanar imaging possible and it is used in navigated spinal surgery [14], pelvic operations [15], and for fractures of several extremeties [16–19].

* Correspondence: JanDirk.Theopold@medizin.uni-leipzig.de
[1]Department of Orthopedics, Trauma and Plastic Surgery, University of Leipzig, Liebigstrasse 20, 04103 Leipzig, Germany
Full list of author information is available at the end of the article

Thus, the purpose of this study was to determine the AP views that are necessary to detect primary screw perforation of the humeral head under a controlled "in-vitro" setup. The secondary goal was to investigate the accuracy of perforation detection via multiplanar reconstructions using a mobile 3D image intensifier.

Methods

Specimen selection and preparation

Twelve paired human humeri were harvested from embalmed cadavers (two male and four female, mean age 76.8 years [range, 52–91 years]). All donors had given prior direct consent that their cadavers could be used for educational purposes or for research projects at the Institutes for Anatomy. Institutional review board approval was not required for this study. The specimens were dissected free of soft tissue, and biplanar radiographs were used to ascertain any bone abnormalities in the proximal humerus. Specimens with previous proximal humeral fractures, other underlying pathologic changes, or surgical intervention were excluded from the study.

Five 1.8 mm K-wires were guided into anterior, superior-anterior, inferior, superior-posterior, and posterior positions using a locking plate with a targeting device (Winsta PH, Axomed, Freiburg, Germany), which ensured a reproducible placement of the K-wires. The wire placement was performed by a single surgeon experienced in shoulder surgery (JT).

Each proximal humerus was positioned horizontally to ensure the maximum projection of the greater humeral tuberosity on a two-dimensional AP view. The perforations were verified by confirming them visually (Fig. 1).

Fluoroscopic imaging and detection of perforation

Image acquisition was initiated by performing a fluoroscopy scan with the mobile Ziehm Vision FD Vario 3D© (Ziehm Imaging GmbH, Nurnberg, Germany). The motorized fluoroscope features a variable isocentric C-arm

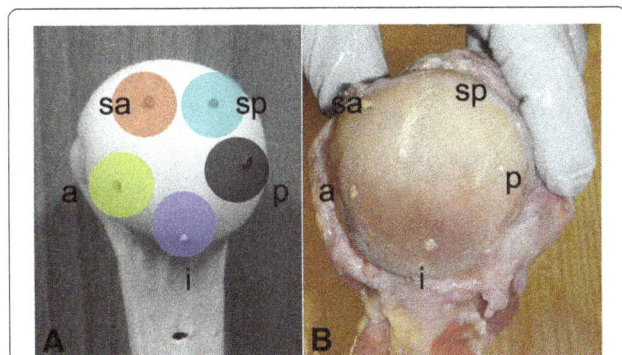

Fig. 1 Regions of articular K-wire perforation; **a** schematic view on a synbone and **b** subchondral placement of K-wires in a specimen in the following positions: a = anterior, sa = superior-anterior, i = inferior, sp = superior-posterior, and p = posterior

design and collects 110 fluoroscopic images during a 135° arc of rotation around an anatomic region of interest. Its isocenter is held in place to allow for the movements of the C-arm cantilever. This readjustment is automated.

Each fluoroscopic image was analyzed (MagicWeb VA60C_0212, Visage Imaging GmbH Berlin, Germany) by three of the authors (JT, PH, KW) and K-wire perforation was documented for all five positions (Fig. 2).

As each image corresponds to a 1.23° step and the perforation was visible in consecutive images, the "angle of visible perforation" (AVP) for each K-wire was calculated by multiplying the number of images with visible perforation (NVP) by 1.23: AVP = NVP*1.23.

The neutral position was set to 0° which matched the classical AP view of the shoulder joint and corresponded to fluoroscopy image number 73. An external rotation (ER) of 45° corresponded to image number 37, while an internal rotation (IR) of 45° corresponded to image number 110. The analysis of K-wire perforation was performed within a 90° range (45° IR to 45° ER; image 37–110; $n = 73$ images). The number and percentage of detected perforating screws were grouped and analyzed for each of the two series of AP views: 30° IR – 0°–30° ER and 45° IR – 0°–45° ER.

All 110 of the fluoroscopic images were then converted into multiplanar CT-like reconstructions using the Ziehm software version 5.63 (Ziehm Imaging GmbH, Nurnberg, Germany). On the workstation, each wire was identified in coronal, axial, and sagittal views (Fig. 3). The correct placement of each K-wire was verified and each K-wire perforation was characterized as "detected" or "not detected". K-wires that did not match the aforementioned inclusion criteria were excluded from further analysis.

The fluoroscopy images, the multiplanar reconstructions and the specimen of the non-detected perforations were subsequently reevaluated. This revealed a secondary displacement of four wires. One K-wire did not perforate the subchondral bone. Three further K-wire perforations were visible in all 110 images. The analysis of the specimen revealed a secondary K-wire dislocation. For all remaining k-wires the initial placement was confirmed.

Statistics

All data were collected in a computerized database. The data was analyzed by means of descriptive statistics (SPSS, version 20, Chicago, IL, USA). A chi square test was used to test differences in the number of visible perforations in the different positions. Cronbach's Alpha statistic was used to evaluate inter-observer error in image analysis. The significance level was set to $p < 0.05$.

Results

Detection of perforation

All 56 K-wire perforations (100%) were detected on the fluoroscopy images of the 12 specimens (Table 1). A

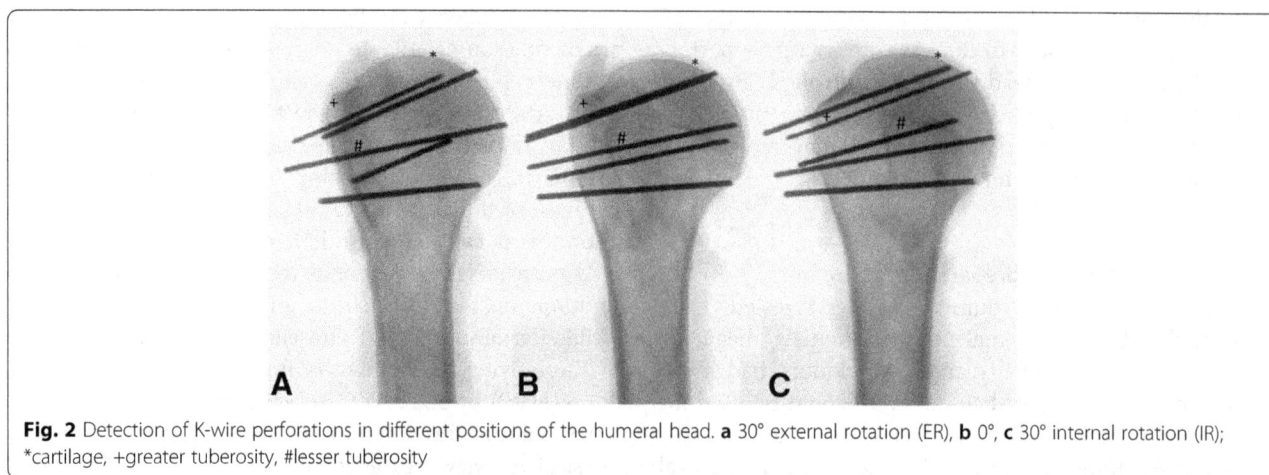

Fig. 2 Detection of K-wire perforations in different positions of the humeral head. **a** 30° external rotation (ER), **b** 0°, **c** 30° internal rotation (IR); *cartilage, +greater tuberosity, #lesser tuberosity

high inter-observer reliability of 0.93 (Cronbach's Alpha) was found. The perforating K-wires of the 12 specimens were detected at an angle of visible perforation (AVP) of mean 29.3° (between 45° IR and 15.7° IR) in the anterior position, 48.3° (between 45° IR and 3.3° ER) in the superior-anterior position, 47.3° (between 25° IR and 22.4° ER) in the inferior position, 69.3° (between 28.2° IR and 41.1° ER) in the superior-posterior position, and 35.8° (between 7.3° ER and 43.1° ER) in the posterior position (Fig. 4).

On the series of fluoroscopy images in the standard neutral position at 30° internal rotation, and at 30° external rotation, perforations of all K-wires ($n = 56$) were detected. Twenty-nine (51.8%) of them were detected in one AP view, 22 (39.3%) in two AP views, and five (8.9%) in three AP views.

In the "45° IR – 0°–45° ER" series, one perforation was not detected (1.8%, one posterior K-wire), while 35 (62.5%) of them were detected in one AP view, 19 (33.9%) in two AP views, and one (1.8%) in three AP views. The one perforation that was not detected in this series was only visible at an angle of 26.8° ER to 36.7° ER. Therefore, the view in 45° ER did not detect the perforating screw.

Significantly more perforations were detected in 30° ER compared to 45° ER ($p = 0.041$). There were no significant differences between the other AP views ($p > 0,05$).

All K-wire perforations (100%, $n = 56$) were detected in the multiplanar reconstructions and the coronal reconstruction offered the best visibility (Fig. 3).

Discussion

The principal findings of this study show that a combination of three AP views – neutral, 30° internal rotation, and 30° external rotation – permit the identification of 100% of articular perforations in an in-vitro setup. Additionally, coronal reconstruction of a 3D fluoroscopic scan provided a 100% rate of detection of the perforating K-wires.

The use of locking plates in the surgical treatment of proximal humerus fractures is associated with an unexpectedly high rate of screw cutouts and revision surgery [9]. Biomechanical studies have emphasized the value of anchoring screws in the subchondral bone of the humeral head to improve implant stability [20, 21]. However, the spherical shape of the proximal humerus and the limited tactile sensation of its soft cancellous bone make it difficult to determine an accurate screw length, and reported rates of intraoperative screw

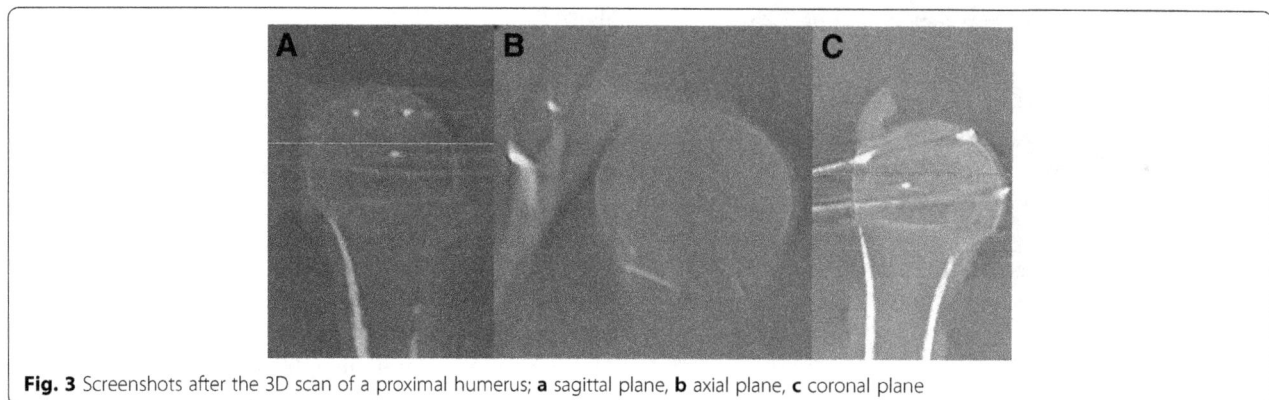

Fig. 3 Screenshots after the 3D scan of a proximal humerus; **a** sagittal plane, **b** axial plane, **c** coronal plane

Table 1 Number (%) of detected K-wire perforations in different AP views

Location of perforation	Arm position				
	45° ER	30° ER	0°	30° IR	45° IR
Superior-posterior	6/9	9/9	8/9	3/9	2/9
Superior-anterior		1/12	7/12	12/12	12/12
Anterior			2/11	11/11	11/11
Posterior	10/12	12/12	3/12		
Inferior	1/12	5/12	11/12	4/12	3/12
Total (n = 56)	17 (30.4%)	27 (48.2%)*	31 (55.4%)	30 (53.6%)	28 (50%)

*significantly more perforations were detected in 30° external rotation (ER) compared to 45° ER (p = 0.041)

penetration are high. Iatrogenic screw penetration, even if recognized and corrected before leaving the operating room, may lead to late failure [11].

The protocol for using locking plates and the attention placed on the technical aspects of applying them have been emphasized in the past [11, 22]. Nevertheless, only a few studies have investigated the potential for optimizing the recognition of early or late stage screw perforation [23, 24].

Complications following proximal humerus fracture surgery may likely be a result of inadequate use of intra-operative radiographs or fluoroscopy [25]. Accordingly, the use of routine intraoperative fluoroscopy to confirm hardware placement and a stable anatomical reduction are recommended. The anteroposterior view is a key component of a basic shoulder series. Often, two AP projections are obtained, namely one with the arm in an

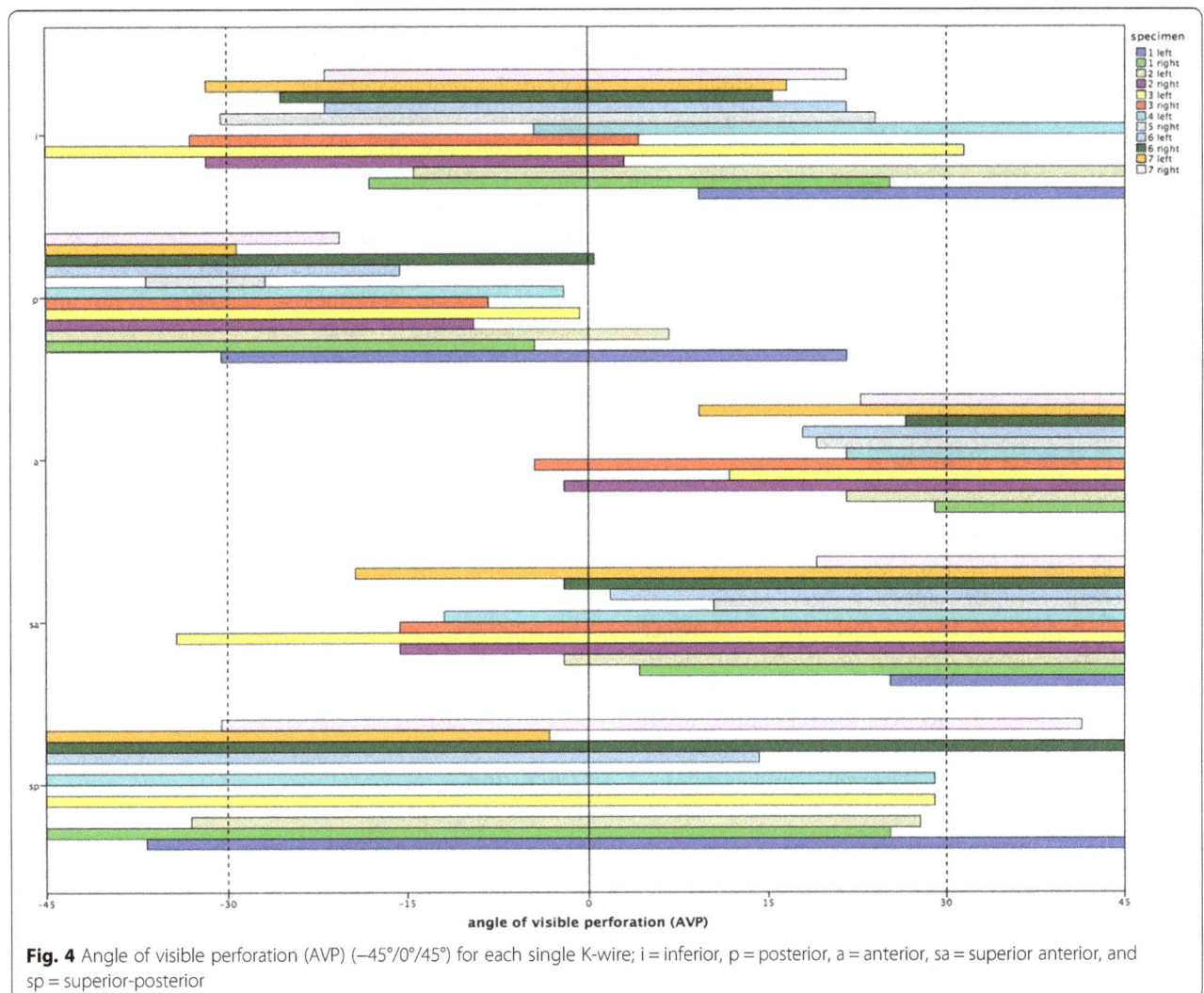

Fig. 4 Angle of visible perforation (AVP) (−45°/0°/45°) for each single K-wire; i = inferior, p = posterior, a = anterior, sa = superior anterior, and sp = superior-posterior

external rotation and one in an internal rotation [26]. Nevertheless, the algorithm for adequate intraoperative imaging remains inconsistent. Bengard and Gardner suggested placing the arm at 20° to 30° flexion and 80° to 90° internal rotation to aid in visualizing the difficult-to-assess posterosuperior region of the humeral head [11]. However, in contrast to our study they did not provide experimental data to corroborate their suggestion. Spross et al. identified a combination of four projections to account for all cut outs and to establish the correct screw position [23]. In a cadaver study, they determined that the axial view with 30° abduction was the best radiographic projection (76% sensitivity), and that a combination of four views (APIR/AP0°/APER/ax30°) had a sensitivity of 100%. They too examined a combination of the external rotation, neutral position and internal rotation (sensitivity 96%), though the degree of internal rotation (sling position) appeared variable. With intraoperative 3D fluoroscopy and multiplanar reconstruction standardized imaging with CT-like quality can be obtained. At the same time the findings of our study suggest that the investigated procedure holds the potential to detect 100% of primary screw perforations as one of the most common intraoperative complications. Recently, Lowe et al. described the use of a combination of nine fluoroscopic images to identify eight of nine intra-articular screws with a sensitivity of 100% [24]. Their recommendation to use nine C-arm views to evaluate screw placement may be realistic under in-vitro conditions with standardized placement of the screws.

Moreover, all screws may be scrutinized under fluoroscopy in varying degrees of internal and external rotation in order to verify that there is no need for intra-articular hardware [12].

We suggest the use of intraoperative 3D scans to detect 100% of screw perforations independent of screw placement. The advantage of the intraoperative fluoroscopic 3D scan compared to conventional live fluoroscopy is the defined number of images together with multiplanar reconstruction. Moreover, the operating personnel can leave the operating room which reduces the radiation exposure. For the analyzed five screw configuration at least four determined images (30° IR, 30° ER, AP, axial) are needed to examine all screws properly. Finding the right plane involves several control images especially as an exact axial plane is not reproducible with certainty. Altogether this would lead again to a higher amaount of radiation exposure at least for the personnel in the operating room.

The important role of intraoperative multiplanar imaging after osteosynthesis is supported by the high rate of immediate corrections for 11–39% of other regions of the body [16, 18, 19, 27]. Hence, the additional medical benefit seems undisputed [28].

In a feasibility study of the intraoperative use of a mobile 3D C-arm with multiplanar imaging for operating on acute proximal humerus fractures in 20 patients, screw replacements due to perforation or subchondral positioning were performed in 25% of cases [29]. Overall, the complication and revision rates due to technical errors after locking plate osteosynthesis [30, 31] may be drastically reduced if flaws were discovered intraoperatively. The question of whether or not the making of intraoperative corrections using 3D scans leads to superior immediate and long-term functional results has not yet been sufficiently investigated for other joints [32].

Our study has the same inherent weakness of many cadaveric studies. However, the mean age of the cadavers used in our study was 76.8 years, corresponding to the typical age of patients undergoing surgery after proximal humerus fractures. In addition, the results of our study are only valid for the tested plate design with the five screw configuration and are not generalizable. Other proximal humeral plate systems and screw configurations would need separate testing to determine the necessary X-ray views for the detection of all perforations. Whereas most implant designs have at least eight options for screw placement, a screw configuration with five screws has been chosen for the present study. This is in accordance with Erhardt et al. [33] who suggested that at least five screws in the humeral head fragment are necessary for the stabilization of proximal humeral fractures. The screw configuration that was used was defined by the angle stable locking plate and the necessary targeting device. Nevertheless, additional X-ray images may be necessary for other screw configurations [23, 24] and plate designs. Despite the positive aspect of our findings, namely the successful identification of all screw perforations with three AP views, additional X-ray images are often required to properly assess reduction and fixation. Therefore, the intraoperative 3D scan with multiplanar reconstruction is optimal in that it detects all perforations, independent of the screw configuration, and provides critical information regarding reduction and fixation. Finally, the radiation exposure of the intraoperative 3D scan may be a major concern, though in comparison to computed tomography, the radiation dose is significantly reduced. However, to our knowledge comparative data are not available in the literature.

Conclusion

In order to reveal all of the intraoperative and postoperative screw perforations in a "five screw configuration", conventional AP images should be established in both the neutral positions (0°), at 30° internal rotation and 30° external rotation. Alternatively, the intraoperative 3D scan with multiplanar reconstructions enables a 100% rate of detection of the screw perforations.

Abbreviations
3D: Three-dimensional; AP: Anterior-posterior; AVP: Angle of visible perforation; CT: Computed tomography; ER: External rotation; IR: Internal rotation; K-Wire: Kirschner wire; NVP: Number of images with visible perforation

Acknowledgements
We acknowledge support from the German Research Foundation (DFG) and Universität Leipzig within the program.

Funding
No Funding.

Authors' contributions
Data collection: JT, KW BM, CF, PH. Data analysis: JT, KW, CJ, PH. Drafting manuscript: JT, KW, BM, CF, CJ, PH. Approving final version: JT, KW, BM, CF, CJ, PH. JT and PH takes responsibility for the integrity of the data.

Competing interests
The authors declare that they have no competing interests.

Disclosures
All authors state that they have no conflict of interest and disclose all restrictions on full access for all authors to all raw data.

Author details
[1]Department of Orthopedics, Trauma and Plastic Surgery, University of Leipzig, Liebigstrasse 20, 04103 Leipzig, Germany. [2]Institute of Anatomy, University of Leipzig, Liebigstrasse 13, 04103 Leipzig, Germany.

References
1. Tepass A, Weise K, Rolauffs B, Blumenstock G, Bahrs C. Treatment of proximal humeral fractures in Germany. Unfallchirurg. 2015;118(9):772–9.
2. Chen H, Ji X, Zhang Q, Liang X, Tang P. Clinical outcomes of allograft with locking compression plates for elderly four-part proximal humerus fractures. J Orthop Surg. 2015;10(1):114.
3. Ockert B, Siebenbürger G, Kettler M, Braunstein V, Mutschler W. Long-term functional outcomes (median 10 years) after locked plating for displaced fractures of the proximal humerus. J Shoulder Elbow Surg. 2014;23(8):1223–31.
4. Oh HK, Cho DY, Choo SK, Park JW, Park KC, Lee JI. Lessons learned from treating patients with unstable multifragmentary fractures of the proximal humerus by minimal invasive plate osteosynthesis. Arch Orthop Trauma Surg. 2015;135(2):235–42.
5. Brorson S, Rasmussen JV, Frich LH, Olsen BS, Hróbjartsson A. Benefits and harms of locking plate osteosynthesis in intraarticular (OTA Type C) fractures of the proximal humerus: A systematic review. Injury. 2012;43(7):999–1005.
6. Brunner F, Sommer C, Bahrs C, Heuwinkel R, Hafner C, Rillmann P, et al. Open reduction and internal fixation of proximal humerus fractures using a proximal humeral locked plate: A prospective multicenter analysis. J Orthop Trauma. 2009;23(3):163–72.
7. Jost B, Spross C, Grehn H, Gerber C. Locking plate fixation of fractures of the proximal humerus: analysis of complications, revision strategies and outcome. J Shoulder Elbow Surg. 2013;22(4):542–9.
8. Kettler M, Biberthaler P, Braunstein V, Zeiler C, Kroetz M, Mutschler W. Treatment of proximal humeral fractures with the PHILOS angular stable plate. Unfallchirurg. 2006;109(12):1032–40.
9. Owsley KC, Gorczyca JT. Displacement/Screw Cutout After Open Reduction and Locked Plate Fixation of Humeral Fractures. J Bone Joint Surg. 2008;90(2):233–40.
10. Südkamp N, Bayer J, Hepp P, Voigt C, Oestern H, Kääb M, et al. Open Reduction and Internal Fixation of Proximal Humeral Fractures with Use of the Locking Proximal Humerus Plate. J Bone Joint Surg. 2009;91(6):1320–8.
11. Bengard MJ, Gardner MJ. Screw depth sounding in proximal humerus fractures to avoid iatrogenic intra-articular penetration. J Orthop Trauma. 2011;25(10):630–3.
12. Barlow JD, Sanchez-Sotelo J, Torchia M. Proximal Humerus Fractures in the Elderly Can Be Reliably Fixed With a "Hybrid" Locked-plating Technique. Clin Orthop Relat Res. 2011;469(12):3281–91.
13. Björkenheim J-M, Pajarinen J, Savolainen V. Internal fixation of proximal humeral fractures with a locking compression plate A retrospective evaluation of 72 patients followed for a minimum of 1 year. Acta Orthop. 2004;75(6):741–5.
14. Jarvers J-S, Katscher S, Franck A, Glasmacher S, Schmidt C, Blattert T, et al. 3D-based navigation in posterior stabilisations of the cervical and thoracic spine: problems and benefits. Results of 451 screws. Eur J Trauma Emerg Surg. 2011;37(2):109–19.
15. Behrendt D, Mütze M, Steinke H, Koestler M, Josten C, Böhme J. Evaluation of 2D and 3D navigation for iliosacral screw fixation. Int J Comput Assist Radiol Surg. 2012;7(2):249–55.
16. Atesok K, Finkelstein J, Khoury A, Peyser A, Weil Y, Liebergall M, et al. The use of intraoperative three-dimensional imaging (ISO-C-3D) in fixation of intraarticular fractures. Injury. 2007;38(10):1163–9.
17. Geerling J, Kendoff D, Citak M, Zech S, Gardner MJ, Hufner T, et al. Intraoperative 3D Imaging in Calcaneal Fracture Care-Clinical Implications and Decision Making. J Trauma. 2009;66(3):768–73.
18. Kendoff D, Citak M, Gardner MJ, Stübig T, Krettek C, Hüfner T. Intraoperative 3D Imaging: Value and Consequences in 248 Cases. J Trauma. 2009;66(1):232–8.
19. Richter M, Geerling J, Zech S, Goesling T, Krettek C. Intraoperative three-dimensional imaging with a motorized mobile C-arm (SIREMOBIL ISO-C-3D) in foot and ankle trauma care: a preliminary report. J Orthop Trauma. 2005;19(4):259–66.
20. Hepp P, Lill H, Bail H, Korner J, Niederhagen M, Haas NP, et al. Where Should Implants Be Anchored in the Humeral Head? Clin Orthop Relat Res. 2003;415:139–47.
21. Liew ASL, Johnson JA, Patterson SD, King GJW, Chess DG. Effect of screw placement on fixation in the humeral head. J Shoulder Elbow Surg. 2000;9(5):423–6.
22. Thanasas C, Kontakis G, Angoules A, Limb D, Giannoudis P. Treatment of proximal humerus fractures with locking plates: a systematic review. J Shoulder Elb Surg. 2009;18(6):837–44.
23. Spross C, Jost B, Rahm S, Winklhofer S, Erhardt J, Benninger E. How many radiographs are needed to detect angular stable head screw cut outs of the proximal humerus–a cadaver study. Injury. 2014;45(10):1557–63.
24. Lowe JB, Monazzam S, Walton B, Nelson E, Wolinsky PR. How to use fluoroscopic imaging to prevent intraarticular screw perforation during locked plating of proximal humerus fractures: A cadaveric study. J Orthop Trauma. 2015;29(10):e401–7.
25. Smith AM, Mardones RM, Sperling JW, Cofield RH. Early complications of operatively treated proximal humeral fractures. J Shoulder Elbow Surg. 2007;16(1):14–24.
26. Goud A, Segal D, Hedayati P, Pan JJ, Weissman BN. Radiographic evaluation of the shoulder. Eur J Radiol. 2008;68(1):2–15.
27. Rübberdt A, Feil R, Stengel D, Spranger N, Mutze S, Wich M, et al. The clinical use of the ISO-C3D imaging system in calcaneus fracture surgery. Unfallchirurg. 2006;109(2):112–8.
28. Hüfner T, Stübig T, Gösling T, Kendoff D, Geerling J, Krettek C. Cost-benefit analysis of intraoperative 3D imaging. Unfallchirurg. 2007;110(1):14–21.
29. Hepp P, Theopold J, Jarvers J-S, Marquaß B, von Dercks N, Josten C. Multiplanar reconstruction with mobile 3D image intensifier. Unfallchirurg. 2014;117(5):437–44.
30. Hepp P, Theopold J, Osterhoff G, Marquass B, Voigt C, Josten C. Bone quality measured by the radiogrammetric parameter "cortical index" and reoperations after locking plate osteosynthesis in patients sustaining proximal humerus fractures. Arch Orthop Trauma Surg. 2009;129(9):1251–9.
31. Voigt C, Woltmann A, Partenheimer A, Lill H. Management of complications after angularly stable locking proximal humerus plate fixation. Chirurg. 2007;78(1):40–6.
32. Carelsen B, Haverlag R, Ubbink DT, Luitse JSK, Goslings JC. Does intraoperative fluoroscopic 3D imaging provide extra information for fracture surgery? Arch Orthop Trauma Surg. 2008;128(12):1419–24.
33. Erhardt JB, Stoffel K, Kampshoff J, Badur N, Yates P, Kuster MS. The position and number of screws influence screw perforation of the humeral head in modern locking plates: a cadaver study. J Orthop Trauma. 2012;26(10):e188–92.

10

The effect of patient anxiety and depression on motion during myocardial perfusion SPECT imaging

Vassiliki Lyra[1][*], Maria Kallergi[2], Emmanouil Rizos[3], Georgios Lamprakopoulos[1] and Sofia N. Chatziioannou[1,4]

Abstract

Background: Patient motion during myocardial perfusion SPECT imaging (MPI) may be triggered by a patient's physical and/or psychological discomfort. The aim of this study was to investigate the impact of state anxiety (patient's reaction to exam-related stress), trait anxiety (patient's personality characteristic) and depression on patient motion during MPI.

Methods: All patients that underwent MPI in our department in a six-month period were prospectively enrolled. One hundred eighty-three patients (45 females; 138 males) filled in the State-Trait Anxiety Inventory (STAI) and the Beck Depression Inventory (BDI), along with a short questionnaire regarding their age, height and weight, level of education in years, occupation, and marital status. Cardiovascular and other co-morbidity factors were also evaluated. Through inspection of raw data on cinematic display, the presence or absence of patient motion was registered and classified into mild, moderate and severe, for both phases involved in image acquisition.

Results: The correlation of patient motion in the stress and delay phases of MPI and each of the other variables was investigated and the corresponding Pearson's coefficients of association were calculated. The anxiety-motion ($r = 0.43$, $P < 0.0001$) and depression-motion ($r = 0.32$, $P < 0.0001$) correlation results were moderately strong and statistically significant for the female but not the male patients. All the other variables did not demonstrate any association with motion in MPI, except a weak correlation between age and motion in females ($r = 0.23$, $P < 0.001$).

Conclusions: The relationship between anxiety-motion and depression-motion identified in female patients represents the first supporting evidence of psychological discomfort as predisposing factor for patient motion during MPI.

Keywords: Patient motion, Anxiety, Myocardial perfusion SPECT imaging, Artifacts, Depression

Background

Good quality data is crucial in order to achieve high diagnostic accuracy in myocardial perfusion SPECT imaging (MPI) [1–5]. Prior to image processing, raw data should be reviewed for image quality and patient motion. Patient motion is considered the most frequent cause of artefactual defects resulting primarily in false positive results [1, 3].

Patient motion has been simulated and evaluated in a variety of studies using different methods [4–9]. Results have not demonstrated a direct correlation between motion pattern (type and magnitude of motion) and imaging outcome [8]. Different semi-automatic and automatic "motion correction" software has been developed to identify and analyze the patient's (voluntary and involuntary) motion, in order to realign the projection data before image reconstruction [10–16]. However, none of the available software is considered accurate enough to capture both the variety and complexity of patient motion, and as a result, the reconstructed image should be interpreted with caution [16]. Therefore, the best approach regarding patient motion is prevention. "Heart motion", due to involuntary motion, such as "Respiratory motion" [17, 18] and "Upward creep" [19, 20] could potentially be prevented through delay in the initiation of acquisition. In contrast, "heart motion", due to

* Correspondence: vslyra@yahoo.gr; vassilikilyra@gmail.com
[1]2nd Department of Radiology, Nuclear Medicine Section, National and Kapodistrian University of Athens, Attikon Hospital, 1 Rimini St., Athens 12462, Greece
Full list of author information is available at the end of the article

voluntary body movements, could be minimized by preventing patient's discomfort [3, 21]. For this reason, the patient should always be in a comfortable position during imaging [21]. Lumbar and knee supporters could minimize back strain caused by the patient being on supine position with overextended left arm. In addition, the patient should always be informed of the negative effects of motion on diagnosis. Despite these routinely taken precautions, motion problems are not alleviated.

The patient's anxiety has been considered another cause of the patient's psychological and physical discomfort and thus contributing to patient's motion during MPI and other imaging modalities [3]. Anxiety is described as a state of emotional distress and inner turmoil, which may be manifested by nervous behavior and restlessness, muscular tension and other somatic complaints [22–24]. Anxiety-related sympathicotonic and claustrophobic reactions and some anxiety reduction protocols have been evaluated mainly for magnetic resonance imaging examinations [25–30]. The aim of this study is to investigate the impact of *state anxiety* (patient's reaction to exam-related stress), *trait anxiety* (patient's personality characteristic), and *depression* on direct patient motion during myocardial perfusion imaging.

Methods
Patients
Two psychometric instruments were administered to 275 consecutive patients (172 men, 103 women) that underwent MPI in our department within a six-month period. The patients were required to fill-in two questionnaires; the one addressed the level of state and trait anxiety of the patients prior to the procedure and the other the level of depression. Forty-nine patients (17.8 %) did not complete the questionnaires while 43 patients (15.6 %) completed them partially. It is noteworthy that the majority (63 %) of these 92 patients were women, while the majority (62.5 %) of patients who were asked to fill-in the questionnaires were men. All of these 92 patients were excluded from the study (Fig. 1).

One hundred and eighty-three (183) patients, 45 women and 138 men, accurately completed and signed the two questionnaires and their responses were evaluated in this study. Demographic information including age, years of education, occupation, and marital status, and anthropometric variables (weight and height) were also gathered. The body mass index (BMI) was calculated according to the relationship: BMI = weight in Kg/ (height in m)^2. The difference in sample sizes between male and female patients was due to a) the smaller proportion of women who underwent MPI (37.5 %, i.e. 103 out of 275 patients), and b) the higher proportion of women (56.3 %, 58/103) compared to men (19.7 %, 34/172), who either refused to complete the questionnaires or completed them partially.

In preparation for the MPI test, information about the patient's cardiovascular and medical history was gathered. Variables evaluated were the presence of known or suspected coronary artery disease, the presence of left ventricular systolic dysfunction (ejection fraction (EF) ≥50 % or EF < 50 %), as well as other comorbidity factors, such as cancer, serious hematologic disorders, hemodialysis, cerebrovascular disease, complicated

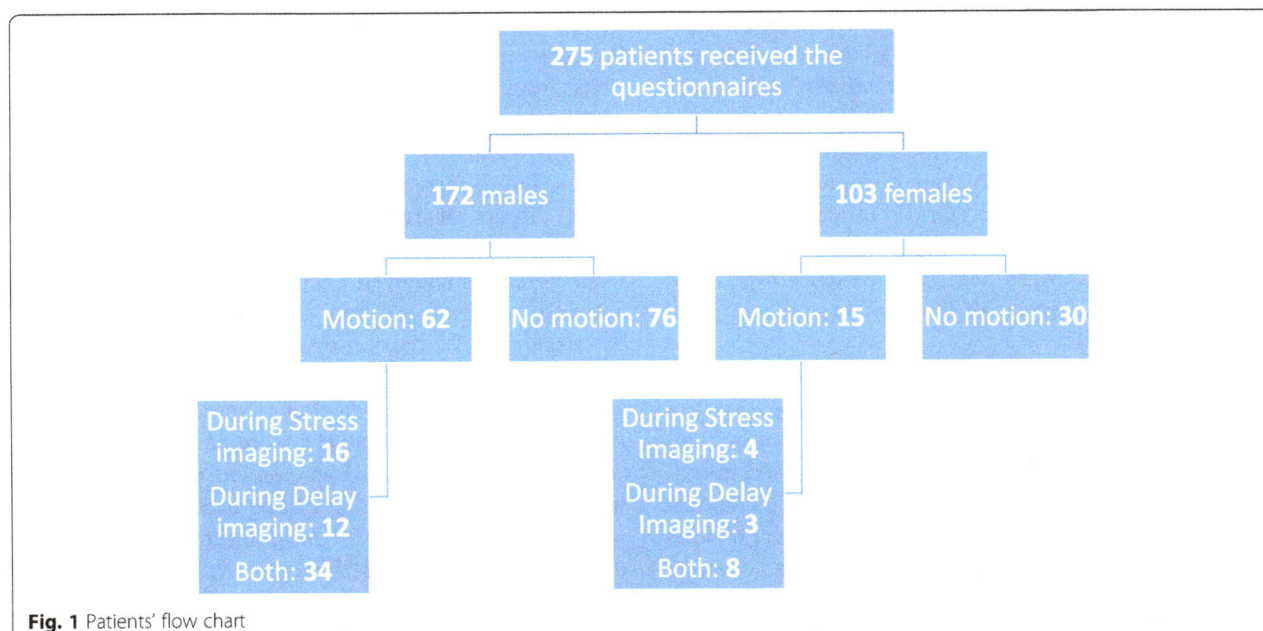

Fig. 1 Patients' flow chart

long standing diabetes mellitus, severe connective tissue disorders, etc.

Psychometric questionnaires

Patients were provided with the first questionnaire and were informed about the succeeding second one, by two physicians of our department, upon arrival. Both physicians had quite similar approach to the patients, in order to minimize interferences.

The *Spielberger's State-Trait Anxiety Inventory* (STAI) [31, 32], is a two-page questionnaire based on a 4-point Likert scale consisting of 40 simple questions on a self-report basis. Theoretically, a 6th grade graduate could readily comprehend and complete them in about 10 min. The STAI measures two types of anxiety: the state anxiety or temporary anxiety about an event, and the trait anxiety or daily anxiety level as a personal characteristic [31, 32]. Namely, the part of state anxiety inventory measures the extent of heightened emotions and overreaction to a situation- a perceived stressor- such as undergoing an MPI imaging. Everyone experience some anxiety, something similar to fear, which is out of proportion to the actual risk involved. The common symptoms of anxiety and fear may include uneasiness, spells of perspiration, bouts of frequent urination and muscular tension, whereas all symptoms can be associated with the release of specific neurohormonal mediators [22, 23].

The part of trait anxiety inventory measures the level of "neuroticism" and unfocused worry which stems from the personality of an individual and induces his stable tendency to respond with anxiety in the anticipation of situations [23, 24]. Higher scores on STAI questionnaire are positively correlated with higher levels of anxiety [31, 32]. Normal values for state anxiety in the Spielberger's healthy population aged 30–59 years, was 38.1 ± 10.1 for females and 37.3 ± 9.8 for males [31]. This questionnaire had been adapted by A. Liakos and S. Giannitsis in the 1980s to suit the Greek population [33], and since, its validity had been re-evaluated by using a random sample of Greek university students and civil servants, with a mean age of 31.71, consisting of 64.8 % females. Mean anxiety state score was 43.21, mean anxiety trait score 42.79 and the resulting STAI score was 86.1 [34].

To maximize time management, the patients were provided with the second questionnaire, known as *Beck Depression Inventory* (BDI) [35, 36], while waiting for the delay phase of MPI. BDI is a commonly used instrument for quantifying levels of depression. It contains a 21 item self-report, each with four possible choices scored on a scale of 0 to 3. Higher total scores indicate more severe depressive symptoms. The standard cutoffs used are [35, 36]: 0–13: minimal depression; 14–19: mild

depression; 20–28: moderate depression; and 29–63: severe depression.

Image acquisition and processing

All patients underwent ergometric (treadmill) or pharmacological (adenosine or dipyridamole) stress. SPECT imaging was performed at 10 min (stress) and 4 h (delay) following intravenous injection of 3 mCi Tl-201. A single-head GE Millennium camera, with a LEGP collimator was used for all cases. Energy window was set at 20 % at 72KeV and 30 % at 167KeV. 32 views of 40 s each, stored in a 64x64 matrix, were acquired for a 180° orbit and a total acquisition time of ~22 min. The pixel size was 6.4 mm. The raw re-projection data was reconstructed by using a filtered backprojection (FBP) algorithm (Butterworth; cutoff frequency, 0.39; power, 10) and an Ordered-Subset Expectation Maximization (OSEM) iterative reconstruction algorithm, on the Xeleris workstation (GE Healthcare).

Detection of patient motion

The analysis of images for patient's motion was based on inspection of the raw data on cinematic display, which was performed by an expert nuclear physician. The absence of motion had to be confirmed on the sinogram image as well [10]. However, motion was regarded as present only when the observer was certain of its existence. Each study was assessed for the presence of visually detectable motion, the type of motion and the grade of motion. The types of patient motion were classified as suggested in the literature [3, 5] in a) bounces (brief up or down movements, observed in <3 frames before returning to the original y-coordinate), b) shifts (up or down movement involving all the remaining frames), c) complex motion (multiple bounces or combination of bounces and shifts), d) lateral movements and translations (rotations of the body around its axis). Patient motion was scored on a scale from 1–3 as *absent* (0), *mild* (1), *moderate* (2) and *severe* (3) depending on the degree and recurrence of motion during rotating cinematic display of raw data. A single subtle event of motion throughout the dataset was identified as mild, while several single events (complex motion) were characterized as severe motion. In case of ambiguity about the largeness of a motion event, distance between lower edge of the image and lowest part of the heart silhouette was compared on the selected frames. Single events of motion, higher than 3 pixels, were characterized as severe. The aforementioned assessment of patient motion was scored for the two sets of raw data, for those of the stress phase called "*Patient Motion Stress*" and for those of the delay phase called "*Patient Motion Delay*" (Fig. 1).

The visual inspection and assessment of motion by one expert was evaluated by repeating the process almost one year after the previous one. In case of a major discrepancy, compared to the previous patient motion evaluation results (patient motion absent instead of present or vice-versa, or a motion score difference of more than 2 points regarding a specific stress or delay phase), the decision was made in cooperation with another nuclear physician expert.

A representative case of "Patient Motion" evaluation and of the corresponding "Motion Artifact" are demonstrated in Fig. 2a and b respectively.

Statistical analysis

Our final database included both qualitative (ordered and unordered) and quantitative (discrete and continuous) types of data. Qualitative variables included *gender, occupation, marital status, major comorbidity, SPECT evaluation, cardiac disease class, patient motion stress,* and *patient motion delay.* Quantitative variables included *education, age, weight, height, BMI, time of cardiac disease*

diagnosis, state anxiety score, trait anxiety score, STAI score (sum of the two anxiety scores), and *BDI score.* The characteristics and the descriptive statistics (mean values and standard deviations) of the study are listed in Table 1.

Our primary interest was the investigation of possible correlations between patient mood and patient motion in the stress and delay phases of MPI. Hence, the Pearson's coefficients of association were determined for pairs of variables.

Associations between categorical variables were also studied by generating 2x2 contingency tables and applying Fisher's two-tailed exact test. The level of significance for all tests was set to 5 %. In the investigation of possible associations, linear or non, between pairs of the variables listed in Table 1, the two variables of motion (Patient Motion Stress & Patient Motion Delay) were considered as *responses* or dependent variables, while all others were considered as *predictors* or independent variables.

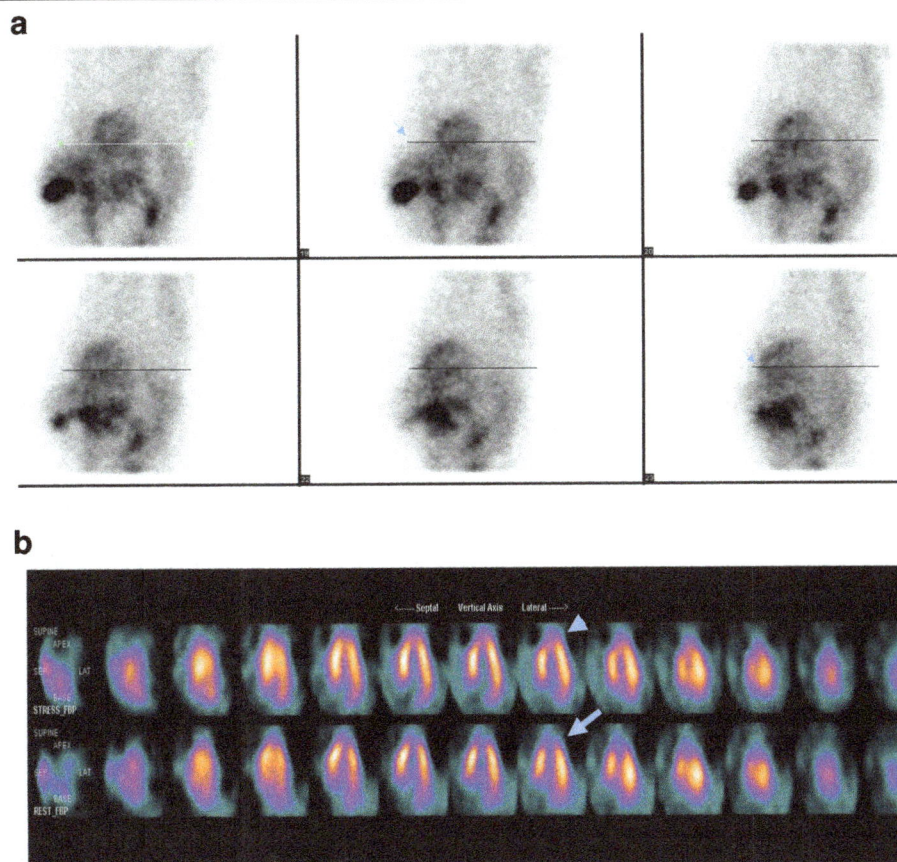

Fig. 2 a From inspection of the raw data (32 planar images) in cinematic display, which were acquired during the "delay phase" of MPI, a downward patient movement was detected. Using tracing lines at the edges of heart silhouette on each of the 32 planar views, the patient's displacement (shift) was confirmed on images 19 to 23 (*arrows*). This is a "Patient Motion Delay" assessment classified as grade 2 (moderately severe motion). **b** The tomographic filtered back projection (FBP) reconstruction of the raw data illustrated on Fig. 2a, revealed a large myocardial apical defect perfusion, which was diagnosed as motion artifact (*arrow*). Conversely, no myocardial apical defect appeared after the tomographic reconstruction of the "stress phase" images (*arrowhead*), since the patient remained motionless during the data acquisition

Table 1 Characteristics of the participants in the MPI motion study

Characteristics of patients	Total patients[a] (183)	Male patients[a] (138)	Female patients[a] (45)
Age (years)	63.3 ± 10.2	62.7 ± 10.1	65.0 ± 10.6
Education (years)	10.7 ± 3.0	11.1 ± 9.2	9.4 ± 2.7
BMI	28.7 ± 4.8	29.1 ± 4.8	27.7 ± 4.9
Occupation (%)			
0 = Homemaker	25 ± 14	0 ± 0	25 ± 56
1 = Retired	89 ± 49	75 ± 54	14 ± 31
2 = Employed	57 ± 31	53 ± 38	4 ± 9
3 = Unemployed	12 ± 7	10 ± 7	2 ± 4
Marital status (%)			
0 = Single	9 ± 5	8 ± 6	1 ± 2
1 = Married	148 ± 81	115 ± 83	33 ± 73
2 = Widow/er	11 ± 6	3 ± 2	8 ± 18
3 = Divorced	15 ± 8	12 ± 9	3 ± 7
Major comorbidity (%)			
0 = No	158 ± 86	120 ± 87	38 ± 84
1 = Yes	25 ± 14	18 ± 13	7 ± 16
Cardiac disease (%)			
0 = Negative	76 ± 42	45 ± 33	31 ± 69
1 = EF ≥50 %	84 ± 46	72 ± 52	12 ± 27
2 = EF < 50 %	23 ± 13	21 ± 15	2 ± 4
Time of cardiac disease diagnosis (years)	2.7 ± 4.3	3.1 ± 4.5	1.5 ± 3.3
SPECT evaluation			
0 = Normal	89 ± 49	53 ± 38	36 ± 80
1 = Mildly abnormal	43 ± 23	38 ± 28	5 ± 11
2 = Moderately abnormal	34 ± 19	30 ± 22	4 ± 9
3 = Severely abnormal	17 ± 9	17 ± 12	0 ± 0
Anxiety state score	41 ± 13.2	38.9 ± 12.9	47.5 ± 12.1
Anxiety trait score	44 ± 9.4	42.5 ± 8.9	48.7 ± 9.4
STAI score	85 ± 21.1	81.3 ± 20.1	96.3 ± 20.3
BDI score	13.6 ± 9.1	12.2 ± 8.0	17.9 ± 10.8
Patient motion stress			
0 = Absent	123 ± 67	90 ± 65	33 ± 73
1 = Mild	20 ± 11	15 ± 11	5 ± 11
2 = Moderate	25 ± 14	19 ± 14	6 ± 13
3 = Severe	15 ± 8	14 ± 10	1 ± 2
Patient motion delay			
0 = Absent	126 ± 69	92 ± 67	34 ± 76
1 = Mild	25 ± 14	19 ± 14	6 ± 13
2 = Moderate	17 ± 9	14 ± 10	3 ± 7
3 = Severe	15 ± 8	13 ± 9	2 ± 4

[a]mean values ± standard deviations

Results

Patients with a basic level of education (22 males, 13 females) required approximately two to three times more than the expected 10 min to complete the STAI and even longer, exceeding half an hour, to complete the BDI questionnaire. The patient motion evaluation had excellent intra-observer agreement (96.1 %, 176/183 patients).

The primary hypothesis of this study was that the patient's pre-scan psychological state, was associated with patient motion during MPI. Hence, the corresponding pairs of variables were studied for possible associations. Table 2 shows the results of the Pearson's coefficient and its P-value for the variables listed in Table 1 for all, male and female patients. The results in Table 2 indicate that there is a strong, statistically significant correlation between patient motion at stress phase and patient motion at delay phase of MPI. There is only a weak but statistically significant association between trait anxiety and patient motion in the delay phase of MPI and between the STAI score and motion in the same phase. With the exception of the motion during the two phases of imaging, only 2-3 % of the variance in one of the variables is accounted for by the variance in the other variable.

Moreover, anxiety was significantly positively correlated with depression both in males ($r = 0.56$; $P < 0.001$) and females ($r = 0.67$; $P < 0.001$) but the women of the study had significantly higher anxiety and depression scores compared to men when taking the MPI test (Table 3). The *two-tailed P-value* for the data in Table 3 is *0.0096*, indicating that the association between the groups (male, female) and the outcomes (trait anxiety scores) are statistically very significant. A similar result was found for the anxiety state scores ($P = 0.0004$), the STAI score ($P = 0.0011$) and the BDI score ($P = 0.0028$).

The most interesting result was that the association between anxiety or depression and motion was statistically significant ($P = 0.0001$) for women but insignificant for men. A higher anxiety STAI score in women was correlated with a moderate risk of motion and this correlation was more evident in the delay phase of MPI ($r = 0.43$). Similarly, a higher BDI score was correlated with a mild to moderate risk of motion ($r = 0.32$) (Table 2). In contrast to the abovementioned observation, a smaller proportion of women moved during image acquisition (33 %, 15/45 females) compared to men (45 %, 62/138 males) while their motion was less severe (13 %, only 2/15 females had a motion score ≥ 3) than that of men (29 %, 18/62 males had a motion score ≥ 3). This is in accordance with what has been described in a previous study [15]. According to Table 4, this difference is not statistically significant for our study, most likely due to population differences (138/183

Table 2 Pearson's correlation coefficient, coefficient of determination, and P-values for selected pairs of variables for all 183 patients and for the 138 males and the 45 females separately

Variables	Pearson's coefficient (r)			Coefficient of determination (r^2)			P-value		
	All	Males	Females	All	Males	Females	All	Males	Females
Motion S/Motion D	0.66	0.64	0.73	0.43	0.41	0.53	<0.0001	<0.0001	<0.0001
State-A/Motion S	0.12	0.12	0.31	0.01	0.01	0.10	0.12	0.12	<0.0001
State-A/Motion D	0.14	0.12	0.42	0.02	0.02	0.17	0.05	0.10	<0.0001
Trait-A/Motion S	0.14	0.14	0.34	0.02	0.02	0.12	0.06	0.07	<0.0001
Trait-A/Motion D	0.16	0.15	0.38	0.03	0.02	0.15	0.03	0.05	<0.0001
STAI/Motion S	0.13	0.14	0.34	0.02	0.02	0.12	0.07	0.07	<0.0001
STAI/Motion D	0.16	0.15	0.43	0.03	0.02	0.18	0.03	0.05	<0.0001
BDI/Motion S	0.04	−0.01	0.32	0.00	0.00	0.10	0.55	0.98	<0.0001
BDI/Motion D	0.07	0.05	0.28	0.01	0.00	0.08	0.32	0.51	<0.0001

Motion S = "Patient Motion Stress", Motion D = "Patient Motion Delay", State-A = "State Anxiety score", Trait-A = "Trait Anxiety score"

patients are men, which is 75 % of the study population). The *two-tailed P-value* for the data in Table 4 is *0.3636* and the association between the two groups of patients and the motion outcome was found not to be statistically significant. Similar results were obtained for the delay phase study ($P = 0.3541$). Finally, to account for population size difference, we matched 42 male to 42 female patients in terms of demographic and physical characteristics. Results were similar for the matched groups, i.e., no statistically significant associations.

Other variables, such as age, education, BMI, occupation, marital status, comorbidity, time and severity of heart disease, were investigated for possible associations with the motion in MPI. Age of the female population of the study was weakly correlated to the motion in the stress phase of imaging ($r = 0.23$; $P < 0.001$). Secondly, these variables were also examined for potential associations with the anxiety and depression results. Only married female patients (73.3 %, 33/45) had a weak but statistically significant correlation to the trait anxiety of these patients ($r = 0.16$; $P = 0.03$). All other associations were not statistically significant.

Discussion

The association of higher state-anxiety scores in patients undergoing MPI, in both males and females has been proved in a previous study [37]. For the first time, to our knowledge, our study investigated the effect of anxiety and depression in patient motion during MPI, whereas common psychometric STAI and BDI questionnaires were used for the assessment. Our hypothesis was that both state and trait anxiety were associated with patient motion during MPI, assuming that patients with state and trait anxiety moved more during imaging than patients with depression. Hence, according to a simplified definition of abovementioned psychological disorders, we hypothesized that anxiety patients who experience tension and uneasiness more frequently [23] should have a higher risk of motion, while depressive patients who more frequently experience fatigue and stillness [38], should have a smaller risk. Finally, since anxiety disorders and depression may co-exist [39–41], only the prevalent condition should affect the patient's motion during data acquisition.

Interestingly, our results in respect to anxiety related motion and depression related motion were statistically significant only in women ($P = 0.0001$) but not in men. A higher anxiety STAI score was moderately correlated to motion. Contrary to our hypothesis, even a high depression BDI score was marginally, but still positively, associated to motion in women (Table 2). Although stillness and immobility are characteristics of melancholic (typical) depressive syndromes, it is also true, that

Table 3 2x2 contingency table for the male and female patients and the trait anxiety assuming the mean score (44) of the entire study population as cutoff point

Group	Outcome		
	Trait-A < 44	Trait-A ≥ 44	Totals
Male	75	63	138
Female	14	31	45
Totals	89	94	183

Trait-A = "Trait Anxiety score"

Table 4 2x2 contingency table for the male and female patients and motion outcome in the stress phase of MPI

Group	Outcome		
	No motion	Motion	Totals
Male	90	48	138
Female	33	12	45
Totals	123	60	183

Patients with motion ratings 1–3 were grouped together under the "Motion" outcome

many depressive patients (atypical depression) experience a feeling of uneasiness and are unable to stay at rest [38, 41], similarly to anxiety disorders.

The significant association of anxiety and depression scores [39–41] and, moreover, the significantly higher anxiety and depression scores in women compared to those in men, observed in our study (Table 3), are in line with the existing literature [31, 42–44]. In general, women present higher rates of anxiety and depression, and the higher rate of diagnosis (more likely report their symptoms and ask medical support) [42, 43] and the different biological (neurohormonal) [45] and social background (e.g. caregiving) [43, 46] have been involved, although the combination of these factors into integrated aetiological models continues to be lacking [47].

In an MRI study [48], the relationship between clinically relevant motion artifacts and pre-scan state anxiety scores was examined. There was no statistical significant relationship ($P = 0.30$) between state anxiety scores and motion artifacts in both men and women, something that is not in line with our results in women. That may be due to the fact, that the end points in both studies were different, since the overall motion was evaluated (75/183 moved) in the present study, while only the motion artifacts were evaluated (19/278 had motion artifacts) in the MRI study.

The presence of less motion in women, as was our initial impression, as demonstrated by a previous study [15], should not appear contradicting to the abovementioned result of a high anxiety score and its positive correlation with motion in women. This actually means, that anxiety and depression do influence the motion of female patients during MPI but do not explain the motion in men. The relative higher rate and higher score of motion in men is an independent variable. None of the other parameters examined, were found to justify motion in men.

Indeed, the anthropometric, demographic and medical information was collected, in our effort to investigate a wider range of variables correlated to the motion or the anxiety and depression scores, in order to provide a better distinction of patients at greater risk for motion.

The occupation and the marital status have been involved to both anxiety and depression, in literature [49]. Married women showed a weak but statistically significant association to the trait anxiety score, which is in accordance to some specialized literature, stating that married women could be more stressed compared to singles [44]. Twenty-two married women in our study, almost half (48.8 %) of our study's population, were elderly housewives or retired, who underwent MPI in order to evaluate an atypical chest pain. They all had a normal MPI. Anxiety could be associated with high rates of medically unexplained symptoms and some women, even without a professional activity, may

experience a greater stress burden due to an important care-giving role to their grandchildren or other family members [46, 50].

Furthermore, an underlying pathology, such as heart failure, may precipitate anxiety and depression, both recently defined as "inflammatory" mood disorders [51–53]. However, our results in respect of heart failure related to motion and of heart failure related to anxiety and depression scores were not statistically significant in men, (almost all our heart failure cases involved men).

A previous study [16] showed that there was no statistically significant association between age and motion. Even though increased age and BMI are factors generally of lack of physical fitness and therefore elementary predisposing factors of patient discomfort which could be aggravated during imaging. However, our study did not demonstrate an overall association between age and motion, too, except for older women who were found to move slightly more. BMI was not found to have an association to patient motion in either men or women.

The strong linear correlation between patient motion at stress and patient motion at delay, confirmed our suspicion that a patient who moved during the first phase was more likely to move during the second phase as well. Therefore, it is of clinical value to examine the raw data upon completion of the first phase, so that if patient motion is detected additional precautions should be taken in order to avoid motion during the second phase. These usually are based on detailed explanation of the acquisition procedure to the patient (even during periods of great workload) and on close observation of the patient during data acquisition and on reminding the patient that he/she needs to remain motionless. In this regard, the effectiveness of an information pamphlet on reducing motion artifacts during MR imaging [54] and the effectiveness of an ameliorate communication between patient and technologist on reducing patients' state anxiety scores during PET/CT imaging [55], have been recently demonstrated.

In summary, the link between mood and motion identified in female patients is the first supporting evidence of anxiety as another elementary factor of patient's cognitive and somatic discomfort during MPI. This is important, since motion is a major cause of falsely positive results in MPI and imaging in general. One could argue that anything that affects the diagnostic accuracy of MPI in women, should be seriously addressed, since many factors, such as smaller heart size, bias of the interpreters, etc., have already been implicated in its lower diagnostic accuracy in this group of patients [56–58].

In our opinion, the identified association between emotional and mental states and motion in women should lead to the development of a suitable questionnaire related patients' prescan state. Its efficacy as motion predictor should be tested on women in a future study. Identifying patients at risk is helpful as deserve a much closer attention to prevent their motion during the long-lasting imaging modalities in general.

Limitations

Motion quantification was not performed in our study. However, the careful visual review of projection images is considered the best way to identify any presence of motion [3, 5]. Moreover, the interobserver reliability of more than 90 % in literature [4] and the intraobserver reliability of more than 96 % in our study are in accordance with the high visual motion assessment reproducibility. Visual inspection is a widely acceptable method for detecting vertical body displacements (parallel to the axis of gantry rotation) even in the order of 3.25 mm (corresponding to half pixel in our study) rather than lateral body displacements (perpendicular to the axis of rotation and detected as a fraction of the actual motion in the particular projection). Several reports suggest that vertical motion is the most common type of motion with greater likelihood in producing clinically important artifacts [5, 6, 16].

Another limitation of our study is the acquisition of the projected images by a single-head camera. Multidetector cameras provide a significant advantage over single-detector systems due to decreased image acquisition times (~15 min compared to ~22 min in our study) and, subsequently, a lower risk of patient movement. However, it should be noted that, in case of motion the effect may be compounded, with a single motion being introduced into the dataset 2 or 3 times. Matsumoto and Germano suggest that the exposure to motion for dual gantries should be neutralized to some degree by increasing the time required for single detector acquisition [13, 14].

An issue was the unexpectedly high amount of time required to fill out the psychometric questionnaires. Another issue was the low level of education in women (31.1 %, 14/45), who were primarily from the agricultural region of the country. It could be possible that these women checked "basic education" in the questionnaire, without even having completed the primary education (primary education became compulsory in '30s but the law was strictly applied only in '70s, when secondary education became compulsory). In that respect, the educational level and the psycho-social background could be the potential factors affecting the high proportion of women who either refused to complete or inaccurately completed the questionnaires. These elderly women might experience a greater insecurity and low self-confidence, hesitating to fill out a questionnaire, since they might be afraid of potential criticism in the event they describe their condition in the questionnaire. Unfortunately, the mode of questionnaire administration, completed by the patient himself as opposed to an interview, could have effect on data quality [59]. So, it may be possible that the routine completion of such questionnaires may interfere with the smooth clinical process and cause substantial delays. An alternative type of simpler questionnaires could be more appropriate for use during clinical practice in an imaging department, which could be distributed and filled out faster and easier.

Conclusions

The association between anxiety-motion and to a lesser degree of depression-motion identified in female patients represents the first supporting evidence of emotional and mental states as predisposing factors for patient's motion during MPI. It may be possible that the utilization of appropriate questionnaires prior to the performance of MPI could discriminate more specifically the group of female patients who deserve a much closer attention to prevent their motion.

Acknowledgements
The authors would like to thank the technologists of Nuclear Medicine Division of our Hospital Radiology Department for their responsibility for giving the instructions and ensuring patients' comfort during imaging, resulting in the accurate implementation of the study.

Funding
No funding was necessary.

Authors' contributions
All authors have participated sufficiently in this work and approved of the final version of the manuscript. VL has been involved in the data collection, review of the literature and in the manuscript drafting overall. GL has participated substantially in the acquisition and quality control of the data. ER has conceived and coordinated the study and has evaluated the psychometric data. MK has performed and drafted the statistical analysis and the interpretation of data and results, and has given important intellectual suggestions. SC has been involved in the conception, design and evaluation of the motion data as well as in the critical revision and the final version of the manuscript.

Authors' information
VL is a nuclear medicine physician and GL is a nuclear medicine physician in training. SC is an associate professor in nuclear medicine with long clinical expertise in nuclear cardiology. MK is a medical health physicist most expertise in imaging. ER is an associate professor in psychiatry with long clinical expertise in anxiety disorders.

Competing interests
The authors declare that they have no competing interests.

Author details
[1]2nd Department of Radiology, Nuclear Medicine Section, National and Kapodistrian University of Athens, Attikon Hospital, 1 Rimini St., Athens 12462, Greece. [2]Department of Medical Instruments Technology, Technological Educational Institution of Athens, TEI, 28 Ag. Spiridona St., Athens 12210, Greece. [3]2nd Department of Psychiatry, National and Kapodistrian University of Athens, Attikon Hospital, 1 Rimini St., Athens 12462, Greece. [4]Nuclear Medicine Section, Biomedical Research Foundation Academy of Athens, BRFAA, 4 Soranou Efesiou St., Athens 11527, Greece.

References

1. Germano G. Technical aspects of myocardial SPECT imaging. J Nucl Med. 2001;42:1499–507.
2. Cooper JA, Neumann PH, McCandless BK. Effect of patient motion on tomographic myocardial perfusion imaging. J Nucl Med. 1992;33:1566–71.
3. Wheat JM, Currie GM. Incidence and characterization of patient motion in myocardial perfusion SPECT: part I. J Nucl Med Technol. 2004;32:60–5.
4. Wheat JM, Currie GM. Impact of patient motion on myocardial perfusion SPECT diagnostic integrity: part II. J Nucl Med Technol. 2004;32:158–63.
5. Prigent FM, Hyun M, Berman DS, Rozanski A. Effect of motion on Tl-201 SPECT studies : a simulation and clinical study. J Nucl Med. 1993;34:1845–50.
6. Cooper JA, Neumann PH, McCandless BK. Detection of patient motion during tomographic myocardial perfusion imaging. J Nucl Med. 1993;34:1341–8.
7. Eisner RL, Noever T, Nowak D, Carlson W, Dunn D, Oates J, et al. Use of cross-correlation function to detect patient motion during SPECT imaging. J Nucl Med. 1987;28:97–101.
8. Friedman J, Berman DS, Van Train K, Garcia EV, Bietendorf J, Prigent F, et al. Patient motion in myocardial SPECT imaging. An easily identified frequent source of artifactual defect. Clin Nucl Med. 1988;13:321–4.
9. Botvinick EH, Zhu Y, O'Connell WJ, Dae MW. A quantitative assessment of patient motion and its effect on myocardial perfusion SPECT images. J Nucl Med. 1993;34:303–10.
10. Fitzgerald J, Danias PG. Effect of motion on cardiac SPECT imaging: recognition and motion correction. J Nucl Cardiol. 2001;8:701–6.
11. O'Connor MK, Kanal KM, Gebhard MW, Rossman PJ. Comparison of four motion correction techniques in SPECT imaging of the heart: a cardiac phantom study. J Nucl Med. 1998;39:2027–34.
12. Leslie WD, Dupont JO, MacDonald D, Peterdy AE. Comparison of motion correction algorithms for cardiac SPECT. J Nucl Med. 1997;38:785–90.
13. Germano G, Chua T, Kavanagh PB, Kiat H, Berman DS. Detection and correction of patient motion in dynamic and static myocardial SPECT using a multi-detector camera. J Nucl Med. 1993;34:1349–55.
14. Matsumoto N, Berman DS, Kavanagh PB, Gerlach J, Hayes SW, Lewin HC, et al. Quantitative assessment of motion artifacts and validation of a new motion-correction program for myocardial perfusion SPECT. J Nucl Med. 2001;42:687–94.
15. Bai C, Maddahi J, Kindem J, Conwell R, Gurley M, Old R. Development and evaluation of a new fully automatic motion detection and correction technique in cardiac SPECT imaging. J Nucl Cardiol. 2009;16:580–9.
16. Massardo T, Jaimovich R, Faure R, Muñoz M, Alay R, Gatica H. Motion correction and myocardial perfusion SPECT using manufacturer provided software. Does it affect image interpretation? Eur J Nucl Med Mol Imaging. 2010;37:758–64.
17. Kovalski G, Israel O, Keidar Z, Frenkel A, Sachs J, Alzhari H. Correction of heart motion due to respiration in clinical myocardial perfusion SPECT scans using respiratory gating. J Nucl Med. 2007;48:630–6.
18. Redgate S, Barber DC, Abdallah AM, Wendy TB. Using a registration-based motion correction algorithm to correct for respiratory motion during myocardial perfusion imaging. Nucl Med Commun. 2013;34:787–95.
19. Mester J, Weller R, Clausen M, Bitter F, Henze E, Lietzenmayer R, et al. Upward creep of the heart in exercise Tl-201 SPECT: clinical relevance and a simple correction method. Eur J Nucl Med. 1991;18:184–90.
20. Karakalioglu AO, Jata B, Kilic S, Arslan N, Ilgan S, Ozguven MA. A physiologic approach to decreasing upward creep of the heart during myocardial perfusion imaging. J Nucl Med Technol. 2006;34:215–9.
21. Cooper JA, McCandless BK. Preventing patient motion during tomographic myocardial perfusion imaging. J Nucl Med. 1995;36:2001–5.
22. Endler NS, Kocovski NL. State and trait anxiety revisited. J Anxiety Disord. 2001;15:231–45.
23. Öhman A. Fear and anxiety: Evolutionary, cognitive and clinical perspectives. Handbook of emotions. 2nd ed. Lewis M, Haviland-Jones JM, editors. NY: The Guilford Press; 2000: 573–93.
24. Sylvers P, Lilienfeld SO, Laprairie JL. Differences between trait fear and trait anxiety: implications for psychopathology. Clin Psychol Rev. 2011;31:122–37.
25. Meléndez JC, McCrank E. Anxiety related reactions associated with magnetic resonance imaging examinations. JAMA. 1993;270:745–7.
26. Selim MA. Effect of pre-instruction on anxiety levels of patients undergoing magnetic resonance imaging examination. East Med Health J. 2001;7:519–25.
27. Grey SJ, Price G, Mathews A. Reduction of anxiety during magnetic resonance imaging: a controlled trial. Magn Reson Imaging. 2000;18:351–5.
28. Harris LM, Cumming SR, Menzies RG. Predicting anxiety in magnetic resonance imaging scans. Int J Behav Med. 2004;11:1 7.
29. Enders J, Zimmermann E, Rief M, Martus P, Klingebiel R, Asbach P, et al. Reduction of claustrophobia during magnetic resonance imaging: methods and design of the "CLAUSTRO" randomized controlled trial. BMC Med Imaging. 2011;11:4 [http://www.biomedcentral.com/1471-2342/11/4].
30. Tischler V, Bronjewski E, O'Connor K, Calton T. MRI scanning for research: the experiences of healthy volunteers and patients with remitted depressive illness. Mental Health Rev J. 2009;14:23–30.
31. Spielberger CD, Gorsuch RL, Lushene R, Vagg PR, Jacobs GA. Manual for the state-trait anxiety inventory. Palo Alto: Consulting Psychologists press; 1983.
32. Tilton SR. Review of the STAI inventory. News Notes. 2008;48:1–3.
33. Liakos A, Giannitsi S. The reliabiland validity of the modified Greek anxiety scale of Spielberger. Encephalos. 1984;21:71–6 (text in Greek).
34. Anagnostopoulou T, Kioseoglou G. The modified Greek anxiety scale of Spielberg: a study on a larger sample of healthy population. Psychometric tools in Greece. Athens 2002: Greek Letters (text in Greek).
35. Beck AT, Steer RA, Garbin MG. Psychometric properties of the Beck depression inventory: twenty-five years of evaluation. Clin Psych Rev. 1988;8:77–100.
36. Richter P, Werner J, Heerlein A, Kraus A, Sauer H. On the validity of the Beck depression inventory. A review. Psychopatology. 1998;31:160–8.
37. Tamam MO, Bagcioglu E, Mulazimoglu M, Tamam L, Ospacaci T. Evaluation of anxiety and depression in patients prior to myocardial perfusion scintigraphy. Int J Psychiatry Clin Pract. 2012;16:93–7.
38. American Psychological Association. Diagnostic and statistical manual of mental disorders, DSV-IV-TR. Washington, DC: American Psychiatric Publishing, Inc; 2000. p. 419–22.
39. Clark DA, Steer RA, Beck AT, Snow D. Is the relationship between anxious and depressive cognitions and symptoms linear or curvilinear? Cogn Ther Res. 1996;20:135–54.
40. Beekman AT, de Beurs E, van Balkom AJ, Deeg DJ, van Dyck R, van Tilburg W. Anxiety and depression in later life: co-occurrence and communality of risk factors. Am J Psychiatry. 2000;157:89–95.
41. Das-Munshi J, Goldberg D, Bebbington PE, Bhugra DK, Traolach SB, Dewey ME, et al. Public health significance of mixed anxiety and depression: beyond current classification. Br J Psychiatry. 2008;192:171–7.
42. Anxiety and depression association of America (ADAA). Depression. [http://www.adaa.org/understanding-anxiety/depression. Updated October 2015].
43. Mental Health Foundation. The fundamental facts 2007. Gender differences. [www. mentalhealth.org.uk/sites/default/files/fundamental_facts_2007.pdf].
44. American Psychological Association (APA): Stress Survey 2010; Stress by Gender. [www.apa.org/news/press/releases/stress/2010/gender-stress.aspx].
45. Valentino RJ, Bangasser D, Van Bockstaele EJ. Sex-based stress signaling: the corticotropin-releasing factor receptor as a model. Mol Pharmacol. 2013; 83:737–45.
46. Mental Health Foundation. Women and Mental Health. [www.mentalhealth.org.uk/a-to-z/w/women-and-mental-health].
47. Piccinelli M, Wilkinson G. Gender differences in depression: critical review. Br J Psych. 2000;177:486–92.
48. Dantendorfer K, Amering M, Bankier A, Helbich T, Prayer D, Youssefzadeh S, et al. A study of the effects of patient anxiety, perceptions and equipment on motion artifacts in MRI. Magn Reson Imaging. 1997;15:301–6.
49. Teasdal EL. Workplace stress. Psychiatry. 2006;5:251–4.
50. Hadfield JC. The health of grandparents raising grandchildren: a literature review. J Gerontol Nurs. 2014;40:32–42. doi:10.3928/00989134-20140219-01.
51. Cavanagh J, Mathias C. Inflammation and its relevance to psychiatry. Adv Psychiatr Treat. 2008;14:248–55.
52. American Psychological Association (APA) 2012: Latest APA survey reveals deepening concerns about connection between chronic disease and stress. [www.apa.org/news/press/releases/2012/01/chronic-disease.aspx].
53. Parissis JT, Adamopoulos S, Rigas A, Kostakis G, Karatzas D, Venetsanou K, et al. Comparison of circulating proinflammatory cytokines and soluble apoptosis mediators in patients with chronic heart failure with versus without symptoms of depression. Am J Cardiol. 2004;94:1326–8.
54. Ali SH, Modic ME, Mahmoud SH, Jones SE. Reducing clinical MRI motion degradation using a prescan patient information pamphlet. AJR. 2013;200:630–4.
55. Acuff SN, Bradley YC, Barlow P, Osborne DR. Reduction of patient anxiety in PET/CT imaging by improving communication between patient and technologist. J Nucl Med Technol. 2014;42:211–7.
56. Hansen C, Crabbe D, Rubin S. Lower diagnostic accuracy of Tl-201 SPECT myocardial perfusion imaging in women: an effect of smaller chamber size. JACC. 1996;28:1214–9.

11

Correlation between degenerative spine disease and bone marrow density: a retrospective investigation

Astrid Ellen Grams[1][*] ⓘ, Rafael Rehwald[2], Alexander Bartsch[1], Sarah Honold[1], Christian Franz Freyschlag[3], Michael Knoflach[4], Elke Ruth Gizewski[1] and Bernhard Glodny[2]

Abstract

Background: Spondylosis leads to an overestimation of bone mineral density (BMD) with dual-energy x-ray absorptiometry (DXA) but not with quantitative computed tomography (QCT). The correlation between degenerative changes of the spine and QCT-BMD was therefore investigated for the first time.

Methods: One hundred thirty-four patients (66 female and 68 male) with a mean age of 49.0 ± 14.6 years (range: 19–88 years) who received a CT scan and QCT-BMD measurements of spine and hip were evaluated retrospectively. The occurrence and severity of spondylosis, osteochondrosis, and spondylarthrosis and the height of the vertebral bodies were assessed.

Results: A negative correlation was found between spinal BMD and number of spondylophytes ($\rho = -0.35$; $p < 0.01$), disc heights ($r = -0.33$; $p < 0.01$), number of discal air inclusions ($\rho = -0.34$; $p < 0.01$), the number of Schmorl nodules ($\rho = -0.25$; $p < 0.01$), the number ($\rho = -0.219$; $p < 0.05$) and the degree ($\rho = -0.220$; $p < 0.05$) of spondylarthrosis. Spinal and hip BMD correlated moderately, but the latter did not correlate with degenerative changes of the spine. In linear regression models age, osteochondrosis and spondylarthrosis were factors influencing spinal BMD.

Conclusion: Degenerative spinal changes may be associated with reduced regional spinal mineralization. This knowledge could lead to a modification of treatment of degenerative spine disease with early treatment of osteopenia to prevent secondary fractures.

Keywords: Muskoskeletal imaging, Quantitative computed tomography, Degenerative spine disease, Bone marrow density, Osteopenia, Osteoporosis

Background

Data from prior studies are inconclusive with respect to the relationship between bone mineral density (BMD) and degenerative changes of the spine. In the few studies conducted to date, dual-energy x-ray absorptiometry (DXA) has been compared with either x-ray or magnetic resonance imaging studies. In some cases there was a positive [1, 2], in others a negative [3, 4] or no relationship [5] with each other. It is known that the presence of spondylophytes, one component of degenerative spine disease, impairs DXA-BMD measurements in the spine;

BMD is systematically overestimated [6]. This overestimation from adjacent dense structures can be avoided by applying quantitative computed tomography (QCT) [7]. Other advantages of this method are that conventional CT scanners can be used, cortical and trabecular BMD can be differentiated, and size-independent, volumetric BMD data can be gained [8]. This leads to advantages in the assessment of changes in bone density over time [8]. Moreover, the bone density can also be calculated from examinations that are not conducted for this purpose, for example from cardiac computed tomographies [9]. The disadvantages are the greater radiation dose – at least in measurements of the spine – for QCT compared with DXA, the lack of data about the prognostic value with respect to future fractures, and the

* Correspondence: astrid.grams@i-med.ac.at
[1]Department of Neuroradiology, Medical University of Innsbruck, Anichstraße 35, A-6020 Innsbruck, Austria
Full list of author information is available at the end of the article

lack of applicability of the WHO criteria regarding the T-score for diagnosing osteoporosis [8]. Although QCT-BMD values, unlike DXA measurements, are not influenced by adjacent dense structures, the method has not yet been used to examine potential relationships between BMD and degenerative changes of the spine itself.

Therefore, the aim of this study was to investigate the possible relationship between different measurable morphological changes of degenerative spine disease detected by CT and the BMD measured by QCT from the same data set.

Methods

In this study, 134 patients (66 female and 68 male) with a mean age of 49.0 ± 14.6 years (range: 19–88 years) who received a CT scan and a quantitative computed tomography BMD measurement of the thoracolumbar spine and the hip were evaluated retrospectively. The study was approved by the Ethics Committee of the Medical University of Innsbruck (Reference number: AN2014-0106335/4.19).

Patients were selected from a cohort of 1249 patients who received a CT scan of the trunk between the years 2007 and 2014 as well QCT-BMD measurements of the thoracolumbar spine and the hip. The patients of this population were examined by CT scan due to chronic back pain. Patients with ankylosing spondylosis, other inflammatory diseases such as psoriasis, fractures, plasmacytoma, multiple myeloma, monoclonal gammopathy, and suspected tumor disease ($n = 1114$) were excluded from the study. None of the selected patients suffered from any of the aforementioned diseases or had any visible bony changes such as fractures, except for degenerative spine disease.

The CT scans were acquired on a LightSpeed 16 or a LightSpeed VCT scanner (General Electric, GE Healthcare, Chalfont St Giles, Buckinghamshire, UK), the latter since 2012. A tube voltage of 120 kV was used in all scans, coupled with automatic adaptation of the current to a predetermined noise factor. Data were acquired in 2.5 mm slice thicknesses. There were always 0.625-mm slice thicknesses available in a bone algorithm, as well coronal and sagittal reconstructions of a slice thickness and a slice interval of 3.0 mm.

Measurements were made by two pairs of observers (AB, SH; AEG, BG). The subjects were selected by two experienced, board-certified radiologists (AEG, BG). To evaluate spondylosis, the number and type of spondylophytes were counted in the entire spine and classified as "marginal spondylophytes" or as "hyperostotic spondylophytes" [10] (Fig. 1a, b). For the assessment of osteochondrosis, the heights of the discs were measured and the number of air inclusions in the discs was counted, as well as the number of Schmorl nodules and sclerotic endplates between the 12th thoracic and the first sacral vertebra. To evaluate spondylarthrosis, the number and severity of degenerative changes of the facet joints between the 12th thoracic and the first sacral vertebra were noted according to a previously published method [11] (Fig. 1c, d), and classified as "normal joint", "narrowed joint space = stage 1", "narrowed joint space and sclerosis or hypertrophy of the facet = stage 2" and "narrowed joint space, sclerosis and spondylophytes = stage 3". Additionally the heights of the vertebral bodies between the 12th thoracic and the first sacral vertebra were measured.

The QCT-BMD was measured in at least three segments of the thoracolumbar spine between the 11th thoracic and the 3rd lumbar segment (Fig. 2a). To do this, a region of interest was marked in the center of the

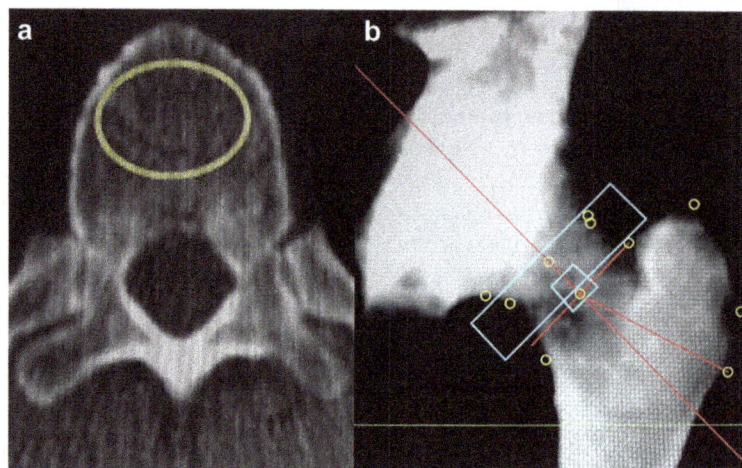

Fig. 1 QCT BMD measurements. Examples for quantitative computed tomography bone marrow density measurements in the spine (**a**) and the femur (**b**)

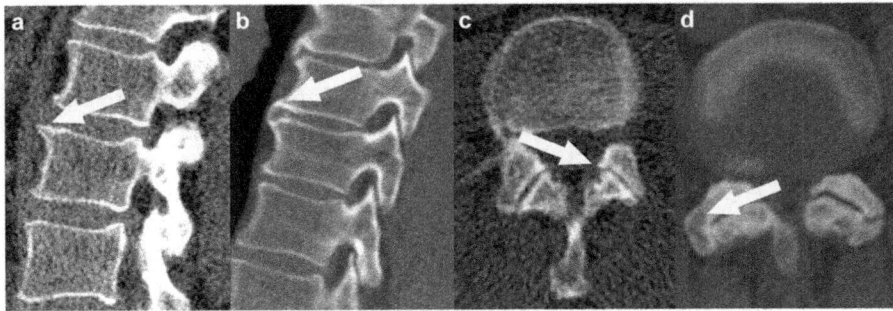

Fig. 2 Examples for degenerative spine disease. Examples of marginal (**a**) and hyperostotic (**b**) spondylophytes, as well as spondylarthrosis grade 1 (**c**) and 3 (**d**); arrows are pointing at the pathologies

vertebral body at a distance of 2–3 mm from the cortex [9], in which the trabecular BMD was calculated in mg/cm^3 of hydroxylapatite. Enostoses, cortical bone, sclerotic zones, and Schmorl nodules were excluded. If this was not possible, an adjacent vertebral body was used. Then the mean of the three vertebral bodies was formed. The practice guidelines of the American College of Radiologists [12] were followed.

Using the femur on one side, the BMD was calculated from the trabecular BMD of the trochanter major, the femoral neck, and the intertrochanteric region (Fig. 2b) in the corresponding ROIs, taking the volume into consideration. For measuring the spinal column and the femur, a Mindways QA phantom (QA Phantom Model 3, Mindways, San Francisco, CA, USA) was used in conjuction with the corresponding software (QCT PRO version 4.2.3, Mindways, San Francisco, CA, USA).

For statistical evaluation, the software Excel (Office 2013, Microsoft, Redmond, WA, USA), GraphPad Prism 6 (GraphPad Software, Inc., La Jolla, CA, USA), and SPSS (IBM SPSS Statistics for Windows, Version 22.0.. IBM Corp, Armonk, NY, USA) were used.

Distributions were tested for normality using the Kolmogorov-Smirnov test. Depending on the result, either the Spearman (ρ) or the Pearson (r) test was used for correlation analyses. Comparisons between three or more groups were made using the Kruskal-Wallis test in combination with Dunn's post hoc test or a one-way ANOVA together with a Bonferroni correction, as appropriate. Finally, different linear regression models were fitted to the target variables "BMD". This was carried out first including all variables, then using stepwise forward selection technique. A $p < 0.05$ was regarded to be significant.

Results

Women displayed a mean spinal QCT-BMD of $256.6 \pm 41.6 \ mg/cm^3$, men a mean BMD of $252.56 \pm 50.03 \ mg/cm^3$. A significant negative correlation was found between BMD and age ($r = -0.62; p > 0.01$). Mean results for the measured

pathologies of the entire population classified by gender are given in Table 1.

Significant positive correlations ($p < 0.01$ each) were found between patient age and the number of spondylophytes ($r = 0.53$), the disc height ($r = 0.25$), the number of discs showing air inclusions ($\rho = 0.43$), the number of endplates affected by Schmorl nodules ($\rho = 0.25$), and the number of facet joints showing spondylarthrosis ($\rho = 0.33$). A slight, but significant negative correlation was found between age and vertebral body height ($r = -0.18; p < 0.05$).

Spinal BMD was found to be significantly lower in patients with spondylophytes, compared to patients without spondylophytes (Fig. 3), but not in patients with spondylarthrosis compared to patients without spondylarthrosis (Fig. 4). The type of spondylophytes was irrelevant.

There were significantly negative correlations between the number of spondylophytes, disc height, the number

Table 1 Observed pathologies by gender

Pathology	All patients	Female	Male
Spondylosis deformans			
Spondylophytes spine	10.55 ± 15.48	10.12 ± 14.02	10.97 ± 16.87
Grade 1	7.76 ± 11.78	7.48 ± 10.97	8.03 ± 12.59
Grade 2	2.38 ± 4.39	2.21 ± 3.82	2.54 ± 4.90
Grade 3	0.41 ± 1.41	0.42 ± 1.38	0.40 ± 1.45
Osteochondrosis			
Disc height (mm)	8.91 ± 1.59	8.51 ± 1.4	9.30 ± 1.68
Air inclusions	0.43 ± 0.99	0.52 ± 1.10	0.35 ± 0.88
Schmorl nodules	1.49 ± 2.28	1.48 ± 2.14	1.50 ± 2.42
Endplate sclerosis	0.12 ± 0.49	0.11 ± 0.43	0.13 ± 0.54
Spondylarthrosis			
Highest grade	0.43 ± 0.87	0.56 ± 0.99	0.29 ± 0.71
Average grade	0.09 ± 0.25	0.11 ± 0.27	0.07 ± 0.23
Number	0.61 ± 1.51	0.74 ± 1.67	0.49 ± 1.33
Vertebral body height (mm)	28.14 ± 1.63	27.55 ± 1.54	28.72 ± 1.52

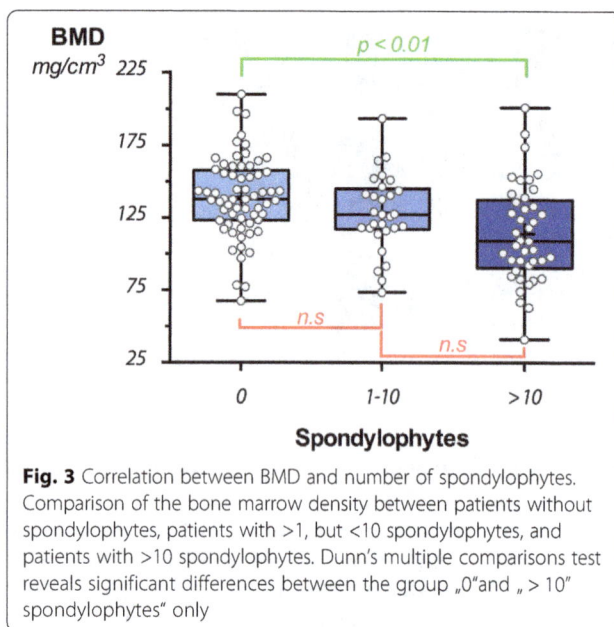

Fig. 3 Correlation between BMD and number of spondylophytes. Comparison of the bone marrow density between patients without spondylophytes, patients with >1, but <10 spondylophytes, and patients with >10 spondylophytes. Dunn's multiple comparisons test reveals significant differences between the group „0"and „ > 10" spondylophytes" only

of discs showing air inclusions, the number of endplates affected by Schmorl nodules, and the number of facet joints showing spondylarthrosis and the BMD of the spine (Table 2).

BMD of the spine correlated significantly with the BMD of the hip ($r = 0.45$; $p < 0.01$). However, correlations between the BMD of the hip and the degenerative changes of the spine were weaker (Schmorl nodules and disk height), insignificant, or absent (Table 2).

In linear regression models age, osteochondrosis and spondylarthrosis were factors with a negative influence on the spine BMD (Table 3).

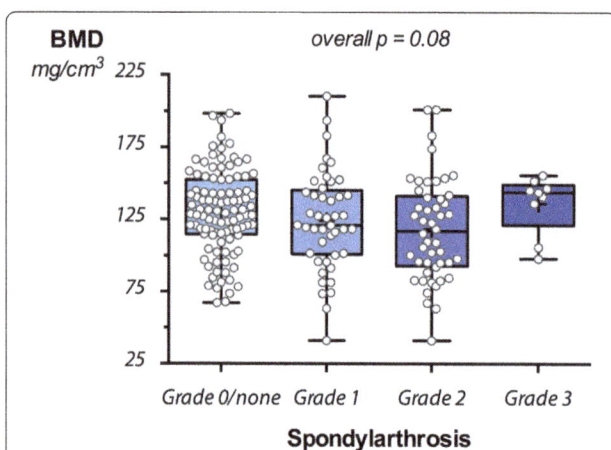

Fig. 4 Correlation between BMD and grade of spondylarthrosis. Comparison of the bone marrow density measurements between patients without spondylarthrosis, patients with grade 1, grade 2, and grade 3 spondylarthrosis. The differences were not significant

Discussion

In theory, degenerative intervertebral disc disease leads to adaptive changes of the adjacent bone with decreased density of the trabecular core and increased density of the cortical vertebral walls [13]. In this study, we were able to underline this hypothesis by finding a lower BMD with increasing severity of degenerative changes in the spine. Due to the fact that the number and degree of degenerative changes correlate inversely with the BMD of the spine, but except for osteochondrosis in terms of the number of Schmorl nodules and disc height not with the BMD of the femur, the loss of BMD may be a local epiphenomenon of the degenerative processes.

In an earlier study it was shown that the height of the discs correlates positively with the spinal DXA-BMD in premenopausal women [4]. However, studies investigating spondylophyte formation [1, 14, 15] or disc degeneration [16] found an increasing DXA-BMD with increasing degenerative changes, such as presence of spondylophytes. In view of the present results, showing a negative association of BMD with degenerative spine disease, the studies cited may be interpreted in a new way; a decrease of disc height as an early stage of detectable degeneration does not appear to affect DXA-BMD, whereas more advanced changes such as spondylophytes occurring later in the degenerative process do [6, 17]. The BMD measured using QCT seems to be more sensitive for slight demineralization [8] going along with early degenerative changes. With the progress of the degeneration and volume loss of the intervertebral disc, the affected segment becomes unstable in a later state, and the adjacent ligaments become loose. This instability can lead to abnormal stress, which can result in releasing nitrogen from the tissue due to a transient negative pressure. The visible air inclusions in the discs or joint spaces are a marker for instability, and consequently are accompanied by demineralization as well.

Degenerative spondylophytes, which are formed as a bracing reaction due to instability, are not associated with an increase of DXA-BMD, as has been previously assumed [1, 2], but with a decrease. This can be explained by several effects. Spondylophytes, as densely calcified structures, may lead to the systematic overestimation of DXA-BMD. Moreover, tilting or rotation of the vertebral bodies occurs with advanced degenerative changes, which could result in further overestimation of the adjacent bone mineral density from DXA-BMD due to summation effects [6]. This overestimation can be avoided with QCT as ROIs can be placed in selected areas and therefore cortical or adjacent structures are not included into the area of measurement [7]. Volumetric, size-independent BMD data can be gained, and cortical and trabecular BMD can be differentiated [8].

Table 2 Correlations of degenerative changes of the sine with spinal and hip BMD

Pathology	Normal distribution[a]	Correlation with BMD spine	p	Correlation with BMD hip	p
Spondylosis deformans					
Spondylophytes spine	no	−0.349	<0.01	−0.077	n.s.
Grade 1	no	−0.341	<0.01	−0.072	n.s.
Grade 2	no	−0.345	<0.01	−0.048	n.s.
Grade 3	no	−0.197	<0.05	0.003	n.s.
Osteochondrosis					
Disc height (mm)	yes	−0.332	<0.01	−0.307	<0.01
Air inclusions	no	−0.341	<0.01	−0.113	n.s.
Schmorl nodules	no	−0.246	<0.01	−0.176	0.046
Endplate sclerosis	no	0.147	0.09	0.085	n.s.
Spondylarthrosis					
Highest grade	no	−0.223	<0.01	−0.080	n.s.
Average grade	no	−0.220	<0.05	−0.077	n.s.
Number	no	−0.219	<0.05	−0.072	n.s.
Vertebral body height (mm)	yes	0.139	0.11	0.008	n.s.

[a]Kolmogorov-Smirnov test, if normal distribution assumed: Pearson correlation coefficient, if not: Spearman correlation (ρ)

In agreement with the literature [5], weak or no correlations between hip QCT-BMD and disc degeneration parameters were found, but a significant correlation was found between the QCT-BMDs of the hip and the spine. This can be interpreted to be an indication that the negative correlation between the degenerative changes of the spine and the BMD could be a local phenomenon. However, due to the retrospective design of this study, it is not possible to identify demineralization as a consequence of the progression of degeneration. Only a longitudinal, prospective observational study would be suitable for this.

A basic limitation of the study is the retrospective design. No information about medication was available in the examined population, so the BMD of the spine could have been influenced from unknown intake of bisphosphonates, for example. Although patients with obvious bony manifestations of diseases were excluded, it is conceivable that disease-associated changes such as micrometastases may have influenced these results. Another limitation is that QCT requires a higher radiation dose than other BMD methods. In the investigated study population, BMD was acquired to estimate the risk of a fracture only when a disease with affection of the bone

was suspected and not for study reasons. This is why only about 11 % of the entire population was selectable, as they did not feature bony changes due to their suspected disease or they did not suffer from the suspected disease. The last limitation is that estimation errors of absolute BMD values may have occurred using QCT as well. We did not examine possible reasons for such effects. However, as the focus of our work lay on the detection of relative changes of BMD in the context of degenerative processes, systematic estimation errors are supposed to be of minor importance only.

The results of the present study will have to be proven in prospective investigations or in a population who received both DXA-BMD and QCT-BMD, especially due to the results that partially contradicted the earlier DXA studies. More detailed research on a larger patient population would be useful for better understanding the entire process of demineralization along with degenerative alterations.

Conclusion

The results of the present study show that degenerative changes of the spine, from loss of disc height to formation of spondylophytes, are accompanied by demineralization of the bone. The lack or insignificance of associations between degenerative changes of the spine and the BMD of the femur, and at the same time moderate associations between the BMD of the spine and of the hip itself may be interpreted to be an indication that degenerative changes of the spine could be the cause of local BMD loss. However, this assumption can be proven only in a longitudinal prospective study.

Table 3 Linear Regression model (stepwise method)

	Beta	Sig.
Dependent: BMD spine		
Patient age (years)	−0.571	<0.001
Osteochondrosis (Disc height)	−0.202	0.002
Spondylarthrosis (Number)	−0.162	0.016

This knowledge may entail modifications of therapy for degenerative spine disease in the future, for example in the earlier initiation of osteoporosis therapy, in order to improve the prevention of serious sequelae for patients with degenerative spine disease.

Abbreviations
ANOVA: analysis of variance; BMD: bone mineral density; CT: computed tomography; DXA: dual-energy x-ray absorptiometry; QCT: quantitative computed tomography; r: Pearson's r; WHO: World Health Organization; ρ: Spearman rho.

Competing interests
The authors declare that they have no competing interests.

Authors' contributions
AEG and BG are the authors mainly responsible for this study. They developed the idea and were responsible for the study design, data acquisition and analysis, image preparation, the writing and revision of the draft and final manuscript. RR contributed to the critical revision of the study, the statistical analysis, image post-processing and the intense revision of the final manuscript. AB and SH were responsible for the data acquisition, the literature search and the writing of the draft. CF revised the draft and the manuscript from a neurosurgical point of view. MK revised the draft and manuscript from a neurological point of view. ERG was responsible for the writing and revision of the draft with special regard to a neuroradiological point of view. All authors agreed to be accountable for all aspects of the work in ensuring that questions related to the accuracy or integrity of any part of the work are appropriately investigated and resolved. All authors gave final approval of the version to be published.

Funding
No funding was received for this study.

Author details
[1]Department of Neuroradiology, Medical University of Innsbruck, Anichstraße 35, A-6020 Innsbruck, Austria. [2]Department of Radiology, Medical University of Innsbruck, Anichstraße 35, A-6020 Innsbruck, Austria. [3]Department of Neurosurgery, Medical University of Innsbruck, Anichstraße 35, A-6020 Innsbruck, Austria. [4]Department of Neurology, Medical University of Innsbruck, Anichstraße 35, A-6020 Innsbruck, Austria.

References
1. Miyakoshi N, Itoi E, Murai H, Wakabayashi I, Ito H, Minato T. Inverse relation between osteoporosis and spondylosis in postmenopausal women as evaluated by bone mineral density and semiquantitative scoring of spinal degeneration. Spine. 2003;28(5):492–5.
2. Kinoshita H, Tamaki T, Hashimoto T, Kasagi F. Factors influencing lumbar spine bone mineral density assessment by dual-energy X-ray absorptiometry: comparison with lumbar spinal radiogram. Journal of orthopaedic science : official journal of the Japanese Orthopaedic Association. 1998;3(1):3–9.
3. Lee BH, Moon SH, Kim HJ, Lee HM, Kim TH. Osteoporotic profiles in elderly patients with symptomatic lumbar spinal canal stenosis. Indian journal of orthopaedics. 2012;46(3):279–84.
4. Baron YM, Brincat MP, Calleja-Agius J, Calleja N. Intervertebral disc height correlates with vertebral body T-scores in premenopausal and postmenopausal women. Menopause international. 2009;15(2):58–62.
5. Wang YX, Kwok AW, Griffith JF, Leung JC, Ma HT, Ahuja AT, et al. Relationship between hip bone mineral density and lumbar disc degeneration: a study in elderly subjects using an eight-level MRI-based disc degeneration grading system. Journal of magnetic resonance imaging : JMRI. 2011;33(4):916–20.
6. Rand T, Seidl G, Kainberger F, Resch A, Hittmair K, Schneider B, et al. Impact of spinal degenerative changes on the evaluation of bone mineral density with dual energy X-ray absorptiometry (DXA). Calcif Tissue Int. 1997;60(5):430–3.
7. Li N, Li XM, Xu L, Sun WJ, Cheng XG, Tian W. Comparison of QCT and DXA: osteoporosis detection rates in postmenopausal women. Int J Endocrinol. 2013;2013:895474.
8. Adams JE. Quantitative computed tomography. Eur J Radiol. 2009;71(3):415–24.
9. Budoff MJ, Hamirani YS, Gao YL, Ismaeel H, Flores FR, Child J, et al. Measurement of thoracic bone mineral density with quantitative CT. Radiology. 2010;257(2):434–40.
10. Freyschmidt J, Brossmann J, Wiens J, Sternberg A. Spinal Column. In: Freyschmidt's,Koehler/Zimmer, Borderlands of Normal and Early Pathological Findings in Skeletal Radiography, vol. 5. Stuttgart: Thieme; 2002. p. 671–731.
11. Pathria M, Sartoris DJ, Resnick D. Osteoarthritis of the facet joints: accuracy of oblique radiographic assessment. Radiology. 1987;164(1):227–30.
12. ACR–SPR–SSR Practice Parameter for the Performance of Quantitative Computed Tomography (QCT) Bone Densitometry. Accesed on February 6th 2016. [http://www.acr.org/~/media/ACR/Documents/PGTS/guidelines/QCT.pdf]
13. Homminga J, Aquarius R, Bulsink VE, Jansen CT, Verdonschot N. Can vertebral density changes be explained by intervertebral disc degeneration? Med Eng Phys. 2012;34(4):453–8.
14. Fujita T, Ohue M, Fujii Y, Miyauchi A, Takagi Y. Intra-individual variation in lumbar bone mineral density as a measure of spondylotic deformity in the elderly. J Bone Miner Metab. 2003;21(2):98–102.
15. Oishi Y, Shimizu K, Katoh T, Nakao H, Yamaura M, Furuko T, et al. Lack of association between lumbar disc degeneration and osteophyte formation in elderly japanese women with back pain. Bone. 2003;32(4):405–11.
16. Wang YX, Griffith JF, Ma HT, Kwok AW, Leung JC, Yeung DK, et al. Relationship between gender, bone mineral density, and disc degeneration in the lumbar spine: a study in elderly subjects using an eight-level MRI-based disc degeneration grading system. Osteoporosis international : a journal established as result of cooperation between the European Foundation for Osteoporosis and the National Osteoporosis Foundation of the USA. 2011;22(1):91–6.
17. Paiva LC, Filardi S, Pinto-Neto AM, Samara A, Marques Neto JF. Impact of degenerative radiographic abnormalities and vertebral fractures on spinal bone density of women with osteoporosis. Sao Paulo medical journal = Revista paulista de medicina. 2002;120(1):9–12.

12

Registration error of the liver CT using deformable image registration of MIM Maestro and Velocity AI

Nobuyoshi Fukumitsu[1*], Kazunori Nitta[2], Toshiyuki Terunuma[1], Toshiyuki Okumura[1], Haruko Numajiri[1], Yoshiko Oshiro[1], Kayoko Ohnishi[1], Masashi Mizumoto[1], Teruhito Aihara[1], Hitoshi Ishikawa[1], Koji Tsuboi[1] and Hideyuki Sakurai[1]

Abstract

Background: Understanding the irradiated area and dose correctly is important for the reirradiation of organs that deform after irradiation, such as the liver. We investigated the spatial registration error using the deformable image registration (DIR) software products MIM Maestro (MIM) and Velocity AI (Velocity).

Methods: Image registration of pretreatment computed tomography (CT) and posttreatment CT was performed in 24 patients with liver tumors. All the patients received proton beam therapy, and the follow-up period was 4–14 (median: 10) months. We performed DIR of the pretreatment CT and compared it with that of the posttreatment CT by calculating the dislocation of metallic markers (implanted close to the tumors).

Results: The fiducial registration error was comparable in both products: 0.4–32.9 (9.3 ± 9.9) mm for MIM and 0.5–38.6 (11.0 ± 10.0) mm for Velocity, and correlated with the tumor diameter for MIM ($r = 0.69$, $P = 0.002$) and for Velocity ($r = 0.68$, $P = 0.0003$). Regarding the enhancement effect, the fiducial registration error was 1.0–24.9 (7.4 ± 7.7) mm for MIM and 0.3–29.6 (8.9 ± 7.2) mm for Velocity, which is shorter than that of plain CT ($P = 0.04$, for both).

Conclusions: The DIR performance of both MIM and Velocity is comparable with regard to the liver. The fiducial registration error of DIR depends on the tumor diameter. Furthermore, contrast-enhanced CT improves the accuracy of both MIM and Velocity.

Institutional review board approval: H28-102; July 14, 2016 approved.

Keywords: Deformable image registration, Rigid image registration, Liver, Proton beam therapy

Background

The various organs of the human body are often deformed by irradiation. Reirradiation is sometimes conducted to treat new lesions that might occur. Before reirradiation is performed, it is vital to confirm the region irradiated by previous radiotherapy to avoid excess irradiation to the normal tissue as this could cause severe adverse effects. Primary liver tumors tend to recur inside the liver after treatment, and metastasis from other organs also makes it highly possible that new lesions will occur inside the liver. A substantial number

of patients, therefore, require reirradiation to treat recurrence of cancer in the liver [1].

Thus, image registration is a particularly important issue for treating patients with liver tumors, even though, since the advent of particle beam radiotherapy, irradiated lesions are now well controlled [2–5]. To conduct image registration, an important problem must be considered: after irradiation, the irradiated area including the tumor is shrunk and the nonirradiated area is shifted and sometimes enlarged or shrunk, thus causing remarkable deformation of the liver in most patients [6]. This issue can be addressed by using deformable image registration (DIR), and a number of software products are now on the market. The use of DIR for applications and assessment of previously delivered irradiation doses

---
* Correspondence: fukumitsun@yahoo.co.jp
[1]Proton Medical Research Center, University of Tsukuba, 1-1-1, Tennoudai, Tsukuba, Japan
Full list of author information is available at the end of the article

is clinically expected to protect the normal liver tissue from receiving harmfully large doses of irradiation [7].

Several DIR algorithms exist, and DIR can be broadly classified into two categories: (1) intensity-based methods, which use a variety of image intensity metrics such as the gray scale, and (2) feature-based methods, which use specific image features such as contours [8]. Transformation models include optical flow-based equations [9], the "Demons" equation [10], B-splines [11], and thin-plate splines [12]. In most registration algorithms, the balance between image similarity and accurate matching of the local features on the one hand and deformation smoothness on the other hand is crucial to accurately measure the deformation [13]. The technique for evaluating the spatial accuracy of DIR involves landmark tracking [14] or contour or structure comparisons [15].

In recent years, advanced software equipped with the function of DIR has been developed for research purposes, and some of them are also available for clinical use. MIM Maestro (MIM Software Inc., OH, USA) (MIM) and Velocity AI (Velocity Medical Solutions, GA, USA) (Velocity) are the two most widely used in Japan and worldwide 2 of the 3 most widely used commercially available software products that can perform DIR and assist radiotherapy planning. In MIM, the DIR algorithm is intensity-based, free form cubic spline interpolation with essentially unlimited degrees of freedom [13]. MIM can dramatically deform the image, while, in cases with little contrast, it might lead to unreasonable deformation of the image. In Velocity, a B-spline deformable model is used [13]. Velocity uses standardized image intensity and has a smoothing and regularization function derived from the B-spline method. Although both software products are relatively new, some reports on their features and differences have been already been published. In brief, these are that MIM has the advantage in terms of small fields but sometimes produces registration error because of image noise, and Velocity has the advantage in terms of large fields. So far, there is no strong evidence for which software is superior [8, 13, 16].

We examined the spatial accuracy of DIR of MIM and Velocity after irradiation in the preliminary stage of deformation of the dose distribution in reirradiated liver tumors.

Methods

We retrospectively reviewed patients who had received proton beam therapy (PBT) at our institute. All the study procedures involving human participants were conducted in accordance with the ethical standards of the institutional research committee and with the 1964 Helsinki declaration and its later amendments or comparable ethical standards. All the treatments were

discussed at inhospital conferences, and informed consent was obtained from all the individual participants included in the study. The study received institutional review board approval (H28-102). We selected those patients who had a metallic material such as a fiducial marker or surgical clip (herein called *metallic marker*) already implanted very close to the liver tumor before PBT. We examined 24 consecutive patients treated between 2009 and 2014 (20 men, 4 women; aged 52–84 years). The most common disease was hepatocellular carcinoma (18 patients), followed by liver metastasis (5 patients) and intrahepatic bile duct carcinoma (1 patient). Fiducial markers for previous PBT were present in 21 patients, and surgical clips, in 3 patients. At our institute, abdominal computed tomography (CT) for diagnosis is usually not taken after metallic marker implantation, so these 21 patients had come to our hospital to receive PBT for new lesions in the liver. Twenty-two patients underwent irradiation for single lesions, and 2 patients, for 2 lesions. The total tumor diameter was 10-69 (median: 35) mm. The tumor was located in the left lobe in 5 patients, in the right lobe in 15 patients, and in both lobes in 4 patients. The distance between the tumor and the metallic marker was 5-33.7 (median: 12.0) mm. The total irradiation dose was 50-74 GyE in 22-37 fractions (Table 1).

Contrast-enhanced CT with the breath-holding technique was taken before and after treatment. The duration between PBT and posttreatment CT was 4-14 (median: 10) months. CT with a matrix resolution of 512*512 and a slice thickness of 5 mm was used. We used both plain and contrast-enhanced CT in our image analysis. For the patients who had dynamic contrast-enhanced CT, we used portal venous-phase CT. We performed rigid image registration (RIR) and then DIR of the pretreatment CT images. During the registration process, the priority area of calculation was manually designated to cover the whole liver. The fiducial registration error was assessed by examining the dislocation of the metallic marker from its position in the posttreatment CT and that in the deformed pretreatment CT images. We used the point at which the metallic density was the highest as the position of the metallic marker. The same process was performed using MIM (version 6.5.2) and Velocity (version 3.1.0).

The fiducial registration errors of MIM and Velocity were compared using both plain and contrast-enhanced CT and a paired t test. The Pearson product moment correlation was performed to examine the correlation between the fiducial registration error of RIR and DIR. Simple linear regression analysis was performed to examine the correlation between tumor diameter and fiducial registration error. Probability values below 0.05 were considered significant.

Table 1 Characteristic of the patients

Number	Disease	materials	Dislocation MIM (plain)	MIM (enhance)	Velocity (plain)	Velocity (enhance)	Tumor location	Tumor diameter	tumor-material distance	Dose (GyE/fr)	Duration (months)	Remark
1	HCC	marker	0.40	1.00	0.50	1.00	S8	35	11.5	72.6/22	9.4	
2	IHBDC	clip	3.00	2.30	18.00	14.30	S3	45	14.2	74/37	14.2	
3	meta	marker	6.70	8.70	9.20	7.70	S7	30	16.1	72.6/22	10.9	
4	HCC	clip	4.70	2.10	4.00	3.10	S4	20	5.2	72.6/22	10.3	
5	HCC	marker	1.80	2.10	4.60	0.30	S4/8	30	7.2	50/25	5.5	
6	meta	marker	15.20	8.20	20.50	4.50	S8	60	8.7	72.6/22	7.2	at
7	HCC	marker	8.20	5.40	22.30	20.40	S4/8	50	10.8	72.6/22	6.2	pl
8	meta	marker	1.30	1.60	4.00	2.20	S6	25	13.2	60/30	10.0	
9	HCC	marker	4.70	4.70	4.80	7.30	S7	25	5.2	50/25	10.9	
10	HCC	marker	1.80	2.20	1.90	2.00	S4	24	5.4	72.6/22	7.8	
11	HCC	marker	0.40	1.20	6.30	9.7	S5	35	5.7	50/25	12.1	
12	HCC	marker	18.10	19.10	4.70	16.60	S7	56	8.3	72.6/22	8.9	as
13	HCC	marker	22.90	5.90	18.30	12.50	S8	30	9.5	50/25	11.2	as
14	meta	marker	11.10	14.60	5.50	5.20	S4/8	47	9.6	60/30	7.2	pl
15	HCC	marker	32.90	18.90	21.40	13.80	S8	60	10.3	72.6/22	11.9	as
16	HCC	marker	11.30	2.30	10.70	7.70	S7	15	12.4	60/30	10.3	
17	HCC	marker	2.10	3.10	1.30	2.60	S1/4	35	14.9	60/30	8.0	as
18	HCC	marker	15.50	20.00	12.50	10.80	S7/8	38	16.1	72.6/22	6.5	
19	HCC	marker	0.80	1.20	3.40	3.10	S5/8	35	16.5	74/37	10.1	at
20	HCC	marker	0.70	2.00	9.70	9.00	S8	10	19.1	60/15	6.8	
21	HCC	marker	2.60	2.90	6.80	6.30	S1	24	30.9	72.6/22	8.7	
22	HCC	marker	29.60	24.90	38.60	55/8	68	68	32.8	52.8/16	4.2	as
23	HCC	marker	24.60	20.80	30.70	19.10	S6,S8	69	33.0	70/35,66/10	12.7	as
24	meta	clip	3.00	2.50	3.20	4.60	S1,S5/8	40	33.7	45/15,72.6/22	13.4	

Abbreviations: *HCC* hepatocellular carcinoma, *IHBDC* intrahepatic bile duct carcinoma, *GyE/fr* Gray equivaent/fractions, *at;* atelectasis appearance during follow-up, *as* ascites appearance or increased during follow-up, *pl* pleural effusion appearance during follow-up, *as* ascites appearance or increased during follow-up
Duration means the interval to the post treatment CT. All unit of length is mm

Results

In the plain CT, the fiducial registration error was 0.4–32.9 (9.3 ± 9.9) mm for MIM and 0.5–38.6 (11.0 ± 10.0) mm for Velocity. The fiducial registration error was less for MIM in 16 patients and for Velocity in 8 patients; overall however, the results for both MIM and Velocity were similar ($P = 0.18$). In the contrast-enhanced CT, the fiducial registration errors for MIM (1.0–24.9 [7.4 ± 7.7] mm) and Velocity (0.3–29.6 [8.9 ± 7.1] mm) were also similar ($P = 0.22$) (Fig. 1a). As for the enhancement effect, the fiducial registration errors for MIM and Velocity were significantly shorter than they were in the plain CT ($P = 0.04$, for both). (Fig. 1b).

With regard to the fiducial registration error, DIR was significantly correlated with RIR for both MIM ($r = 0.62$, $P = 0.001$) and Velocity ($r = 0.9$, $P = 3.3 \times 10^{-9}$) in the plain CT (Fig. 2a). In the contrast-enhanced CT, DIR was also significantly correlated with RIR for both MIM ($r = 0.66$, $P = 0.0004$) and Velocity ($r = 0.84$, $P = 3.6 \times 10^{-7}$). The fiducial registration error was significantly correlated with the tumor diameter for both MIM ($r = 0.69$, $P = 0.002$) and Velocity ($r = 0.68$, $P = 0.0003$) in the plain CT. In the contrast-enhanced CT, the fiducial registration error was also significantly correlated with the tumor diameter for both MIM ($r = 0.75$, $P = 2.8 \times 10^{-5}$) and Velocity ($r = 0.63$, $P = 9 \times 10^{-5}$). The tumor diameter predicted to produce a 10-mm fiducial registration error was 39.4 mm for

MIM and 35.5 mm for Velocity in the plain CT and 45.6 mm for MIM and 42 mm for Velocity in the contrast-enhanced CT (Fig. 2b).

The tumor-marker distance did not differ according to the classification of the tumor location. However, cases in which the tumor in the right lobe had a trend toward the tumor-marker distance became large (Table 2).

Figure 3 shows a case in which the fiducial registration error was small and similar for both MIM and Velocity. Figure 4 shows the cases that showed the biggest discrepancies between MIM and Velocity in terms of the fiducial registration error. Figure 5 shows the cases in which the DIR results were greatly affected by the contrast enhancement effect. All the deformed images showed slice levels that corresponded to the location of the metallic marker on the posttreatment CT.

Discussion

We compared the capabilities of MIM and Velocity. At first, we considered the advantages of MIM. Although the fiducial registration error of DIR correlated with that of RIR both for MIM and for Velocity, there were some differences in the degree of fiducial registration error. As shown in Fig. 2(a), the correlation coefficient for Velocity was 0.9, which is an extremely strong correlation, whereas for MIM it was 0.62, which is only a moderate correlation. Figure 4(a) shows the case with the largest

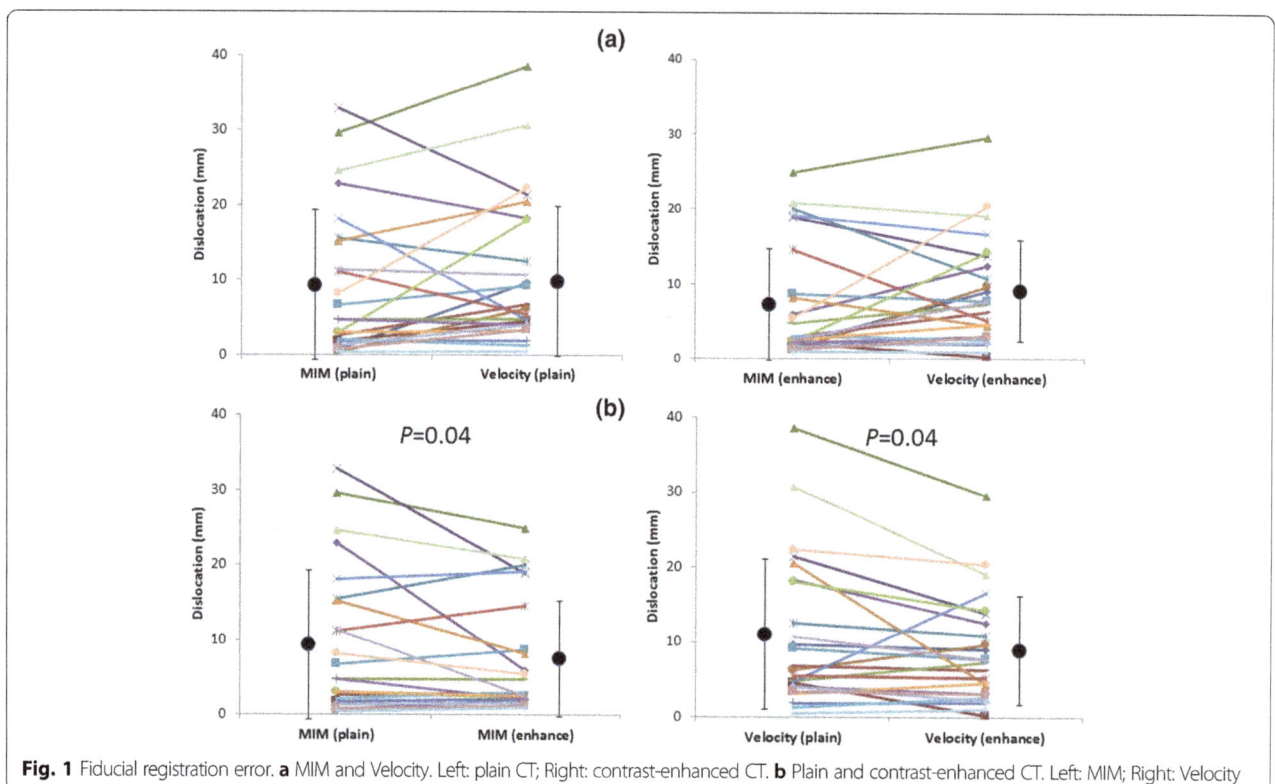

Fig. 1 Fiducial registration error. **a** MIM and Velocity. Left: plain CT; Right: contrast-enhanced CT. **b** Plain and contrast-enhanced CT. Left: MIM; Right: Velocity

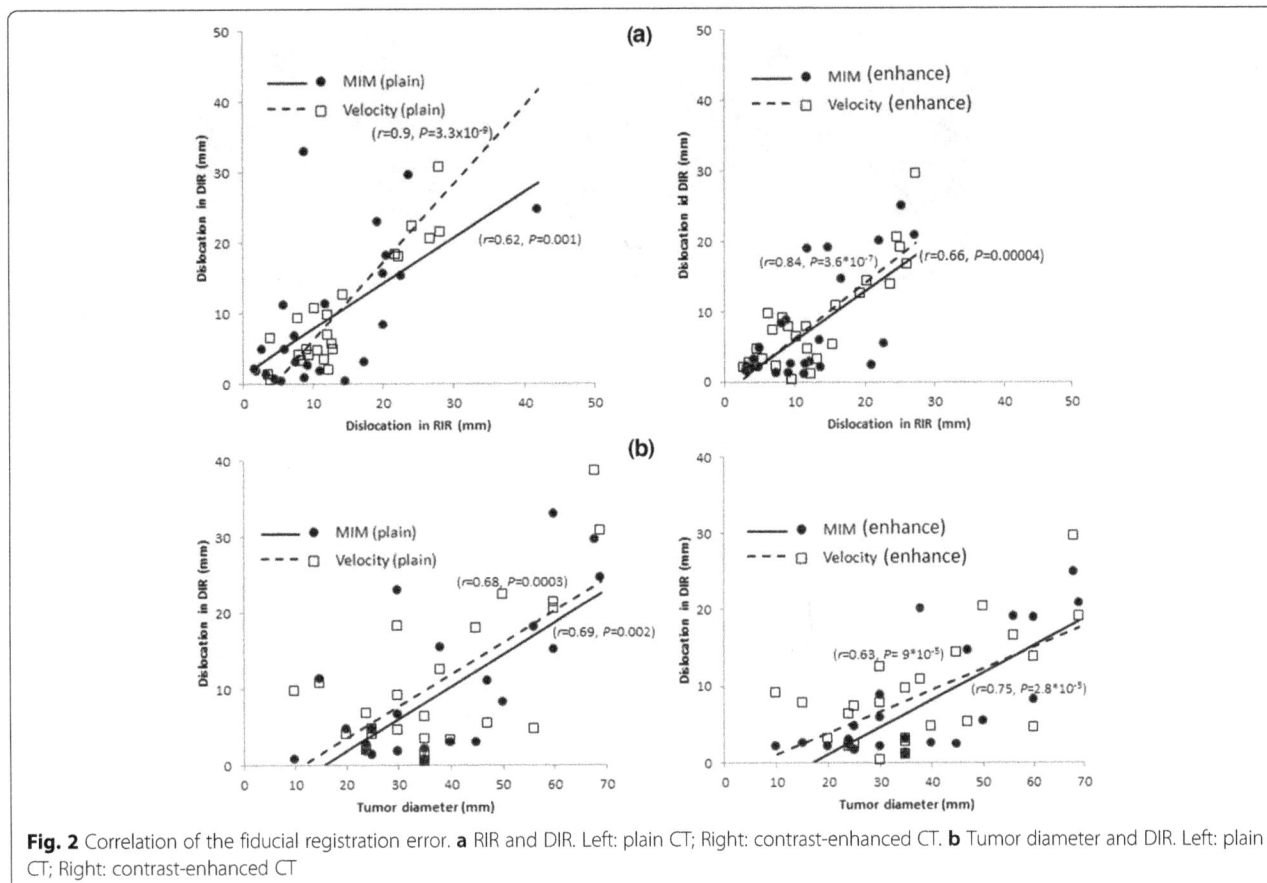

Fig. 2 Correlation of the fiducial registration error. **a** RIR and DIR. Left: plain CT; Right: contrast-enhanced CT. **b** Tumor diameter and DIR. Left: plain CT; Right: contrast-enhanced CT

difference in fiducial registration error between Velocity and MIM. The metallic marker could not be found in the axial, coronal, or sagittal image in the RIR process of both MIM and Velocity. However, during the DIR process, MIM could correctly identify the location in which the metallic marker was observed in any of the directional images. In contrast, the DIR process of Velocity shifted the location to a position in which the metallic marker was not observed in any of the directional images. Yeo et al reported that the magnitude of deformation has a much larger effect on the accuracy of registration than does the complexity of deformation [17]. Our results suggest that the DIR process in

Velocity seems to be more dependent on the RIR, while MIM has a greater ability to modify during the process of DIR. Next, we considered the advantages of Velocity. As shown in Fig. 4(b) of an irradiated tumor in the right lobe, MIM showed an unnaturally deformed low-density tumor, especially in the coronal image, whereas Velocity showed the natural shape of the tumor. Previous studies have shown that MIM produces beautiful image similarity but may produce nonphysical deformation fields, while Velocity produces smooth, physically plausible deformation fields [18]. It seems that MIM has higher flexibility and causes excellent overall spatial accuracy; although it tends to deform forcibly. This could

Table 2 Cases with large tumor marker distance

MIM (plain)			MIM (enhance)			Velocity (palin)			Velocity (enhance)		
T. M. D. (mm)	T. L.	T. D. (mm)	Dis. (mm)	Loc.	T. D. (mm)	Dis. (mm)	Loc.	T. D. (mm)	Dis. (mm)	Loc.	T. D. (mm)
22.9	S8	30	20.0	S7/8	38	21.4	S8	60	20.4	S4/8	50
24.6	S6,S8	69	20.8	S6, S8	69	22.3	S4/8	50	29.6	S5/8	68
29.6	S5/8	68	24.9	S5/8	68	30.7	S6, S8	69			
32.9	S8	60				38.6	S5/8	68	68		

Abbreviations: *T. M. D.* tumor marker distance, *T. L* tumor location, *T. D* tumor diameter

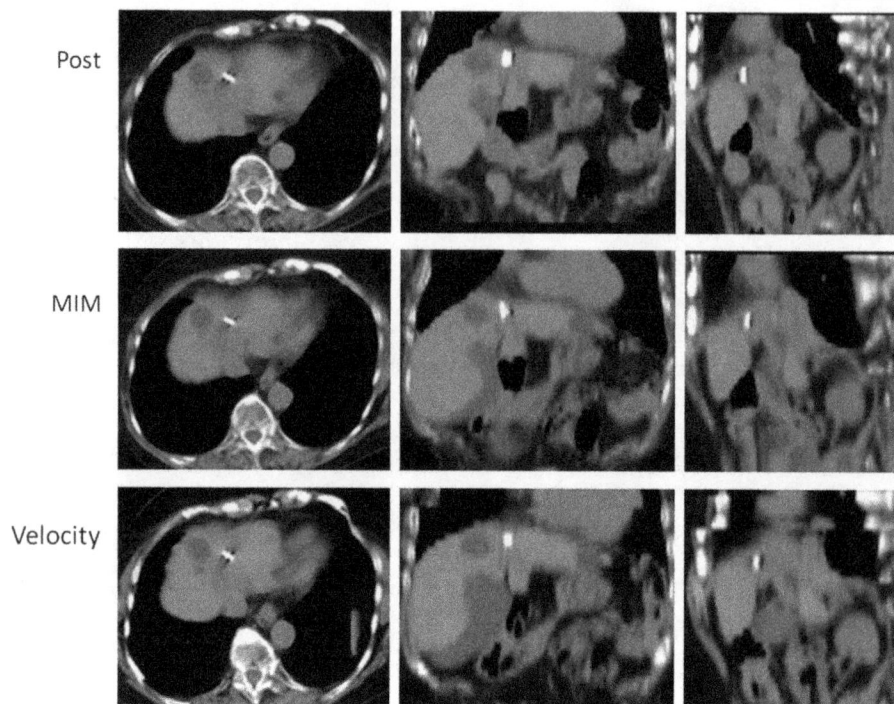

Fig. 3 A case with a small registration error for both MIM and Velocity. Proton beams at 72.6 GyE were delivered to the tumor in S4 7.8 months before. The fiducial registration error was 1.8 mm in MIM and 1.9 mm in Velocity, the shortest among all the patients

sometimes cause unreasonable DIR and diminish the ability to transfer contours.

As shown in Fig. 1(a), although the fiducial registration errors of MIM and Velocity were similar overall, they were not necessary closely correlated, and for some patients either MIM or Velocity had a distinct advantage. Some previous studies reported that it is hard to decide which software is impartially superior to others in terms of DIR accuracy [8, 13, 18]. Our results also demonstrate that the superiority of DIR accuracy for the liver varies by patient, making it difficult to state which software is better. It is generally understood that DIR will work well with feature-rich images in which there is little or no ambiguity between corresponding points in the source and target images. The liver is one of the organs that have a relatively homogeneous Hounsfield unit (HU) and a lack of morphological characteristics. Therefore, one important objective of this study was to determine how well these software products can perform DIR in low-contrast organs such as the liver. We analyzed the portal vein phase image, which enhances a greater number of vessels. As we expected, contrast-enhanced CT could accomplish on average 1.9-mm less fiducial registration error than could plain CT in MIM. Moreover, Velocity could also, on average, accomplish a

2.1-mm enhancement effect, as shown in Fig 1(b). In addition, the enhancement effect could change the deformation pattern. As shown in Fig. 5, the vector went toward the right posterior direction in the plain CT; by contrast, the vector circled in a clockwise direction in the contrast-enhanced CT of MIM. Similarly, in the plain CT, the vector moved slightly backwards only in the peripheral region of the liver, whereas in the contrast-enhanced CT of Velocity, the vector moved forward through most of the regions of the liver. We are convinced that in the DIR of both MIM and Velocity, enhancement-derived contrast not only works toward spatial accuracy but also changes the deformation pattern, such as the linear and rotational directions.

We used a metallic marker to calculate the image registration accuracy because it is difficult to measure the registration error of the tumor itself and because precise contouring of the whole liver by distinguishing the liver from the porta hepatis is not completely reproducible in each study. It is feasible to calculate the fiducial registration error at multiple points in each patient. However, in the daily clinical setting, the number of implanted metallic markers is usually 1 or 2. Therefore, we selected only the patients whose metallic materials were close to the tumor. In this

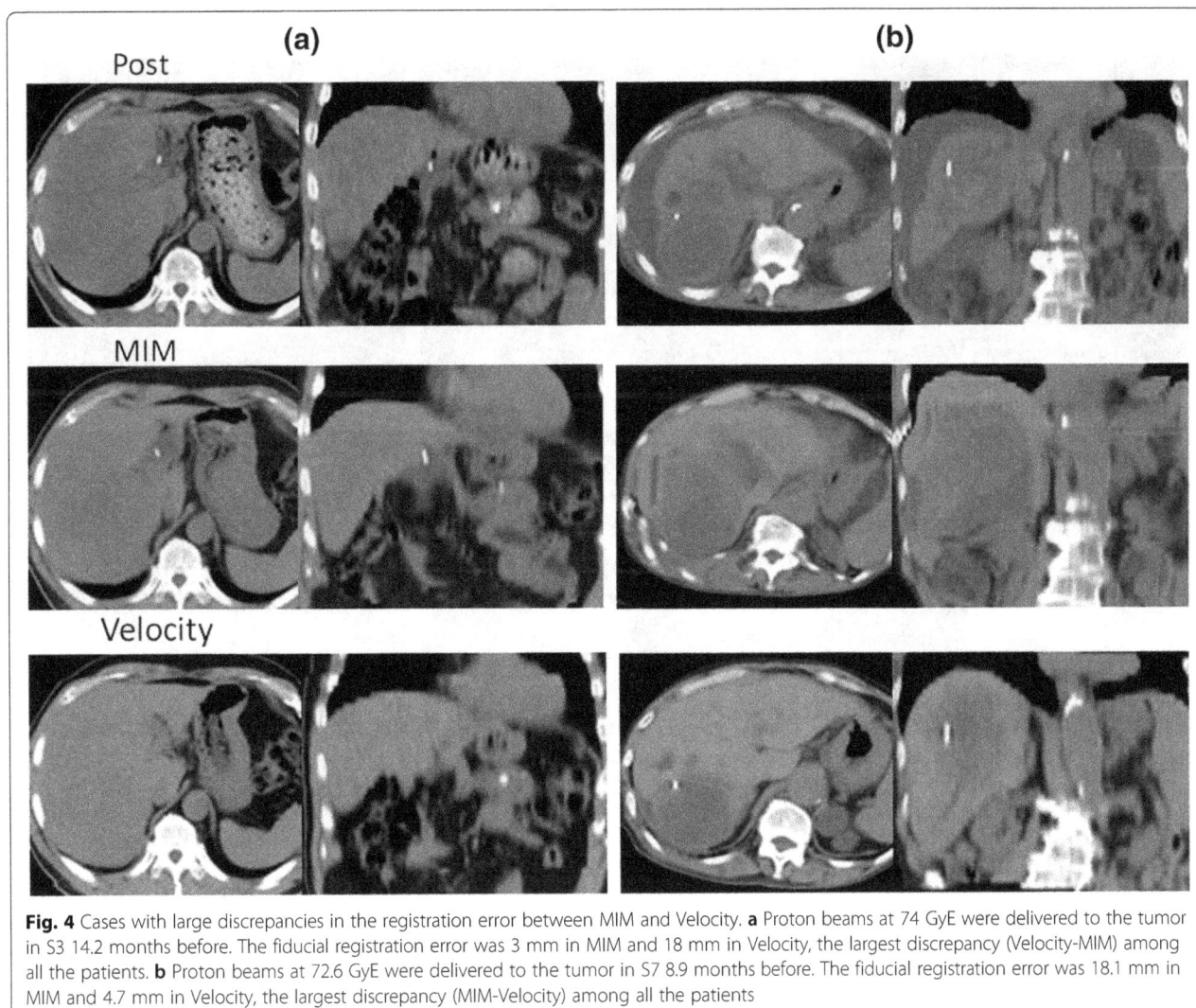

Fig. 4 Cases with large discrepancies in the registration error between MIM and Velocity. **a** Proton beams at 74 GyE were delivered to the tumor in S3 14.2 months before. The fiducial registration error was 3 mm in MIM and 18 mm in Velocity, the largest discrepancy (Velocity-MIM) among all the patients. **b** Proton beams at 72.6 GyE were delivered to the tumor in S7 8.9 months before. The fiducial registration error was 18.1 mm in MIM and 4.7 mm in Velocity, the largest discrepancy (MIM-Velocity) among all the patients

study, the metallic markers were implanted close to the tumor, with a range of 5–33.7 (median: 12.0) mm. Thus, we consider the metallic markers to act as surrogates of the fiducial registration error in DIR. There may be criticism that the high HU of the metallic markers could have affected the image registration. However, in all the patients, the metallic artifact was so small when compared with the large volume of the liver, and therefore, we think that the accuracy of the image registration is seldom affected by the artifact. Moreover, we routinely compare and conduct image registration of CTs with tiny metallic markers already implanted. Therefore, this analysis reflects the conditions of the daily clinical setting, and we consider that analysis using CT with implantation of tiny metallic markers is clinically allowable.

Both MIM and Velocity have rapidly expanded the market for such types of software, and new software products have been manufactured or are planned for manufacture to meet the demand for high-precision radiotherapy. It is expected that several types of commercial-based software products equipped with the DIR function will be developed, not only for examination of previous radiotherapy planning, but also for use in adaptive radiotherapy. In this study, we investigated the registration error by using clinical data. However, it is also important to investigate and validate the registration error by using phantoms. We are considering a phantom study as the next step to prove the registration error that we concluded in this clinical study.

Conclusion

For image registration of the liver, the DIR performances of MIM and Velocity are similar overall. However, which software is the better option varies according to the patient. The spatial accuracy of DIR depends on the

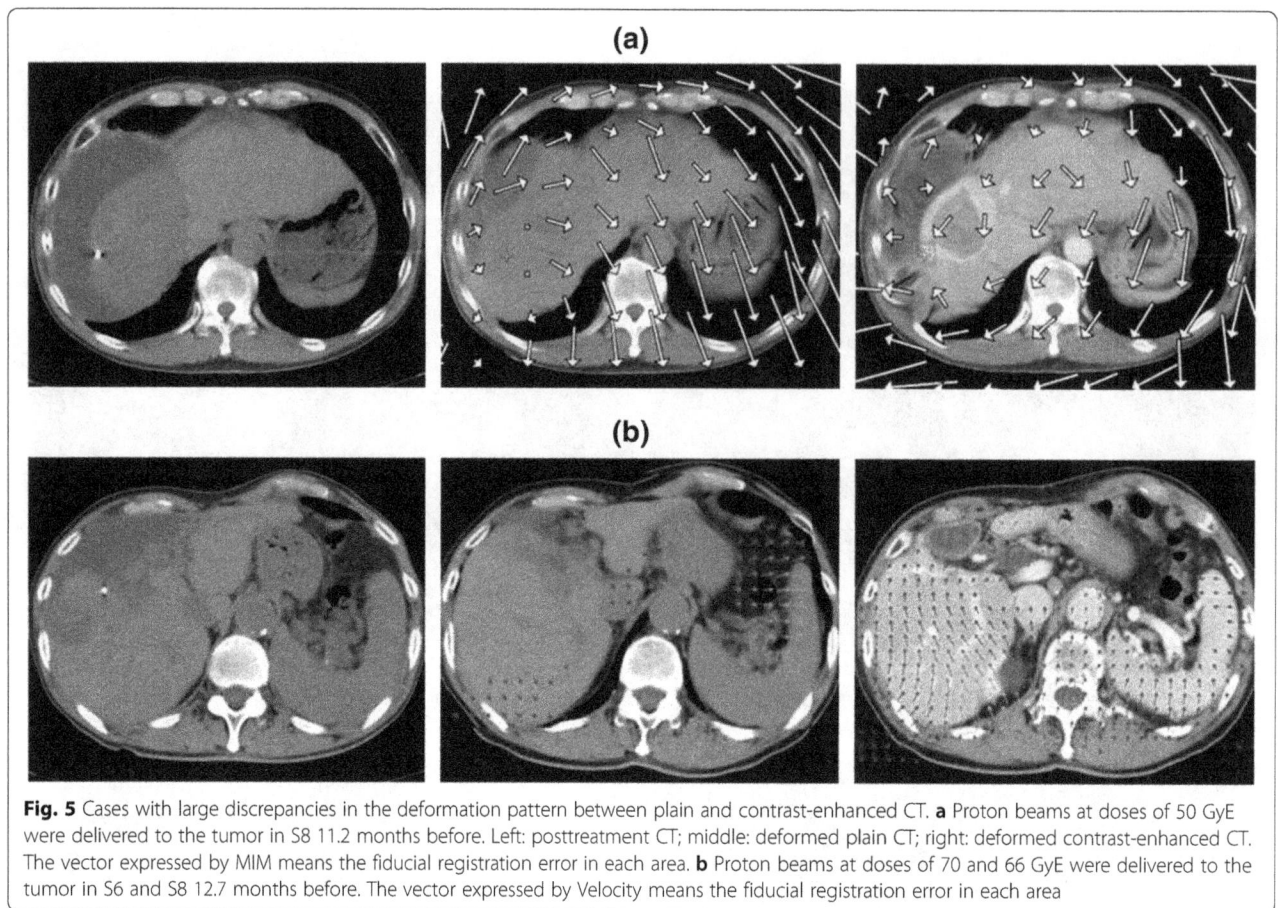

Fig. 5 Cases with large discrepancies in the deformation pattern between plain and contrast-enhanced CT. **a** Proton beams at doses of 50 GyE were delivered to the tumor in S8 11.2 months before. Left: posttreatment CT; middle: deformed plain CT; right: deformed contrast-enhanced CT. The vector expressed by MIM means the fiducial registration error in each area. **b** Proton beams at doses of 70 and 66 GyE were delivered to the tumor in S6 and S8 12.7 months before. The vector expressed by Velocity means the fiducial registration error in each area

accuracy of RIR and also on the tumor diameter. Finally, contrast-enhanced CT improves the accuracy of both MIM and Velocity.

Abbreviations
CT: (Computed tomography): image used by computer-processed combinations of many X-ray images; DIR: (Deformable image registration): image registration technique with deformation; HU: (Hounsfield unit): A quantity commonly used in CT to express CT numbers in a standardized and convenient form; MIM: (MIM Maestro): name of software; PBT: (Proton beam therapy): a type of radiotherapy using proton beams; RIR: (Rigid image registration): image registration technique horizontally and rotationally without deformation; Velocity: (Velocity AI): name of software

Acknowledgements
We really appreciate Thomas Mayers and Flaminia Miyamasu, Medical English Communications Center, University of Tsukuba, for grammatical revision of the manuscript.

Funding
None.

Author's contributions
NF carried out manuscript writing. KN carried out data analysis of Velocity. TT carried out data analysis of MIM. TO supported data analysis. HN carried out clinical examinations. YO participated in the design of the study. KO carried out clinical examinations. MM participated in the design of the study. TA carried out clinical examinations. HI supported statistical analysis. KT supported to draft the manuscript. HS supported data analysis. All authors read and approved the final version of the manuscript.

Competing interests
The authors declare that they have no competing interests.

Author details
[1]Proton Medical Research Center, University of Tsukuba, 1-1-1, Tennoudai, Tsukuba, Japan. [2]Division of Radiology, Ibaraki Prefectural Central Hospital, 6528, Koibuchi, Kasama, Japan.

References
1. Hashimoto T, Tokuuye K, Fukumitsu N, Igaki H, Hata M, Kagei K, Sugahara S, Ohara K, Matsuzaki Y, Akine Y. Repeated proton beam therapy for hepatocellular carcinoma. Int J Radiat Oncol Biol Phys. 2006;65(1):196–202.
2. Bush DA, Kayali Z, Grove R, Slater JD. The safety and efficacy of high-dose proton beam radiotherapy for hepatocellular carcinoma: a phase 2 prospective trial. Cancer. 2011;117(13):3053–9.
3. Fukumitsu N, Sugahara S, Nakayama H, Fukuda K, Mizumoto M, Abei M, Shoda J, Thono E, Tsuboi K, Tokuuye K. A prospective study of hypofractionated proton beam therapy for patients with hepatocellular carcinoma. Int J Radiat Oncol Biol Phys. 2009;74(3):831–6.
4. Mizumoto M, Okumura T, Hashimoto T, Fukuda K, Oshiro Y, Fukumitsu N, Abei M, Kawaguchi A, Hayashi Y, Ookawa A, et al. Proton beam therapy for hepatocellular carcinoma: a comparison of three treatment protocols. Int J Radiat Oncol Biol Phys. 2011;81(4):1039–45.
5. Qi WX, Fu S, Zhang Q, Guo XM. Charged particle therapy versus photon therapy for patients with hepatocellular carcinoma: a systematic review and meta-analysis. Radiother Oncol. 2015;114(3):289–95.
6. Ahmadi T, Itai Y, Onaya H, Yoshioka H, Okumura T, Akine Y. CT evaluation of hepatic injury following proton beam irradiation: appearance, enhancement, and 3D size reduction pattern. J Comput Assist Tomogr. 1999;23(5):655–63.

7. Fukumitsu N, Hashimoto T, Okumura T, Mizumoto M, Tohno E, Fukuda K, Abei M, Sakae T, Sakurai H. Investigation of the geometric accuracy of proton beam irradiation in the liver. Int J Radiat Oncol Biol Phys. 2012;82(2):826–33.

8. Wognum S, Heethuis SE, Rosario T, Hoogeman MS, Bel A. Validation of deformable image registration algorithms on CT images of ex vivo porcine bladders with fiducial markers. Med Phys. 2014;41(7):071916.

9. Yang D, Chaudhari SR, Goddu SM, Pratt D, Khullar D, Deasy JO, El Naqa I. Deformable registration of abdominal kilovoltage treatment planning CT and tomotherapy daily megavoltage CT for treatment adaptation. Med Phys. 2009;36(2):329–38.

10. Wang H, Dong L, Lii MF, Lee AL, de Crevoisier R, Mohan R, Cox JD, Kuban DA, Cheung R. Implementation and validation of a three-dimensional deformable registration algorithm for targeted prostate cancer radiotherapy. Int J Radiat Oncol Biol Phys. 2005;61(3):725–35.

11. Wen N, Glide-Hurst C, Nurushev T, Xing L, Kim J, Zhong H, Liu D, Liu M, Burmeister J, Movsas B, et al. Evaluation of the deformation and corresponding dosimetric implications in prostate cancer treatment. Phys Med Biol. 2012;57(17):5361–79.

12. Vasquez Osorio EM, Hoogeman MS, Bondar L, Levendag PC, Heijmen BJ. A novel flexible framework with automatic feature correspondence optimization for nonrigid registration in radiotherapy. Med Phys. 2009;36(7):2848–59.

13. Kirby N, Chuang C, Ueda U, Pouliot J. The need for application-based adaptation of deformable image registration. Med Phys. 2013;40(1):011702.

14. Castillo R, Castillo E, Guerra R, Johnson VE, McPhail T, Garg AK, Guerrero T. A framework for evaluation of deformable image registration spatial accuracy using large landmark point sets. Phys Med Biol. 2009;54(7):1849–70.

15. Wognum S, Bondar L, Zolnay AG, Chai X, Hulshof MC, Hoogeman MS, Bel A. Control over structure-specific flexibility improves anatomical accuracy for point-based deformable registration in bladder cancer radiotherapy. Med Phys. 2013;40(2):021702.

16. Nie K, Chuang C, Kirby N, Braunstein S, Pouliot J. Site-specific deformable imaging registration algorithm selection using patient-based simulated deformations. Med Phys. 2013;40(4):041911.

17. Yeo UJ, Supple JR, Taylor ML, Smith R, Kron T, Franich RD. Performance of 12 DIR algorithms in low-contrast regions for mass and density conserving deformation. Med Phys. 2013;40(10):101701.

18. Singhrao K, Kirby N, Pouliot J. A three-dimensional head-and-neck phantom for validation of multimodality deformable image registration for adaptive radiotherapy. Med Phys. 2014;41(12):121709.

13

Applying a computer-aided scheme to detect a new radiographic image marker for prediction of chemotherapy outcome

Yunzhi Wang[1*], Yuchen Qiu[1], Theresa Thai[2], Kathleen Moore[2], Hong Liu[1] and Bin Zheng[1]

Abstract

Background: To investigate the feasibility of automated segmentation of visceral and subcutaneous fat areas from computed tomography (CT) images of ovarian cancer patients and applying the computed adiposity-related image features to predict chemotherapy outcome.

Methods: A computerized image processing scheme was developed to segment visceral and subcutaneous fat areas, and compute adiposity-related image features. Then, logistic regression models were applied to analyze association between the scheme-generated assessment scores and progression-free survival (PFS) of patients using a leave-one-case-out cross-validation method and a dataset involving 32 patients.

Results: The correlation coefficients between automated and radiologist's manual segmentation of visceral and subcutaneous fat areas were 0.76 and 0.89, respectively. The scheme-generated prediction scores using adiposity-related radiographic image features significantly associated with patients' PFS ($p < 0.01$).

Conclusion: Using a computerized scheme enables to more efficiently and robustly segment visceral and subcutaneous fat areas. The computed adiposity-related image features also have potential to improve accuracy in predicting chemotherapy outcome.

Keywords: Computer-aided detection (CAD), Quantitative image feature analysis, Prediction of chemotherapy outcome, Clinical image markers for cancer prognosis prediction

Background

Due to the cancer heterogeneity, patient response to a specific therapeutic treatment varies significantly. In order to improve cancer treatment efficacy, the recent Precision Medicine Initiative calls for developing a new cancer treatment strategy that takes individual variability into account [1]. This requires using effective biomarkers to more accurately characterize patients and/or predict clinical outcome of the patients in participation of the targeted chemotherapy. Although many cancer genomic biomarkers have been discovered [2], which aim to optimally select the targeted therapies to treat cancer patients [3], using existing biomarkers to determine a specific therapeutic treatment strategy for

individual patients remains a clinically difficult task because 1) many biomarkers are only applicable to a small group of patients [4, 5], 2) genomic tests are often invasive and expensive [6] and 3) most genomic biomarkers have lower specificity [7]. Therefore, radiographic imaging tests are still important in cancer diagnosis and prognosis assessment. However, reading and interpreting medical images in the clinical imaging facilities has several limitations including the large inter-reader variability and the lack of methods to quantitatively assess useful image features.

In order to overcome these limitations, developing new quantitative image feature analysis methods to increase the discriminatory power in predicting cancer risk and prognosis has attracted wide research interest and efforts recently [8–10]. For example, using the new concept of "Radiomics," some researchers believed that one can use the quantitative image features computed from

* Correspondence: yunzhi.wang-1@ou.edu
[1]School of Electrical and Computer Engineering, University of Oklahoma, Norman, OK 73019, USA
Full list of author information is available at the end of the article

medical images including computed tomography (CT) and magnetic resonance imaging (MRI) to build new predictive models to phenotype gene-protein signatures and/or genomic biomarkers. As a result, using quantitative feature analysis has potential to produce new clinical markers to better assist cancer diagnosis and prognosis assessment [11, 12]. However, a prerequisite of developing a reliable quantitative image feature analysis approach is developing an accurate automated image segmentation scheme, which remains a challenging task. Although researchers have previously developed and tested many different computerized schemes to detect and segment different types of suspicious lesions or anatomic structures depicting on different types of medical images, selecting and/or applying which segmentation algorithms depends on the specific application tasks.

Recently, much research effort has been spent on the development of image processing based clinical decision support systems. For example, we previously investigated the feasibility of applying quantitative image feature analysis methods to identify image markers for assisting prediction of prognosis and treatment efficacy of several different types of cancers, which include breast [13], lung [14], and ovarian cancer patients [15, 16]; Ramirez et al. tested an image parameter selection and support vector machine based framework for improving early detection of Alzheimer's disease [17]; Olsen et al. developed an image-processing based system to enable dental caries detection [18]. In existing image based decision support systems for prognosis and treatment assessment of ovarian cancer, all of the previous studies only computed image features from the segmented tumors from either CT or MR images. For example, Qiu et al. extracted image features related to tumor volume, density and variance for predicting clinical benefit of treating ovarian cancer at early stage [15]; Tan et al. applied a B-spline based image registration process to identify or track tumor changes and assess treatment response [16]. However, besides tumor-related image features, the patients' overall health condition and other non-tumor related image features may also be important to indicate how the patients will respond to (or receive benefit or not from) the chemotherapy. For example, angiogenesis played a fundamental role in the pathogenesis of epithelial ovarian cancer (EOC) with higher vascular endothelial growth factor (VEGF) expression. It promotes tumor growth, ascites and metastasis [19]. Thus, a bevacizumab-based therapy that targets the angiogenesis-specific pathways has been developed and tested to treat EOC patients in the clinical trials [20–22], which indicated that some EOC patients received benefit with increased progression-free survival (PFS) or overall survival (OS) [21], while some others did not receive any benefit with shorter PFS and OS [20]. Because of the high toxicity and other harmful side effects of using bevacizumab-based chemotherapy [23], it is important to rationally select who are most likely to receive the benefit from bevacizumab or other antiangiogenic therapies among the EOC patients [24]. Among the image feature based clinical markers, a recent study has shown that the ratio of visceral fat areas (VFA) and subcutaneous fat areas (SFA) has been recognized as potentially useful features to predict clinical outcome of bevacizumab-based chemotherapy [25]. However, manually segmenting VFA and SFA in a large number of CT image slices is quite tedious and often inconsistent due to the intra- and inter-reader variability.

In order to overcome the difficulty of manual segmentation and improve consistency and efficiency of SFA and VFA segmentation, we proposed and developed a new computer-aided image feature analysis scheme to automatically segment and quantify the entire volume of the VFA and SFA computed from the abdominal CT images of the EOC patients. We compared the correlation between the fat areas (VFA and SFA) segmented by the automated scheme on volumetric CT image data and a radiologist on one selected CT image slice of each testing case. In addition, to test the potential clinical utility of applying this automated scheme to predict prognosis or treatment efficacy of the EOC patients based on new quantitative image feature analysis method, we also built two logistic regression models using the image features computed from the segmented VFA and SFA and assess the feasibility of applying the new computerized scheme to identify and/or select EOC patients who are most likely to get benefit from receiving the bevacizumab-based chemotherapy.

Methods

In this study, a retrospectively collected image dataset that involves CT images of 32 patients was assembled based on our Institutional Review Board (IRB) approved data collection and study protocol. All patients were diagnosed and treated with advanced Stage III and IV epithelial ovarian cancer (EOC) in our University Medical Center. For each patient, the contrast enhanced perfusion CT image scans were performed post the primary cyto-reductive surgery and prior to the chemotherapy initiation. All the perfusion CT images were scanned and produced using a GE LightSpeed VCT 64-detector or a GE Discovery 600 16-detector CT machine. As an established testing protocol in our University Medical Center, X-ray power output of the CT machine was set at 120 kVp and a variable range from 100 to 600 mA depending on body size of the patient. In each examination, 100 cc contrast agent of Isovue 370 was intravenously injected using a standard power injector with a rate of 2-3 cc/second before starting CT image scanning.

As a standard procedure, each patient also received chemotherapy of bevacizumab (175 mg/kg) plus pacli-taxel (175 mg/m2), and plus carboplatin AUC 6 with a follow-up maintenance bevacizumab. In addition, we collected the PFS and OS data of all 32 patients in the dataset. Among these patients, mean age is 59.5 years old, mean weight is 70 kg along with a mean body mass index (BMI) of 26.1, and the median PFS and OS were 28.9 and 40.8 months, respectively.

For each of the EOC patients, perfusion CT was per-formed to scan from lung to pelvis, which crosses the entire abdomen region (as illustrated in Fig. 1). In each case, an upper and a lower boundary were manually placed to mark and select a CT scanning range in the entire abdomen scanning region. The upper bound of the selected CT image slices is just located below the lung area, while the lower bound of the region is just placed above the umbilicus level of a patient.

We then developed and applied a computer-aided image processing scheme to (1) detect and segment vis-ceral fat area (VFA) and subcutaneous fat area (SFA) on the masked or selected abdominal CT image slices, and (2) compute volumes of VFA and SFA, as well as the fat density distribution related image features. Figure 2 shows a flow diagram of our computer-aided scheme in detecting and segmenting VFA and SFA with the follow-ing four image processing steps.

First, the scheme was used to detect and segment a body trunk region from the background including air and CT bed depicting on each CT image slice as shown in Fig. 3a. This was done using a previously developed and tested algorithm of automated CT image segmenta-tion [26]. In this method, an operating threshold of −140 HU (determined by previous experiments) is applied to generate a body trunk related mask. Using this thresh-old, the scheme scans the images from four edges of the CT image slice line-by-line in four different directions

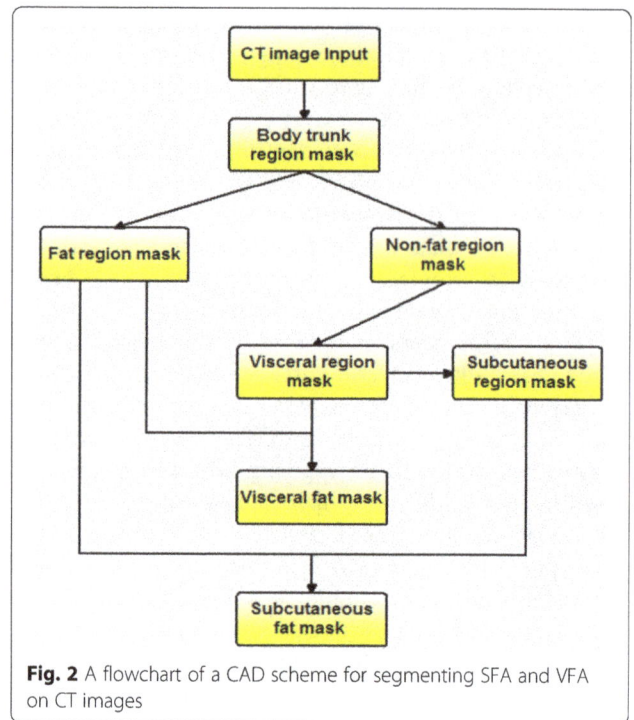

Fig. 2 A flowchart of a CAD scheme for segmenting SFA and VFA on CT images

namely, from top to bottom, from bottom to top, from left to right, and from right to left, to determine the pixels of the mask boundary. Specifically, in each linear scan, the scheme scans each pixel along the line and keeps moving forward until it hits a pixel, which has a HU value greater than the predetermined threshold. The scheme then defines this pixel as a boundary pixel of a body trunk mask and the scan along this line stops. Once the body trunk mask was defined (as shown in Fig. 3b, it is straightforward to apply this mask on the CT image slice to segment the body section and remove other air background and CT bed sections from the image slice (Fig. 3c).

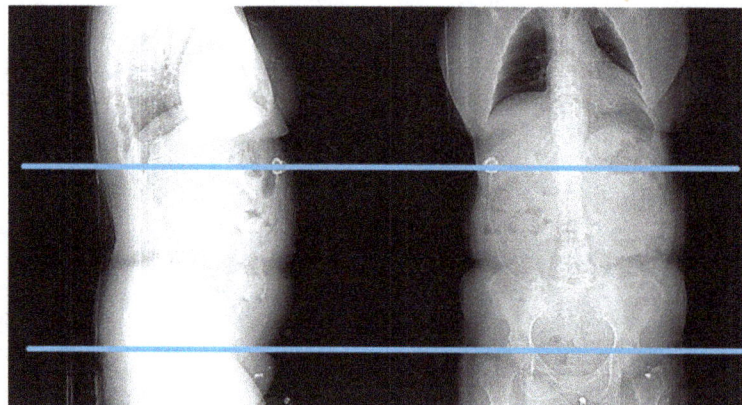

Fig. 1 Illustration of CT image scanning range (between two horizontal bars) selected by the CAD scheme to segment VFA and SFA and compute the corresponding image features

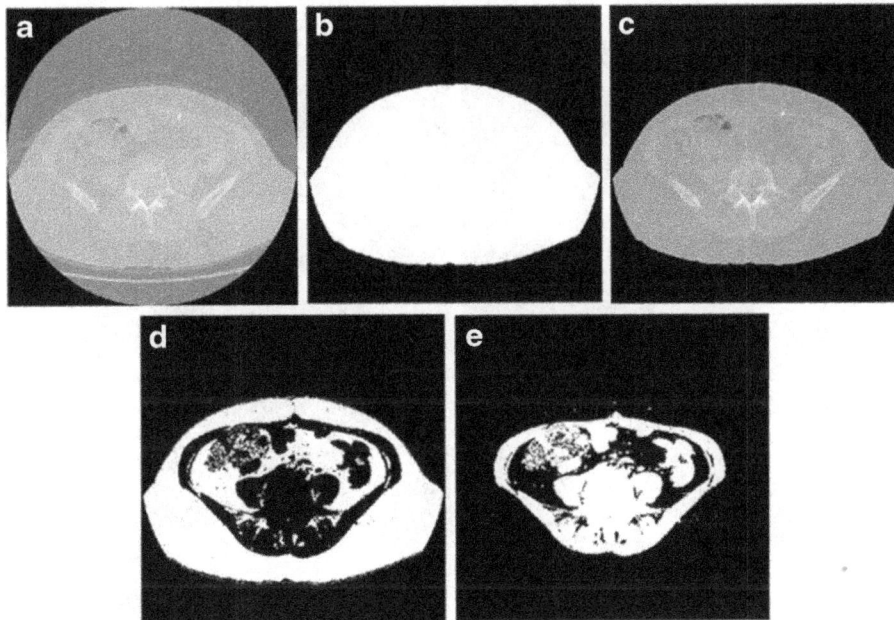

Fig. 3 An example of applying our CAD scheme to segment a CT image slice. **a** An original CT image, **b** a CAD-generated body trunk mask, **c** segmented body region, **d** a CAD-generated fat region mask, and **e** a CAD-generated non-fat region mask

Second, since CT numbers of the fat pixels range from −140 HU to −40 HU as defined in the previous study [27], these two values are used by the scheme as two operating thresholds to define and segment the body region within the body trunk mask placed on the CT image. The scheme then generates two new masks to cover the fat and non-fat regions as represented by white pixels in Fig. 3d and e, respectively.

Third, in attempt to detect between VFA and SFA regions, the scheme applies several image processing algorithms to the non-fat region mask and then produces a new visceral region mask [28]. As shown in an example of Fig. 4, a 4-pixel connected labelling algorithm was applied to the non-fat region mask. The scheme removes the connected regions with sizes smaller than a predefined threshold (e.g., 200). As a result, all small and isolated pixels located inside the SFA region were discarded. The scheme then applies a morphological dilation operation with a spherical kernel to the non-fat image region. This process breaks the potential connection between SFA and VFA regions in some CT slices. Last, the scheme creates a visceral region mask by performing a hole-filling algorithm to cover all non-fat structures after a morphological erosion operation (e.g., Fig. 4d).

Fourth, the scheme defines (1) a VFA mask by performing an "AND" logic operator between the fat region mask (e.g., Fig. 3d) and the visceral region mask (e.g., Fig. 4d) and (2) a SFA mask by performing another "AND" logic operator between the fat region mask and body truck mask (e.g., Fig. 3c minus the visceral region mask). After

completing the above image processing steps, the scheme is able to classify all image pixels in fat region mask as either the subcutaneous fat pixels or the visceral fat pixels.

Last, these four image processing steps are iteratively performed on all CT slices in the preselected abdominal section of each patient. Our computer-aided scheme was applied to process all 32 cases in our dataset to detect and segment VFA and SFA regions. Although in many previous studies, the manually traced segmentation results were often used as "ground truth" to evaluate accuracy of the automated segmentation, the manually traced boundaries typically suffer from significant inter-reader variability and results in the lower reproducibility [29]. To balance this limitation, we took two approaches and two criteria to evaluate segmentation accuracy of our CAD scheme. First, for each case, SFA and VFA were also manually segmented and measured by a radiologist on one cross-sectional CT image slice visually selected at the umbilicus level using the previous standard method reported in the literature [27]. We then computed the correlation coefficient between the manually segmented SFA/VFA and CAD-segmented/measured SFA/VFA, which is the first evaluation criterion used in this study. Second, since we recognized that the "ground-truth" provided by one radiologist may not be reliable, our ultimate goal is to assess whether we can use quantitative fat or adiposity-related image features that are computed from the automatically segmented VFA and SFA to predict prognosis or clinical outcome of the patients in participation of the targeted chemotherapy.

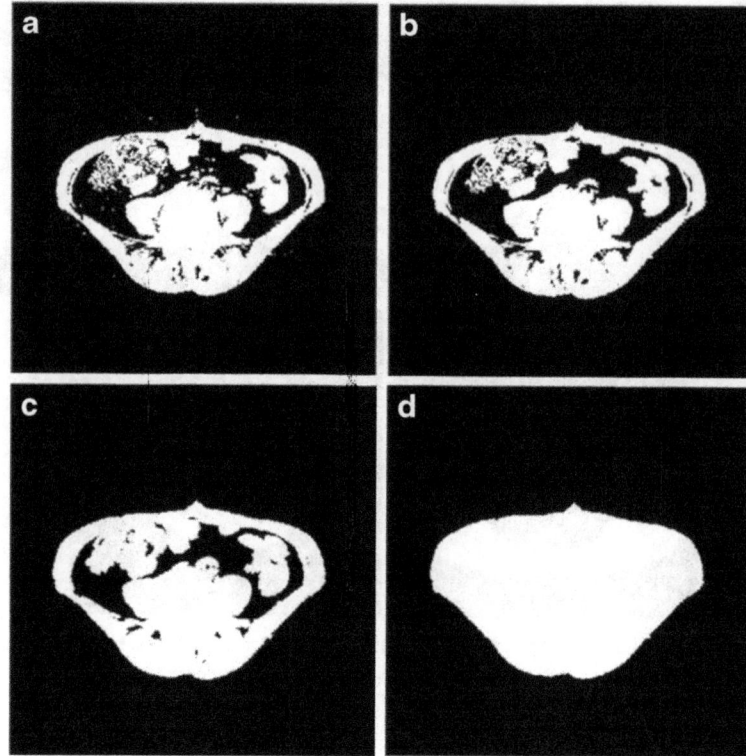

Fig. 4 Illustration of defining a visceral region mask, **a** A mask of non-fat area, **b** after removing the small and isolated regions using a pixel labeling algorithm, **c** after a morphological dilation operation, and **d** a mask to cover the entire visceral region

Therefore, our second evaluation criterion is the accuracy of predicting clinical outcomes of the patients using the computed fat image features.

Thus, to predict clinical outcome of the patients, we applied our computer-aided scheme to compute seven image features from the entire segmented CT image slices, which include (1) the ratio (or percentage) of either VFA or SFA volumes as comparing to the whole body volume (size) computed from all scheme-processed CT image slices in the targeted abdominal section, (2) the mean and standard deviation of the CT HU number (pixel value) of the VFA and SFA, and (3) the ratio between the segmented volume between SFA and VFA. In summary, combining with the pre-measured body mass index (BMI) of each patient, we built an image feature pool that includes eight features: f_1 – BMI, f_2 – Ratio between SFA and the whole body size; f_3 – Ratio between VFA and the whole body size; f_4 – Mean CT number of the segmented SFA volume; f_5 – Standard deviation of the CT number of all SFA-related pixels; f_6 – Mean CT number of the segmented VFA volume; and f_7 – Standard deviation of the CT number of all VFA-related pixels.

Next, we applied logistic regression approaches or models that combine BMI and the computed quantitative features to predict patient's clinical outcome (PFS or OS). Since a logistic regression based statistical classification model can use or combine two or more continuous variables (or features) to generate binary outcomes that indicate which class the observations (or test samples) belong to [30], we in this study built and optimized two multiple logistic regression classifiers or models to predict PFS and OS of the EOC patients, respectively. For this purpose, PFS and OS values of 32 patients were divided into two classes by using the median PFS and OS value of these 32 patients as the threshold. Two classes then indicate "long" and "short" survival (for both indices of PFS and OS). Specifically, we divided 16 cases into "long" survival and 16 cases into "short" survival classes based on the actually clinical outcome data of these 32 patients. Then, a logistic regression based statistical prediction model was trained and performed to classify these 32 testing cases into these two "long" and "short" survival classes based on the scheme (or model) generated prediction scores.

In order to identify optimal feature set and eliminate un-correlated features to build each model, we applied a Sequential Forward Floating Selection (SFFS) [31] feature subset selection algorithm to identify and select the feature subset with high discriminatory power. In order to minimize the training bias of the logistic regression model, the model performance was trained and tested using a leave-one-case-out (LOCO) based cross-validation method [32]. Specifically, in each model training and testing iteration, the scheme selects 31 cases to train the model and uses one remaining case to test the remaining. SFFS was performed on the training cases to select a subset of features and logistic regression was optimized using these selected features. The evaluation index used in this training and testing process is an area under a receiver operating characteristic (ROC) curve (AUC), which is computed using a maximum likelihood data analysis based ROC curve fitting program (ROCKT, http://metz-roc.uchicago.edu/MetzROC/software, University of Chicago). After building an optimal prediction model, we compared the classification accuracy to a null binomial distribution $B(\eta, \rho)$ and investigated the significance of the classification performance over a random guess level. Here η is the total observations and ρ is a random guess accuracy (i.e. 0.5). Meanwhile, the classification or prediction accuracy after adding image features was also compared with that using BMI feature only.

Results

Figure 5 shows two images that are marked with the segmented VFA and SFA regions depicting on two abdominal CT image slices of interest, which are acquired from two EOC patients in which one patient has substantially higher SFA ratio (a) than another patient (b). Figure 6 shows two scatter plots of the manually segmented SFA/VFA volumes (in cm^2) and the CAD-segmented/measured SFA/VFA percentage (in %) among all 32 cases in our dataset. The computed correlation coefficients between manual and automated data are 0.886 for SFA and 0.726 for VFA, respectively, which shows a relatively higher correlation of the SFA and VFA segmented between a radiologist and our CAD scheme.

Table 1 summarized the performance of applying the two logistic regression based statistical prediction models to classify the EOC patients in our dataset into two classes of "long" and "short" survival based on the known clinical outcome criteria of both PFS and OS of the patients. It demonstrated that the classification accuracy of PFS was significantly greater ($p < 0.01$) than a binomial null distribution with chance level (i.e. 0.5) accuracy, while the difference is not significant for the logistic regression model used to predict OS. Table 2 ranked the importance of the features for predicting PFS according to their frequencies of being selected by SFFS in the LOO process. It shows that quantitative features were more frequently selected by SFFS and thus possibly more discriminative for predicting PFS than BMI.

Table 3 includes and compares two confusion matrixes when using (1) BMI and (2) quantitative features selected by SFFS. When using BMI, 18 of 32 cases were predicted or classified into the correct classes with an overall classification accuracy of 56.3 %. Both positive and negative predictive values are 56.3 % (9/16). After building a logistic regression model using SFFS-selected image features, the overall new model classification accuracy increased to 87.5 % (28/32), which represents a 55.6 % increase as comparing to using BMI only. The results show that the feasibility of using the computed quantitative image features to provide valuable supplementary or complementary information to help increase accuracy in predicting or assessing clinical outcome of the patients treating with chemotherapy.

Discussion

Identifying quantitative image feature based clinical markers that correlate well with the patients' clinical outcome is important to establish an optimal personalized cancer treatment strategy and/or develop precision medicine in the future. For this purpose, many studies have been performed by a number of research groups including our group to explore, identify and compute different image feature analysis based clinical markers

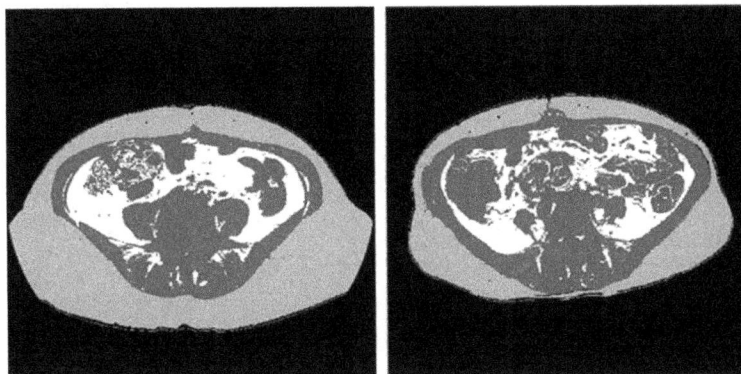

Fig. 5 Two examples showing the segmentation of VFA and SFA in four CT image slices. In these two images, SFA is shown in *light gray* color, VFA is represented by *white* color, and *dark gray* color masks other human organs and/or structures

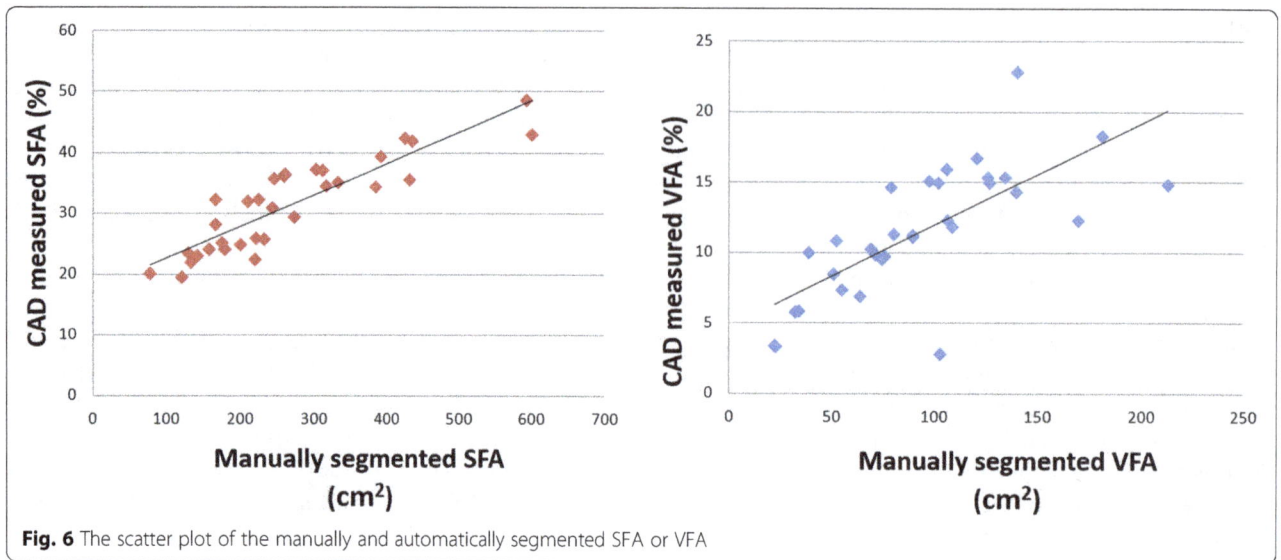

Fig. 6 The scatter plot of the manually and automatically segmented SFA or VFA

[13–18]. This study is different from the previous studies in this field (e.g., Radiomics). We demonstrated that the image features computed from non-tumor regions could also provide important and/or supplemental information to assist predicting response of cancer patients to the chemotherapy. Although this study only predicted whether the EOC patients can benefit from receiving the bevacizumab-based chemotherapy, the new computer-aided image processing scheme provides a new quantitative image marker that is also applicable to analyze PFS or OS of EOC patients without receiving maintenance bevacizumab therapy [33] and/or many other different types of cancer patients underwent similar chemotherapy because the angiogenesis and/or vascular endothelial growth factor (VEGF) expression play a fundamental role in the pathogenesis of many types of cancers. Thus, accurately or quantitatively assessment of SFA and VFA is important to determine whether and how the cancer patients should be optimally treated using bevacizumab or other against angiogenesis related chemotherapy.

Since accurate SFA and VFA segmentation is the first step to develop a reliably quantitative image feature analysis approach, which will determine the accuracy of the computed image features as well as the final model prediction results, we developed a simple, computationally efficient and robustly performed scheme to segment SFA and VFA from the volumetric CT image data. Our

scheme applies four image processing steps based on the modified region growing algorithms to define a number of corresponding masks that cluster and classify the pixels of each CT image slice into four categories namely, (1) outside the body, (2) SFA, (3) VFA and (4) other human internal organs. We applied this automated image segmentation scheme to all 32 cases in our dataset and visually examined the segmentation results. We did not visually identify any significant segmentation errors in this dataset. We also asked an experienced radiologist to manually segment/trace the SFA and VFA boundary on one CT image of each case using the method reported in the literature [25]. We then computed and compared the correlation coefficients between the manual and automated segmentation results in both SFA and VFA. The relatively higher correlation as shown in Fig. 6 indicates that automated scheme could be used to replace the manual segmentation. Although due to the lack of accurate "ground-truth," it is often difficult to evaluate the absolute region segmentation accuracy of using an automated scheme, using the computer-aided image segmentation scheme has several advantages to

Table 1 Summary of performance in classifying the two classes of "longer" and "shorter" survival using the multiple logistic regression models

Clinical Outcomes	Prediction accuracy	p-value over null hypothesis	AUC	95 % confidence interval
PFS	0.875	9.65×10^{-6}	0.827	(0.634,0.938)
OS	0.531	0.43	0.505	(0306,0.702)

Table 2 Rank of features according to the frequencies of being selected by SFFS for predicting PFS

Feature ID	Frequency of Selection
f_2	23/32
f_6	8/32
f_3	2/32
f_4	2/32
f_1	0/32
f_5	0/32
f_7	0/32

Table 3 Comparison of two computed confusion matrixes between using BMI and SFFS-selected image features to classify patients into two "longer" and "shorter" PFS classes

PFS class	BMI		SFFS-selected features	
	Long	Short	Long	Short
Long	9	7	15	1
Short	7	9	3	13

yield high efficient and also avoid inter-reader variability. In another aspect, changes of parameters in the segmentation model only affect the segmentation results of a small percentage of selected CT slices. As a result, measurement from multiple CT slices may provide more robust and accurate results than from a single CT slice.

We also tested the performance of using a number of image features computed from the automatically segmented SFA and VFA regions from CT images to classify the patients into the "long" and "short" survival class groups after receiving the bevacizumab-based chemotherapy. We applied a simple logistic regression based statistical data analysis method to build prediction models and demonstrated that the model-prediction scores have a statistically significant association with the PFS of the EOC patients. It is also quite encouraging to observe from the study results that using the computed SFA and VFA image features yielded substantially higher prediction accuracy than using BMI (as shown in Table 3). Since BMI is computed from height and weight from the patients and is the most commonly used measurement of adiposity in current clinical practices, our results demonstrated that the quantitative features may provide supplementary and useful information other than BMI. This is a more important evidence to support the potentially clinical utility of applying our CAD-based automated SFA and VFA segmentation scheme. Using the CAD scheme, we are able to compute not only the size or volume of SFA and VFA similar to the previous manual method [25], and also other related image features (i.e., the CT number distribution, which relates to the heterogeneity of the SFA and VFA). This is also an importantly potential advantage of developing and applying our CAD scheme.

Despite the promising results, this is a preliminary study with several limitations. First, the dataset size is small and CT images were collected from a single medical institution (or a single CT imaging acquisition protocol). Thus, the 95 % confidence intervals of the AUC values as shown in Table 1 are relatively large. To overcome this issue, further studies and better cross-validation using the new independent datasets are needed before this computer-aided image processing scheme can be accepted and integrated into the advanced quantitative image feature analysis schemes to more accurately predict clinical outcome of EOC patients

underwent bevacizumab or other types of chemotherapy. Second, the selection of multiple CT slices belonging to abdomen part was manually processed, which was time-consuming and may introduce inter and intra reader variability. Therefore, further studies will focus on developing automated framework for CT slices selection. Third, due to the limited dataset, the scheme-generated classification scores only significantly associate with PFS, but not OS of EOC patients receiving maintenance bevacizumab based chemotherapy in this study. Further efforts (e.g. extract more features or collect a larger dataset) are required to validate whether OS is significantly related to adiposity characteristics of EOC patients.

Conclusion

In this study we developed and applied a new computer-aided image segmentation scheme to segment SFA and VFA regions from the volumetric CT image data. We also trained and tested logistic regression models to combine a number of quantitative image features computed from the segmented VFA and SFA regions. Using the leave-one-case-out cross-validation method, our experimental results showed that using this new computer-aided scheme or prediction model enabled to generate a new radiographic image feature marker, which could help more accurately predict which EOC patients are most likely to benefit from receiving maintenance bevacizumab-based chemotherapy than using the traditional BMI based approach. Meanwhile, we also recognized the limitations of this study and identified future research tasks or directions. In summary, we believe that this is a valid technology development study, which demonstrated the feasibility of developing and providing clinical researchers a new computer-aided image processing tool to quantitatively assess a potentially important radiographic image-marker and investigate its association with clinical outcome of cancer patients underwent variety of chemotherapy treatment.

Acknowledgements
This work was supported in part by Grant R01 CA197150 from the National Cancer Center, National Institutes of Health and Grant HR15-016 from the State of Oklahoma Center for the Advancement of Science and Technology. The authors also acknowledge the support received from the Peggy and Charles Stephenson Cancer Center, University of Oklahoma.

Authors' contributions
YW and Dr. YQ developed image processing algorithms, did data analysis and wrote the initial draft of the manuscript. Dr. TT and Dr. KM provided image datasets and truth file, participated in design of this study protocol, and provided clinical advises. Dr. HL and Dr. BZ provided advises of study design and helped write the manuscript. All authors read and approved the final manuscript.

Competing interest
The authors declare that they have no competing interests.

Author details
[1]School of Electrical and Computer Engineering, University of Oklahoma, Norman, OK 73019, USA. [2]Health Science Center of University of Oklahoma, Oklahoma City, OK 73104, USA.

References

1. Collins FS, Varmus H. A new initiative on precision medicine. N Engl J Med. 2015;372(9):793–5.

2. Chiarle R, Voena C, Ambrogio C, Piva R, Inghirami G. The anaplastic lymphoma kinase in the pathogenesis of cancer. Nat Rev Cancer. 2008;8(1):11–23.

3. Goetsch CM. Genetic tumor profiling and genetically targeted cancer therapy. In: Seminars in oncology nursing: 2011. Philadelphia, USA: WB Saunders; 2011. p. 34–44.

4. Hagen AI, Kvistad KA, Maehle L, Holmen MM, Aase H, Styr B, Vabø A, Apold J, Skaane P, Møller P. Sensitivity of MRI versus conventional screening in the diagnosis of BRCA-associated breast cancer in a national prospective series. Breast. 2007;16(4):367–74.

5. Kobayashi S, Boggon TJ, Dayaram T, Jänne PA, Kocher O, Meyerson M, Johnson BE, Eck MJ, Tenen DG, Halmos B. EGFR mutation and resistance of non–small-cell lung cancer to gefitinib. N Engl J Med. 2005;352(8):786–92.

6. Herper M, Gene test for Pfizer cancer drug to cost $1,500 per patient, Forbes 8/29/2011; www.forbes.com/sites/matthewherper/2011/08/29/gene-test-for-pfizer-cancer-drug-to-cost-1500-per-patient. Accessed 29 Aug 2011.

7. Diamandis EP. Mass spectrometry as a diagnostic and a cancer biomarker discovery tool opportunities and potential limitations. Mol Cell Proteomics. 2004;3(4):367–78.

8. Bhooshan N, Giger M, Edwards D, Yuan Y, Jansen S, Li H, Lan L, Sattar H, Newstead G. Computerized three-class classification of MRI-based prognostic markers for breast cancer. Phys Med Biol. 2011;56(18):5995.

9. Lambin P, Rios-Velazquez E, Leijenaar RT, Carvalho S, van Stiphout RG, Granton P, Zegers CM, Gillies R, Boellard R, Dekker A. Radiomics: extracting more information from medical images using advanced feature analysis. Eur J Cancer. 2012;48(4):441–6.

10. Tan M, Pu J, Cheng S, Liu H, Zheng B. Assessment of a four-view mammographic image feature based fusion model to predict near-term breast cancer risk. Ann Biomed Eng. 2015;43(10):2416–28.

11. Aerts HJ, Velazquez ER, Leijenaar RT, Parmar C, Grossmann P, Carvalho S, Bussink J, Monshouwer R, Haibe-Kains B, Rietveld D. Decoding tumour phenotype by noninvasive imaging using a quantitative radiomics approach. Nat Commun. 2014;5:4006.

12. Kumar V, Gu Y, Basu S, Berglund A, Eschrich SA, Schabath MB, Forster K, Aerts HJ, Dekker A, Fenstermacher D. Radiomics: the process and the challenges. Magn Reson Imaging. 2012;30(9):1234–48.

13. Aghaei F, Tan M, Hollingsworth AB, Zheng B. Applying a new quantitative global breast MRI feature analysis scheme to assess tumor response to chemotherapy. J. Magn. Reson. Imaging. 2016. DOI: 10.1002/jmri.25276

14. Emaminejad N, Qian W, Guan Y, Tan M, Qiu Y, Liu H, Zheng B. Fusion of quantitative image and genomic biomarkers to improve prognosis assessment of early stage lung cancer patients. IEEE Trans Biomed Eng. 2016;63(5):1034–43.

15. Qiu Y, Tan M, McMeekin S, Thai T, Ding K, Moore K, Liu H, Zheng B. Early prediction of clinical benefit of treating ovarian cancer using quantitative CT image feature analysis. Acta Radiologica. 2015. doi:10.1177/0284185115620947

16. Tan M, Li Z, Qiu Y, McMeekin SD, Thai TC, Ding K, Moore KN, Liu H, Zheng B. A new approach to evaluate drug treatment response of ovarian cancer patients based on deformable image registration. IEEE Trans Med Imaging. 2016;35(1):316–25.

17. Ramírez J, Górriz J, Salas-Gonzalez D, Romero A, López M, Álvarez I, Gómez-Río M. Computer-aided diagnosis of Alzheimer's type dementia combining support vector machines and discriminant set of features. Inf Sci. 2013;237:59–72.

18. Olsen GF, Brilliant SS, Primeaux D, Najarian K: An image-processing enabled dental caries detection system. In: Complex Medical Engineering, 2009 CME ICME International Conference on: 2009: NJ, USA: IEEE; 2009. p. 1–8.

19. Abulafia O, Triest WE, Sherer DM. Angiogenesis in primary and metastatic epithelial ovarian carcinoma. Am J Obstet Gynecol. 1997;177(3):541–7.

20. Burger RA, Brady MF, Bookman MA, Monk BJ, Walker JL, Homesley HD, Fowler J, Greer BE, Boente M, Fleming GF. Risk factors for GI adverse events in a phase III randomized trial of Bevacizumab in first-line therapy of advanced ovarian cancer: a gynecologic oncology group study. J Clin Oncol. 2014;32(12):1210–7.

21. Burger RA, Brady MF, Rhee J, Sovak MA, Kong G, Nguyen HP, Bookman MA. Independent radiologic review of the gynecologic oncology group study 0218, a phase III trial of Bevacizumab in the primary treatment of advanced epithelial ovarian, primary peritoneal, or fallopian tube cancer. Gynecol Oncol. 2013;131(1):21–6.

22. Perren TJ, Swart AM, Pfisterer J, Ledermann JA, Pujade-Lauraine E, Kristensen G, Carey MS, Beale P, Cervantes A, Kurzeder C. A phase 3 trial of bevacizumab in ovarian cancer. N Engl J Med. 2011;365(26):2484–96.

23. Teoh D, Secord AA. Antiangiogenic therapies in epithelial ovarian cancer. Cancer Control. 2011;18(1):31–43.

24. Guiu B, Petit JM, Bonnetain F, Ladoire S, Guiu S, Cercueil J-P, Krausé D, Hillon P, Borg C, Chauffert B. Visceral fat area is an independent predictive biomarker of outcome after first-line bevacizumab-based treatment in metastatic colorectal cancer. Gut. 2010;59(3):341–7.

25. Slaughter KN, Thai T, Penaroza S, Benbrook DM, Thavathiru E, Ding K, Nelson T, McMeekin DS, Moore KN. Measurements of adiposity as clinical biomarkers for first-line bevacizumab-based chemotherapy in epithelial ovarian cancer. Gynecol Oncol. 2014;133(1):11–5.

26. Leader JK, Zheng B, Rogers RM, Sciurba FC, Perez A, Chapman BE, Patel S, Fuhrman CR, Gur D. Automated lung segmentation in X-ray computed tomography: development and evaluation of a heuristic threshold-based scheme 1. Acad Radiol. 2003;10(11):1224–36.

27. Yoshizumi T, Nakamura T, Yamane M, Waliul Islam AHM, Menju M, Yamasaki K, Arai T, Kotani K, Funahashi T, Yamashita S. Abdominal fat: Standardized technique for measurement at ct 1. Radiology. 1999;211(1):283–6.

28. Liou T-H, Chan WP, Pan L-C, Lin P, Chou P, Chen C-H. Fully automated large-scale assessment of visceral and subcutaneous abdominal adipose tissue by magnetic resonance imaging. Int J Obes. 2006;30(5):844–52.

29. Stroom J, Blaauwgeers H, van Baardwijk A, Boersma L, Lebesque J, Theuws J, van Suylen R-J, Klomp H, Liesker K, van Pel R. Feasibility of pathology-correlated lung imaging for accurate target definition of lung tumors. Int J Radiat Oncol Biol Phys. 2007;69(1):267–75.

30. Hosmer Jr DW, Lemeshow S. Applied logistic regression. Hoboken: John Wiley & Sons; 2004

31. Pudil P, Ferri F, Novovicova J, Kittler J: Floating search methods for feature selection with nonmonotonic criterion functions. In: In Proceedings of the Twelveth International Conference on Pattern Recognition, IAPR: 1994. NJ, USA: IEEE; 1994.

32. Li Q, Doi K. Reduction of bias and variance for evaluation of computer-aided diagnostic schemes. Med Phys. 2006;33(4):868–75.

33. Wang Y, Thai T, Moore K, Ding K, McMeekin S, Liu H, Zheng B. Quantitative measurement of adiposity using CT images to predict the benefit of bevacizumab-based chemotherapy in epithelial ovarian cancer patients. Oncol Letter. 2016;12:680–6.

14

Magnetic resonance enterography changes after antibody to tumor necrosis factor (anti-TNF) alpha therapy in Crohn's disease: correlation with SES-CD and clinical-biological markers

Luca Pio Stoppino[1]*, Nicola Della Valle[2], Stefania Rizzi[1], Elsa Cleopazzo[1], Annarita Centola[1], Donatello Iamele[1], Christos Bristogiannis[1], Giuseppe Stoppino[3], Roberta Vinci[1] and Luca Macarini[1]

Abstract

Background: In recent years, the use of MRI in patients with Crohn's disease (CD) has increased. However, few data are available on how MRI parameters of active disease change during treatment with anti-TNF and whether these changes correspond to symptoms, serum biomarkers, or endoscopic appearance. The aim of this study was to determine the changes over time in MRI parameters during treatment with anti-TNF in patients with CD, and to verify the correlation between MRI score, endoscopic appearance and clinical-biological markers.

Methods: We performed a prospective single centre study of 27 patients with active CD (18 males and 9 females; median age of 27,4 ys; age range, 19–49). All patients underwent ileocolonoscopy and MRI at baseline and 26 weeks after anti-TNF therapy. Endoscopic severity was graded according to the Simple Endoscopic Score for Crohn's Disease (SES-CD) and Magnetic Resonance Index of Activity (MaRIA) was calculated. Patients underwent clinical evaluation (CDAI) and the C-reactive protein (CRP) level was measured. The associations between variables were assessed with Pearson's bivariate correlation analysis.

Results: A total of 135 intestinal segments were studied. The median patient age was 27,4 years, 67 % were male and the mean disease duration was 6,1 years. For induction of remission, 18 patients were treated with infliximab and 9 with adalimumab. The mean SES-CD and MaRIA scores significantly changed at week 26 (SES-CD: 14,7 ± 8,9 at baseline vs. 4,4 ± 4,6 at 26 weeks - $p < 0.001$; MaRIA: 41,1 ± 14,8 at baseline vs. 32,8 ± 11,7 at 26 weeks - $p < 0.001$). Also the CDAI and serum levels of CRP decreased significantly following treatment ($p < 0.001$). The overall MaRIA correlated with endoscopic score and with clinical activity (CDAI) both at baseline and at week 26 ($p < 0.05$). The correlation between overall MaRIA and CRP was significant only at week 26 ($p < 0.001$).

Conclusions: The MaRIA has a good correlation with SES-CD, a high accuracy for prediction of endoscopic mucosal healing and is a reliable indicator to monitor the use of TNF antagonists in patients with CD.

Keywords: Crohn's disease, Magnetic resonance enterography, Anti-TNF drugs, Simple Endoscopic Score for Crohn's Disease

* Correspondence: luca.stoppino@unifg.it
[1]Division of Diagnostic Imaging, Department of Surgical Sciences, University of Foggia, Viale Luigi Pinto n.1, Foggia 71122, Italy
Full list of author information is available at the end of the article

Background

Crohn's disease (CD) is a disabling transmural and segmental chronic inflammatory bowel disease (IBD) with a relapsing and remitting course. Its inflammatory lesions can affect the entire gastrointestinal (GI) tract leading to various intestinal (internal and external fistulas, intestinal strictures, abdominal and perianal abscesses) and extra-intestinal manifestations [1].

Although its aetiology is still unknown considerable progress has been made in the understanding of the molecular mediators and mechanisms of tissue injury. Current treatment protocols, based on the use of drugs with a gradually increasing strength of action, are aimed at modulating the complex inflammatory events leading to intestinal injury [2].

The proinflammatory cytokine Tumor Necrosis Factor (TNF) alpha is a key mediator of inflammation associated with CD [3] and the recent development of antibody to TNF alpha (anti-TNF) drugs has led to significant improvements in the medical treatment of these patients [4, 5].

These antagonists of TNF-alpha, i.e. infliximab (IFX) and adalimumab (ADA), are effective in inducing as well as maintaining clinical remission in patients with moderately-to-severely active CD disease who are refractory to traditional treatments (corticosteroids and immunosuppressive drugs). Complete disappearance of mucosal ulcerations is associated with favourable outcome, and after initiation with anti-TNF, mucosal healing (MH) leads to a decrease both in relapse rates and in disease related hospitalization, reducing the need for surgery [6].

Unfortunately, the proven clinical efficacy of anti-TNF drugs is contrasted with the elevated frequency of premature relapses on discontinuing treatment once maintained remission of the disease is achieved [7]. This phenomenon is attributed to the persistence of inflammatory activity despite an apparent positive clinical response [8]. In fact, CD is a typically transmural disease and its activity can be difficult to accurately evaluate. Therefore, for assessing CD activity, for tailoring therapy, and for measuring treatment response, objective determination of inflammatory activity should be essential. The gold standard for assessment of luminal inflammation in CD is endoscopy with biopsies, which can evaluate MH but it is invasive, exposes patients to inherent procedural risks, and is unable to assess the mid-small intestine [9]. Symptom-based disease activity indexes are subjective by design and often unreliable [10].

Cross-sectional imaging can serve as an alternative or an adjunct to ileocolonoscopy to evaluate therapeutic response and transmural healing. Computed tomographic and magnetic resonance enterography have been reported to be useful modalities for the evaluation of luminal inflammation and extra intestinal complications in CD. MRI can be performed without radiation exposure,

making it the preferred imaging technique for the evaluation of CD [11]. To our knowledge the effects of the biological agents on transmural inflammation and their resulting imaging are largely unknown.

The primary aim of this study was to, therefore, determine the changes over time in MRI parameters during treatment with anti-TNF in patients with CD. Secondary aim is to examine whether radiologic response to anti-TNF treatment correlates with endoscopic appearance and clinical-biological markers.

Methods

Patients

Between April 2012 and April 2015, 27 outpatients diagnosed with CD according to the Lennard-Jones criteria (Table 1) [12], were prospectively studied at single centre. The patient cohort comprised 18 males and 9 females, with a median age of 27,4 years (age range, 19–49). The median disease duration was 6,1 years (mean SD, 2,2). Inclusion criteria were age ≥ 18, moderate-to-severe intestinal disease (Crohn's Disease Activity Index – CDAI - score > 220 points) and elevated C-reactive protein (CRP) level (>5 mg/l). Exclusion criteria were active or latent tuberculosis, contraindications for MR, treatment with more than 15 mg of systemic corticosteroids (prednisone equivalent) within the 2 weeks prior to baseline MRI, documented abdominal abscess or internal fistula as well as medical contraindications for anti TNF therapy.

Table 1 Lennard-Jones anatomic criteria for the diagnosis of CD recognizable by clinical, radiological and pathologic examination

	Clinical/ endoscopy	X-ray	Biopsy	Resected specimen
Mouth to anus				
Upper gut	+	+	+	+
Anus	+		+	+
Discontinuous	+	+	+	+
Transmural inflammation				+
Fissure		+		+
Abscess	+	+		+
Fistula	+	+		+
Fibrosis/Stenosis	+	+		+
Lymphoid				
Ulcers			+	+
Aggregates			+	+
Mucin Retention			+	
Granuloma			++	++

[a]A diagnosis of Crohn's disease requires 3 positive findings, or one positive finding with granulomas on histology

The anti-TNF treatment consisted of administering an induction regimen, either with IFX or ADA in the case of patients who had previously been treated with IFX and who had presented complications in its administration. The induction regimen for IFX consisted of administering three intravenous doses of 5 mg/Kg in weeks 0, 2 and 6, and maintenance every 8 weeks thereafter. The induction regimen for ADA consisted of an 160 mg subcutaneous injection as an initial dose, followed by 80 mg after 2 weeks and 40 mg every other week thereafter [5]. After obtaining written informed consent, endoscopy (reference standard), clinical-biological assessment and MRI were performed in all patients prior to the first anti-TNF drugs infusion and at week 26. Ileocolonoscopy and MRI were performed within a maximum interval of 7 days and the time gap between these tests and the start-end of anti-TNF therapy was to a maximum of 3 days.

Endoscopic examination

Ileocolonoscopy was considered the reference standard for the evaluation of IBD extension and severity. In all cases endoscopy was performed under anaesthesia by experienced endoscopist in IBD (NDV) using standard equipment (CV-180; Olympus, Japan) and following the standard protocol used in clinical practice (colonic cleansing with 4 L polyethylene glycol plus low-fiber diet 3 days before). The length of terminal ileum evaluated on colonoscopy ranged from 5 to 15 cm. Quantification of endoscopic lesions was calculated globally and per segment using the Simple Endoscopic Score for Crohn's Disease (SES-CD). For accuracy of endoscopic data collection, endoscopist completed the SES-CD on a predefined scoring sheet immediately after finishing the procedure.

For the grading of endoscopic findings with SES-CD, the bowel was divided into 5 segments: terminal ileum; right, transverse, and left colon; and rectum. Four endoscopic variables in the 5 segments were scored from 0 to 3 [13]. The variable "presence and size of ulcers" was scored 0 when no ulcers were present, 1 for small ulcers (diameter, 0.1–0.5 cm), 2 for medium-sized ulcers (diameter, 0.5–2 cm), and 3 for large ulcers (>2 cm). The variable "extent of ulcerated surface" was scored 0 when no ulcers were present, 1 when extent was <10 %, 2 when extent was 10 % to 30 %, and 3 when extent was >30 %. The variable "extent of affected surface" was scored 0 if none, 1 when <50 %, 2 when 50 % to 75 %, and 3 when >75 %. The variable "presence and type of narrowing" was scored 0 when no narrowing was present, 1 for a single passable narrowing, 2 for multiple passable narrowed areas, and 3 for a non-passable narrowing. The

resulting score was (Table 2): SES-CD = sum of all variables – 1,4 × number of affected segments.

The SES score can range from 0 to 60, with a higher score indicating more severe disease. Investigator reporting the endoscopic lesions was blinded to the results of the MRI examination.

Magnetic resonance enterography

All MRI examinations were performed in the supine position with a 1.5 T magnet (Achieva, Philips Medical System, Eindhoven, The Netherlands) equipped with a phased-array-16-elements coil. 1 h prior to MRI, all patients received orally 1000–1500 ml of iso-osmotic PEG solution, which was freshly prepared by dissolving in water a granular powder containing PEG (58.32 g), sodium sulphate (5.69 g) sodium bicarbonate (1.69 g), sodium chloride (1.46 g) and potassium chloride (0.74 g) (Selg 1000, Promefarm, Milan, Italy). In order to ensure an adequate intestinal distension, a coronal T2 scan was performed after 30 min after oral contrast administration. If the minimum diameter of the small bowel loops was 15 mm o larger, the bowel distension was judged satisfactory and MRI was continued after intravenous administration of 20 mg N-butylscopolamine (Buscopan, Boringher Ingelheim, Ingelheim am Rhein, Germany) in order to suppress small bowel peristalsis and avoid motion artifacts.

Then, the acquisition protocol outlined in Table 3 was performed. 3D T1-weighted high-resolution isotropic volume excitation (THRIVE) before and 30–40s, 70–90s and 120–140 s after intravenous administration of 0.2 ml/kg body weight of gadolinium chelate (Gd-DTPA, Magnevist, Schering AG, Germany) and finally a T1-weighted water selective (WATS) fat-saturated sequence in the axial plane late after injection were acquired.

Image analysis was performed by one experienced radiologist (LPS) and one junior radiologist (SR) using a dedicated postprocessing workstation (ViewForum, Philips Medical System, Eindhoven, The Netherlands). To

Table 2 Scoring sheet for SES-CD

	Ileum	Right colon	Transverse colon	Left colon	Rectum	SUM
Presence and size of ulcers						+
Extent of ulcerated surface						+
Extent of affected surface						+
Presence and type of narrowing						=
Sum of all variables						TOT
Affected segments	☐	☐	☐	☐	☐	

TOT – 1.4 × (number of affected segments) = SES-CD

Table 3 MRE protocol

	T2-TSE	T2 SPAIR	DUAL FFE	BFFE	Gd-DTPA THRIVE	T1 WATS
Plane	Axial	Axial	Axial	Coronal	Coronal (3D)	Axial
Slices thickness (mm)	5	5	5	4	1.5	5
FOV (mm)	450x450	400x400	450x450	400x400	420x420	450x450
TR (ms)	1200	1200	140	3,7	2.3	346
TE (ms)	80	80	4,6/2,3	1,9	4.7	6.6
Flip angle	90	90	80	40	10	70

allow comparison with endoscopic score, the same division into segments was considered. The small and large bowel were examined to detect the segment with the most severe lesions on the basis of the following criteria: bowel wall thickness (mm), presence of mucosal ulcers (defined as deep depressions in the mucosal surface), presence of mural oedema (hyperintensity on T2-weighted sequences of the bowel wall relative to the signal of the psoas muscle), presence of enlarged regional mesenteric lymph nodes, presence of fistula or abscess, and relative contrast enhancement (RCE) of the intestinal wall. Quantitative measurements of wall signal intensity (WSI) were obtained from the areas with the greatest thickening [region of interest (ROI)] before and after intravenous injection of gadolinium (70 s). RCE was calculated according to the following formula: RCE = [(WSI postgadolinium – WSI pregadolinium)/(WSI pregadolinium)] × 100 × (SD noise pregadolinium/SD noise postgadolinium). As defined by Rimola et al. [14, 15] for measurement of therapeutic response by means of MRI and to allow comparison with the reference standard (SES-CD), the MaRIA in each segment was calculated according to the following formula: 1.5 × wall thickening (mm) + 0.02 × RCE (relative contrast enhancement) + 5 × oedema + 10 × ulcers.

The global MaRIA score was calculated as the sum of the MaRIA in ileum, right colon, transverse colon, left colon-sigmoid and rectum.

Response assessment

In order to quantify disease activity the SES-CD and the MaRIA were calculated at baseline and 26 weeks after treatment initiation. MH was defined as the absence of mucosal ulcerations at week 26 in patients who had mucosal lesions endoscopically confirmed at baseline [16]. The endoscopic response was defined as a decrease from baseline in SES-CD score of at least 5 points and at least 50 % [17] with a complete endoscopic remission (MH) when SES-CD score ≤ 2 [18]. In MRI examinations the MH was defined as the complete disappearance of intestinal lesions at week 26, while the radiologic response was

defined as an overall MaRIA score reduction of at least 9.7 points.

In addition, the response to treatment was assessed both clinically as well as biologically by calculating the CDAI and the nephelometric determination of the serum concentration of CRP. The CDAI is a numerical calculation derived from the sum of products from a list of 8 items (Table 4), and multiplied by weighting factors for each item to define the severity of "disease activity" in patients with CD [19]. Three categories were identified to define the clinical-biological response: (a) Lack of response when the CDAI and CRP levels increased or did not change; (b) Partial response when the CDAI decreased by more than 70 points and CRP levels decreased but did not restore to normal and (c) Remission when the CDAI was lower than 150 points and CRP levels were normal.

Statistical analysis

Quantitative variables are given as means and standard deviation (SD) and proportions are expressed as percentages and 95 % confident intervals (CIs). Differences in quantitative measures were tested by Student's test. The associations between continuous variables were evaluated with Pearson's bivariate correlation analysis. To determine the best cut-off value both of the overall MaRIA and of the Δ MaRIA scores for predicting endoscopic remission (SES-CD score ≤ 2) receiver operating characteristic (ROC) curves were calculated. Inter-observer agreement between paired evaluations of MR by two radiologists (LPS and SR) was performed with Pearson correlation coefficient.

Table 4 CDAI items and weighting factors

Item (daily sum per week)	Weighting factor
Number of liquid or very soft stools	2
Abdominal pain score in one week (rating, 0–3)	5
General well-being (rating, 1–4)	7
Sum of physical findings per week:	20
Arthritis/arthralgia	
Mucocutaneous lesions (e.g. erythema nodosum, aphthous ulcers)	
Iritis/uveitis	
Anal disease (fissure, fistula, etc.)	
External fistula (enterocutaneous, vesicle, vaginal, etc.)	
Fever over 37.8 °C	
Antidiarrheal use	30
Abdominal mass (no = 0, equivocal = 2, yes = 5)	10
47 minus hematocrit (males) or 42 minus hematocrit 6 (females)	6
1-x (1-body weight divided by a standard weight)	1

The Statistical Package for the Social Sciences (version 21, SPSS Inc, Chicago, Ilinnois, USA) was used to describe and analyse the data, considering values of $p < 0.05$ as significant.

Results

27 consecutive patients were included in the study for a total of 135 segments explored by ileocolonoscopy and then evaluated by MRI. Baseline characteristics of the patients are given in Table 5. Before the administration of the anti-TNF treatment, all patients had a CDAI > 220 points, a CRP level greater than 5 mg/l and a SES-CD > 3. For induction of remission, 18 patients (67 %) were treated with IFX and 9 (33 %) with ADA.

The correlation between overall SES-CD and overall MaRIA was good at baseline ($p = 0.03$) and very high at week 26 ($p < 0.001$) (Fig. 1).

A significant correlation between overall MaRIA and CDAI, including both baseline and week 26, was observed ($p = 0.03$; $p < 0.001$, respectively). The correlation between overall MaRIA and CRP was significant only at week 26 (baseline: $p = 0.4$; week 26: $p < 0.001$). A significant correlation of the Δ MaRIA score was observed with Δ SES-CD ($p < 0.001$), Δ CDAI ($p < 0.001$) and Δ CRP ($p < 0.001$).

The administration of the anti-TNF drug induced endoscopic response in 16 patients (59 %) and among these a complete disease remission/MH (SES-CD ≤ 2) occurred in 13 patients (48 %). 10 patients (37 %) showed a stable or slightly lower SES-CD compared to baseline. Only 1 patient (4 %) had a SES-CD slightly increased at the end of the study.

Using a cut-off point of 30.8 the overall MaRIA was found to have a high accuracy for prediction of endoscopic MH (SES-CD score ≤ 2) with an area under the ROC curve of 0.967, sensitivity of 93 % and specificity of 77 % (Fig. 2). At week 26 the overall MaRIA score was < 30.8 in 13 patients (48 %; Fig. 3).

Table 5 Baseline characteristics of the patients

Patients $n = 27$	
M/F	18/9
Age at diagnosis [median]	27,4
Disease duration [years, mean (SD)]	6,1 (2,2)
Disease location	
-Rectum	0
-Sigmoid/Left colon	9
-Transverse colon	3
-Right colon	3
-Ileum	27
Anti-TNF drugs	
-IFX	18
-ADA	9

A Δ MaRIA score ≥ 9.7 had a good diagnostic accuracy for predicting endoscopic remission/MH with sensitivity of 77 % and specificity of 57 % (area under the curve 0.580; 95 % CI: 0.634–0.944). At week 26 the overall MaRIA score decreased of at least 9.7 points in 10 patients (37 %) while increased in 4 patients (15 %). In the remaining 13 patients (48 %) the overall MaRIA score decreased by less than 9.7 points compared to baseline (Fig. 4).

Clinical-biological assessment of therapeutic response demonstrated that a CDAI < 150 at week 26 was achieved in 12 patients (44 %) and CRP levels restored to normal in 21 patients (78 %). At week 26, CRP levels reduced in 6 patients (22 %) and 3 patients (12 %) had a CDAI decrease of more than 70 points, defined as a partial response. Lack of response with CDAI increased or not changed was observed in remaining 12 patients (44 %). No patients showed an increase of CRP levels.

The results of the endoscopic, MRI and clinical-biological changes induced by the treatment are shown in Table 6.

In terms of endoscopy and MRI, there was a statistically significant reduction both in SES-CD and in MaRIA score ($p < 0.001$). Also the CDAI and serum levels of CRP decreased significantly following treatment ($p < 0.001$).

We observed high interobserver agreement for the overall MaRIA score both at baseline and at week 26 (κ = 0.93, s.e. = 0.88; κ = 0.95, s.e. = 0.98, respectively). Accuracy rates for the overall MaRIA score were 92 % at baseline and 96 % at the end of the study.

Discussion

Since the beginning of anti-TNF therapy, MH has become an important predictor of long-term disease outcome in IBD. MH during scheduled anti-TNF therapy reduces need for surgery and hospital treatment significantly [20]. Accordingly, the assessment of therapeutic efficacy requires close monitoring of the mucosa and the bowel wall. To date, ileocolonoscopy remains the gold standard for assessing disease remission in CD, and in the present study we prefer to use the SES-CD since it is a reproducible index for this evaluation [13, 21], easier and faster to calculate than Crohn's Disease Endoscopic Index of Severity (CDEIS). In fact CDEIS, although it has proven to be a reliable and reproducible marker of MH in a number of therapeutic trials [22–24], is rather time consuming and elaboration of the score requires analogue scale transformation. These characteristics make CDEIS unsuitable for everyday clinical practice and also its use can be complex in clinical trials. Nevertheless, endoscopy remains an invasive procedure with potential complications [25], can be felt as a problem by

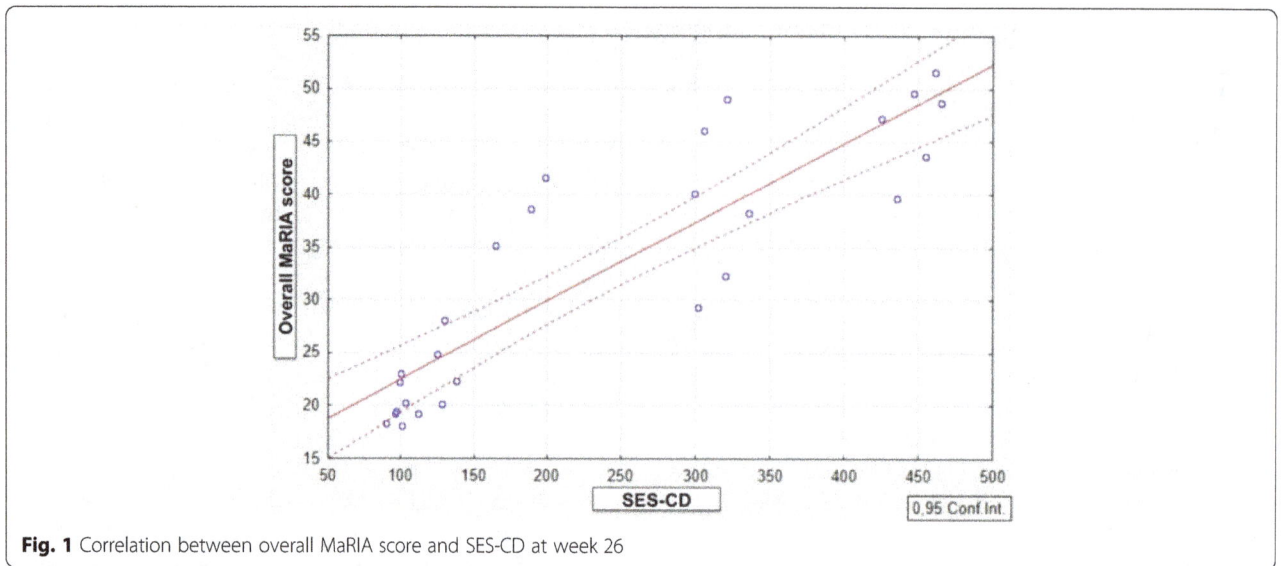

Fig. 1 Correlation between overall MaRIA score and SES-CD at week 26

CD patients and does not reflect the overall burden of the disease [26].

As the small bowel is difficult to reach with conventional endoscopy, several non-invasive tools have been developed in the last two decades in the investigation of CD. MRI is probably to date the best alternative, owing to its nonionizing characteristics and high performances especially in detecting signs of intestinal inflammation [27]. In particular, MRI has great potentials in characterization of the CD, being able to assess parameters such as parietal thickening, hypervascularity (comb signs), mesenteric fibro-fatty proliferation and others [11]. Since CD is a trans-mural disease, the use of MRI represent an important step in the diagnostic, therapeutic and prognostic management of the disease, because the mucosal lesions assessable by endoscopy represents only the tip of the inflammatory process. These findings call for revision of the current understanding of "intestinal healing" in the treatment of CD. MRI may be in fact employed to determine

microscopic structural wall changes, including edema and fibrosis, hypervascularity, capillary permeability, and likely, in the next years, specific molecular abnormalities, extending beyond the concept of "mucosal healing" [27].

Recently Rimola and co-workers developed the MaRIA score, which is able to assess inflammation in ileal and colonic CD [14, 15]. The MaRIA score is a validated index for describing the severity of inflammation, but it is not a gold standard for describing CD, which is much more complex. Despite this limitation, MRI in CD can be considered as the most validated tool for evaluating inflammation.

In our study, we evaluated MRI findings, before and after medical therapy with anti-TNF, and the correlation between endoscopic assessments, clinical-biological responses and MRI modifications. The first study assessing the responsiveness of MRI in patients with CD was published in 1999 [28]. In this small study, 8 patients with active CD were examined before and after treatment

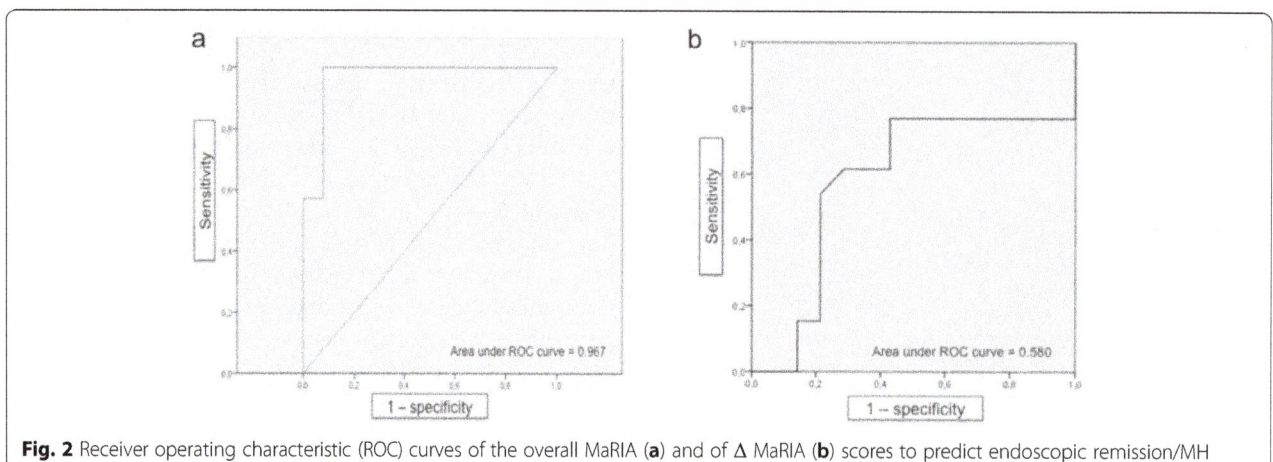

Fig. 2 Receiver operating characteristic (ROC) curves of the overall MaRIA (**a**) and of Δ MaRIA (**b**) scores to predict endoscopic remission/MH

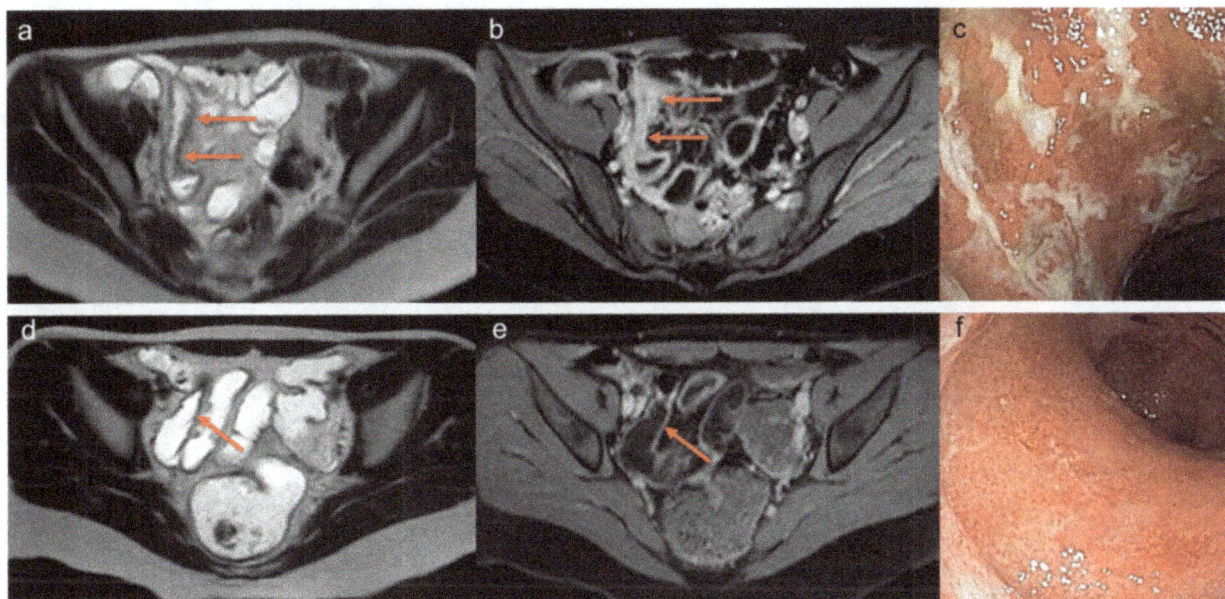

Fig. 3 Patient with CD of the terminal ileum in treatment with IFX. At baseline, MRI (**a** and **b**) detected moderate inflammatory lesions of the terminal ileum, with wall thickening accompanied by oedema, irregularity of the mucosal surface and hyperenhancement after intravenous contrast administration (Overall MaRIA score = 49). Baseline endoscopy of the same segment confirmed the presence of serpiginous, longitudinal ulcerations (**c**; SES-CD = 20). At week 26, the terminal ileum achieved healing at both MRI (**d** and **e**; Overall MaRIA score = 19,2; Δ MaRIA score = 29,8) and endoscopy (**f**; SES-CD = 0)

with corticosteroids using low-field magnetic resonance (1.0 T). The MRI parameters that showed a significant reduction during treatment were contrast enhancement ($p < 0.001$) and wall thickness ($p = 0.03$), which is in agreement with the results of the current study.

More recently, Ordas et al. [29] performed a prospective multicentre study of 48 patients with active CD, examining patients who underwent ileocolonoscopy and MRI at baseline and 12 weeks after treatment with steroid or tumor necrosis factor inhibitor (specifically ADA). The primary end points for the study were determining the accuracy of MRI in identifying ulcer healing (defined as the disappearance of ulcers on endoscopic exam) and the endoscopic remission (quantified using CDEIS <3.5). MRI had a high diagnostic accuracy for both predicting endoscopic ulcer healing, with sensitivity of 75 % and specificity of 80 %, and endoscopic remission, with sensitivity of 83 % and specificity of 84 %. Our data showed similar MRI diagnostic accuracy for predicting endoscopic remission/MH with a higher sensitivity (93 %) and a slightly lower specificity (77 %). These comparable results were obtained in spite of our study was a single centre using a 1.5 T MR unit while the Ordas was a multicentre study performed with 3.0 T scanner, which should have a better signal and higher spatial resolution. Moreover, the results were not influenced despite the use of different endoscopic indexes, different therapeutic strategies and the lack of colon distension by instillation of water through a rectal catheter.

Similar to our study, Van Assche and co-workers [30] recruited only anti-TNF-naïve patients in a multicentric and prospective trial evaluating the effects of IFX therapy on MRI ileal CD lesions. This pilot study included 15 patients that were studied at baseline, 2, and 26 weeks after starting IFX induction and maintenance therapy. The authors concluded that normalization of MRI findings is rare after IFX therapy. This is apparently discrepant with the observations of the current study, in which normalization of MRI findings paralleled endoscopic and clinical responses. The reasons for this discrepancy might include the fact that the study by Van Assche et al. used a different activity index and it only assessed ileal disease in a limited sample size.

In the current study a prospective series of patients with ileo-colonic CD was assessed in which a 59 % rate of endoscopic partial or complete response was achieved using an anti-TNF induction therapy. This percentage is similar to those described in the literature [31]. In our series, a reduction of the overall MaRIA score was found in 48 % of patients and a significant improvement in Δ MaRIA score was found in 37 % of patients following the treatment. A complete disappearance of MRI alterations was found only in 5 patients. As expected, the MRI improvement was significantly related to the endoscopic and the clinical-biological response in such a way that it only occurred in patients who responded to the treatment. These data support the reliability of MRI as

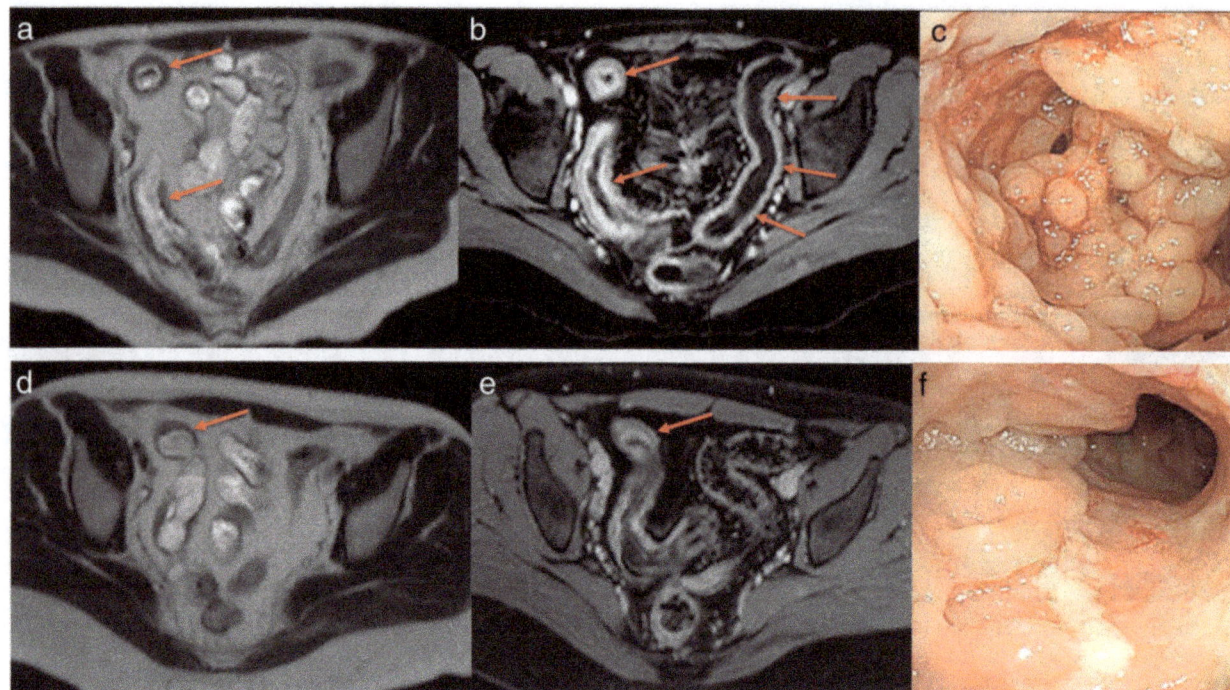

Fig. 4 Patient with CD of the distal ileum, left and transverse colon in treatment with IFX. At baseline, MRI (**a** and **b**) detected severe inflammatory lesions of the terminal ileum, with marked wall thickening accompanied by oedema, extensive irregularity of the mucosal surface and stratified hyperenhancement after intravenous contrast administration. A moderate wall thickening of the left colon is also present with hyperenhancement after intravenous contrast administration (Overall MaRIA score = 62,7). Baseline endoscopy at the distal ileum revealed the presence of stricturing, cobblestone appearance of the mucosal surface (**c**; SES-CD = 33). At week 26, the distal ileum continues to present at MRI a moderate wall thickening with mild hyperenhancement after intravenous contrast administration (**d** and **e**; Overall MaRIA score = 52,6; Δ MaRIA score = 10,1) Endoscopy of the same segment shows irregular longitudinal ulcers (**f**; SES-CD = 10)

a tool in assessing response to treatment in-patient with CD.

This study has its limitations. In a purely observational design, our endoscopic end-points MRI, laboratory and clinical findings present the outcome of a heterogeneous CD patient group during treatment with anti-TNF in real-life clinical practice. Confounding relevant factors are our use of both ADA and IFX and their varying dosages and the small proportion of CD patients.

Conclusions

In conclusion, our data demonstrate that MaRIA have a high correlation both with SES-CD and with clinical-biological activity of the disease. According to Tielbeek et al. [32], MRI is a valid and reliable technique to monitor the use of TNF antagonists in clinical practice and it provides an accurate measure for prediction of endoscopic MH in patients with CD.

Abbreviations
ADA: adalimumab; anti-TNF: anti-tumour necrosis factor-α antibodies; CD: Crohn's disease; CDAI: Crohn's Disease Activity Index; CDEIS: Crohn's Disease Endoscopic Index of Severity; CI: confidence interval; CRP: C-reactive protein; CTE: computed tomography enterography; IBD: inflammatory bowel disease; IFX: infliximab; IL: interleukin; MH: mucosal healing; MRI: magnetic resonance imaging; PEG: polyethylene glycol; RCE: relative contrast enhancement; ROC: curve receiver operator characteristic curve; SD: standard deviation; SES-CD: Simple Endoscopic Score for Crohn's Disease; TNFα: tumour necrosis factor-α; WSI: wall signal intensity.

Competing interests
The study was not sponsored by public or industrial funding. None of the authors has a conflict of interest to declare.

Authors' contributions
LPS is responsible for drafting the manuscript. LPS and NDV are responsible for the study design. SR, EC, AC and DI are responsible for the data

Table 6 Endoscopic, MRE, clinical and biological changes induced by anti-TNF treatment

	Pre-treatment	Post-treatment
SES-CD [mean (SD)]	14,7 (8,9)	4,4 (4,6)
Overall MaRIA [mean (SD)]	41,1 (14,8)	32,8 (11,7)
CDAI [mean (SD)]	423,7 (71,1)	238,5 (140,1)
CRP [(mg/l) mean (SD)]	25,1 (23,6)	4,6 (5,6)

acquisition. LPS and SR are responsible for the data analysis. LPS, CB, GS and RV are responsible for revising the manuscript. LM gives final approval of the version to be published. All authors have read and approved the manuscript.

Author details

[1]Division of Diagnostic Imaging, Department of Surgical Sciences, University of Foggia, Viale Luigi Pinto n.1, Foggia 71122, Italy. [2]Division of Gastroenterology, Department of Surgical Sciences, University of Foggia, Viale Luigi Pinto n.1, Foggia 71122, Italy. [3]Division of Gastroenterology, Department of Surgical Sciences, Azienda Sanitaria Locale Provincia di Foggia, Piazza della Libertà n.1, Foggia 71122, Italy.

References

1. Baumgart DC, Sandborn WJ. Inflammatory bowel disease: clinical aspects and established and evolving therapies. Lancet. 2007;369:1641–57.
2. Travis SP, Stange EF, Lemann M, et al. European Crohn's and Colitis Organisation. European evidence-based consensus on the diagnosis and management of Crohn's disease: current management. Gut. 2006;55 Suppl 1:i16–35.
3. Breese E, McDonald TT. TNF alpha secreting cells in normal and diseased human intestine. Adv Exp Med Biol. 1995;371:821–4.
4. Rutgeerts P, Van Assche G, Vermeire S. Optimizing anti-TNF treatment in inflammatory bowel disease. Gastroenterology. 2004;126:1593–610.
5. Clark M, Colombel JF, Feagan BC, et al. American Gastroenterological association consensus development conference on the use of biologics in the treatment of inflammatory bowel disease, june 21–23, 2006. Gastroenterology. 2007;133:312–39.
6. Rutgeerts P, Feagan BG, Lichtenstein GR, et al. Comparison of scheduled and episodic treatment strategies of infliximab in Crohn's disease. Gastroenterology. 2004;126:402–13.
7. Dome'nech E, Hinojosa J, Nos P, et al. Clinical evolution of luminal and perianal Crohn's disease after inducing remission with infliximab: how long should patients be treated? AlimentPharmacol Ther. 2005;22:1107–13.
8. Lichtenstein GR, Abreu MT, Cohen R, Tremaine W. American Gastroenterological Association Institute technical review on corticosteroids, inmunomoduladors, and infliximab in inflammatory bowel disease. Gastroenterology. 2006;130:940–87.
9. Terheggen G, Lanyi B, Schanz S, et al. Safety, feasibility, and tolerability of ileocolonoscopy in inflammatory bowel disease. Endoscopy. 2008;40:656–63.
10. Freeman HJ. Limitations in assessment of mucosal healing in inflammatory bowel disease. World J Gastroenterol. 2010;16:15–20.
11. Macarini L, Stoppino LP, Centola A, et al. Assessment of activity of Crohn's disease of the ileum and large bowel: proposal for a new multiparameter MR enterography score. Radiol Med. 2013;118:181–95.
12. Lennard Jones JE. Classification of inflammatory bowel disease. Scand J Gastroenterol. 1989;24 suppl 170:2–6.
13. Daperno M, D'Haens G, Van Assche G, et al. Development and validation of a new, simplified endoscopic activity score for Crohn's disease: the SES-CD. Gastrointest Endosc. 2004;60:505–12.
14. Rimola J, Rodriguez S, Garcia-Bosch O, et al. Magnetic resonance for assessment of disease activity and severity in ileocolonic Crohn's disease. Gut. 2009;58:1113–20.
15. Rimola J, Ordas I, Rodriguez S, et al. Magnetic resonance imaging for evaluation of Crohn's disease: validation of parameters of severity and quantitative index of activity. Inflamm Bowel Dis. 2011;17:1759–68.
16. Colombel JF, Sandborn WJ, Reinisch W, et al. Infliximab, azathioprine, or combination therapy for Crohn's disease. N Engl J Med. 2010;362:1383–95.
17. Ferrante M, Noman M, Vermeire S, et al. Evolution of endoscopic activity scores under placebo therapy in Crohn's disease. Gastroenterology. 2010;138:S358.
18. Moskovitz DN, Daperno M, Van Assche G, et al. Defining and validating cut-offs for the simple endoscopic score for Crohn's disease. Gastroenterology. 2007;132:S1097.
19. Winship DH, Summers RW, Singleton JW, et al. National cooperative Crohn's disease study: study design and conduct of the study. Gastroenterology. 1979;77:829–42.
20. Schnitzler F, Fidder H, Ferrante M, et al. Mucosal healing predicts long-term outcome of maintenance therapy with infliximab in Crohn's disease. Inflamm Bowel Dis. 2009;15:1295–301.
21. Ferrante M, Colombel JF, Sandborn WJ, et al. Validation of endoscopic activity scores in patients with Crohn's disease based on a post-hoc analysis of data from SONIC. Gastroenterology. 2013;145:978–86.
22. Modigliani R, Mary JY, Simon JF, et al. Clinical, biological, and endoscopic picture of attacks of Crohn's disease. Evolution on prednisolone. Groupe d'Etude therapeutique des affections inflammatoires digestives. Gastroenterology. 1990;98:811–8.
23. Landi B, Anh TN, Cortot A, et al. Endoscopic monitoring of Crohn's disease treatment: a prospective, randomized clinical trial. The groupe d'Etudes therapeutiques des affections inflammatoires digestives. Gastroenterology. 1992;102:1647–53.
24. Cellier C, Sahmoud T, Froguel E, et al. Correlations between clinical activity, endoscopic severity, and biological parameters in colonic or ileocolonic Crohn's disease. A prospective multicentre study of 121 cases. The groupe d'Etudes therapeutiques des affections inflammatoires digestives. Gut. 1994;35:231–5.
25. Buisson A, Chevaux JB, Hudziak H, et al. Colonoscopic perforations in inflammatory bowel disease: a retrospective study in a French referral centre. Dig Liver Dis. 2013;45:569–72.
26. Pariente B, Cosnes J, Danese S, et al. Development of the Crohn's disease digestive damage score, the Lémann score. Inflamm Bowel Dis. 2011;17:1415–22.
27. Baumgart DC, Sandborn WJ. Crohn's disease. Lancet. 2012;6736:1–16.
28. Madsen SM, Thomsen HS, Schlichting P, et al. Evaluation of treatment response in active Crohn's disease by low-field magnetic resonance imaging. Abdom Imaging. 1999;24:232–9.
29. Ordas I, Rimola J, Rodriguez S, et al. Accuracy of magnetic resonance enterography in assessing response to therapy and mucosal healing in patients with Crohn's disease. Gastroenterology. 2014;146:374–82.
30. Van Assche G, Herrmann KA, Louis E, et al. Effects of infliximab therapy on transmural lesions as assessed by magnetic resonance enteroclysis in patients with ileal Crohn's disease. J Crohns Colitis. 2013;7:950–7.
31. Rutgeerts P, Van Assche G, Vermeire S. Review article: infliximab therapy for inflammatory bowel disease–seven years on. Aliment Pharmacol Ther. 2006;23:451–63.
32. Tielbeek JA, Lowenberg M, Bipat S, et al. Serial magnetic resonance imaging for monitoring medical therapy effects in Crohn's disease. Inflamm Bowel Dis. 2013;19:1943–50.

15

Abdominal ultrasound-scanning versus non-contrast computed tomography as screening method for abdominal aortic aneurysm – a validation study from the randomized DANCAVAS study

Mads Liisberg[1,2]* , Axel C. Diederichsen[2,3,4] and Jes S. Lindholt[1,2,4]

Abstract

Background: Validating non-contrast-enhanced computed tomography (nCT) compared to ultrasound sonography (US) as screening method for abdominal aortic aneurysm (AAA) screening.

Methods: Consecutively attending men ($n = 566$) from the pilot study of the randomized Danish CardioVascular Screening trial (DANCAVAS trial), underwent nCT and US examination. Diameters were measured in outer-to-outer fashion. Sensitivity and specificity were done testing each modality against each other as reference standard. Measurements were tested for correlation, variance in diameters, and mean differences were tested using paired t-test.

Results: Due to logistics, 533 underwent *both* nCT and US. In four patients, aortae could not be visualized with US, and two of these had an AAA (>30 mm) as diagnosed by nCT. Using nCT 30 (5.7%, 95% CI: 4.2;7.5%) AAA were found. US failed to detect 9 of these, but diagnosed 3 other cases, resulting prevalence by US was 4.5% (95% CI: 3.0;6.6%). Additionally, 5 isolated iliac aneurysms (≥20 mm) (0.9%, 95% CI: 0.3;2.2%) were discovered by nCT.
US performed reasonably, with sensitivity ranging from 57.1–70.4%, specificity however, ranged higher 99.2–99.6%. Comparably nCT performed with sensitivity ranging from 82.6–88.9%, nCTs specificity however ranged from 97.7–98.4%. Analysis showed good correlations with no tendency to increasing variance with increasing diameter, and no significant differences between nCT and US with means varying slightly in both axis.

Conclusions: nCT seems superior to US concerning sensitivity, and is able to detect aneurysmal lesions not detectable with US. Finally, the prevalence of AAA in Denmark seems to remain relatively high, in this small pilot study group.

Background

Screening for abdominal aortic aneurysm (AAA) based upon abdominal aortic ultrasound sonography (US) has proven beneficial, cost-effective, which partly is the reason why US-based screening programs have been implemented in several countries [1–3]. However as reported by the MASS trial [3], AAA related deaths do occur

years after screening programs finding normal aortas in the attenders. This might be prevented by rescreening, although intervals for rescreening in normal aortas have yet to be established. Following this, the reduced AAA specific mortality by screening is only about 50%, which contrasts with reported attendance rates close to 80% [4]. The specific causes are unknown - it could be, that those in high risk do not attend, or down to false negative findings, incidental development, a combination, or mistaken recorded cause of death.

Today two modalities are utilized to assess the infrarenal aortic diameter (IAD) to diagnose AAA, namely

* Correspondence: Mads@liisberg.eu
[1]Department of Cardiothoracic and Vascular Surgery, Odense University Hospital, Cardiovascular Centre of Excellence (CAVAC), Sdr. Boulevard 29, Afd. T - Forskerreden, 5000 Odense C, Denmark
[2]Elitary Research Centre of Individualised Treatment of Arterial Diseases (CIMA), Odense University Hospital, Odense C, Denmark
Full list of author information is available at the end of the article

US and computed tomography (CT), each with their own benefits, and drawbacks.

As a screening modality for AAA, US has become accepted, because it is easy to operate, cheap and with an estimated sensitivity and specificity close to 100% [5]. This however, was based upon the size distribution in the population, and observed intervariation of US measurements. In reality, US has never been validated as a screening modality for AAA, it has only been validated when AAA was present, and even when present with significant interobserver variability [6–8]. Adding to this, some infrarenal aortas are difficult to visualize due to intestinal gas and/or adiposity [9].

Using non-contrast CT scanning as an alternative screening method for AAA might be more reliable, and offer other screening potentials as coronary calcifications, thoracic- and iliac lesions. Because CT scanners are becoming widely available and perform better with each iteration, while using less radiation due to modern iterative reconstruction algorithms, effectively enabling CT to be a valid screening modality.

Contrast enhanced CT-scans are known to be more precise, probably with 100% sensitivity and specificity, but have not been tested as a screening tool. Additionally, it would expose the examined individuals not only for radiation, but potential nephrotoxic contrast. Contrast enhanced CT-scans are not widely available, time consuming and thus expensive, making it a less rational screening modality.

Nearly half the population in the Western world dies due to cardiovascular diseases (CVD), mainly due to ischemic heart disease. Focusing on traditionally risk markers like hypertension, hypercholesterolemia and diabetes screening and intervention have been tested in randomized setups, and proven insufficient [10]. The question is whether detection of asymptomatic arterial lesions could lead to a better risk stratification and intervention. Low dose non-contrast-enhanced cardiac CT scan quantifying the degree of coronary arterial calcification, and has been proven to be one of the best predictors of future cardiac events [11, 12], and might be the tool for future screening and intervention. If such a scan is expanded to include the chest and abdomen, thoracic as well as abdominal aortic aneurysms would be exposed, but the question is whether infrarenal aorta will be sufficiently visualized. This question arises from the modern low dosage scans used in cardiac CT which might not visualize the infrarenal aorta sufficiently.

Consequently, in the pilot study of the randomized Danish CardioVascular Screening trial (DANCAVAS trial) men underwent screening for AAA by both US and non-contrast-enhanced CT scanning (nCT) [13, 14]. The aim of this study, is to validate nCT as a comparable modality to US in a AAA screening setting.

Methods

Design

Population based cross-sectional study within a population based multicenter randomized screening trial. All Danish citizens are given a unique civil registration number at birth, with which we are able to track all their interactions with the Danish health institutions (e.g. hospital admissions, drug prescriptions etc.). Through this registry 45.000 men will be randomly selected based on their age, and geographic location, to correspond to our screening sites. A third of the selected men will be invited to our cardiovascular screening program, whilst the remaining two thirds will be followed through the registries. There are no exclusion criteria for the participants in this study. This article will only be analyzing data from primary attenders the pilot study, consisting of 956 invitees, of which 566 attended primarily.

Participants

The DANCAVAS trial is an ongoing multicenter trial with Danish screening sites in Odense, Svendborg, Vejle and Silkeborg. Ethical approval was obtained by the Southern Denmark Region Committee on Biomedical Research Ethics (S-20140028) and the Data Protection Agency, and registered in ISRCTN (DOI 10.1186/ISRCTN12157806) [13]. The study protocol was reviewed and approved by the institutional review board, all participants were given written and oral information about the study, and written consent was obtained from each participant.

The primary aim is to investigate whether combined advanced cardiovascular screening will prevent death and cardiovascular events, and whether the likely health benefits are cost effective.

One-third of 45.000 will be invited a screening examinations at one of the 4 locations. The screening will include: (1) nCT scan to detect coronary artery calcification above the corresponding age median, and aortic/iliac aneurysms, (2) Brachial and ankle blood pressure index to detect peripheral arterial disease and hypertension, (3) an assessment of the CT monitored heart rhythm to detected atrial fibrillation, and (4) a measurement of the cholesterol and plasma glucose levels. Up-to-date cardiovascular preventive treatment is recommended in case of positive finding. Positive AAA findings is defined as infra renal aortic diameter ≥30 mm, and iliac aneurysms are defined as ≥20 mm.

In Odense, men aged 65–74 were consecutively invited to participate in the DANCAVAS *pilot* screening program in the autumn 2014, with *no exclusion criteria*. In total, 956 were invited and 566 attended initially when this validation study took place.

Imaging

Medical students, received training by an experienced vascular surgeon, before being allowed to evaluate participants used a GE Logiq E9 with a C1-5-D or C1-6-D transducer to perform all ultrasound abdominal aortic measurements. Using the cinematic function, the maximal systolic outer-to-outer diameter was measured in the anterior-posterior (AP) and transverse plane [15, 16]. The US examinations were blinded to the results from the nCT examinations carried out consecutively, and vice versa.

Low dose nCT were performed with a Siemens Somatom Definition Flash: spiral scan with a pitch of 3.2 (Flash), 100 kV tube voltage, 90 mAs, collimation of 128 x 0.6 mm, Safire 3 and slice thickness 5 mm from the thoracic aorta, to the common femoral arteries. Trained radiographers, using Siemens Syngo.via, evaluated the resulting CT-images. In case of an obvious aneurysm, the diameters were measured outer to outer, measurements were in the axis of the aorta for both AP/transverse planes. In case of no aneurysms the outer to outer dimensions of the abdominal aorta was measured in a transversal and an anterior-posterior plane just above the bifurcation of the aorta. Diameters of the iliac arteries were noted in case of aneurysm.

Statistical analysis

Data was initially merged in a 2x2 table (Tables 1A-C) and sensitivity and specificity was calculated, using each method as reference standard for the other. Sensitivity and specificity as well as predictive values are presented in percentages for ease of interpretation, their confidence intervals are 'exact' Clopper-Pearson confidence intervals.

The data was mainly analyzed as suggested by Bland and Altman [17]. First data was examined for normal-distribution, this was found to be true, although diameters slightly shifted to the left graphically. Secondly, data were examined by plotting the results from nCT against US. Systematic differences between the two methods were tested by paired t-test. Statistical analysis was carried out using SPSS 22 (IBM Corp. Released 2013. IBM SPSS Statistics for Windows, Version 22.0. Armonk, NY: IBM Corp.) and Stata 14 (StataCorp. 2015. Stata Statistical Software: Release 14. College Station, TX: StataCorp LP.).

Results

Visibility and prevalence

533 men, mean age 69.4 years ±2.51 (1SD), underwent *both* nCT and US, additionally 4 (0.7%) of these were

Table 1 A-C, Title: Cross tabulation of results used for sensitivity calculations

		CT AP		
		0	1	Total
US AP	0	495	8	503
	1	4	19	23
Total		499	27	526

		CT Trans		
		0	1	Total
US Trans	0	499	12	511
	1	2	16	18
Total		501	28	529

		CT AAA		
		0	1	Total
US AAA	0	493	9	502
	1	3	21	24
Total		496	30	526

Legend: US/CT AP – 0 denotes an AP diameter of <30 mm; 1 denotes an AP diameter of >30 mm
US/CT Trans - 0 denotes a Transverse diameter of <30 mm; 1 denotes a Transverse diameter of >30 mm
US/CT AAA – 0 denotes any US measurements <30 mm; 1 denotes any measured diameter >30 mm

unable to be assessed satisfyingly by US, due to adiposity and/or intestinal gas, these were excluded from the calculations completely. Two of the 4 US invisible cases had an AAA diagnosed by nCT sized 32 mm and 42 mm, respectively. Consequently, 529 underwent both nCT and US. Thirty AAA were discovered using nCT, resulting in an occurrence of 5.7% (95% CI: 4.2;7.5%). US failed to identify 9 of these aneurysms, which were measured to be 27.4–42.8 mm in AP and 27.3–40.5 mm in the transverse plane with nCT (Fig. 1a and b).

US diagnosed 24 AAA (4.5% (95% CI: 3.0;6.6%)), 3 of which were not identified by nCT, these were found to be 30.2–31.8 mm in AP plane and 19.8–44.6 mm in the transverse plane using US, these were however measured by nCT to range from 18.3–19.7 mm in both planes (Fig. 2).

Unfortunately, the US examinations were not stored, but the CT scans were. Two senior consultants reexamined the nCT scans of the 12 conflicting findings blinded by knowledge of which test modality was used to diagnose the aneurysm. They uniformly classified all

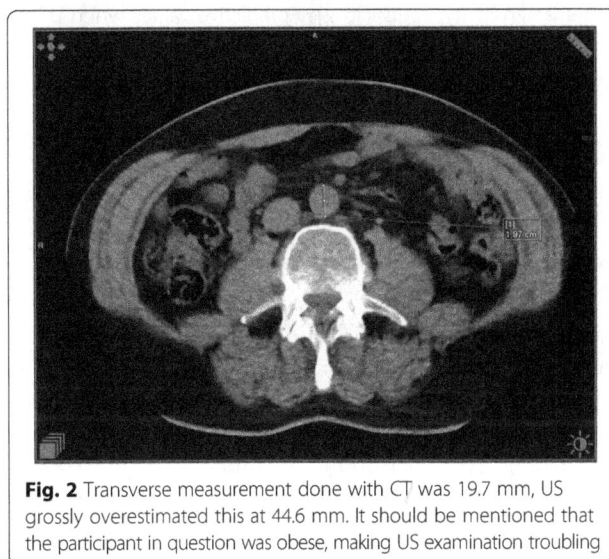

Fig. 2 Transverse measurement done with CT was 19.7 mm, US grossly overestimated this at 44.6 mm. It should be mentioned that the participant in question was obese, making US examination troubling

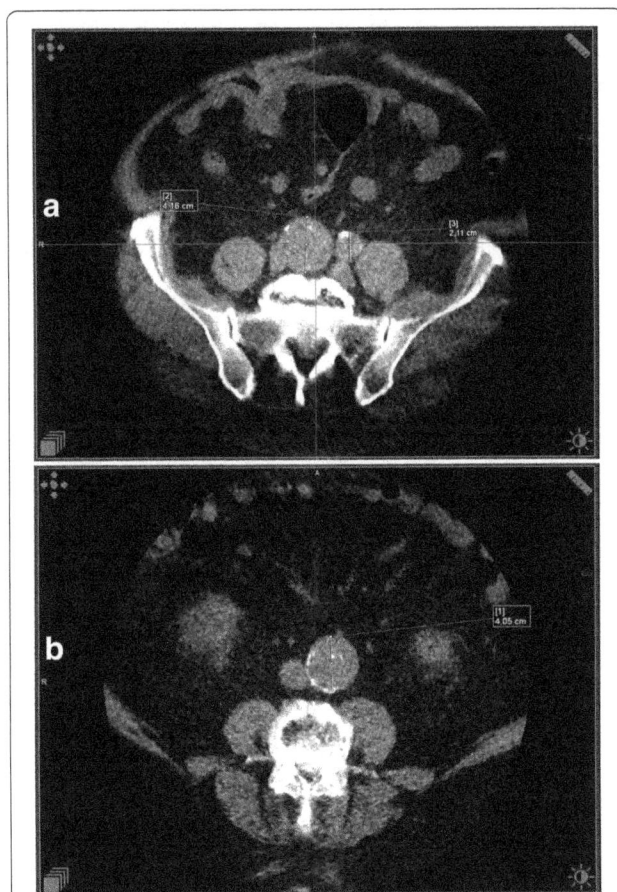

Fig. 1 a Shows AAA measured 41.6 mm and a.iliaca aneurisms measuring 21.1 mm. **b** False Negative US finding, was measured to be 25.7 mm in the transverse with US, however nCT measured it was found to be 40.5 mm

the 9 cases only diagnosed by nCT as AAA, and none of the 3 AAA diagnosed by US scans.

In addition, 5 isolated iliac aneurysms (≥20 mm) (0.9%, 95% C.I.: 0.3;2.2%) were discovered by nCT, – none of these were discovered by US, which were also validated by senior consultants.

Sensitivity, and specificity and predictive values

Each modality was used as a reference standard for the other to analyze sensitivity and specificity respectively. Iliac aneurysms were not included as positive findings, when calculating sensitivity and specificity.

US performed with a modest sensitivity ranging from 57.1% (95% C.I.: 37.2;75.5%) to 70.4% (95% C.I.: 49.8;86.3%), with high specificity ranging from 99.2% (95% C.I.: 97.9;99.8%) to 99.6% (95% C.I.: 98.6;99.9%) (Table 2).

nCT performed better with a sensitivity ranging from 82.6% (95% C.I.: 61.2;95.1%) to 88.9% (95% C.I.: 65.3;98.6%). Concerning specificity, nCT fared comparably to US with a specificity of 97.7% (95% C.I.: 95.9;98.8%) to 98.4% (95% C.I.: 96.9;99.3%) (Table 3).

Expert review in those cases where US found an aneurysm, and nCT however did not, resulted in nCT sensitivity of 100% (95% C.I: 88.4;100%) and equally with a specificity of 100% (95% C.I.: 99.3;100%).

Analysis of discrepancies concerning diameter

Comparing all measurements including AAA, mean diameters in CT^{ap} and US^{ap} measurements show means of 21.3 and 21.2 mm respectively, with standard deviations of 5.3 and 5.0 (paired mean difference -0.05 ± -3.16 (SD), $p = 0.70$). The same applies for the measurements for the transverse plane showing CT^{trans} and US^{trans} means of 21.6 and 21.3 mm respectively, along with

Table 2 Sensitivity, Specificity and predictive values when US compared to nCT as reference standard CT

	Sensitivity	95% CI	Specificity	95% CI	PV+	95% CI	PV-	95% CI
AP	0.7037	0.5;0.86	0.9920	0.98;0.99	0.8261	0.68;0.97	0.9841	0.68;0.97
Trans	0.5714	0.37;0.76	0.9960	0.99;0.99	0.8889	0.65;0.98	0.9765	0.96;0.99
AAA	0.7000	0.51;0.85	0.9940	0.98;0.99	0.8750	0.68;0.97	0.9821	0.97;0.99

For each measured plane, the sensitivity and specificity values and their corresponding 95% CI interval is presented. Additionally, positive and negative predictive values are included, with their 95% CI interval
AP: Cases are participants with a anterior posterior mesurement of >30 mm
TRANS: Cases are participants with a transverse measurement of >30 mm
AAA: Cases are particpants with measurement in any plane of >30 mm

standard deviations of 5.5 and 5.1 (paired mean difference -0.28 ± -3.67 (SD), $p = 0.08$).

Pearson's correlation analysis of the measured diameter by the two modalities showed good agreement concerning AP measurement (Rho = 0.81, $p < 0.0001$) and to a close extent concerning transverse measurements (Rho = 0.75, $p < 0.0001$) (Fig. 3a and b). Bland-Altman plots [14] presenting the difference vs. the mean of the measured diameter in both planes showed apparently, no tendency to increasing difference with increasing diameter in either planes (Fig. 4a and b). However, Pearson's correlation analysis of the difference versus the mean diameter was r = 0.114 ($p = 0.0088$) concerning AP measurements, and r = 0.083 ($p = 0.0569$) concerning transverse diameter indicating a minor increasing difference by increasing maximal aortic diameter in both planes.

Comparing mean AAA diameters in CT^{ap} and US^{ap} measurements show means of 38.1 and 34.7 mm respectively, with standard deviations of 9.7 and 10.5 (paired mean difference -3.3 ± 5.8 (SD), $p = 0.004$). The same applies for the measurements for the transverse plane showing CT^{trans} and US^{trans} means of 38.6 and 34.2 mm respectively, along with standard deviations of 9.5 and 9.9 (paired mean difference -4.39 ± 8.17 (SD), $p = 0.006$). Pearson correlation analysis of the measured diameter by the two modalities showed only a modest agreement concerning AP (r = 0.7508, p < 0.0001) and transverse measurements (Rho = 0.7008, p < 0.0001). Pearson correlation analysis of the difference versus the mean diameter was Rho = 0.1853 (p < 0.0001) and r = 0.1203 ($p = 0.0055$) concerning AP and transverse diameter, respectively. Bland-Altman plots examining the recorded AAA cases, showed increased difference between the used modalities with increasing diameters (Fig. 5a and b).

Discussion

This is the first direct comparison of screening for AAA with non-contrast CT versus US. nCT was found to have superior sensitivity compared to US, and similar specificity. Our study is hampered by the lack of a real reference modality such as contrast CT, or contrast MRi. However, this was not included in the primary protocol because of the lack of feasibility to include such a modality. It was therefore decided that the modalities would be held up against each other, as reference standards, since neither had been validated as a AAA screening modality.

This study shows that in a screening setting, nCT has improved sensitivity over US. However, there is still a great deal of clinical evidence favoring US as a method, due to the reduced costs availability, and high specificity.

When aorta is visible utilizing US, it showed reasonable sensitivity for US with nCT being superior over US. Both modalities had a comparable high specificity. In addition, isolated iliac aneurysms are not likely to be detected by US, because AAA screening does not include the iliac arteries when using US. Consequently, as a screening tool for AAA, nCT seems acceptably valid, which is coherent with our hypothesis. In addition, it adds to the shortcomings of current AAA screening programs, because it is able to include the iliac arteries as well. Whether it too is acceptable as part of a multifaceted screening offer, we cannot conclude, as re-invitations, and final attendance rates are not yet available. It should be noted, that the pilot study was troubled by some preventable mishaps, with random lacking ultra sound devices, and not being able to review the US images being the most important issues. However, these issues would probably not have changed the final results of this study, but are worth mentioning.

Table 3 Sensitivity, Specificity and predictive values when CT compared to US as reference standard[a]

	SENSITIVITY	95% CI	SPECIFICITY	95% CI	PV+	95% CI	PV-	95% CI
AP	0.8261	0.61;0.95	0.9841	0.97;0.99	0.7037	0.5;0.86	0.9920	0.98;0.99
TRANS	0.8889	0.65;0.99	0.9765	0.96;0.99	0.5714	0.37;0.76	0.9960	0.99;0.99
AAA	0.8750	0.68;0.97	0.9821	0.97;0.99	0.7000	0.51;0.85	0.9940	0.98;0.99

[a]AP : Cases are participants with a anterior posterior mesurement of >30 mm
TRANS: Cases are participants with a transverse measurement of >30 mm
AAA: Cases are particpants with measurement in any plane of >30 mm

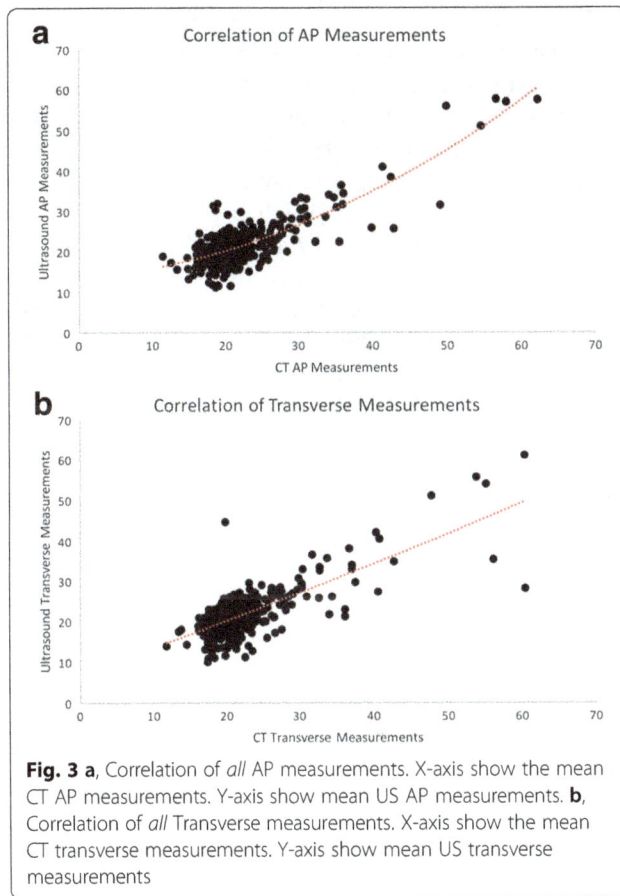

Fig. 3 a, Correlation of *all* AP measurements. X-axis show the mean CT AP measurements. Y-axis show mean US AP measurements. **b**, Correlation of *all* Transverse measurements. X-axis show the mean CT transverse measurements. Y-axis show mean US transverse measurements

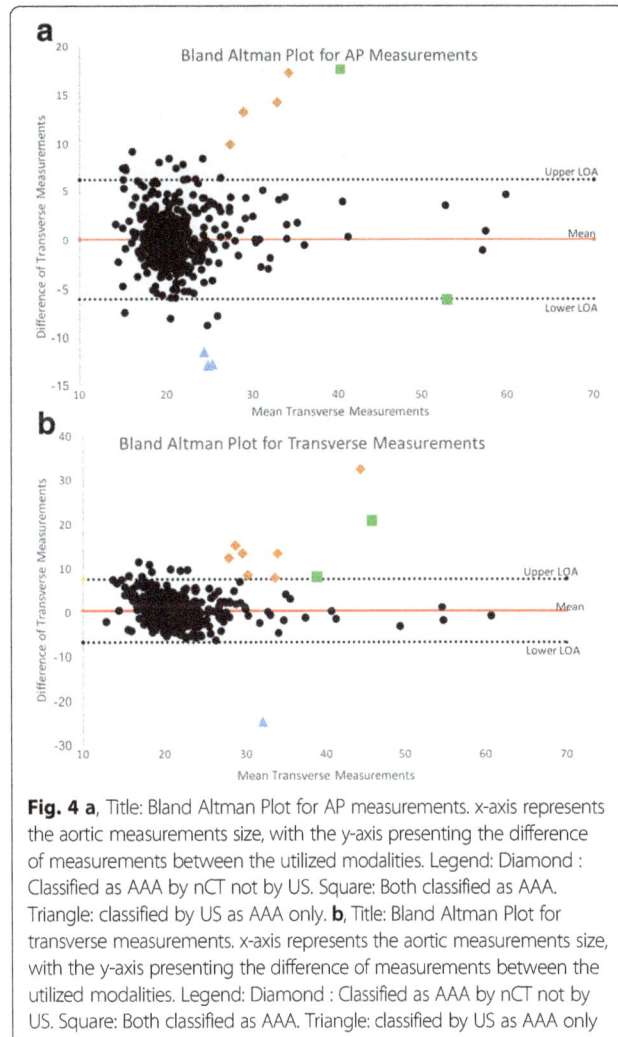

Fig. 4 a, Title: Bland Altman Plot for AP measurements. x-axis represents the aortic measurements size, with the y-axis presenting the difference of measurements between the utilized modalities. Legend: Diamond : Classified as AAA by nCT not by US. Square: Both classified as AAA. Triangle: classified by US as AAA only. **b**, Title: Bland Altman Plot for transverse measurements. x-axis represents the aortic measurements size, with the y-axis presenting the difference of measurements between the utilized modalities. Legend: Diamond : Classified as AAA by nCT not by US. Square: Both classified as AAA. Triangle: classified by US as AAA only

A possible limitation of this study is the lack of a truly accurate reference standard, which in this case would be 3D contrast enhanced CT scans, but this was not feasible nor ethically responsible to include.

Only men were invited to participate in this study, and this could be argued as a limitation, however, men are at increased risk solely because of their gender why a cardiovascular screening program would be targeted at men. However, a subgroup of women will be invited, to evaluate the potential cost-benefit of expanding the screening program to include women.

Although, nCT showed a comparable specificity to US, we cannot conclude that this should be the reference standard for screening for AAA as it is not widely available causing longer travel distances with assumable lower attendance, is time consuming and thus expensive. Nevertheless, nCT was able to detect more AAA (prevalence 5.7% versus 4.5%) and iliac aneurysms compared to US. This could – at least partially – explain the relatively low reduction in aneurysm related death in US-based randomized screening trials. nCT may thus be more efficient and perhaps a cost-effective alternative in a screening scenario, this however requires more data than currently available. This is especially true if repeated US scans are required to improve sensitivity to a

comparable level of CT, since only one repetition of a US scan, closes the cost-gap between US and CT.

The medical students were trained in US, but have not undergone the same magnitude of screening as ultrasonographers and other health care personnel conducting AAA screening. On the other hand, equipment with better-quality resolution, than portable scanners can offer was used. IAD was measured outer-to-outer, to be comparable to the UK screening program which also measures IAD in this fashion. The majority (7 of 9) of the AAA not detected by US but having visible aortas were found to be ectatic (>25 mm), while two were normal < 25 mm. These might have been detected by later 5-year interval, if introduced, since half of ectatic cases develop true AAA within 5 years [2]. This is due to true incidental cases or false negative findings. Those detected as ectatic by US but positive with nCT may be false positives, this could question whether rescreening five years after non-contrast screening will be beneficial [18]. However, they hardly make out the 50% reported to

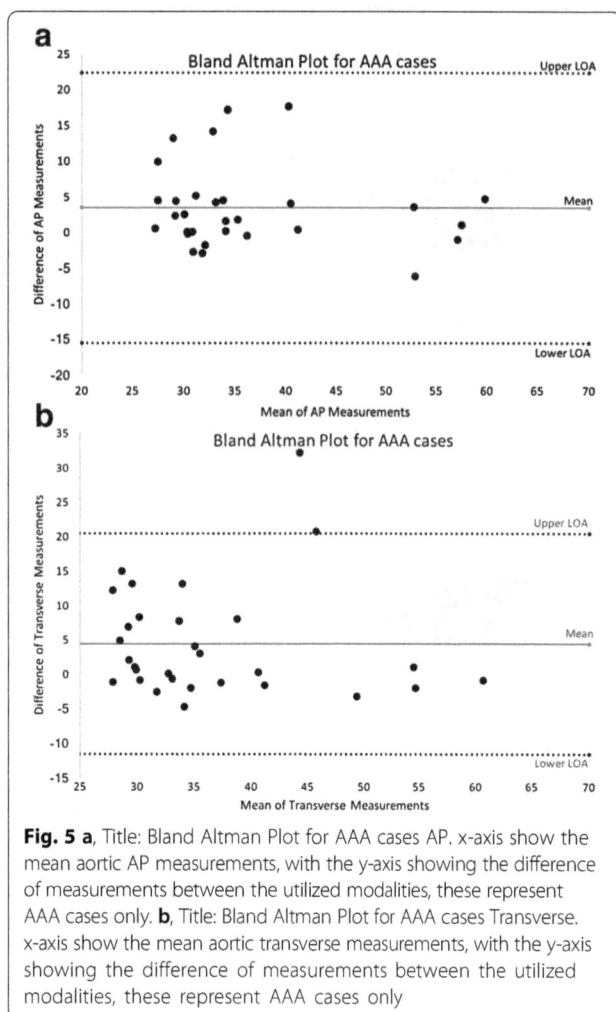

Fig. 5 a, Title: Bland Altman Plot for AAA cases AP. x-axis show the mean aortic AP measurements, with the y-axis showing the difference of measurements between the utilized modalities, these represent AAA cases only. **b**, Title: Bland Altman Plot for AAA cases Transverse. x-axis show the mean aortic transverse measurements, with the y-axis showing the difference of measurements between the utilized modalities, these represent AAA cases only

develop an AAA in this subgroup of the male population [2]. Consequently, DANCAVAS will re-invite this group after five years. Additionally, it could be argued that the 3 cases found by US and not by nCT, are actually false positives, thus making nCT appear less precise than it essentially is.

While US is an acceptable screening modality, it does have some shortcomings, mainly patients with a large waist circumference or intestinal gas diameters become difficult to asses properly, there are of course certain maneuvers to improve the assessment, but in a screening scenario these are not feasible.

We theorized that calcification would improve the validity of the non-contrast CT, but have not recorded any aortic calcification quantification. Consequently, we used two indirect signs of calcification as the coronary artery calcification score and ankle brachial index. The coronary artery calcification score correlated significantly positively with the difference of the measurements. However, this could be due to confounding from a clear positive correlation between coronary artery calcification score

and waist circumference, as the other indirect calcification marker, lowest measured ankle brachial index, did not correlate with the observed differences.

As an epidemiological sub finding, this study also gave a modern estimate on the prevalence of AAA in Denmark in men, which does not seem to decline as reported in UK and Sweden [19]. The prevalence of AAA in Denmark remains relatively high. US based prevalence on Fyn (DANCAVAS 2014) is almost similar to the prevalence of 4.2% detected in the Viborg County (1994–98) [20] and higher than the prevalence of 3.3% detected in the VIVA trial (2008–11) in the Mid region of Denmark [21]. However, it should be noted that this is a small sample, and as the DANCAVAS trial continues, the AAA prevalence will be reported with increased certainty.

Using low dose nCT for screening purposes will ultimately result, in increased radiation exposure to those participating. However, screening for AAA is a one-time event, which in combination with the advances made with modern CT-scanners reduces this risk greatly, making the risk negligible in these elderly males [22]. Thus, making nCT a worthwhile modality, since it allows for a more thorough CVD screening than US does, while not inducing illnesses. Additionally, there may be incidental findings further improving disease prevention, this however would require the participant's approval. This was not a part of this study, however, if a suspicious found was made by accident, the participant was informed and referred to the relevant specialties.

It is worth noting, that there is a secondary benefit to a reliable screening method, because of the psychological impact a false positive or negative result will have on the participant. This is especially important, when screening for common and potentially lethal diseases.

Conclusions

Low-dose nCT scanning seems to be more sensitive than US, screening for AAA, making it a possible tool for a larger scale screening program.

Expanding the screening to not only include AAA but also generally for CVDs, nCT may become truly beneficial, because it enables evaluations of the aortic and iliac vessels in their entire length, as well as evaluating any arcane lesions to the coronary arteries, thus providing more information about the patient's possible risks – this however requires additional research.

Abbreviations

AAA: Abdominal Aortic Aneurysm; AP: Anterior-Posterior; CVD: Cardiovascular disease; DANCAVAS: The randomized Danish CardioVascular Screening trial; IAD: Infrarenal aortic diameter; nCT: Non-contrast-enhanced computed tomography; US: Ultrasound

Acknowledgements
Jannie L. Poulsen (1,2), Jonas O. Krogh (2), Lars M Rasmussen (2), Lærke M. Kvist (2), Marie Salling (2), Mette S. Sørensen (2), Nikolaj Jangaard (2), Thomas V. Kvist (2), for assisting with participant enrollment.

Funding
This work was supported by Research council of Odense University Hospital, Research council of Region Southern Denmark, Danish Research Council, Danish Heart Foundation and Helsefonden.

Authors' contributions
JSL and ACD were responsible for the design, planning and funding of this study. ML analyzed, interpreted the data, and wrote the manuscript. All authors edited, and finalized the manuscript. All authors have read and approved the final version of the manuscript.

Competing interests
None of the authors have anything to declare.

Presentation information
This study was presented in the AAA forum at the British Vascular Societies Annual Scientific Meeting 2015 11–13 November, Bournemouth United Kingdom. The study was also presented in the open plenary forum at the Danish Vascular Society Annual Meeting 2015 23–24 October, Aarhus Denmark.

Author details
[1]Department of Cardiothoracic and Vascular Surgery, Odense University Hospital, Cardiovascular Centre of Excellence (CAVAC), Sdr. Boulevard 29, Afd. T - Forskerreden, 5000 Odense C, Denmark. [2]Elitary Research Centre of Individualised Treatment of Arterial Diseases (CIMA), Odense University Hospital, Odense C, Denmark. [3]Department of Cardiology, Odense University Hospital, Odense C, Denmark. [4]OPEN, Odense Patient data Explorative Network, Odense University Hospital, Odense C, Denmark.

References
1. Kim LG, Thompson SG, Briggs AH, Buxton MJ, Campbell HE. How cost-effective is screening for abdominal aortic aneurysms? J Med Screen. 2007;14:46–52.
2. Preventive Services Task Force US. Screening for abdominal aortic aneurysm: recommendation statement. Ann Intern Med. 2005;142:198–202.
3. Thompson SG, Ashton HA, Gao L, Scott RA. MASS study group. Screening men for abdominal aortic aneurysm: 10 year mortality and cost effectiveness results from the randomised multicentre aneurysm screening study. BMJ. 2009;338:b2307.
4. Cosford PA, Leng GC, Thomas J. Screening for abdominal aortic aneurysm Cochrane database of systematic reviews. Cochrane Database Syst Rev. 2007;2:CD002945.
5. Wilmink AB, Forshaw M, Quick CR, Hubbard CS, Day NE. Accuracy of serial screening for abdominal aortic aneurysms by ultrasound. J Med Screen. 2002;9(3):125–7.
6. Hartshorne TC, McCollum CN, Earnshaw JJ, Morris J, Nasim A. Ultrasound measurement of aortic diameter in a national screening programme. Eur J Vasc Endovasc Surg. 2011;42(2):195–9.
7. Jaakkola P, Hippelainen M, Farin P, Rytkonen H, Kainulainen S, Partanen K. Interobserver variability in measuring the dimensions of the abdominal aorta: comparison of ultrasound and computed tomography. Eur J Vasc Endovasc Surg. 1996;12(2):230–7.
8. Wanhainen A, Bergqvist D, Bjorck M. Measuring the abdominal aorta with ultrasonography and computed tomography - difference and variability. Eur J Vasc Endovasc Surg. 2002;24(5):428–34.
9. Long A, Rouet L, Lindholt JS, Allaire E. Measuring the maximum diameter of native abdominal aortic aneurysms: review and critical analysis. Eur J Vasc Endovasc Surg. 2012;43(5):515–24.
10. Jørgensen T, Jacobsen RK, Toft U, Aadahl M, Glümer C, Pisinger C. Effect of screening and lifestyle counselling on incidence of ischaemic heart disease in general population: Inter99 randomised trial. BMJ. 2014;348:g3617.
11. Polonsky TS, McClelland RL, Jorgensen NW, Bild DE, Burke GL, Guerci AD, et al. Coronary artery calcium score and risk classification for coronary heart disease prediction. JAMA. 2010;303(16):1610–6.
12. Erbel R, Mohlenkamp S, Moebus S, Schmermund A, Lehmann N, Stang A, et al. Coronary risk stratification, discrimination, and reclassification improvement based on quantification of subclinical coronary atherosclerosis: the Heinz Nixdorf recall study. J Am Coll Cardiol. 2010;56(17):1397–406.
13. The Danish Cardiovascular Screening Trial (DANCAVAS). www.isrctn.com/ISRCTN12157806. Accessed 5 Jan 2017.
14. Diederichsen AC, Rasmussen LM, Søgaard R, Lambrechtsen J, Steffensen FH, Frost L, et al. The Danish cardiovascular screening trial (DANCAVAS): study protocol for a randomized controlled trial. Trials. 2015;16:554. doi:10.1186/s13063-015-1082-6.
15. Bredahl K, Eldrup N, Meyer C, Eiberg JE, Sillesen H. Reproducibility of ECG-gated ultrasound diameter assessment of small abdominal aortic aneurysms. Eur J Vasc Endovasc Surg. 2013;45(3):235–40.
16. Grondal N, Bramsen MB, Thomsen MD, Rasmussen CB, Lindholt JS. The cardiac cycle is a major contributor to variability in size measurements of abdominal aortic aneurysms by ultrasound. Eur J Vasc Endovasc Surg. 2012;43(1):30–3.
17. Bland J, Altman D. Statistical methods for assessing agreement between two methods of clinical measurement. Lancet. 1986;1(8476):307–10.
18. Sprouse LR, Meier GH, LeSar CJ, DeMasi RJ, Sood J, Parent FN, et al. Comparison of abdominal aortic aneurysm diameter measurements obtained with ultrasound and computed tomography: is there a difference? J Vasc Surg. 2003;38(3):466–71.
19. Choke E, Vijaynagar B, Thompson J, Nasim A, Bown MJ, Sayers RD. Changing epidemiology of abdominal aortic aneurysms in England and wales: older and more benign? Circulation. 2012;125(13):1617–25.
20. Lindholt JS, Juul S, Fasting H, Henneberg EW. Screening for abdominal aortic aneurysms: single centre randomised controlled trial. BMJ. 2005;330(7494):750.
21. Lindholt JS, Juul S, Fasting H, Henneberg EW. Preliminary ten year results from a randomised single centre mass screening trial for abdominal aortic aneurysm. Eur J Vasc Endovasc Surg. 2006;32(6):608–14.
22. Pedersen C, Thomsen CF, Hosbond SE, Thomassen A, Mickley H, Diederichsen AC. Coronary computed tomography angiography - tolerability of β-blockers and contrast media, and temporal changes in radiation dose. Scand Cardiovasc J. 2014;48(5):271–7.

16

Development of a morphology-based modeling technique for tracking solid-body displacements: examining the reliability of a potential MRI-only approach for joint kinematics assessment

Niladri K. Mahato[1,2*], Stephane Montuelle[2], John Cotton[1,3], Susan Williams[1,2], James Thomas[1,4] and Brian Clark[1,2,5]

Abstract

Background: Single or biplanar video radiography and Roentgen stereophotogrammetry (RSA) techniques used for the assessment of *in-vivo* joint kinematics involves application of ionizing radiation, which is a limitation for clinical research involving human subjects. To overcome this limitation, our long-term goal is to develop a magnetic resonance imaging (MRI)-only, three dimensional (3-D) modeling technique that permits dynamic imaging of joint motion in humans. Here, we present our initial findings, as well as reliability data, for an MRI-only protocol and modeling technique.

Methods: We developed a morphology-based motion-analysis technique that uses MRI of custom-built solid-body objects to animate and quantify experimental displacements between them. The technique involved four major steps. First, the imaging volume was calibrated using a custom-built grid. Second, 3-D models were segmented from axial scans of two custom-built solid-body cubes. Third, these cubes were positioned at pre-determined relative displacements (translation and rotation) in the magnetic resonance coil and scanned with a T_1 and a fast contrast-enhanced pulse sequences. The digital imaging and communications in medicine (DICOM) images were then processed for animation. The fourth step involved importing these processed images into an animation software, where they were displayed as background scenes. In the same step, 3-D models of the cubes were imported into the animation software, where the user manipulated the models to match their outlines in the scene (rotoscoping) and registered the models into an anatomical joint system. Measurements of displacements obtained from two different rotoscoping sessions were tested for reliability using coefficient of variations (CV), intraclass correlation coefficients (ICC), Bland-Altman plots, and Limits of Agreement analyses.

Results: Between-session reliability was high for both the T_1 and the contrast-enhanced sequences. Specifically, the average CVs for translation were 4.31 % and 5.26 % for the two pulse sequences, respectively, while the ICCs were 0.99 for both. For rotation measures, the CVs were 3.19 % and 2.44 % for the two pulse sequences with the ICCs being 0.98 and 0.97, respectively. A novel biplanar imaging approach also yielded high reliability with mean CVs of 2.66 % and 3.39 % for translation in the x- and z-planes, respectively, and ICCs of 0.97 in both planes.

(Continued on next page)

* Correspondence: nm620511@ohio.edu
[1]Ohio Musculoskeletal and Neurological Institute, Ohio University, Athens, OH 45701, USA
[2]Department of Biomedical Sciences, Ohio University, Athens, OH 45701, USA
Full list of author information is available at the end of the article

(Continued from previous page)

Conclusions: This work provides basic proof-of-concept for a reliable marker-less non-ionizing-radiation-based quasi-dynamic motion quantification technique that can potentially be developed into a tool for real-time joint kinematics analysis.

Keywords: MRI, Stereophotogrammetry, Scientific rotoscoping, Dynamic sequence, Back pain

Background

Visualization of skeletal elements is central to three-dimensional (3-D) kinematic analysis of joint motion. Indirect methods based on tracking surface landmarks (using reflective markers attached to the skin surface) within a calibrated volume (stereophotogrammetry) can contain artifacts (errors of transformation) due to integumentary displacements relative to actual skeletal motion [1–5]. Direct visualization of bony elements during joint motion are typically accomplished *via* fluoroscopy or cineradiography. Unfortunately, both of these techniques require the use of ionizing radiation, and outcomes from these techniques are restricted mostly to two-dimensional (2-D) analyses as the majority of these systems use single-plane imaging [6, 7]. Emergence of the roentgen stereophotogrammetry (RSA) technique has enabled *in-vivo* measurement of complex 3-D skeletal kinematics from a series of radiographs acquired with biplanar, orthogonal fluoroscopy [1, 8, 9]. Although this technique is accurate, it commonly requires surgical implantation of markers in bones [2, 9–12], although model-based RSA techniques have recently begun to appear in the literature [13–15].

Recording a series of joint-motion images using x-ray fluoroscopy and then manually superimposing 3-D models of the same skeletal elements to match corresponding outlines in the x-ray images has been used to quantify *in-vivo* joint motion. [7, 16–18]. More recently, Gatesy *et al.* reported using the scientific rotoscoping (SR) motion analysis technique, which involves biplanar fluoroscopy to image skeletal movements, creation of 3-D models of joint skeleton from high-resolution computed tomography (CT) scans, followed by model-to-image matching and registration (rotoscoping) performed over several frames of images yielding skeletal motion animation and 3-D kinematic data [6, 19–21]. SR was developed from the X-Ray Reconstruction of Moving Morphology (XROMM) motion quantification technique, which tracks implanted markers digitized in biplanar fluoroscopic images captured within a calibrated imaging volume, instead of utilizing the model superimposition technique [6]. Though accurate, both SR and XROMM techniques require corrections of geometrical distortions in images prior to the animation [11, 12, 22–24]. While x-ray-based motion analysis techniques like SR, XROMM, and RSA are clearly novel and advanced, their translation to clinical

research (i.e., human subjects research) has been limited due to health-related concerns associated with the radiation exposure [25–29].

From a clinical research perspective, understanding *in vivo* skeletal motion is of interest to both scientists and clinicians [30–32]. More specifically, x-ray-based diagnostic imaging techniques measuring human inter-vertebral displacements have focused mostly on imaging the spine at static end-of-range positions [32–40]. However, qualitative and quantitative assessments of spinal motion have been enhanced by quantitative radiographic techniques that track displacements of pre-assigned co-ordinate points of specific anatomic locations on ortho-graphic spinal images and by real-time joint-motion evaluation with XROMM-like techniques (using CT/magnetic-resonance-imaging-based 3-D models) and RSA (with per-operative implanted vertebral markers) in human subjects [22, 28, 38, 41–47]. Regrettably, these approaches still require exposure to ionizing radiation and, at times, require marker implantation on the bones.

Magnetic resonance imaging (MRI), when used for quantifying inter-vertebral motion, has mostly been restricted to the analysis of end-of-range sagittal-plane displacements [48–50]. However, dynamic cine-phase contrast (cine-PC) or fast-phase contrast (fast-PC) imaging with ultra-fast gradient echo sequences have been employed for evaluating joint kinematics, especially in ankle, knee, or shoulder motion [51–57]. The main approach for these techniques has been the use of pulse sequences that permit volume extraction from full 3-D motion datasets at selected time points along the range of motion (ROM). However, these techniques can be time-consuming. Additionally, the use of cine-PC sequences require a repeated, cyclic, velocity-controlled motion to be performed at the joint of interest during scanning to make the motion synchronized with velocity-encoded motion capture [57, 58]. Also, these images have low resolution and may present motion artifacts [56, 58, 59]. More recently, the combined use of segmented 3-D anatomical models (from high resolution, ~15 mins duration, static axial scans) registered to low resolution, volumetric images acquired at different joint positions using high speed (~40 sec) T_1 sequences has been reported [57]. Although such techniques acquire multi-position data with much greater speed, the segmentation of these low-resolution images still require multi-slice images of the experimental quasi-dynamic joint positions. Accordingly, recent advancements in these methods have focused on the acquisition of faster and fewer slices of joint motion (without compromising image resolution) for model-to-image registration and without reducing the accuracy of the technique (time-accuracy tradeoff).

Currently, no modeling techniques exist for quantification of inter-vertebral joint displacements using single-plane or orthogonal magnetic-resonance (MR) image templates for 3-D model registration. Accordingly, our long-term goal is to develop a 3-D model-based technique that permits fast dynamic MR imaging of the human lumbar spine using an open-bore weight-bearing musculoskeletal MRI. Our study focuses on the lumbar spine as low back pain (LBP) is one of the most common reasons for seeking medical care world-wide and accounts for over 3.7 million physician visits per year in the United States alone [60–64]. As such, LBP is arguably one of the most debilitating and costly health disorders, and the development of technologies to aid scientists and clinicians in better understanding the etiology of LBP—as well as in monitoring the effects of therapeutic interventions— is desperately needed.

As a first step towards our long-term goal, we present in this article our initial research and development findings for an MRI-only protocol involving imaging (using a standard T_1 and a fast contrast-enhanced MRI sequences), a series of pre-determined displacements between solid-body models, 3-D models (segmenting T_1 weighted axial scans), and a morphology-based rotoscoping strategy for animation and quantification of the displacements. The use of the contrast-enhanced sequence will allow us, firstly, to test the feasibility and reliability of its use as a fast imaging tool and secondly, to compare its outcome with that of the standard high-resolution T_1 images. The feasibility and reliability of this MRI-based technique is discussed here, and we anticipate further developing this technique into a motion-assessment tool for the lumbar spine and other di-arthrodial joints.

Methods

General overview of the experimental design

The experiment involved scanning a pair of wooden cubes placed at pre-determined positions (displacement trials) relative to each other in a custom-calibrated coil of an open-MRI system (0.3 Tesla; Esaote G-scan Brio, Genoa, Italy). Additional axial images of the solid cubes were acquired and segmented using the AVIZO software (Hillsboro, OR, USA) to create 3-D virtual models of the cubes. Next, the MR images of the displacement trials and the 3-D cube models were transferred into an animation software (AutoDesk MAYA, San Rafael, CA, USA); and animations of these displacement trials were performed to quantify the relative motion incurred by the solid bodies. The technique involved four principal steps (Fig. 1a). First, the imaging volume of the MRI coil was calibrated using a custom-built grid (Fig. 2a). Second, 3-D models were segmented out from axial scans of the solid-body cubes (Fig. 2b ii-v). Third, the solid bodies were positioned at pre-determined displacements relative to each other in the MRI coil and scanned (Fig. 2b i); and the digital imaging and communications in medicine (DICOM) images were pre-processed into gray-scale TIF format. Fourth, these images were imported into the animation software using calibration data acquired from the grid used in the first step. These images were displayed as a series of background scenes in the animation environment (Fig. 2c & d i-iii). Next, the 3-D models were imported into the animation software and manually manipulated by the user to "register" the models to their outlines visible in the background

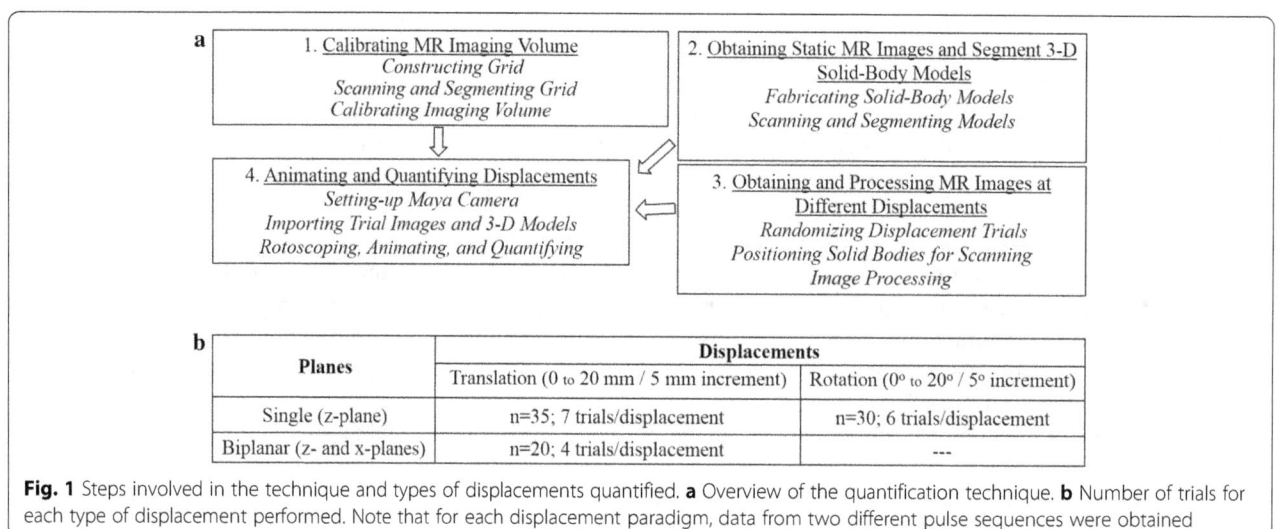

Planes	Displacements	
	Translation (0 to 20 mm / 5 mm increment)	Rotation (0° to 20° / 5° increment)
Single (z-plane)	n=35; 7 trials/displacement	n=30; 6 trials/displacement
Biplanar (z- and x-planes)	n=20; 4 trials/displacement	---

Fig. 1 Steps involved in the technique and types of displacements quantified. **a** Overview of the quantification technique. **b** Number of trials for each type of displacement performed. Note that for each displacement paradigm, data from two different pulse sequences were obtained

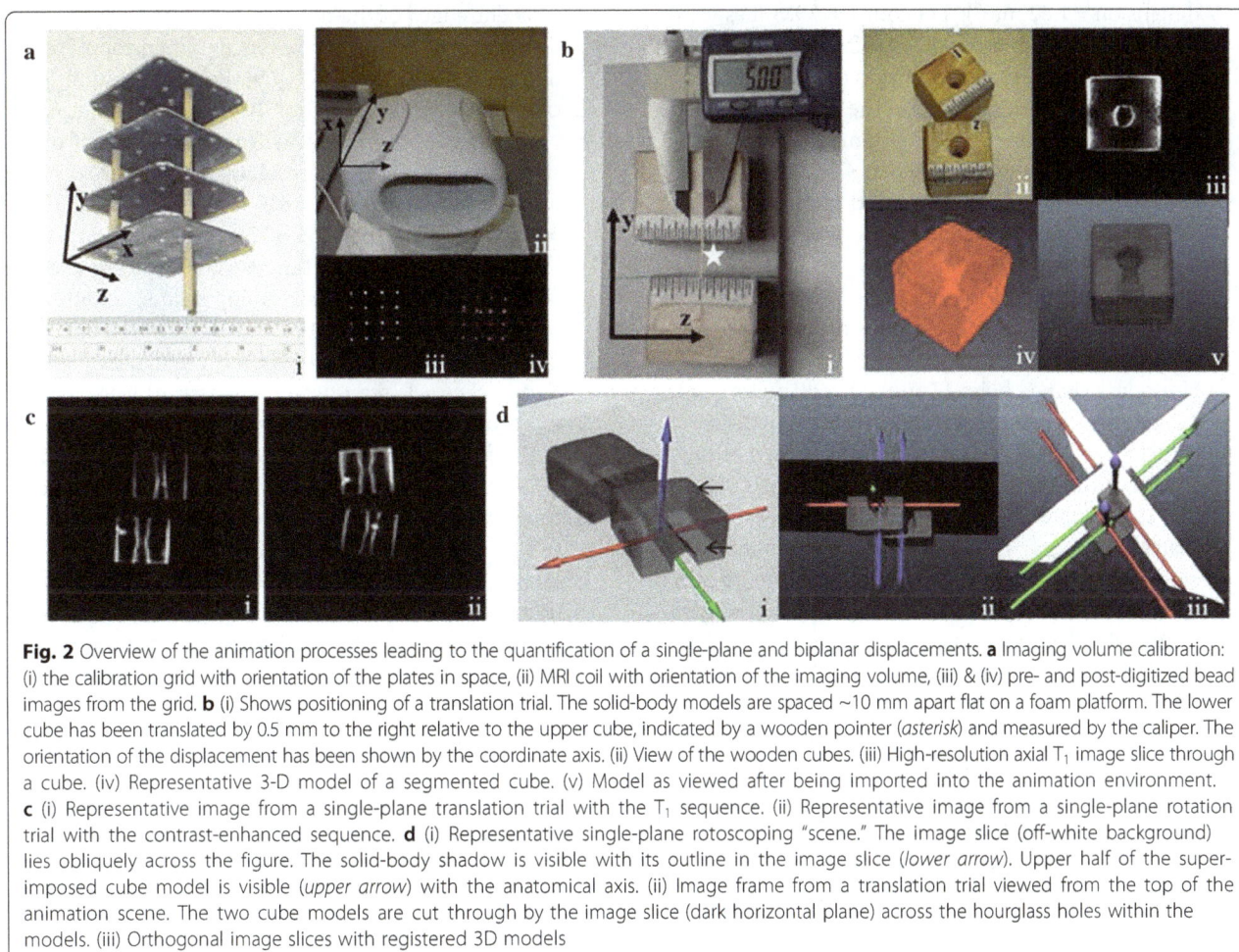

Fig. 2 Overview of the animation processes leading to the quantification of a single-plane and biplanar displacements. **a** Imaging volume calibration: (i) the calibration grid with orientation of the plates in space, (ii) MRI coil with orientation of the imaging volume, (iii) & (iv) pre- and post-digitized bead images from the grid. **b** (i) Shows positioning of a translation trial. The solid-body models are spaced ~10 mm apart flat on a foam platform. The lower cube has been translated by 0.5 mm to the right relative to the upper cube, indicated by a wooden pointer (*asterisk*) and measured by the caliper. The orientation of the displacement has been shown by the coordinate axis. (ii) View of the wooden cubes. (iii) High-resolution axial T_1 image slice through a cube. (iv) Representative 3-D model of a segmented cube. (v) Model as viewed after being imported into the animation environment. **c** (i) Representative image from a single-plane translation trial with the T_1 sequence. (ii) Representative image from a single-plane rotation trial with the contrast-enhanced sequence. **d** (i) Representative single-plane rotoscoping "scene." The image slice (off-white background) lies obliquely across the figure. The solid-body shadow is visible with its outline in the image slice (*lower arrow*). Upper half of the superimposed cube model is visible (*upper arrow*) with the anatomical axis. (ii) Image frame from a translation trial viewed from the top of the animation scene. The two cube models are cut through by the image slice (dark horizontal plane) across the hourglass holes within the models. (iii) Orthogonal image slices with registered 3D models

images (Fig. 2c & d). Lastly, inter-cube translational and rotational displacements were calculated using this technique. All measurements required for fabricating the grid and solid-body cubes and for measuring the experimental displacements during scanning were performed by a digital caliper (sensitivity = 0.02 mm) (Global Industrial, Port Washington, NY, USA). The details of each step are described below.

1. Calibrating the MR Imaging Volume: The volume of the MRI coil was calibrated using a custom-built calibration grid (Fig. 2a). Four square Perspex fiber plates (area = 80 mm^2; thickness = 2 mm) (Modular-Movement Tray-Set, Games Workshop/NG, UK) were serially stacked with a distance of 30 mm between each plate with three wooden dowels drilled across the plates and glued at all their contact points for stability. Before fixing the dowels, sixteen holes, each 2 mm in diameter, were drilled into each plate in a 4X4 array. Adjacent holes were drilled 20 mm apart from each other. Each hole was fitted with a 2-mm-diameter water bead using a small amount of glue. Three additional beads were embedded into two adjacent plates to define x, y, and z coordinates of the grid (Fig. 2a) [65]. The x- and z-axes were located in the same plane representing the plane of the grid plates, whereas the y-axis extended perpendicular to the plane of grid plates (Fig. 2a). These coordinates were assigned as per the joint coordinate system (JCS) defined by the Standardization and Terminology Committee of the International Society of Biomechanics for studying inter-vertebral motion [65]. To facilitate visualization of the beads in the MR images, the grid was submerged in a 1 % saline solution for 30 s and then air dried for 2 min prior to scanning. The y-axis of the grid was placed along the longer axis of the MRI coil bore (DPA Wrist Coil, Esaote, Genoa, Italy). Four non-contiguous axial 3-mm-thick slices were acquired parallel to and across the grid in a way that each slice image included a single plate with all the 16 beads of a plate in view using a Fast Spin Echo T_2 sequence (repetition time [TR] = 7810 ms, time to echo [TE] = 120 ms, field of view [FOV] = 200 x 200, Matrix = 256 × 256; resolution = 0.78 mm; voxel

dimension = 1.82 mm^3). The four DICOM files were then transferred to the AVIZO software, where all the beads were segmented and images of all segmented individual plates were stored in the TIF format using Photoshop software (Adobe Systems Inc., San Jose, California) for later use in Step 4. Additionally, the surface rendition of the segmented beads representing a composite view of the entire grid was saved as an .OBJ file for digitization in Step 4.

2. Constructing and Segmenting the Solid-Body Cubes: Two solid-body cubes, with sides measuring ~40 mm, were cut from a wood block (Fig. 2b). Hourglass shaped holes (7-mm base diameters) were drilled through the center of both cubes with a stepped-cone drill. These holes were drilled to create a distinct morphological feature within the cubes and to facilitate the rotoscoping and model-to-scene matching process in a later step. The cubes measured close to the average transverse dimensions of the first lumbar vertebral body in humans, and the hourglass feature simulated the appearance of the vertebral canal in a motion segment [19, 66–68]. Adjacent edges of the cubes were marked with a 20-mm scale with 1.0 mm graduations (Fig. 2b). A neutral position was defined as zero displacement between the mid-lines of the scales. The relative positions between these mid-lines on the scales were manipulated by the user to perform the translation trials with a range of 20 mm in either direction of the neutral position. The opposite sides of the cubes were marked with a protractor to measure inter-cube rotations on both sides of a 0° neutral position at increments of 5° through 90° of rotational displacement. Additionally, 3-D cube models were manually segmented in AVIZO using contiguous high resolution (pixel = 0.78 mm) axial T$_1$ weighted scans (TR = 810 ms, TE = 30 ms, FOV = 200 × 200, Matrix = 256 × 256) (Fig. 2b).

3. Displacement Trials: The solid-body cubes were immersed in ~1 % saline for 30 s, wiped dry, and positioned within the MR coil. The long axes of the hourglass-shaped holes in both the cubes were placed along the y-axis of the imaging volume and scanned in the neutral position. The single-plane translations and rotations were performed in the z-plane of the imaging volume. The axis for the rotation trials was formed by the x-plane. The cubes were placed and fixed by double-sided tape on a flat foam platform in the coil to avoid shifting during scans. After scanning the neutral position, the platform was pulled out of the coil; and the cubes were re-positioned for the next trail, with the displacements verified by the Vernier caliper before the platform was re-positioned inside the MRI coil (Fig 2b). A gap of ~10 mm was maintained between

adjacent edges of the cubes during translation, a distance representing the average dimension of a human lumbar disc space [69]. For the rotation trials, the center of rotation (COR) of the rotating cube was kept 50 mm away from the center of the stationary cube. A high-resolution (0.78 mm) T$_1$ weighted sequence (TR = 810 ms, TE = 30 ms, FOV = 220 × 220, Matrix = 256 × 256, slices = 3, gap = 0, thickness = 5 mm, scan time = ~2 mins/scan) and a fast contrast-enhanced streaming sequence with resolution 0.98 mm (2D hybrid contrast enhanced streaming sequence [2D HYCE S]; thickness = 8 mm, slice = 1, scan time = ~10 s/scan) were used to acquire single-slice images of displaced positions in the mid-sagittal (zy-) plane with the central core of both cubes in view (Fig. 2c). The trials included translations between 0.0–20 mm in 5 mm increments (n = 35 trials; 7 trials/displacement) and rotations ranging between 0° to 20° in 5° increments (n = 30 trials; 6 trials/displacement) on both sides of the neutral position (Table 1). Biplanar translations were scanned in static positions after the cubes were displaced both in the z- and x-planes through a range of 5 mm increments in a 0.0 to 20 mm range (n = 20; 4 trials/displacement). All trials were number-coded and randomly performed in three separate scanning sessions each designated for translational, rotational, and biplanar trials, respectively. For the biplanar trials, additional orthogonal slices were acquired with the central parts of both cubes in view.

4. Animation of the Imaging Volume and Quantification in MAYA [6, 21, 70]: The MAYA software was used to create the animation environment. The environment essentially represented the calibrated MR imaging volume. The software also provided a "camera-view" for the user to view the cube models and the background scene in the calibrated animation environment (Fig. 2d). The user manually manipulated the 3-D models to match and register them to their outlines seen in the background scenes. The steps for creating the animation environment are as follows:

(a) Creating a MAYA framespec File [6]:

The composite grid .OBJ file created in Step 1 was transferred to MAYA, all the beads were serially numbered according to their actual positions in the grid system, and the centroid points for each segmented bead was calculated by the program. Next, the values of the coordinate points for each bead centroid were calculated in the context of all other beads, representing the entire grid volume. The x, y, and z values of all bead coordinate points were merged together to generate the MAYA 'framespec' file to be used for the next step of grid digitization.

Table 1 Mean values and standard deviations, between-session average coefficient of variation (CV) and intra-class correlation coefficients (ICC) for the solid-body displacements

		Scanned Displacements	Mean±SD for S1	Mean±SD for S2	Mean CV (%)	ICC (95 % CI)
Single (z-) plane	Translation in T_1 (n=7/displacement)	0.0 mm	0.90±0.64 mm	0.73±0.47 mm	14.63	0.99 (0.98–0.99)
		5.0 mm	5.53±0.32 mm	5.30±0.44 mm	1.07	
		10.0 mm	11.60±0.41 mm	11.30±0.45 mm	2.80	
		15.0 mm	15.01±0.54 mm	15.27±0.52 mm	1.22	
		20.0 mm	20.84±0.43 mm	21.13±0.53 mm	1.81	
	Translation in 2D HYCE S (n=7/displacement)	0.0 mm	1.09±0.69 mm	1.32±0.65 mm	13.50	0.97 (0.98–0.99)
		5.0 mm	5.34±0.75 mm	5.20±0.40 mm	4.68	
		10.0 mm	10.35±0.59 mm	10.97±0.59 mm	4.12	
		15.0 mm	14.70±1.05 mm	15.20±0.60 mm	2.39	
		20.0 mm	19.79±0.72 mm	20.25±0.44 mm	1.61	
	Rotation in T_1 (n=6/displacement)	0°	0.21±0.18°	0.22±0.13°	2.29	0.98 (0.97–0.99)
		5°	5.43±0.77°	4.89±0.64°	7.41	
		10°	10.14±0.95°	10.38±0.75°	1.67	
		15°	14.44±1.22°	15.15±1.72°	3.37	
		20°	20.60±0.59°	20.95±0.64°	1.19	
	Rotation in 2D HYCE S (n=6/displacement)	0°	0.11±0.05°	0.12±0.09°	7.59	0.98 (0.97–0.99)
		5°	5.08±0.11°	5.01±0.06°	1.10	
		10°	10.39±0.17°	10.56±0.35°	1.17	
		15°	14.92±0.35°	15.20±0.21°	1.30	
		20°	20.20±0.63°	20.51±0.42°	1.05	
Biplanar (z- & x-planes)	Translation in 2D HYCE S z-plane (n=4/displacement)	0.0 mm	0.65±0.31 mm	0.92±0.61 mm	3.61	0.97 (0.98–0.99)
		5.0 mm	5.44±0.42 mm	5.03±0.32 mm	6.15	
		10.0 mm	10.54±0.59 mm	11.29±0.61 mm	4.84	
		15.0 mm	14.99±0.31 mm	14.71±0.99 mm	1.32	
		20.0 mm	20.94±0.89 mm	21.39±0.98 mm	1.51	
	Translation in 2D HYCE S x-plane (n=4/displacement)	0.0 mm	0.88±0.52 mm	0.83±0.41 mm	3.95	0.97 (0.98–0.99)
		5.0 mm	5.33±0.33 mm	5.12±0.45 mm	2.80	
		10.0 mm	11.40±0.28 mm	10.95±0.50 mm	2.82	
		15.0 mm	15.06±0.48 mm	15.58±0.40 mm	2.41	
		20.0 mm	20.88±0.58 mm	21.27±0.69 mm	1.32	

SD, standard deviation; CV, coefficient of variation; 95 % CI, lower and upper confidence intervals, S1: Session 1, S2: Session 2

(b) Digitizing the Beads:

A MEL-script (MAYA Embedded Language-script) command was run in Matlab. An image of a grid plate previously segmented in AVIZO and stored in a TIF format in Step 1 was opened using the Matlab program, and all beads in the plate were digitized serially by clicking over their central points. Next, the framespec file created in the previous step was loaded into the program to yield the Direct Linear Transformation (DLT) coefficient values for the concerned plate [6, 21]. All four plates were digitized sequentially to generate the DLT coefficient value for each plate image. The program allowed automated corrections for minimization of errors and to contain coefficient values ≤ 1 [21]. This step was repeated for all four plates, and each step yielded a plate coefficient value and a "xyz point" .csv file specific to the concerned digitized plate. The data points of the xyz-point files from all the four plates were collated to generate a common "four-plate xyz point" .csv file for the grid [65]. Next, the four-plate xyz-point and the framespec files were loaded into the Matlab program using the MEL-script. One of the segmented plate-images were opened in the Matlab and re-digitized. The four-plate xyz-point file was loaded into the program, and the MEL-script was re-run to generate a "MayaCam".csv file that was used to re-create the MR imaging within the animation software and to create the camera-view for the user.

(c) Rotoscoping, Animation, and Quantification: The animation scene was created using the MayaCam file. After the animation environment was created, the background scene was introduced by importing the TIF format images of the trials into MAYA (Fig. 2c & d). These images were clustered into a series of frames, with each series representing a specific trial type. Next, the two 3-D cube models were imported into MAYA using a scaling factor of 0.1 (from segmentation environment in mm to the animation environment in cm). The models were manipulated with the computer mouse and keyboard functions to achieve maximum geometrically alignment and match between the 3-D model and corresponding image outlines in the background scene. The sharp external boundaries and outlines of the hourglass silhouettes within the solid bodies were utilized to facilitate the model-to-scene match (Fig. 2c & d). This process was called rotoscoping. Once rotoscoping in the first frame of the scene (neutral position in the series) was achieved, an Anatomical Joint Axis (AJX) was assigned to the solid bodies. The image of the background scene was then advanced to the next frame and the rotoscoping repeated; this process was repeated for all remaining trial images. For the biplanar translations, two orthogonal camera views were created to provide background scenes of displacements from two different, the x- and z-plane, perspectives (Fig. 2d). Although the animation software generated solid-body motion data for all rotoscoped image frames in all six degrees of freedom, only applicable single-plane measures were extracted for analysis and reporting. Two sessions (S1 and S2) of rotoscoping and displacement quantification were performed separately for translational, rotational, and biplanar motion by a single observer (NKM). All trials were number coded, and the rater was blinded to the displacement type and the pulse sequence used for the scan. The AJX created in Session 1 was used for rotoscoping in the corresponding Session 2. The approximate time for rotoscoping (Step 4(c)) a series of image frames representing a specific trial type, e.g., a seven-translation series, in this study was ~40 min including matching of the neutral position at the start and extracting displacement data from the series at the end.

Statistical analysis

Test–retest reliability for the outcomes involving the T_1 and 2D HYCE S sequences from the two sessions were determined by coefficient of variation (CV), t-test, intra-class correlation coefficients (ICC) (two-way random effects model with a single measure of reliability), and 95 % limits of agreement (LOA) analyses. Variability between the outcomes from a single displacement quantified in two different sessions was analyzed using CV. For example, if a particular displacement was quantified as 11.5 mm in Session 1 and 10.8 mm in Session 2, the CV was calculated as: Standard Deviation of the two sessions divided by the mean of the two sessions times 100. Thus, for this example, the CV = (0.5/11.15) × 100 = 4.44 %. The sessions were performed at an interval of one week. Additionally, we used dependent sample t-tests to compare the values between testing sessions.

The ICC was calculated using a (2, 1) two-way random effects model with a single measure of reliability computed over the variance observed in the two sessions. A (2, 1) model was chosen as it allows the determination of any existing systematic bias. The statistical software SPSS (SPSS Inc., Version 21.0, Chicago, IL, USA) was used to calculate the ICC. The main objective of the statistical analysis was to ascertain the reliability of this technique. The relative reliability was assessed by calculating the ICC, which assesses the reproducibility of a measurement relative to a sample of repeated measurements. The absolute stability of a measure typically defines the contribution of the main-error component in the observed variance. To fully understand the absolute stability or reliability of a measure, it is essential to understand the contribution of different components of the measurement error [71, 72]. Accordingly, the measurement error was broken into two components. The first component was defined as the systematic bias, and the second was termed the random error. The systematic bias denoted the contribution of any learning effect on the part of the assessor in explaining the between-session variability of the data, whereas the random error explained a biological or mechanical effect [72, 73]. The first step was to generate Bland-Altman plots using the between-session means and differences data. The correlation (R^2) between the absolute differences and the means of the between-session values was calculated to determine the spread of the dependent variable. R^2 values between 0 and 0.1 represented homoscedasticity, suggesting that there was no correlation between the size of the error and the size of the measured variable. Heteroscedasticity was considered to be present with R^2 values > 0.1 and indicated that the degree of error increased with increase in the values of the measured variable along the scale, e.g., the error term increased as the technique attempted to measure larger displacements (translation/rotation) in the experiment [71–74]. Finally, the ratio LOA was calculated for verification of the absolute reliability of the measure using the following equation: ratio LOA = [(SDdiffs/AVGmeans) × 1.96] × 100, where *SDdiffs* was defined as the Standard Deviation of the difference of scores (Session 1 and Session 2), *AVGmeans* represented the average of the mean scores (Session 1and Session 2) for each measurement, and the factor 1.96 specified the inclusion of 95 % of observations of the differences in scores. The ratio LOA was interpreted as the highest percentage by which two tests will differ due to measurement error in either the positive or negative direction [72].

Results
Summary of results
Descriptive statistics and CV and ICC reliability measures obtained from the T_1 and 2D HYCE S images for each type of displacement are provided in Table 1. A high degree of between-session reliability was observed for both the T_1 and the contrast-enhanced dynamic pulse sequences. Specifically, the average CVs for translation were 4.31 % and 5.26 % for the two pulse sequences, respectively, while the ICCs were 0.99 for both sequences. For rotation measures, the CVs were 3.19 % and 2.44 % for the two pulse sequences with the ICCs being 0.98 and 0.97, respectively. A novel biplanar imaging approach also yielded high reliability, with mean CVs of 3.39 % and 2.66 % noted for translation in the z- and x-plane, respectively, along with ICCs of 0.97 in both planes. Additionally, all but one displacement variables showed homoscedastic relationships with the Bland-Altman's LOA analysis of the between-session measurements and demonstrated a relatively low degree of systematic bias.

Translation trials
Analysis of the between-session measurements of each of the two sequences, applying a paired sample 2-tailed *t*-test, did not show any significant differences in means between the T_1 ($p > 0.98$) and the 2D HYCE S ($p > 0.84$) pulse sequences. The reliability of the measured variables demonstrated high levels of consistency, with the T_1 sequence having CVs ranging from 1.1 to 14.63 % and an ICC of 0.99. For the 2D HYCE S sequence, the CVs ranged from 1.6 to 13.5 %, and the ICC was also 0.99. The Bland-Altman plot with 95 % confidence interval (±1.96*standard deviation [SD]) analysis of the between-session data showed that all cases had a test-retest difference within ±1.24 mm (mean/bias = 0.02 mm) and ±1.59 mm (mean/bias = -0.34 mm) for the T_1 and the 2D HYCE S sequences, respectively (Fig. 3a). The LOA analysis for translation indicated a relatively low degree of systematic bias in the between-session

differences ($p = 0.98$ and 0.84) and a homoscedastic relationship between the differences and averages of the between-session measurements for both T_1 and the 2D HYCE S pulse sequences respectively ($R^2 = 0.07$ and $R^2 = 0.03$) (Fig. 3a). The homoscedasticity indicated that the random errors did not increase with the increase of the measured displacement values. The follow-up ratio LOA analysis demonstrated a systematic bias in the order of 0.02 and -0.34 and random error of ±14.14 and ±13.68 for the T_1 and 2D HYCE S sequences, respectively. The ratio LOA analysis for translation suggested that the between-session measurement errors obtained with the technique did not exceed 14.15 % and 13.34 % in either the positive or negative direction with the use of T_1 and the 2D HYCE S pulse sequences, respectively.

Rotation trials
Analysis of the between-session measurements of the two sequences applying a paired sample 2-tailed *t*-test did not show any significant mean differences for the T_1 ($p > 0.94$) and the 2D HYCE S ($p > 0.96$) sequences. The reliability of the measured variables demonstrated high levels of consistency, with the T_1 sequence having CVs ranging from 1.2 to 7.6 % and an ICC of 0.98. For the 2D HYCE S sequence, the CVs ranged from 1.05 to 7.6 %, and the ICC was 0.98. The Bland-Altman plot with 95 % confidence interval (±1.96*SD) analysis of the between-session data showed that all cases had a test-retest difference within ±1.27° (mean/bias = -0.14°) and ±0.65° (mean/bias = 0.09°) for the T_1 and the 2D HYCE S sequences, respectively. The LOA analysis for the rotation trials indicated a relatively low degree of systematic bias in the between-session differences ($p = 0.94$ and 0.96) and a homoscedastic relationship between the differences and averages of the between-session measurements for both T_1 and the 2D HYCE S pulse sequences respectively ($R^2 = 0.06$ and 0.04) (Fig. 3b). A homoscedastic relationship indicated that the random errors did not increase with the increase of the measured values. The follow-up ratio LOA analysis indicated a systematic bias in the order of -0.15 and -0.09 and random error of ±14.55 and ±20.10 for the T_1 and 2D HYCE S sequences, respectively. The ratio LOA analysis for rotation suggested that the between-session measurement errors obtained with the technique did not exceed 14.40 % and 20.01 % in either the positive or negative direction using the T_1 and the 2D HYCE S pulse sequences, respectively.

Comparing outcomes between the pulse sequences
Analysis of the difference between the averages of Session 1 and Session 2 translations obtained by T_1 and 2D HYCE S pulse sequences did not show any significant

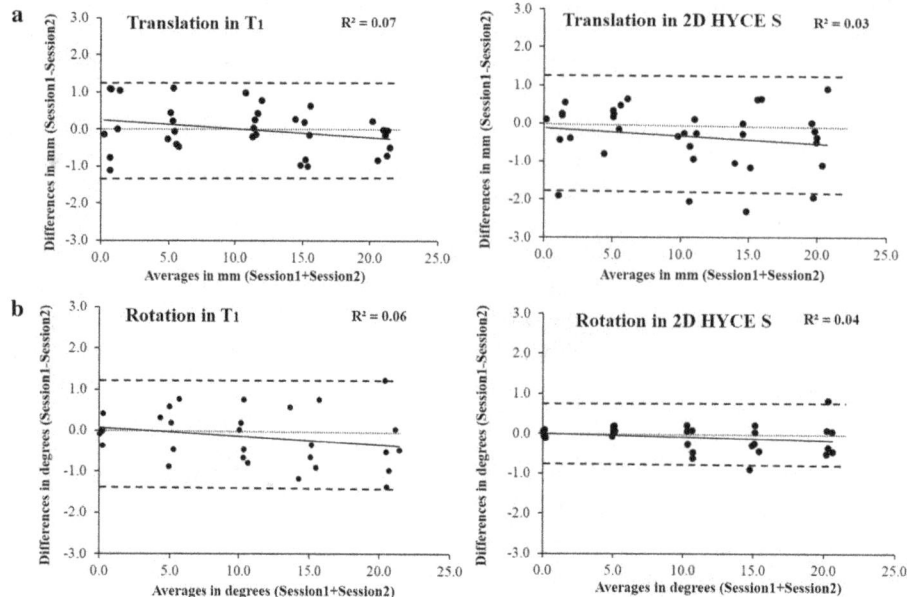

Fig. 3 Bland–Altman plots of translation (**a**) and rotation (**b**) trials for each sequence. **a**: Plots of the translation displacements quantified with the two sequences. The dashed lines representing the 95 % confidence interval of test-retest differences for all translations show that the between-session differences were within ±1.24 mm (mean/bias = 0.02 mm) and ±1.59 mm (mean/bias = -0.34 mm) for the T_1 (left) and the 2D HYCE S (right) sequences, respectively. **b**: Plots of the rotation displacements quantified with the two sequences. The dashed lines representing the 95 % confidence interval of all rotations show that the test-retest differences were within ±1.27° (mean/bias = -0.14°) and ±0.65° (mean/bias = 0.09°) for the T_1 (left) and the 2D HYCE S (right) sequences, respectively. The central narrow line denotes zero difference mark. The dark line at the center represents the trend line. Homoscedasticity (R^2 values < 0.1) indicated that the between-session differences in the measurements did not increase with an increase in the magnitude of the measured displacement. Heteroscedasticity was represented by R^2 values > 0.1, indicating that the between-session differences in the measurements increased with an increase in the magnitude of the measured displacement

results using an independent sample 2-tailed t-test (p = 0.83). The Bland-Altman plot with 95 % confidence interval (±1.96*SD) analysis of the between-sequence data showed a test-retest difference within ±1.50 mm (mean/bias = 0.35 mm) (Fig. 4a). A small heteroscedastic relationship observed in the translation measures indicated that the T_1 vs 2D HYCE S between-sequence difference in measured translations increased with assessments of larger magnitudes of translation (R^2 = 0.24). The follow-up ratio LOA analysis demonstrated a systematic bias in the order of 0.354 and random error of ±13.41. The ratio LOA analysis for translation suggested that between-sequence measurement errors were within 13.77 % in either the positive or negative direction.

Analysis of the difference between the averages of Session 1 and Session 2 rotations obtained by T_1 and 2D HYCE S pulse sequences did not show any significant results using an independent sample 2-tailed t-test (p = 0.98). The Bland-Altman plot with 95 % confidence interval (±1.96*SD) analysis of the between-sequence data showed a test-retest difference within ±0.95° (mean/bias = 0.02°) (Fig. 4a). A homoscedastic relationship observed in the rotation measures indicated that the between-sequence random errors did not increase with assessments of larger magnitudes of translation

(R^2 = 0.03). The follow-up ratio LOA analysis demonstrated a systematic bias in the order of 0.03 and random error of ±14.28. The LOA ratio analysis for rotation suggested that the between-sequence measurement errors with the T_1 and 2D HYCE S pulse sequences were within 14.31 % in either the positive or negative direction.

Biplanar trials

Analysis of the between-session measurements with a paired sample 2-tailed t-test did not show any significant difference for the z- (p = 0.79) and x (p = 0.73) planes. The reliability of the measured variables demonstrated high levels of consistency, with the z-plane having CVs ranging from 1.51 to 6.15 % and an ICC of 0.97. The CVs for the x-plane measurements ranged from 1.32 to 3.95 %, and the ICC was 0.97. The Bland-Altman plot with the 95 % confidence interval (±1.96*SD) analysis of the biplanar between-session data showed that all displacements had a test-retest difference within ±1.41 mm (mean/bias = -0.04 mm) and ±2.70 mm (mean/bias = 0.12) for the x- and z-planes, respectively (Fig. 4b). The LOA analysis for the biplanar trials demonstrated a relatively low degree of systematic bias in the between-session differences (p = 0.79 and 0.73) and a systematic bias in the order of -0.04 and -0.01 and random error of

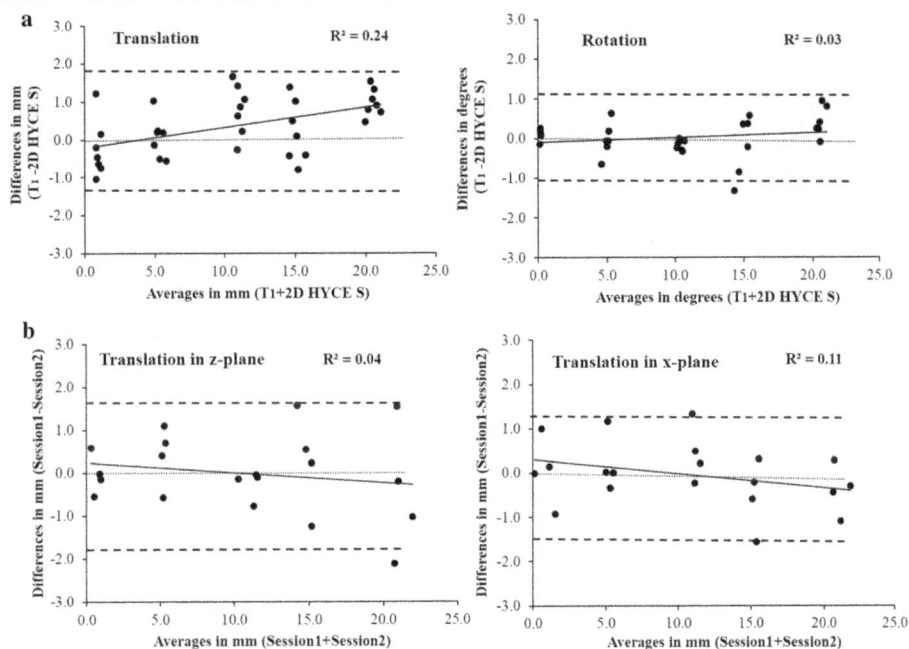

Fig. 4 Bland-Altman plots comparing outcomes between T_1 and the 2D HYCE S sequences (**a**). Plots of the bi-planar translation quantified with the 2D HYCE S sequence (**b**). **a**. Plots comparing outcomes using T_1 and the 2D HYCE S sequences. The dashed lines representing the 95 % confidence intervals show that the between-session differences in the measurements obtained with the T_1 and the 2D HYCE S sequences fell within ±1.85 mm (mean/bias = 0.35 mm) for translations (left) and within ±0.95° (mean/bias = 0.02°) for all rotations (right) quantified. **b**. Bland–Altman plots for biplanar translations. The dashed lines representing the 95 % confidence intervals show that the test-retest differences for translations fell within ±1.77 mm (mean/bias = -0.01 mm) and ±1.41 mm (mean/bias = -0.04 mm) for the z- and x-planes, respectively. The central narrow line denotes zero difference mark. The dark line at the center represents the trend line. Homoscedasticity (R^2 values < 0.1) indicated that the random errors did not increase with an increase in the magnitude of the measured values. Homoscedasticity (R^2 values < 0.1) indicated that the differences in the measurements did not increase with the increase in the magnitude of the measured displacement. Heteroscedasticity was represented by R^2 values > 0.1, indicating that the differences in the measurements increased with the increase in the magnitude of the measured displacement

±10.87 and ±21.03 for the z- and for the x-planes, respectively. The ratio LOA analysis for translation suggested that the between-session measurement errors obtained with the technique did not exceed 21.03 % and 10.76 % in either the positive or negative direction for the x- and z-planes, respectively. The ratio LOA analysis for the biplanar translation trials showed a homoscedastic relationship between the differences and averages of the between-session measurements for the z-plane (R^2 = 0.04), indicating that the random errors did not increase with the increase of the measured values. The x-plane data, however, showed a marginal heteroscedastic relationship (R^2 = 0.11), indicating that the random errors did marginally increase with the increase of the measured values (Fig. 4b).

Discussion

In this study, we describe a novel MRI-based approach that is conceptually similar to some fluoroscopy-based modeling protocols with the major difference of not requiring exposure to ionizing radiation, which has obvious implications for clinical research [6, 18, 19]. While this is the first step in the development of an MRI-based

protocol of this nature, our initial work indicates that this technique has promise as we have successfully developed a logical and rational approach to the quantification of motion and have also demonstrated relative and absolute reliability. Below we discuss our findings within the context of the extant literature as well as our future directions.

As stated above, the primary innovation of this work is that it represents an MRI-only, morphology-based modeling technique for tracking solid-body displacements, which is similar to fluoroscopy-based approaches, such as RSA, SR, and XROMM, and static x-ray-based techniques. The scope of application of these fluoroscopy-based techniques is limited due to the ionizing radiation exposure. For instance, obtaining serial measures involving significant radiation exposure over time in research studies requiring oversight by an institutional review board (or other analogous committees charged with approving, monitoring and reviewing biomedical research involving humans) could raise questions about the cost-to-benefit ratio, particularly in light of the Institute of Medicine's recommendation on avoiding unnecessary medical radiation throughout life [26, 28]. Accordingly, we believe that an MRI-only-based modeling technique for investigating joint kinematics has significant advantages, particularly for the advancement of clinical research.

Available MRI modeling techniques have usually applied multi-slice imaging of the objects of interest to capture the experimental displacements introduced into these objects in the scanning environment. Our study has uniquely attempted a morphology-based single-plane and an orthogonal imaging protocol to quantify experimentally induced displacements in our models. Additionally, we have used a fast-scanning protocol with dynamic contrast-enhanced pulse sequence and compared its outcome to a standard high-resolution T_1 imaging. Both these methods have demonstrated high-levels of reliability in quantifying displacements in objects within the MR imaging volume. These findings provide basic proof-of-concept for the notion that a reliable non-ionizing-radiation-based motion quantification technique can potentially be used to characterize a quasi-static visualization of joint kinematics from a single and biplanar approach. The use of dynamic sequence and image processing can be further explored to attempt quantification of joint kinematics in synchronized motion. Additionally, while our single-plane technique does not objectively address detecting out-of-plane motion, inclusion of the orthogonal imaging in the biplanar approach helps manual positioning of the model to match the corresponding out-of-plane shifts of the image silhouettes.

While our initial development results are promising, our study has some limitations. First, we have used static two-dimensional imaging for quantification purposes; and we do not know whether comparable levels of reliability would have been observed if the dynamic pulse sequence were used to scan the solid-bodies in real-time during an un-synchronized motion with subsequent quantification of these images using the technique reported here. The approach we chose was based on technology currently available; to our knowledge, an MRI-compatible device that would permit real-time manipulation of motion is not commercially available, and the custom development of such a device would require significant resources. Second, the current approach required manual segmentation and post-processing, which is very time intensive. Accordingly, we do not know how the use of semi-automatic protocols or automatic iterative segmentation algorithms would have changed our results. Third, while we reported high levels of reliability for a novel biplanar imaging modality (i.e., quantification of motion in two planes, or coupled motion), the orthogonal images obtained for this analysis were not acquired simultaneously (i.e., an image slice was first acquired in one plane and then acquired for the corresponding orthogonal plane) due to the inherent limitation of MR

imaging to do so. While this is not necessarily a limitation of the current work, it could pose a limitation for future work that seeks to acquire simultaneous multi-planar images of motion. Lastly, we only assessed reliability and did not assess accuracy. We are currently conducting experiments that will assess accuracy of our technique in a porcine spine model.

Conclusion

In summary, this work provides basic proof-of-concept for a reliable non-ionizing-radiation-based marker-less imaging technique that can potentially be used to quantify quasi-dynamic displacements between joint elements. Additionally, this morphology-based MRI-only technique could be explored further as a tool for real-time joint kinematics analysis.

Abbreviations
RSA: roentgen stereophotogrammetry; MRI: magnetic resonance imaging; 2D HYCE S: Two-Dimensional Hybrid Contrast Enhanced Streaming Sequence; CV: coefficient of variation; DICOM: digital imaging and communications in medicine; ICC: intraclass correlation coefficient; LOA: limits of agreement; SR: scientific rotoscoping; XROMM: X-Ray Reconstruction of Moving Morphology; AJX: anatomical joint axis; FOV: field of view.

Competing interests
The authors declare that they have no competing interests.

Authors' contributions
NM conceived the study idea and design, performed image acquisition, data analysis, drafting and revision of manuscript. SM supported in designing the study, development of technical strategy, draft of manuscript. JC provided inputs on data analysis and drafting of manuscript. SW helped with the study design and to draft and revise the manuscript. JT assisted with study design and in editing the manuscript. BC contributed with data analysis, major edits on original manuscript and the revision. All authors read and approved the revisions and the final version of the manuscript.

Acknowledgement
All MEL scripts and animation related software tools were used from XROMM resources developed at and made available by the Brown University, RI, USA.

Source of funding
This work was supported by the American Osteopathic Association (AOA) Research Grant # 13-08-682.

Author details
[1]Ohio Musculoskeletal and Neurological Institute, Ohio University, Athens, OH 45701, USA. [2]Department of Biomedical Sciences, Ohio University, Athens, OH 45701, USA. [3]Department of Mechanical Engineering, Ohio University, Athens, OH 45701, USA. [4]School of Rehabilitation and Communication Sciences, Ohio University, Athens, OH 45701, USA. [5]Department of Geriatric Medicine, Ohio University, Athens, OH 45701, USA.

References
1. Cappozzo A et al. Human movement analysis using stereophotogrammetry. Part 1: theoretical background. Gait Posture. 2005;21(2):186–96.
2. Della Croce U et al. Human movement analysis using stereophotogrammetry. Part 4: assessment of anatomical landmark misplacement and its effects on joint kinematics. Gait Posture. 2005;21(2):226–37.
3. Reinschmidt C et al. Effect of skin movement on the analysis of skeletal knee joint motion during running. J Biomech. 1997;30(7):729–32.

4. Cereatti A, Della Croce U, Cappozzo A. Reconstruction of skeletal movement using skin markers: comparative assessment of bone pose estimators. J Neuroeng Rehabil. 2006;3:7.

5. Chiari L et al. Human movement analysis using stereophotogrammetry. Part 2: instrumental errors. Gait Posture. 2005;21(2):197–211.

6. Brainerd EL et al. X-ray reconstruction of moving morphology (XROMM): precision, accuracy and applications in comparative biomechanics research. J Exp Zool A Ecol Genet Physiol. 2010;313(5):262–79.

7. Yamazaki T et al. Improvement of depth position in 2-D/3-D registration of knee implants using single-plane fluoroscopy. IEEE Trans Med Imaging. 2004;23(5):602–12.

8. Axelsson P, Karlsson BS. Intervertebral mobility in the progressive degenerative process. A radiostereometric analysis. Eur Spine J. 2004;13(6):567–72.

9. Selvik G. Roentgen stereophotogrammetric analysis. Acta Radiol. 1990;31(2):113–26.

10. Bojan AJ et al. Three-dimensional bone-implant movements in trochanteric hip fractures: Precision and accuracy of radiostereometric analysis in a phantom model. J Orthop Res. 2015;33(5):705–11.

11. Bey MJ et al. Accuracy of biplane x-ray imaging combined with model-based tracking for measuring in-vivo patellofemoral joint motion. J Orthop Surg Res. 2008;3:38.

12. Martin DE et al. Model-based tracking of the hip: implications for novel analyses of hip pathology. J Arthroplasty. 2011;26(1):88–97.

13. Lai JY et al. A new registration method for three-dimensional knee nearthrosis model using two X-ray images. Comput Methods Biomech Biomed Engin. 2010;13(2):265–78.

14. Hurschler C et al. Comparison of the model-based and marker-based roentgen stereophotogrammetry methods in a typical clinical setting. J Arthroplasty. 2009;24(4):594–606.

15. Bey MJ et al. Validation of a new model-based tracking technique for measuring three-dimensional, in vivo glenohumeral joint kinematics. J Biomech Eng. 2006;128(4):604–9.

16. Dial KP, Goslow GE, Jenkins FA. The Functional-Anatomy of the Shoulder in the European Starling (Sturnus-Vulgaris). J Morphol. 1991;207(3):327–44.

17. Jenkins Jr FA, Dial KP, Goslow Jr GE. A cineradiographic analysis of bird flight: the wishbone in starlings is a spring. Science. 1988;241(4872):1495–8.

18. Zhu Z et al. The accuracy and repeatability of an automatic 2D-3D fluoroscopic image-model registration technique for determining shoulder joint kinematics. Med Eng Phys. 2012;34(9):1303–9.

19. Baier DB, Gatesy SM. Three-dimensional skeletal kinematics of the shoulder girdle and forelimb in walking Alligator. J Anat. 2013;223(5):462–73.

20. Gatesy SM, David BB. The Origin of the Avian Flight Stroke: A Kinematic and Kinetic Perspective. Paleobiology. 2005;31(3):382–399.

21. Gatesy SM et al. Scientific rotoscoping: a morphology-based method of 3-D motion analysis and visualization. J Exp Zool A Ecol Genet Physiol. 2010; 313(5):244–61.

22. Anderst WJ, Vaidya R, Tashman S. A technique to measure three-dimensional in vivo rotation of fused and adjacent lumbar vertebrae. Spine J. 2008;8(6):991–7.

23. Tashman S et al. Dynamic function of the ACL-reconstructed knee during running. Clin Orthop Relat Res. 2007;454:66–73.

24. Schueler BA. The AAPM/RSNA physics tutorial for residents: general overview of fluoroscopic imaging. Radiographics. 2000;20(4):1115–26.

25. Latini G et al. Reproductive effects of low-to-moderate medical radiation exposure. Curr Med Chem. 2012;19(36):6171–7.

26. Kesavachandran CN, Haamann F, Nienhaus A. Radiation exposure of eyes, thyroid gland and hands in orthopaedic staff: a systematic review. Eur J Med Res. 2012;17:28.

27. Hricak H et al. Managing radiation use in medical imaging: a multifaceted challenge. Radiology. 2011;258(3):889–905.

28. Mellor FE, Thomas P, Breen A. Moving back: The radiation dose received from lumbar spine quantitative fluoroscopy compared to lumbar spine radiographs with suggestions for dose reduction. Radiography. 2014;20(3):251–7.

29. Boice Jr JD, Mandel JS, Doody MM. Breast cancer among radiologic technologists. JAMA. 1995;274(5):394–401.

30. Licciardone JC, Gatchel R, Dagenais S. Assessment and management of back pain. JAMA Intern Med. 2014;174(3):478–9.

31. Freddolini M, Strike S, Lee RY. Stiffness properties of the trunk in people with low back pain. Hum Mov Sci. 2014;36:70–9.

32. Hasegewa K et al. Biomechanical evaluation of segmental instability in degenerative lumbar spondylolisthesis. Eur Spine J. 2009;18(4):465–70.

33. Pearcy MJ, Bogduk N. Instantaneous axes of rotation of the lumbar intervertebral joints. Spine (Phila Pa 1976). 1988;13(9):1033–41.

34. Gertzbein SD et al. Centrode characteristics of the lumbar spine as a function of segmental instability. Clin Orthop Relat Res. 1986;208:48–51.

35. Panjabi MM. Clinical spinal instability and low back pain. J Electromyogr Kinesiol. 2003;13(4):371–9.

36. Dvorak J et al. Clinical validation of functional flexion-extension roentgenograms of the lumbar spine. Spine (Phila Pa 1976). 1991;16(8):943–50.

37. McGill SM, Cholewicki J. Biomechanical basis for stability: an explanation to enhance clinical utility. J Orthop Sports Phys Ther. 2001;31(2):96–100.

38. Passias PG et al. Segmental lumbar rotation in patients with discogenic low back pain during functional weight-bearing activities. J Bone Joint Surg Am. 2011;93(1):29–37.

39. Weiler PJ, King GJ, Gertzbein SD. Analysis of sagittal plane instability of the lumbar spine in vivo. Spine (Phila Pa 1976). 1990;15(12):1300–6.

40. Yeager MS, Cook DJ, Cheng BC. Reliability of computer-assisted lumbar intervertebral measurements using a novel vertebral motion analysis system. Spine J. 2014;14(2):274–81.

41. Shin JH et al. Investigation of coupled bending of the lumbar spine during dynamic axial rotation of the body. Eur Spine J. 2013;22(12):2671–7.

42. Tan Y et al. Kinetic magnetic resonance imaging analysis of lumbar segmental mobility in patients without significant spondylosis. Eur Spine J. 2012;21(12):2673–9.

43. Yao Q et al. Motion characteristics of the lumbar spinous processes with degenerative disc disease and degenerative spondylolisthesis. Eur Spine J. 2013;22(12):2702–9.

44. Pearcy MJ. Stereo radiography of lumbar spine motion. Acta Orthop Scand Suppl. 1985;212:1–45.

45. Pearcy MJ, Hindle RJ. New method for the non-invasive three-dimensional measurement of human back movement. Clin Biomech (Bristol, Avon). 1989; 4(2):73–9.

46. Schneider G, Pearcy MJ, Bogduk N. Abnormal motion in spondylolytic spondylolisthesis. Spine (Phila Pa 1976). 2005;30(10):1159–64.

47. Yang JS et al. Dynamic Radiographic Results of Different Semi-Rigid Fusion Devices for Degenerative Lumbar Spondylolisthesis: "Dynamic Rod" vs. "Dynamic Screw Head". Turk Neurosurg. 2016;26(2):268–73.

48. Keorochana G et al. Effect of sagittal alignment on kinematic changes and degree of disc degeneration in the lumbar spine: an analysis using positional MRI. Spine (Phila Pa 1976). 2011;36(11):893–8.

49. Lee SH, Daffner SD, Wang JC, Davis BC, Alanay A, Kim JS. The change of whole lumbar segmental motion according to the mobility of degenerated disc in the lower lumbar spine: a kinetic MRI study. Eur Spine J. 2014. doi:10. 1007/s00586-014-3277-z.

50. Chung SS et al. Effect of low back posture on the morphology of the spinal canal. Skeletal Radiol. 2000;29(4):217–23.

51. Rebmann AJ, Sheehan FT. Precise 3D skeletal kinematics using fast phase contrast magnetic resonance imaging. J Magn Reson Imaging. 2003;17(2): 206–13.

52. Behnam AJ, Herzka DA, Sheehan FT. Assessing the accuracy and precision of musculoskeletal motion tracking using cine-PC MRI on a 3.0 T platform. J Biomech. 2011;44(1):193–7.

53. Ward SR et al. Assessment of patellofemoral relationships using kinematic MRI: Comparison between qualitative and quantitative methods. J Magn Reson Imaging. 2002;16(1):69–74.

54. Quick HH et al. Real-time MRI of joint movement with TrueFISP. J Magn Reson Imaging. 2002;15(5):710–5.

55. Shellock FG et al. Kinematic magnetic resonance imaging of the joints: techniques and clinical applications. Magn Reson Q. 1991;7(2):104–35.

56. Clarke EC et al. A non-invasive, 3D, dynamic MRI method for measuring muscle moment arms in vivo: demonstration in the human ankle joint and Achilles tendon. Med Eng Phys. 2015;37(1):93–9.

57. Fellows RA et al. Repeatability of a novel technique for in vivo measurement of three-dimensional patellar tracking using magnetic resonance imaging. J Magn Reson Imaging. 2005;22(1):145–53.

58. Fellows RA et al. Magnetic resonance imaging for in vivo assessment of three-dimensional patellar tracking. J Biomech. 2005;38(8):1643–52.

59. d'Entremont AG et al. Do dynamic-based MR knee kinematics methods produce the same results as static methods? Magn Reson Med. 2013;69(6):1634–44.

60. Whitehurst DG et al. Implementing Stratified Primary care Management for low Back Pain: Cost Utility Analysis alongside a Prospective, Population-based, Sequential Comparison Study. Spine (Phila Pa 1976). 2015.

61. Manchikanti L et al. Epidemiology of low back pain in adults. Neuromodulation. 2014;17 Suppl 2:3–10.

62. Schaefer C et al. Pain severity and the economic burden of neuropathic pain in the United States: BEAT Neuropathic Pain Observational Study. Clinicoecon Outcomes Res. 2014;6:483–96.

63. North RB et al. A review of economic factors related to the delivery of health care for chronic low back pain. Neuromodulation. 2014;17 Suppl 2:69–76.

64. March L et al. Burden of disability due to musculoskeletal (MSK) disorders. Best Pract Res Clin Rheumatol. 2014;28(3):353–66.

65. Wu G et al. ISB recommendation on definitions of joint coordinate system of various joints for the reporting of human joint motion–part I: ankle, hip, and spine. International Society of Biomechanics. J Biomech. 2002;35(4):543–8.

66. Cheung JP, Shigematsu H, Cheung KM. Verification of measurements of lumbar spinal dimensions in T1- and T2-weighted magnetic resonance imaging sequences. Spine J. 2014;14(8):1476–83.

67. Ostrofsky KR, Churchill SE. Sex determination by discriminant function analysis of lumbar vertebrae. J Forensic Sci. 2015;60(1):21–8.

68. Rhoad RC et al. A new in vivo technique for three-dimensional shoulder kinematics analysis. Skeletal Radiol. 1998;27(2):92–7.

69. Hong CH et al. Measurement of the normal lumbar intervertebral disc space using magnetic resonance imaging. Asian Spine J. 2010;4(1):1–6.

70. Nyakatura JA, Fischer MS. Three-dimensional kinematic analysis of the pectoral girdle during upside-down locomotion of two-toed sloths (Choloepus didactylus, Linne 1758). Front Zool. 2010;7:21.

71. Clark BC, Cook SB, Ploutz-Snyder LL. Reliability of techniques to assess human neuromuscular function in vivo. J Electromyogr Kinesiol. 2007;17(1): 90–101.

72. Atkinson G, Nevill AM. Statistical methods for assessing measurement error (reliability) in variables relevant to sports medicine. Sports Med. 1998;26(4): 217–38.

73. Bland JM, Altman DG. Statistical methods for assessing agreement between two methods of clinical measurement. Lancet. 1986;1(8476):307–10.

74. Kaya RD, Hoffman RL, Clark BC. Reliability of a modified motor unit number index (MUNIX) technique. J Electromyogr Kinesiol. 2014;24(1):18–24.

17

Diffusion tensor MR imaging characteristics of cerebral white matter development in fetal pigs

Wenxu Qi[1], Song Gao[2], Caixia Liu[3], Gongyu Lan[1], Xue Yang[3] and Qiyong Guo[1*]

Abstract

Background: The purpose of this study was to investigate the anisotropic features of fetal pig cerebral white matter (WM) development by magnetic resonance diffusion tensor imaging, and to evaluate the developmental status of cerebral WM in different anatomical sites at different times.

Methods: Fetal pigs were divided into three groups according to gestational age: E69 ($n = 8$), E85 ($n = 11$), and E114 ($n = 6$). All pigs were subjected to conventional magnetic resonance imaging (MRI) and diffusion tensor imaging using a GE Signa 3.0 T MRI system (GE Healthcare, Sunnyvale, CA, USA). Fractional anisotropy (FA) was measured in deep WM structures and peripheral WM regions. After the MRI scans, the animals were sacrificed and pathology sections were prepared for hematoxylin & eosin (HE) staining and luxol fast blue (LFB) staining. Data were statistically analyzed with SPSS version 16.0 (SPSS, Chicago, IL, USA). A P-value < 0.05 was considered statistically significant. Mean FA values for each subject region of interest (ROI), and deep and peripheral WM at different gestational ages were calculated, respectively, and were plotted against gestational age with linear correlation statistical analyses. The differences of data were analyzed with univariate ANOVA analyses.

Results: There were no significant differences in FAs between the right and left hemispheres. Differences were observed between peripheral WM and deep WM in fetal brains. A significant FA growth with increased gestational age was found when comparing E85 group and E114 group. There was no difference in the FA value of deep WM between the E69 group and E85 group. The HE staining and LFB staining of fetal cerebral WM showed that the development from the E69 group to the E85 group, and the E85 group to the E114 group corresponded with myelin gliosis and myelination, respectively.

Conclusions: FA values can be used to quantify anisotropy of the different cerebral WM areas. FA values did not change significantly between 1/2 way and 3/4 of the way through gestation but was then increased dramatically at term, which could be explained by myelin gliosis and myelination, respectively.

Background

From a simple tubular structure to a mature organ with complete function, the development and evolution of fetal brain is precise and complicated. White matter (WM) development of the intrauterine prenatal fetal brain is closely associated with a variety of nervous and mental diseases in the neonatal phase, early childhood, adolescence, and adulthood [1–10]. By studying and clarifying the intrauterine developmental patterns of

cerebral WM before birth, and deciphering the anatomical and microstructural characteristics of fetal brain at different stages of development, we can not only analyze the procedures and steps of fetal brain developmental processes, but also study brain diseases related to brain development. Diseases such as perinatal brain injury and neonatal hypoxic-ischemic encephalopathy are closely related to cerebral white matter (WM) development [2]. Pigs are the standard animal model for studying neonatal hypoxic-ischemic encephalopathy (HIE) [11–14]. However, the mechanisms of normal fetal cerebral WM development have not been reported.

* Correspondence: guoqiyong2016@163.com
[1]Department of Radiology, Shengjing Hospital, China Medical University, Shenyang 110004, People's Republic of China
Full list of author information is available at the end of the article

Diffusion tensor imaging (DTI) can quantitatively determine the parameters related to the movement direction of water molecules in the cerebral WM. DTI can not only quantitatively analyze the microstructure of cerebral WM, but also has the advantages of three-dimensional imaging of the cerebral WM fiber [15].

The current study utilized conventional MRI T2 structural imaging and DTI to measure the various specific characteristic FA values of different anatomical parts of the cerebral WM in fetal and neonatal pig brain, and used HE staining and LFB (Luxol Fast Blue) myelin staining to study the developmental changes in cerebral WM tissues, in order to determine the correlation between imaging and histology. The study allows preliminary exploration of the intrauterine developmental rules of pig cerebral WM at different stages.

Intrauterine prenatal fetal cerebral WM development is closely related to a variety of neurological and psychiatric diseases at the neonatal phase, early childhood, adolescence, and adulthood [1–10]. To study and clarify the developmental patterns of cerebral WM in the uterus before birth, and to clarify the anatomical and microstructure characteristics of fetal brain during different stages of development, we can not only analyze the procedures and steps of fetal brain developmental processes, but also study the brain diseases related to development. Diseases such as perinatal brain injury and neonatal hypoxic-ischemic encephalopathy are closely related to cerebral WM development [2].

The pig is the standard animal model for studying neonatal hypoxic-ischemic encephalopathy (HIE) [11–14]. However, studies investigating the normal fetal cerebral WM development have not been reported.

The current study utilized conventional MRI T2 structural imaging and DTI to measure the various specific characteristics FA values of different anatomical parts of the cerebral WM in fetal and neonatal pig brain, and used HE staining and FLB myelin staining to study the developmental changes in cerebral WM tissue, to determine the correlation between imaging and histology, thus allowing a preliminary exploration of the intrauterine developmental rules of pig cerebral WM at different stages.

Methods
Animal preparation
This study was conducted on the approval of Ethical Committee at Shengjing Hospital, China Medical University (Permit Number:2014PS153K). Through caesarean section, eight fetal pigs with gestational age of 69 days, and 11 fetal pigs with gestational age of 85 days were obtained from healthy pregnant pigs. Another six neonatal pigs from the

same mother pig, with gestational age of 114 days, were also included in the current study. All the pigs were divided into three groups based on their gestational age, which were named as the E69 group, E85 group, and E114 group.

MRI scanning
MRI scanning was carried out using a 3.0-T MR system (Signa Excite HD; GE Medical Systems, Milwaukee, Wis), with rat coil (5 cm in diameter) used for the E69 and E85 groups, and knee joint coil (15 cm in diameter) used for the E114 group. The conventional T2WI scan parameters were: TR5000 ms, TE80 ms, with layer thickness of 2 mm and interval of 0.3 mm. The SE-EPI sequence was utilized for DTI examination with scanning parameters as follows: TR8000 ms, TE100 ms; scan matrix: 128*128; Field of View: 4–6 cm; layer thickness of 2 mm, and interval of 0.3 mm. Scanning was carried out twice with a diffusion weighting coefficient b value of 0/600 s/mm2 and a gradient field intensity applied at 25 directions. The scanning time was about 12 min.

Specimen preparation
After the MRI examination, the animals were sacrificed immediately with the whole brain quickly collected, then immersed, and fixed in 4% formalin solution. After 72-h fixation, the right and left hemispheres of the specimen were separated, followed by cross-sectional sampling, then embedded in paraffin and sliced.

Regular HE staining
The morphology, quantity and the density of the glia cells, and the density of nervous fibers were evaluated by HE staining of sections. The neurons and glial cells were counted in highpower field (×200) .7 anatomic sites of the deep brain white matter and 4 anatomical sites of superficial brain white matter were selected for each of the brain specimens.

LFB myelin specific staining
The method for LFB staining was: (1) Paraffin slice and alcohol dehydration; (2) staining with LFB, and incubation overnight with 1% LFB dye at 60 °C; (3) differential fixation with 70% alcohol immersion and 0.05% lithium carbonate; (4) washing in water; (5) HE counterstaining; and (6) mounting. The myelin sheaths stained blue using this method.

Post-processing and analysis of the images
Images with conventional scanning
The T2WI image obtained by conventional scanning was analyzed by two experienced neuroradiologists using a double-blind approach. The semiquantitative maturity evaluation score method was as previously described [16]. Two experienced clinicians evaluated the images

separately, with further discussions in cases of differing opinions.

DTI results

Data processing was carried out with GE Workstation Function Tool software (GE Healthcare). Regions of interest (ROIs) in the T2WI map, Colored orientation map, Average DC map and FA map were defined by two experienced radiologists who were not familiar with the gestational age of the study animals, with the FA values of each ROI measured. The ROIs are outlined on T2WI maps,also can be superimposed on the Colored orientation maps, Average DC maps and FA maps at the same time on GE Functool station.

The measuring method was the size of the ROI at a point region of 1 mm2, which was moved within the anatomical position to obtain the highest FA value. The selected ROIs included deep cerebral WM including the anterior limb internal capsule (ALIC), the posterior limb internal capsule (PLIC), the genu corporis callosi (GCC), the splenium corporis callosi (SCC), the periventricular white matter (PV), the optic radiation (OR), the corona radiate (CR), and the superficial white matter regions including the frontal lobe (FL), temporal lobe (TL), parietal lobe (PL), and occipital lobe (OL), as shown in Fig. 1. Measurements were of both sides of the brain.

Statistical analyses

SPSS version 15 (SPSS) was used for data analyses, and $P < 0.05$ was considered statistically significant. All data were expressed as mean ± standard deviation (M ± SD), with paired t-tests used to analyze whether there was a significant difference in the FA values of the same site between the left and right hemispheres. Spearman's rank correlation analysis was used to analyze the correlation coefficient of the gestational age and FA values in different parts of the brain. The differences in FA values among different parts of the brain, or at different gestational ages, were analyzed using univariate ANOVA. The mean values of FA in the deep cerebral WM and the

superficial cerebral WM were calculated. Spearman's rank correlation analyses were utilized to determine the correlation coefficient between the FA value of the fetal cerebral WM and the gestational age. The differences between FA values and the number of neurons and glial cells of the deep and superficial cerebral WM, or at different gestational ages, were analyzed using univariate ANOVA.

Results

Morphological changes

No myelination changes were observed in the E69 group (Fig. 2), and were equivalent to the normal human levels of a gestational age younger than 20 weeks. In the E85 group, low punctate signals indicated myelination in the medulla, caudex cerebri, and at the back of pons in T2WI images, with no myelination in the PLIC and lateral parts of the thalamus. This was equivalent to the human level at 27–35 weeks of gestational age. In the E114 group, a low signal was observed at the spinal cord, extending from the medulla oblongata and dorsal pons, through the medial lemniscus to the cerebral peduncle, thalamic ventral lateral, PLIC, and central part of the corona radiata, consistent with the human level of neonates at 40 weeks of gestational age.

In the germinal matrix (Fig. 3), the E69 group had a low signal in the germinal matrix along the anterior horn, thalamic tail groove, and the posterior horn. The E85 group had a low signal corresponding to the anterior horn and thalamic tail groove, but not the posterior horn, which was equivalent to the human level at 26 weeks of gestational age. In the E114 group, no germinal matrix was observed, corresponding with the human level at older than 34 weeks.

Sulci and gyri (Fig. 4) in the E69 group showed smooth insula with no anterior or posterior temporal sulcus, visible hemisphere cerebral sulcus, and a lateral cerebral fissure separating the frontotemporal and parietal occipital sulcus. In the E85 group, a shallow insular sulcus and gyrus with shallow anterior and posterior temporal sulcus were observed. Fissura calcarina, sulcus

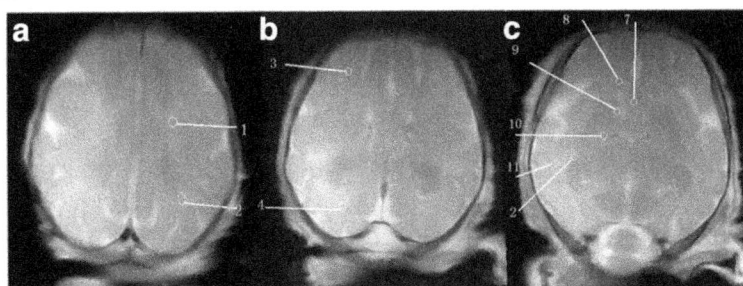

Fig. 1 Fetal brain graph of interest region (from 1 to 12 were the corona radiate, parietal lobe white matter, frontal lobe white matter, occipital lobe white matter, corpus callosum genu, periventricular white matter, the anterior limb internal capsule, white matter of temporal lobe, optic radiation). (**a**) the level of semioval center (**b**) the level of lateral ventricle (**c**) the level of basal nuclei

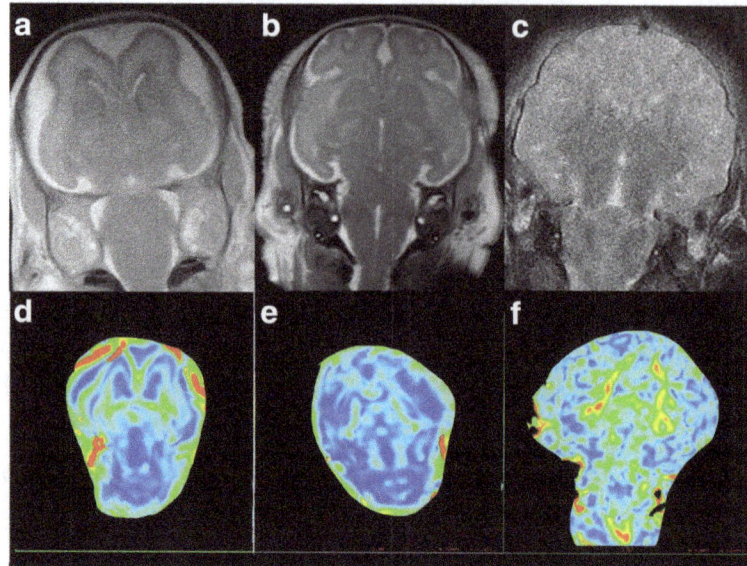

Fig. 2 Basal ganglia T2WI map (**a-c**), FA (**d-f**) (from the left and right are gestational age 69, 85, 114 days respectively) No myelination changes were observed in the E69 group (**a**). In the E85 group, low punctate signals indicated myelination in the medulla, caudex cerebri, and at the back of pons in T2WI images, with no myelination in the PLIC and lateral parts of the thalamus (**b**). In the E114 group, a high signal was observed at the spinal cord, extending from the medulla oblongata and dorsal pons, through the medial lemniscus to the cerebral peduncle, thalamic ventral lateral, PLIC, and central part of the corona radiata (**c**)

ammonis, the anterior central gyrus, the central gyrus, and the posterior gyrus were observed, along with a shallow anterior and posterior frontal gyrus, and anterior and posterior temporal gyrus. In group E114, a deep insular sulcus and gyrus, and deepened anterior and posterior temporal sulci were observed, along with a deep anterior and posterior frontal gyrus, anterior and posterior temporal gyrus, and temporal occipital gyrus, as well as a visible frontotemporal gyrus. The lateral fissure of the brain was almost closed, with the insula covered.

The brain maturity scores of the E69 group, the E85 group, and the E114 group were 1 point, 6 points, and 11 points, respectively, and were approximately equivalent to the levels of the human fetus at 20, 27, and 40 weeks, respectively [16].

DTI data

There were no significant differences in the FA values found between the left and right cerebral hemispheres at the same site using paired t-tests ($P > 0.05$). The average values were calculated for further analyses.

The average FA values of the deep cerebral white matter in the different gestational age groups, including ALIC, PLIC, GCC, SCC, PV, OR, and CR and in the superficial cerebral WM, including Frontal Lobe, Parietal Lobe, Temporal Lobe and Occipital Lobe (Table 1). The FA values of different parts of the brain at the same gestational age were different. For the E114 group, the regions with the highest to lowest FA values were the PLIC, ALIC, SCC, GCC, PV, OR, CR, the occipital, parietal, temporal, and the frontal lobe WM. For the E85

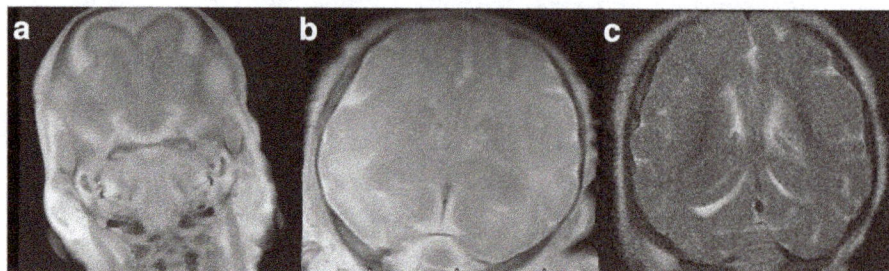

Fig. 3 Germinal matrix T2WI map (**a-c**) (from the left and right are gestational age 69, 85, 114 days respectively) the E69 group had a low signal in the germinal matrix along the anterior horn, thalamic tail groove, and the posterior horn (**a**). The E85 group had a low signal corresponding to the anterior horn and thalamic tail groove, but not the posterior horn (**b**). In the E114 group, no germinal matrix was observed (**c**)

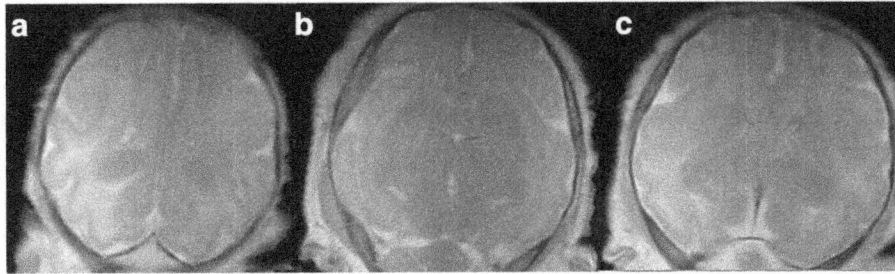

Fig. 4 Cerebral sulcus development T2WI map (**a-c**) (from the left and right are gestational age 69, 85, 114 days respectively) In the E69 group, smooth insula with no anterior or posterior temporal sulcus, visible hemisphere cerebral sulcus, and a lateral cerebral fissure separating the frontotemporal and parietal occipital sulcus (**a**). In the E85 group, a shallow insular sulcus and gyrus with shallow anterior and posterior temporal sulcus were observed. Fissura calcarina, sulcus ammonis, the anterior central gyrus, the central gyrus, and the posterior gyrus were observed, along with a shallow anterior and posterior frontal gyrus, and anterior and posterior temporal gyrus (**b**). In group E114, a deep insular sulcus and gyrus, and deepened anterior and posterior temporal sulci were observed, along with a deep anterior and posterior frontal gyrus, anterior and posterior temporal gyrus, and temporal occipital gyrus, as well as a visible frontotemporal gyrus. The lateral fissure of the brain was almost closed, with the insula covered (**c**)

group, the FA values were (from highest to lowest): PLIC, SCC, PV, OR, ALIC, GCC, CR, occipital, parietal, frontal, and temporal lobe WM. For the E69, the FA values were (from highest to lowest): PLIC, PV, SCC, GCC, ALIC, CR, frontal, parietal, temporal, and occipital lobe WM. During the process of overall development, among the deep cerebral WM, the FA values of the PLIC and SCC were higher, while the value of the OR and CR were lower.

Spearman's rank correlation analyses showed that the FA value of each ROI was positively correlated with gestational age, and the correlation was statistically significant ($P < 0.01$) (Table 2).

The univariate ANOVA analyses of the differences among the FA values of various regions at different gestational ages showed no statistically significant difference in the deep cerebral WM between the E69 group and E85 group, except for the ALIC and SCC ($P > 0.05$). There were no significant differences between the WM of the frontal and temporal lobes ($P > 0.05$). The average

FA values of the deep cerebral WM were higher than those of the peripheral cerebral WM ($P < 0.05$) (Table 3).

Spearman's rank correlation analyses showed that the FA value of each ROI was positively correlated with gestational age, and the correlation was statistically significant ($P < 0.01$) (Table 3). The FA values of the anatomical regions were gradually increased with the gestational age, but at different speeds. The increasing change at the first stage, from the second trimester to late pregnancy, was slow (the deep and peripheral cerebral WM increases were 1.36% and 23.92%, respectively). The increase at the second stage, from the late pregnancy to neonatal stage, was greater (the deep and peripheral cerebral WM increases were 76.2% and 83.2%, respectively).

Univariate ANOVA analyses for the differences in FA values of different parts or different gestational ages showed no significant differences in the deep cerebral

Table 1 The average FA value of different parts of different gestational age

	E69	E85	E114
ALIC	0.214 ± 0.004	0.218 ± 0.011	0.452 ± 0.010
PLIC	0.233 ± 0.008	0.234 ± 0.009	0.587 ± 0.021
GCC	0.216 ± 0.007	0.217 ± 0.032	0.385 ± 0.103
SCC	0.229 ± 0.011	0.234 ± 0.012	0.428 ± 0.014
PV	0.231 ± 0.012	0.231 ± 0.008	0.337 ± 0.023
OR	0.212 ± 0.009	0.220 ± 0.009	0.285 ± 0.011
CR	0.203 ± 0.003	0.206 ± 0.010	0.280 ± 0.015
Frontal Lobe	0.086 ± 0.014	0.090 ± 0.025	0.145 ± 0.026
Temporal Lobe	0.069 ± 0.014	0.078 ± 0.032	0.151 ± 0.022
Parietal Lobe	0.084 ± 0.014	0.097 ± 0.012	0.173 ± 0.015
Occipital Lobe	0.069 ± 0.007	0.118 ± 0.008	0.230 ± 0.006

Table 2 Correlation analysis between FA value and gestational age at different sites

	r	P
ALIC	0.734	0.000
PLIC	0.579	0.002
GCC	0.715	0.000
SCC	0.580	0.002
PV	0.568	0.002
OR	0.760	0.000
CR	0.605	0.001
Frontal Lobe	0.510	0.008
Temporal Lobe	0.581	0.002
Parietal Lobe	0.741	0.000
Occipital Lobe	0.929	0.000

Note: R is the correlation coefficient, $P < 0.05$ has statistical significance

Table 3 Deep brain WM and Superficial brain WM data table

	Deep brain WM		Superficial brain WM		T	P
	Average value	Standard deviation	Average value	Standard deviation		
E69	0.220	0.004	0.077	0.005	57.703	0.000
E85	0.223	0.006	0.095	0.014	25.216	0.000
E114	0.393	0.03	0.175	0.007	16.439	0.000
r	0.715		0.833			
P	0.000		0.000			

Note: R is the correlation coefficient, T is the single factor variance analysis

WM, except between that of the E69 group and the E85 group ($P > 0.05$).

Histological examination of the pig fetal brain tissue
HE staining of the cerebral white matter
HE staining and optical microscopy images of the fetal pig brain at different gestational ages (Fig. 5) demonstrated that the superficial WM neurons in the E69 group were immature with sparse nerve fibers and processes. The deep WM showed pink staining of the cytoplasm, with more mature neurons and sparse nerve fibers.

The nerve fibers of the E85 group were not densely clustered, the density of nerve fibers was not significantly different from that of the E69 group, but had significantly increased neurons. Compared with the E69 group, neurons in the deep cerebral WM of the E85 group were more densely clustered, mature, and close to the normal status, with larger numbers and densities of glia cells, more concentrated neuronal fibers, and increased numbers and lengths of cellular processes (axons or dendrites).

The morphology and numbers of the superficial WM neurons in the E114 group were close to that of the E85 group, but with denser nerve fibers. The morphology of the deep brain WM neurons in the E114 group was not significantly changed compared with the previous stage, but the nerve fibers were thicker and the glial cells

became larger and more complicated, which corresponded with the beginning of myelination.

LFB staining of cerebral white matter
LFB staining of pig brain at different gestational ages (Fig. 6) showed bright blue staining of the myelin sheath visible under optical microscopy. Typical funicular distribution of blue staining was observed in the deep cerebral WM of the E114 group. No blue staining was observed in the deep and superficial cerebral WM of the E69 and E85 groups, or the superficial cerebral WM of the E114 group.

The number of neurons of the superficial WM in E69 group, E85 group, E114 group were $6.38 \pm 3.045, 13.73 \pm 7.029, 16.13 \pm 9.993$, respectively. The number of glial cells of the superficial WM in E69 group, E85 group, E114 group were $11.69 \pm 3.505, 61.98 \pm 23.460, 64.50 \pm 26.203$; respectively. The number of neurons of the deep WM in E69 group, E85 group, E114 group were $9.95 \pm 4.952, 18.81 \pm 9.022, 18.79 \pm 8.446$; respectively. The number of glial cells of the deep WM in E69 group, E85 group, E114 group were $13.50 \pm 4.596, 121.00 \pm 40.811, 116.84 \pm 44.584$, respectively.

Multiple groups means were compared with single factor analysis of variance, and the comparison among groups was performed with SNK method. Based on $\alpha = 0.05$, There was no statistically significant difference in population mean of neurons and glial cells between the

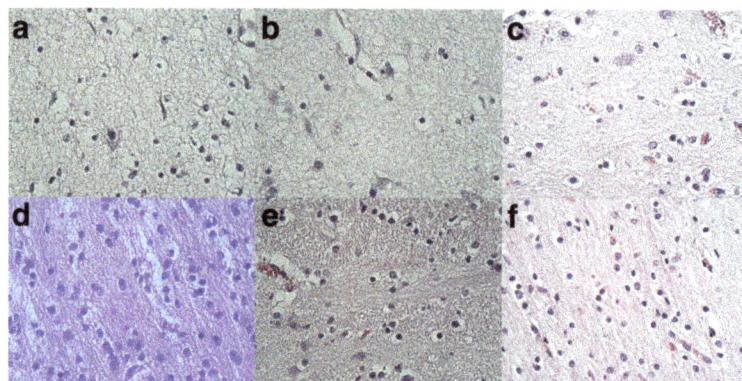

Fig. 5 HE staining 200 times light microscope (from left to right frontal lobe, anterior parts) (**a**, **b**: E69 group; group **c** and **d**:E85; **e**, **f**: E114 group) T

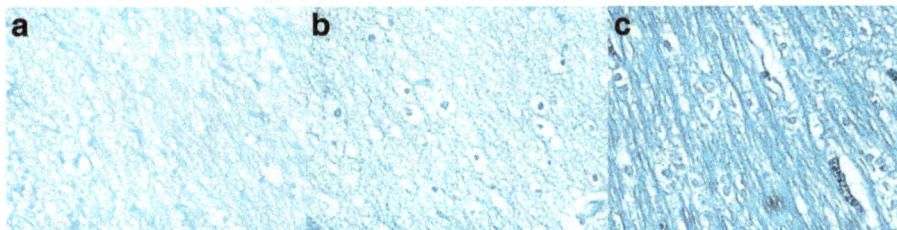

Fig. 6 FLB staining 200 times light microscope (internal cerebral white matter: **a**: E69 group, **b**: E85 group, **c**: E114 group)

E85 group and E114 group, including the deep brain WM and superficial brain WM. In addition, there are significant statistically difference in population mean between any other two groups.

Discussion

DTI study of development animal brain

This study chose to examine the pig brains at gestational ages of 69, 85, and 114 days corresponding to the human gestational weeks of one half, three quarters, and full pregnancy, respectively. Earlier gestational ages, have smaller head diameter, cannot be studied because the unsuited magnetic resonance coil would affect the quality of the images. The data show that T2 images of conventional MRI demonstrated a degree of myelination, degeneration of the germinal matrix, and morphological changes of the brain sulcus roughly corresponding with the human fetal level of 20 weeks, 27 weeks, and 40 weeks. The FA values of the WM were consistent with the DTI study of the fixed primate fetal brain at 90–185 days of gestational age, and had almost the same FA values at all regions of the WM at a gestational age of 90 days, with no significant differences between the deep and superficial WM. At a gestational age of 185 days, the FA values of the WM were higher, especially for the myelinated WM such as the internal capsule [17], which is consistent with our observations and past studies.

There was also a study investigating the DTI changes in cat brain after birth. Although the cats were already born, the development of the myelin sheath was consistent with the intrauterine development of pig and primates; therefore, their FA value changes could also be used as references. The P0 samples showed diffusive WM with low FA values, which had slightly higher local FA values at areas with more concentrated neurons such as the corpus callosum and internal capsule. Along with the development (P35), LBS staining was used to detect myelination in deep cerebral WM, which showed major projection fibers such as primary visual and sensory motor fibers. In these regions, the FA values were highest, with increased FA values at the peripheral WM.

These changes occurred at 1 month after birth, which was also consistent with the process we observed between the second trimesters to full pregnancy [18]. In addition, using the afterbirth development of rats as a reference for the study of human intrauterine development is also useful [3, 19, 20].

The rules of development and FA value changes of fetal cerebral WM DTI can reflect the anatomical and pathological processes of WM fibers, which is a great improvement in imaging methodology, and may also improve the field of WM fiber study [21]. Our results showed that the values of FA increased along with myelination development. Therefore, measuring values can be used as a noninvasive imaging quantitative marker for fetal cerebral WM maturation. The anisotropy of WM fibers is determined by macroscopic and microscopic conditions. First, the microstructural characteristics of the tissues, such as the diameter and density of the fibers, and the degree of the myelination, and then, the macrostructural characteristics of tissues, such as the interconnections among the fiber channels, can be determined. As summarized in previous studies, the histological development related to the rapid changes of FA values of the cerebral WM include increased numbers and densities of neuronal axons, enhanced phosphorylation of nerve fibers, increases in number and maturity of myelin sheaths of nerve fibers, and the expression of myelin basic protein [22, 23].

The differences between the deep WM and the peripheral WM

The current study demonstrated that at various gestational ages, the FA values of the deep cerebral WM in fetal brain were significantly higher than in peripheral WM. Combined with histological examination results, a possible mechanism could be suggested: 1) In terms of axonal fiber arrangement, although the extent of development of the WM in this study is very immature [24], the structure of the deep cerebral WM is significantly more complete and complicated than the superficial WM, where the axons form parallel, compact, and bundled structures during the second trimester (15 to 28 weeks) [25, 26]. At the same time, the superficial

WM of the cortex is very sparse, with scattered axon fibers in the WM. 2) Myelination of the deep cerebral WM starts from the second trimester, and reaches the PLIC at a gestational age of 35 weeks (the latest age evaluated in this study), and can expand to the main deep cerebral WM at the central part, such as in the center of the half oval. The superficial cerebral WM is mainly composed of tissues under the cortex that will develop into the far-end joint, contacting and projecting WM fiber to connect the two hemispheres of the cortex, but will not undergo myelination [22, 27]. 3) Regarding the direction of projections, the direction of the deep cerebral WM is more consistent with the unitary direction of the projection, union, and contact of nerve fibers, with almost no distortion and more concentrated directions. While the superficial part of the cerebral WM is an extension of the deep cerebral WM into the cortex, the direction is more scattered. 4) Regarding the shaft radius, the radius of the scattered fiber is obviously smaller than the radius of the central axis. 5) The deep cerebral WM is also known as dense WM, the structure of which is relatively dense. With dense neurons and lower water content, the FA values of the deep brain WM are high at various developmental phases. However, the superficial cerebral WM neurons are sparse and contain a large amount of extracellular fluid. A previous study [28] concluded that the increase of FA values in brain parenchyma was due to decreased water content in the brain and the convergence of macromolecular materials, which is also consistent with another report [29]. The results of this study showed that the developmental pattern of the cerebral WM is in the order of center to periphery, posterior to anterior, and bottom-up, which has been confirmed by additional studies [30].

Changes of FA in the deepWM during development

The current study demonstrated the temporal variation of the deep cerebral WM in different fetal age groups. FA values did not change significantly between 1/2 way and 3/4 of the way through gestation but was then increased dramatically at term. These findings are consistent with in vivo observations of human intrauterine development [31] and the model based on the hypothesis of premature infant development [29, 32]. Intrauterine brain development studies of 23–38 weeks evaluated the changes in the corticospinal tract, optic radiation, and corpus callosum, while premature infant brain development studies evaluated the postnatal changes of the callosity body, cerebral peduncle, corticospinal tract, spinothalamic tract, internal capsule, radiation, inferior longitudinal fasciculus, and cingulum at 1–4 month after birth. It was found that "axonal organization", "myelin gliosis", and "myelination" corresponded with increased, unchanged, and increased FA values, respectively. The

"axonal organization" manifested as scattered axons transformed into a coherent and clear bundle of nerves. The diffusion direction of water is gradually limited to the direction of the axon (from central to the periphery). The model of the water molecule diffusion direction increases. The "myelin gliosis" manifested as glial cells formed around neurons, which does not change the diffusion direction of the water molecules, and confirms the model of water molecular diffusion direction. During the process of "myelination", the direction of water molecule diffusion is limited to radiation, that is, from peripheral to axons. The "myelin gliosis" is more specifically reflected in the corticospinal tract at 28.5–32.5 weeks, or at 26.3–34.8 weeks, the SCC at 25.6–35.4 weeks, and the GCC from 25 weeks to after birth (38 weeks), suggesting that FA values would not significantly change, consistent with the histological observations [33, 34]. The data correspond to the lack of significant change from 1/2 to 3/4 pregnancy term in the deep cerebral WM, and the dramatic increase from 3/4- to full pregnancy observed in animal studies. The change of FA values during the period of "myelin gliosis" was not obvious, while the dramatic elevation of FA values during "myelination" in the premature infants and neonates has been reported in many studies [35–37]. Myelination is an important factor affecting the increase of FA values. The slow increase of FA values of the superficial cerebral WM may therefore be related to the microstructural development that limits water dispersion, including gradual densification of WM and lowered water content. The data and changes of FA values correspond with our histological findings, indicating that the FA values, reflecting the diffusion tensor anisotropy of magnetic resonance, can quantitatively reflect the level of the intrauterine developmental maturity of the fetal cerebral WM, and the changes of FA values could be used to divide cerebral WM development into different stages. From the perspective of guiding clinical practice, during "myelin gliosis" period, precursors of oligodendrocytes in the WM gradually develop into immature oligodendrocytes, which may correspond to the high-risk time frame (23–32 weeks) of periventricular leukomalacia (PVL). At this stage, the majority of oligodendrocytes is at the phase of advanced oligodendrocyte precursors, which is suspected to be a potential target of PVL [33, 34].

Limitations

Limitations of the current study include: 1) Because the head size of the experimental animals did not match the rat coil, the study time period was set after mid pregnancy. 2) Due to experimental conditions, including limits such as field strength and coil, the quality of animal experimental images need to be improved. Different diameter of the magnetic resonance scan coils and different diameter of the animal heads, using the same scanning parameters may lead to relatively poor quality of T2WI. However, These features included degree of sulcation, extent of visualization of the germinal matrix, extent of myelination can be clearly distinguished,it does not affect the experimental results. 3) The size and location of ROIs have a great influence on the results of FA values. 4) Because the size of the animal's head is small, the structure is not easy to identify, therefore there was less anatomical evaluation.

Conclusions

In conclusion, we showed that FA values of DTI images reflect the anisotropy characteristics of the cerebral microstructural development, which can be used for quantitative analysis of the intrauterine developmental changes of cerebral WM in the fetal pig. The FA values of the deep cerebral WM were higher than that of the superficial cerebral WM, which histologically reflect the higher maturity of the deep cerebral WM when compared with the superficial WM. FA values did not change significantly between 1/2 way and 3/4 of the way through gestation, which were related to the myelin gliosis. However, it was then increased dramatically at term may be closely related to the myelination of nerve fibers.

Abbreviations
ALIC: The anterior limb internal capsule; CR: The corona radiate; DTI: Diffusion tensor imaging; FA: Fractional anisotropy; GCC: The genu corporis callosi; HE: Hematoxylin & eosin; HIE: Hypoxic-ischemic encephalopathy; LFB: Luxol fast blue; MRI: Magnetic resonance imaging; OR: The optic radiation; PLIC: The posterior limb of the internal capsule; PV: The periventricular white matter; ROI: Region of interest; SCC: The splenium corporis callosi; WM: White matter

Acknowledgements
We would like to thank Yue Li for the help with pathology sections.

Funding
This study is financially supported with the Shengjing Hospital but not commercial organization. The funding source has estimated the feasibility of the study, but has no role in the collection, analysis, or interpretation of the data or in the decision to submit the manuscript for publication.

Authors' contributions
QWX and GQY designed and performed the study. QWX acquired and analyzed the data, wrote the paper, GQY reviewed and edited the manuscript; GS, LCX, LGY and YX performed the experiment; all authors read and approved the final manuscript.

Competing interests
The authors declare that they have no competing interests.
This study was conducted on the approval of Ethical Committee at Shengjing Hospital, China Medical University.

Author details
[1]Department of Radiology, Shengjing Hospital, China Medical University, Shenyang 110004, People's Republic of China. [2]Morphology Teaching and Reasearch Section, Liaoning Vocational College of Medcine, Shenyang 110100, People's Republic of China. [3]Department of Obstetrics and Gynecology, Shengjing Hospital, China Medical University, Shenyang 110004, People's Republic of China.

References
1. Huang H, Vasung L. Gaining insight of fetal brain development with diffusion MRI and histology. Int J Dev Neurosci. 2014;32:11–22.
2. Huang H, Zhang J, Wakana S, Zhang W, Ren T, Richards LJ, Yarowsky P, Donohue P, Graham E, van Zijl PC, et al. White and gray matter development in human fetal, newborn and pediatric brains. NeuroImage. 2006;33(1):27–38.
3. Huang H, Yamamoto A, Hossain MA, Younes L, Mori S. Quantitative cortical mapping of fractional anisotropy in developing rat brains. J Neurosci. 2008;28(6):1427–33.
4. Huang H, Xue R, Zhang J, Ren T, Richards LJ, Yarowsky P, Miller MI, Mori S. Anatomical characterization of human fetal brain development with diffusion tensor magnetic resonance imaging. J Neurosci. 2009;29(13):4263–73.
5. Vasung L, Huang H, Jovanov-Milosevic N, Pletikos M, Mori S, Kostovic I. Development of axonal pathways in the human fetal fronto-limbic brain: histochemical characterization and diffusion tensor imaging. J Anat. 2010;217(4):400–17.
6. Huang H. Structure of the fetal brain: what we are learning from diffusion tensor imaging. Neuroscientist. 2010;16(6):634–49.
7. Huang H, Jeon T, Sedmak G, Pletikos M, Vasung L, Xu X, Yarowsky P, Richards LJ, Kostovic I, Sestan N, et al. Coupling diffusion imaging with histological and gene expression analysis to examine the dynamics of cortical areas across the fetal period of human brain development. Cereb Cortex. 2013;23(11):2620–31.
8. Woodward LJ, Anderson PJ, Austin NC, Howard K, Inder TE. Neonatal MRI to predict neurodevelopmental outcomes in preterm infants. N Engl J Med. 2006;355(7):685–94.
9. Takahashi E, Dai G, Rosen GD, Wang R, Ohki K, Folkerth RD, Galaburda AM, Wedeen VJ, Ellen Grant P. Developing neocortex organization and connectivity in cats revealed by direct correlation of diffusion tractography and histology. Cereb Cortex. 2011;21(1):200–11.
10. Takahashi E, Folkerth RD, Galaburda AM, Grant PE. Emerging cerebral connectivity in the human fetal brain: an MR tractography study. Cereb Cortex. 2012;22(2):455–64.
11. Domoki F, Zolei-Szenasi D, Olah O, Toth-Szuki V, Nemeth J, Hopp B, Bari F, Smausz T. Comparison of cerebrocortical microvascular effects of different hypoxic-ischemic insults in piglets: a laser-speckle imaging study. J Physiol Pharmacol. 2014;65(4):551–8.
12. Hoque N, Sabir H, Maes E, Bishop S, Thoresen M. Validation of a neuropathology score using quantitative methods to evaluate brain injury in a pig model of hypoxia ischaemia. J Neurosci Methods. 2014;230:30–6.
13. Ezzati M, Broad K, Kawano G, Faulkner S, Hassell J, Fleiss B, Gressens P, Fierens I, Rostami J, Maze M, et al. Pharmacokinetics of dexmedetomidine combined with therapeutic hypothermia in a piglet asphyxia model. Acta Anaesthesiol Scand. 2014;58(6):733–42.
14. Gang Q, Zhang J, Hao P, Xu Y. Detection of hypoxic-ischemic brain injury with 3D-enhanced T2* weighted angiography (ESWAN) imaging. Eur J Radiol. 2013;82(11):1973–80.
15. Mori S, Zhang J. Principles of diffusion tensor imaging and its applications to basic neuroscience research. Neuron. 2006;51(5):527–39.
16. Vossough A, Limperopoulos C, Putt ME, du Plessis AJ, Schwab PJ, Wu J, Gee JC, Licht DJ. Development and validation of a semiquantitative brain maturation score on fetal MR images: initial results. Radiology. 2013;268(1):200–7.
17. Kroenke CD, Bretthorst GL, Inder TE, Neil JJ. Diffusion MR imaging characteristics of the developing primate brain. NeuroImage. 2005;25(4):1205–13.
18. Takahashi E, Dai G, Wang R, Ohki K, Rosen GD, Galaburda AM, Grant PE, Wedeen VJ. Development of cerebral fiber pathways in cats revealed by diffusion spectrum imaging. NeuroImage. 2010;49(2):1231–40.
19. Watson RE, Desesso JM, Hurtt ME, Cappon GD. Postnatal growth and morphological development of the brain: a species comparison. Birth Defects Res B Dev Reprod Toxicol. 2006;77(5):471–84.
20. Mori S, Itoh R, Zhang J, Kaufmann WE, van Zijl PC, Solaiyappan M, Yarowsky P. Diffusion tensor imaging of the developing mouse brain. Magn Reson Med. 2001;46(1):18–23.

21. Lim KO, Hedehus M, Moseley M, de Crespigny A, Sullivan EV, Pfefferbaum A. Compromised white matter tract integrity in schizophrenia inferred from diffusion tensor imaging. Arch Gen Psychiatry. 1999;56(4):367–74.

22. Haynes RL, Borenstein NS, Desilva TM, Folkerth RD, Liu LG, Volpe JJ, Kinney HC. Axonal development in the cerebral white matter of the human fetus and infant. J Comp Neurol. 2005;484(2):156–67.

23. Huppi PS, Maier SE, Peled S, Zientara GP, Barnes PD, Jolesz FA, Volpe JJ. Microstructural development of human newborn cerebral white matter assessed in vivo by diffusion tensor magnetic resonance imaging. Pediatr Res. 1998;44(4):584–90.

24. Brody BA, Kinney HC, Kloman AS, Gilles FH. Sequence of central nervous system myelination in human infancy. I. An autopsy study of myelination. J Neuropathol Exp Neurol. 1987;46(3):283–301.

25. Rakic P, Yakovlev PI. Development of the corpus callosum and cavum septi in man. J Comp Neurol. 1968;132(1):45–72.

26. ten Donkelaar HJ, Lammens M, Wesseling P, Hori A, Keyser A, Rotteveel J. Development and malformations of the human pyramidal tract. J Neurol. 2004;251(12):1429–42.

27. Price DJ, Kennedy H, Dehay C, Zhou L, Mercier M, Jossin Y, Goffinet AM, Tissir F, Blakey D, Molnar Z. The development of cortical connections. Eur J Neurosci. 2006;23(4):910–20.

28. Mukherjee P, Miller JH, Shimony JS, Philip JV, Nehra D, Snyder AZ, Conturo TE, Neil JJ, McKinstry RC. Diffusion-tensor MR imaging of gray and white matter development during normal human brain maturation. AJNR Am J Neuroradiol. 2002;23(9):1445–56.

29. Dubois J, Hertz-Pannier L, Dehaene-Lambertz G, Cointepas Y, Le Bihan D. Assessment of the early organization and maturation of infants' cerebral white matter fiber bundles: a feasibility study using quantitative diffusion tensor imaging and tractography. NeuroImage. 2006;30(4):1121–32.

30. Gao W, Lin W, Chen Y, Gerig G, Smith JK, Jewells V, Gilmore JH. Temporal and spatial development of axonal maturation and myelination of white matter in the developing brain. AJNR Am J Neuroradiol. 2009;30(2):290–6.

31. Zanin E, Ranjeva JP, Confort-Gouny S, Guye M, Denis D, Cozzone PJ, Girard N. White matter maturation of normal human fetal brain. An in vivo diffusion tensor tractography study. Brain and behavior. 2011;1(2):95–108.

32. Dubois J, Dehaene-Lambertz G, Perrin M, Mangin JF, Cointepas Y, Duchesnay E, Le Bihan D, Hertz-Pannier L. Asynchrony of the early maturation of white matter bundles in healthy infants: quantitative landmarks revealed noninvasively by diffusion tensor imaging. Hum Brain Mapp. 2008;29(1):14–27.

33. Back SA, Luo NL, Borenstein NS, Levine JM, Volpe JJ, Kinney HC. Late oligodendrocyte progenitors coincide with the developmental window of vulnerability for human perinatal white matter injury. J Neurosci. 2001;21(4):1302–12.

34. Back SA, Luo NL, Borenstein NS, Volpe JJ, Kinney HC. Arrested oligodendrocyte lineage progression during human cerebral white matter development: dissociation between the timing of progenitor differentiation and myelinogenesis. J Neuropathol Exp Neurol. 2002;61(2):197–211.

35. Kasprian G, Brugger PC, Weber M, Krssak M, Krampl E, Herold C, Prayer D. In utero tractography of fetal white matter development. NeuroImage. 2008; 43(2):213–24.

36. Bui T, Daire JL, Chalard F, Zaccaria I, Alberti C, Elmaleh M, Garel C, Luton D, Blanc N, Sebag G. Microstructural development of human brain assessed in utero by diffusion tensor imaging. Pediatr Radiol. 2006;36(11):1133–40.

37. Partridge SC, Mukherjee P, Henry RG, Miller SP, Berman JI, Jin H, Lu Y, Glenn OA, Ferriero DM, Barkovich AJ, et al. Diffusion tensor imaging: serial quantitation of white matter tract maturity in premature newborns. NeuroImage. 2004;22(3):1302–14.

18

An improvement of carotid intima-media thickness and pulse wave velocity in renal transplant recipients

Zhaojun Li[1] , Yan Qin[2], Lianfang Du[1] and Xianghong Luo[3*]

Abstract

Background: Renal transplantation can significantly improve the quality of life of patients with end stage renal disease (ESRD) who would otherwise require dialysis. Renal transplant (RT) recipients have higher risks of cardiovascular disease compared with general population. The carotid intima-media thickness (CIMT) and pulse wave velocity (PWV) have been used as the important predicting factor of vascular arteriosclerosis. Therefore, this study was to investigate the improvement of carotid intima-media thickness and pulse wave velocity in renal transplant recipients.

Methods: Thirty-one patients with chronic kidney disease being treated with hemodialysis, 31 renal transplant recipients and 84 healthy control subjects were included to have the clinical evaluations and ultrasonography of bilateral carotid arteries. CIMT and PWV were independently measured by two ultrasonographers using the technique of ultrasonic radiofrequency tracking and correlated with arteriosclerosis risk factors. The progression of CIMT and PWV with age were analyzed by linear regression models, and the slopes of curves were compared using Z test.

Results: Compared with the patients on hemodialysis, the CIMT was significantly lower in renal transplant recipients and healthy control. The PWV were higher in hemodialysis patients and renal transplant recipients than that of the subjects in control group. The progression is CIMT positively corelated with age and cumulative duration in renal transplant recipients and hemodialysis patients. In both hemodialysis patients and renal transplant recipients, age and cumulative time on dialysis were all positively correlated with the increase of PWV as well.

Conclusions: Carotid intima-media thickness and pulse wave velocity is the predicting factors of developing arteriosclerosis, which were improved in renal transplant recipients.

Keywords: Renal transplantation, Carotid intima-media thickness, Arteriosclerosis, Pulse wave velocity

Background

Kidney transplantation is the standard treatment for patients with ESRD because it can significantly prolong the life of the patient, mainly by improving renal function to prevent progression of cardiovascular disease [1]. Advancement in immunosuppressant therapies and surgical techniques have significantly improved RT outcomes with surgical complications decreased from 30 to 10% and rejection rates sharply declined from 50% to less than 10% [2, 3]. Compared with dialysis patients, kidney transplant recipients have a 10-fold reduction in cardiac death [4].

However, although the transplanted kidney improves the renal and cardiac function, renal function is still lower than normal. Compared with the normal population, kidney transplant patients still have a 10-fold higher in cardiac death, and 50 times annual fatal or non-fatal cardiovascular events [1]. The progression of arteriosclerosis is closely related to a variety of risk factors and plays an important role in the development of cardiovascular and cerebrovascular events. [5]. Intima-media thickness (IMT) and pulse wave velocity (PWV) are regarded as the footprints of arteriosclerosis [6, 7]. Although studies reported that decline of IMT may occur in some patients who received renal transplant, few studies have investigated the change of PWV in renal transplant recipients. There we performed this study to assess carotid

* Correspondence: lxh_20050703@sina.com
[3]Department of Echocardiography, Shanghai General Hospital, Shanghai Jiaotong University School of Medicine, No.100 Hai Ning Road, Hongkou District, Shanghai 200080, China
Full list of author information is available at the end of the article

intima-media thickness (CIMT) and PWV in hemodialysis patients and renal transplant recipients, with the purpose of investigating the value of using carotid intima-media thickness (CIMT) and pulse wave velocity (PWV) as the predictive factor of vascular arteriosclerosis.

Methods

Subjects

This study involved 112 consecutive adult ESRD patients (age ≥ 18 years) from May 2015 to December 2016. Among the 112 patients, 50 peritoneal dialysis patients were excluded. All the patients who received the renal transplant had been treated with hemodialysis. Considering the effect of arteriovenous fistulas on arterial stiffness in hemodialysis patients, peritoneal dialysis patients without arteriovenous fistulas were excluded from the study. Thus, the final study subjects comprised of 62 ESRD patients, including 31 patients who received a single renal transplant (renal transplant recipients group) and 31 patients relied on hemodialysis (hemodialysis patients group). All the RT patients received the treatment of immunosuppression, including tacrolimus, steroids and mofetil mycophenolate. The clinical information of the subjects was extracted from our Hospital Renal Transplant database, which had been updated yearly since 1993. 84 sex- and age-matched healthy subjects (55 men and 29 women; age rang, 20–80 years) were recruited as controls. They have no history of chronic kidney disease, and the results for physical and laboratory examinations,including electrocardiography, echocardiography and blood tests of hepatic and renal function, are normal. The study was approved by the Institutional Review Board of Shanghai General Hospital (2014158). Written informed consents were provided by all participants.

Patient demographic characteristics

Demographic characteristics, including age, gender, comorbidities, actual treatment, smoking status, weight and height, were collected from the electronic database of our hospital. Cardiovascular risk factors, including systolic blood pressure (SBP), diastolic blood pressure (DBP), fasting blood glucose (FBG), hemoglobin A1c (HbA1c), total cholesterol (TC), triglyceride (TG), low-density lipoprotein cholesterol (LDL-C) and high-density lipoprotein cholesterol (HDL-C), were recorded for all subjects. Diabetes was diagnosed as fasting plasma glucose levels ≥126 mg/Dl at the time of entry in this study, or if the individual who was undergoing treatment with a hypoglycemic agent or any long-acting insulin, was diagnosed diabetic patients. Hypertension was defined as systolic pressure ≥ 140 mmHg and/or diastolic pressure ≥ 90 mmHg, or continuous on the antihypertensive medications. Subjects were classified as smokers if they had smoked at least one 20-cigarette pack per day in the year before the study. Body mass index

(BMI) was calculated as weight (kg) divided by the square of height (m2). Serum calcium (Ca) and phosphorus (P) were tested. Parathormone (PTH) concentrations were measured with the ELISA method (Diagnostic System Laboratories, Webster, TX, USA).

Carotid ultrasonography

All ultrasonographic measurements were performed by two ultasonographers who were blinded to the clinical data (ZJ Li and LF Du, with 16 and 30 years of experience in ultrasound diagnosis, respectively), as described previously [8]. Ultrasound examinations were conducted with the Mylab Twice ultrasonographic diagnostic system (ESAOTE Medical Systems, Genova, Italy), equipped with a 4–13 MHz linear array transducer and intima-media thickness (QIMT) and arterial stiffness (QAS) quantity software (Fig. 1). After the subject was placed in supine position, the common carotid artery (CCA) was shown in a longitudinal view. The imaging acquisition was focused on 1.5-cm segment proximal to the dilatation of the bifurcation. The anterior and posterior walls were depicted clearly. Following the entry of blood pressure while acquiring the imaging date, with the initiation of QIMT and QAS functions, the RF signals tracking the vascular walls for at least six cardiac cycles. The local carotid systolic pressure (Loc-Psys), diastolic pressure (Loc-Pdia), CIMT and PWV were automatically recorded.

Specifically, PWV was calculated from the following equation:

$$\mathrm{PWV} = \frac{1}{\sqrt{\rho \cdot \mathrm{DC}}} = \sqrt{\frac{D^2 \cdot \Delta P}{\rho \cdot (2 \cdot D \cdot \Delta D + \Delta D^2)}} \qquad [9].$$

Where, D = diastolic diameter, ΔD = change of diameter in systole and DC = distensibility coefficient, ΔP = local pulse pressure, ρ = blood density. PWV is a functional parameter directly affected by arterial wall stiffness. In addition to these hemodynamic parameters, the peak systolic velocity (V_{max}), end diastolic velocity (V_{min}), mean flow velocity (V_{mean}), velocity time integral (VTI), artery S/D ratio, resistance index (RI) and pulsatility index (PI) of the CCA were also recorded by using vascular ultrasound measurement. RI and S/D ratio were calculated using the following formulas:

$$\mathrm{RI} = (V_{max} - V_{min})/V_{max}$$

$$\mathrm{PI} = (V_{max} - V_{min})/V_{mean}$$

$$\mathrm{S/D} = V_{max}/V_{mean}$$

Statistical analysis

Continuous data were expressed as mean ± SD. The one-way analysis of variance analysis and least

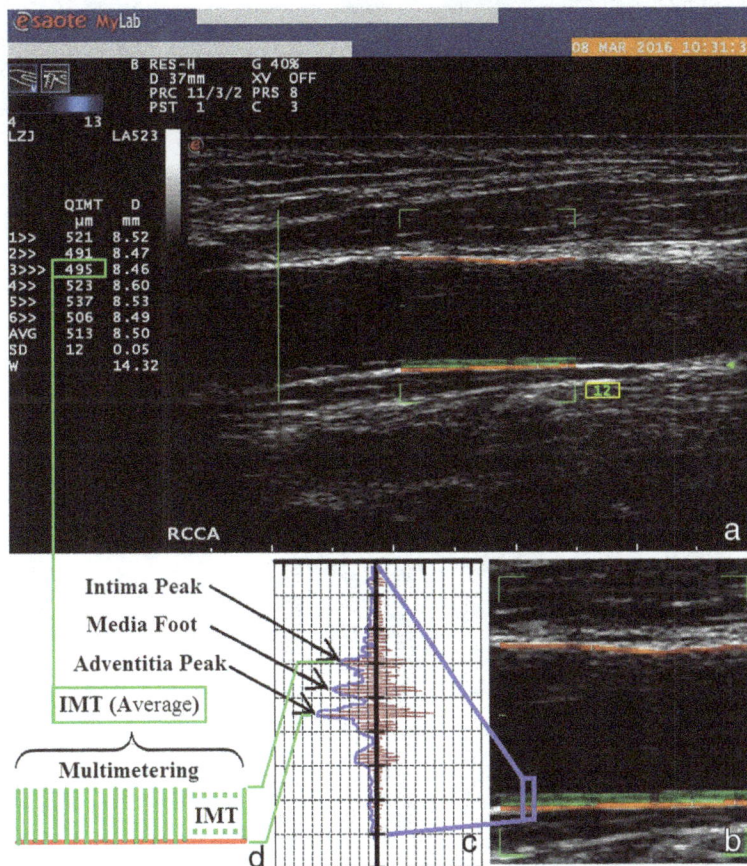

Fig. 1 The Measurement of CIMT and PWV using ultrasonic radiofrequency tracking technique. **a** Analysis of CIMT and PWV using the ultrasound system equipped with the assoated software. **b** Magnification of the region of interest. **c** Ultrasonic RF signal diagram for single IMT point. **d** Assessment of multipoint IMT on segmental carotid artery

significant difference method were used to compare the differences between the groups. The Chi-square test was used for the comparisons of categorical variables between the groups. Repeatability evaluation between the two observers using linear correlation analysis and Bland-Altman Plots. Subsequently, variables related to the carotid morphological were correlation with stiffness parameters by using the stepwise multiple linear regression models. The slops of the CIMT-to-Age and PWV-to-age were determined using linear regression models. Z test was used for the comparison of slopes between groups. The statistical analyses were performed using SPSS 13.0 (SPSS, Chicago, IL) and the statistical significance set at $P < 0.05$.

Results

Characteristics of the subjects

Basic clinical characteristics and laboratory results were described in Table 1. transplant recipients had higher DBP than hemodialysis patients, while no significant difference of SBP between hemodialysis patients and RT patients exist. Level of serum phosphorus was higher in hemodialysis patients, comparing with the transplant recipients and control groups. There was no significant difference of cumulative time on dialysis between the hemodialysis patients group and hemodialysis patients. No difference of age, BMI, TG, TC, LDL-C, HDL-C, FBG, and HbA1c exist among the three groups.

Comparison on repeatability

The median CIMT measured by the two observers were 505 μm (IQR, 397–599 μm) and 526 μm (IQR, 421–594 μm). The median PWV were 7.2 m/s (IQR, 5.4–8.6 m/s) and 7.1 m/s (IQR, 5.4–8.7 m/s), respectively. The ICC for the CIMT and PWV measured by the two observers was 0.93 for PWV (95% confidence interval [CI]: 0.91, 0.94) and 0.95 for CIMT (95% CI: 0.94, 0.98). Combining Bland-Altman and linear correlation analysis in intergroup, the results were further confirmed the measurement of CIMT and PWV was a consistent trend. (Additional file 1: Figures S1-S4).

Table 1 Clinical characteristics of three groups

Variables	Controls ($n = 84$)	Hemodialysis($n = 31$)	RT ($n = 31$)	[a]P Values
Age (years)	58.1 ± 19.9	59.3 ± 17.9	57.9 ± 14.3	0.141
Male, n (%)	55(65)	20(65)	22(71)	0.317
Body-mass index (kg/ m^2)	26.2 ± 4.5	26.0 ± 5.5	24.2 ± 3.5	0.083
Time in predialytic ERSD (mo)	–	70(1–148)	73(1–216)	0.351
Cumulative time on dialysis (mo)	–	24(1–94)	26(1–104)	0.561
Hypertension, n (%)	11(12)	28(90)[†]	25(80)[†]	0.039
Diabetes mellitus, n (%)	11(13)	9(28)[†]	8(27)[†]	0.025
Dyslipidemia, n (%)	4 (5)	2(6)	2(6)	0.676
Smokers, n	4	3	1	0.07
Systolic blood pressure (mmHg)	119.3 ± 15.8	146.9 ± 21.3[†]	145.8 ± 13.5[†]	<0.001
Diastolic blood pressure (mmHg)	77.1 ± 8.3	86.9 ± 13.5[†]	94.3 ± 8.6[†‡]	<0.001
Glycosylated hemoglobin A1c (%)	4.6 ± 0.7	4.7 ± 0.7	4.9 ± 0.6	0.156
Total cholesterol (m mol / L)	6.0 ± 1.2	4.9 ± 1.2	4.5 ± 0.8	0.322
Triglycerides (m mol / L)	1.4 ± 0.7	1.9 ± 0.9	1.4 ± 0.3	0.345
Low-density lipoprotein (m mol / L)	3.1 ± 0.9	2.7 ± 0.9	2.3 ± 0.6	0.224
High-density lipoprotein (m mol / L)	1.2 ± 0.3	1.3 ± 0.3	1.4 ± 0.3	0.432
Fasting glucose (m mol / L)	5.3 ± 1.1	4.6 ± 0.6	4.9 ± 0.7	0.245
Ca (m mol / L)	2.39 ± 0.10	2.40 ± 0.14	2.33 ± 0.19	0.422
P (m mol / L)	1.33 ± 0.12	1.79 ± 0.24†	1.39 ± 0.56[#]	0.003
PTH (pg/ml)	35 ± 26	27 ± 20†	39 ± 22[#]	0.050
ACEI use, n (%)	5(6)	17(56)[†]	20(64)[†]	0.038
Calcium channel antagonist, n (%)	4(5)	16(50)[†]	10(32)[†]	0.032
Diuretics, n (%)	4(5)	12(40)[†]	6(18)[†#]	0.042
Beta-blockers, n (%)	4(5)	12(40)[†]	8(25)[†#]	0.036
Statin use, n (%)	15(18)	11(35)[†]	10(33)[†]	0.046

[a]In three groups, Chi-squared test or ANOVA test was used to compare the distribution of age, gender, BMI, Time in predialytic ERSD, Cumulative time on dialysis, hypertension, hyperlipidemia, diabetes mellitus, Dyslipidemia, smoking, SBP, DBP, HbA1c, TC, TG, LDL, HDL, FBG, Ca, P, and PHT
[*]$P<0.05$, [†]$P < 0.01$ compared with the control group; [#]$P<0.05$, [‡]$P < 0.01$ compared with the hemodialysis group. Data presented as mean (SD) or n (%)

Comparison of carotid structure, function and hemodynamics

The morphologic, functional and hemodynamic analyses result of carotid arteries were provided in Table 2. Compared with the hemodialysis patients group, the CIMT was significantly lower in both the renal transplant group and control group. No significant difference of CIMT was found between the renal transplant recipients and the control group. PWV of both the hemodialysis patients and renal transplant recipients were all higher than that in the control group. No significant difference of PWV was found between the renal transplant group and the hemodialysis patients. Compared with the control group, the V_{max}, PI and S/D were significantly lower in the renal transplant recipients. The three groups showed no significant difference in VTI, V_{min}, V_{mean}, and RI.

Table 2 Comparision of sonographic carotid artery measures in three groups

Variables	Controls (n = 84)	Hemodialysis (n = 31)	RT (n = 31)	[a]P Values
Carotid intima-media thickness (μm)	529.7 ± 131.8	561.9 ± 147.7[*]	480.5 ± 90.3[#]	0.045
Pulse wave velocity (m/s)	6.68 ± 2.25	7.87 ± 2.25[*]	8.05 ± 2.17[†]	0.004
Velocity time integral (m)	0.2 ± 0.1	0.2 ± 0.1	0.2 ± 0.1	0.250
Peak systolic velocity (cm/s)	64.4 ± 19.9	56.6 ± 20.3	49.9 ± 14.5[†]	0.002
End diastolic velocity (cm/s)	16.27 ± 6.5	17.5 ± 10.5	15.9 ± 7.3	0.702
Mean flow velocity (cm/s)	26.9 ± 7.4	27.5 ± 10.1	24.8 ± 7.7	0.388
Pulsatility index	1.8 ± 0.6	1.6 ± 0.7[*]	1.4 ± 0.4[†]	0.003
Resistance index	0.7 ± 0.2	0.7 ± 0.2	0.7 ± 0.2	0.197
S/D ratio	4.3 ± 1.2	4.1 ± 2.1	3.4 ± 0.9[†]	0.017

[a]In three groups, Chi-squared test or ANOVA test was used to compare the distribution of CIMT, PWV, VTI, PSV, EDV, MFV, PI, RI and S/D ratio
[*]$P<0.05$, [†]$P < 0.01$ compared with the control group; [#]$P<0.05$, [‡]$P < 0.01$ compared with the hemodialysis group

Impact of risk factors on CIMT and PWV

CIMT was positively correlated with Age and SBP in both the control group and renal transplant recipients, however negatively correlated with age in hemodialysis patients. In the hemodialysis patients and renal transplant recipients, CIMT was positively correlated with cumulative time on dialysis. No significant correlation between CIMT and SBP was found in the hemodialysis patients (Table 3).

In the control group, PWV were positively correlated with age and SBP ($r = 0.07$ and 0.04, all $P<0.05$), respectively. In both hemodialysis patients and renal transplant recipients, PWV were all positively correlated with age and cumulative time on dialysis (In HD group, $r = 0.07$, 0.53 and In RT group, $r = 0.08$, 0.58, all $P<0.05$), respectively (Table 3).

Tendency of CIMT and PWV with age

The age-CIMT curves of the 3 groups showed that the slopes of curves were 6.357, 4.693, and 2.914 in the control group, the renal transplant recipient group, and the hemodialysis patients group, respectively. The pairwise comparisons showed that the slopes of the age-CIMT curve of the control group was higher than the renal transplant recipient group ($Z = 1.417$, $P = 0.006$) and the hemodialysis patient group ($Z = 2.223$, $P<0.001$), respectively. No significant difference was found between the renal transplant recipient group and the hemodialysis patient group ($Z = 1.038$, $P = 0.723$) (Fig. 2). PWV trended to increase with age and the positive correlation between PWV and age were showed in the 3 groups. Compared with the control group, the age-PWV slope was significantly lower in the hemodialysis patients ($Z = 1.087$, $P = 0.019$. No difference was found between the slope of the age-PWV curve in the renal transplant recipient and that in both control and hemodialysis patients ($Z = 0.6787$, and $P = 0.563$) and between the renal transplant recipients and hemodialysis patients ($Z = 1.307$, $P = 0.818$) (Fig. 3).

Discussion

It remains in debate whether renal transplantation could retard the progression of atherosclerosis in patients with end-stage renal disease. In this study, the technique of ultrasonic radiofrequency tracking was used to quantify the CIMT and PWV, with the recording of up to 50,000 images per second and acquisition of 30–50 samples of one 1–1.5-cm segment of carotid artery, which allows the precise measurement of CIMT and PWV at the micron level and ensures the great repeatability. Our study shows that CIMT and PWV values were lower in age-matched renal transplant recipients than in hemodialysis patients.

A few studies reported the measurement of CIMT using conventional ultrasound in two dimensions and showed that the CIMT increased after renal transplant [10]. Nafar et al. followed up 26 renal transplant recipients and found that the CIMT of carotid arteries increased after renal transplant. This trend of CIMT increase continued during the 2th, 4th, and 6th month ([0.85 ± 0.22], [0.87 ± 0.23], and [0.88 ± 0.24] mm, respectively) post renal transplant [11]. Mitsnefes et al. found that children had higher CIMT after kidney transplant than pre-transplantation ([0.42 ± 0.07] mm vs. [0.38 ± 0.06] mm), and the CIMT value was closely related to SBP [12]. However, in our study, the CIMT was smaller in renal transplant recipients than in hemodialysis patients, and there was no significant difference of CIMT between the renal transplant recipients and the control group. Danielson et al. published their study on the patients with type 1 diabetes after pancreatic islet transplantation [13], showing a significant decrease in CIMT after islet transplantation in individuals with type 1 diabetes. 12 months after transplant, CIMT decreased by 0.062 mm (0.801pre-0.739post = – 0.062 mm). At the time of 50 months after transplant, CIMT significantly decreased by 0.026 mm (0.801pre-0.775post = – 0.026 mm). Their study showed that that the decrease of CIMT was associated with the

Table 3 Multiple linear regression analysis of carotid intima-media thickness, carotid diameter versus cardiovascular risk factors

Variables	Carotid intima-media thickness			Pulse wave velocity		
	Control	HD	RT	Control	HD	RT
	$\beta^a(\beta^b)$	$\beta^a(\beta^b)$	$\beta^a(\beta^b)$	$\beta^a(\beta^b)$	$\beta^a(\beta^b)$	$\beta^a(\beta^b)$
Age	6.91 (0.84)[‡]	−1.40(− 0.19)[†]	2.38 (0.30)[†]	0.07(0.64) [‡]	0.07(0.57) [‡]	0.08 (0.50) [†]
CTD	/	0.39(0.24)[‡]	1.81 (0.23)[†]	/	0.53(0.17)[†]	0.58 (0.21)[†]
PI	−101.42 (−0.37)	−197.74(− 1.14)	162.70(0.78)	− 0.43(− 0.10)	−1.26(− 0.38)	2.12 (0.43)
RI	662.43(0.62)	246.21 (0.49)	− 469.76 (− 0.78)	−0.04(− 0.01)	0.60(0.06)	−9.10 (− 0.67)
EDV	10.84(0.53)[†]	−2.96 (1.14)	− 15.61 (− 0.74)	−0.01(− 0.03)	0.01(0.04)	−0.08 (− 0.23)
MFV	−20.47 (− 0.96)[†]	−9.67 (− 0.70)	14.60 (0.74)	−0.02(− 0.05)	0.01(0.01)	0.04 (0.13)
SBP	−32.38(−0.29)[†]	51.59 (0.90)	− 37.73(− 0.46)[†]	0.04(0.26)[‡]	0.03(0.29)	0.04 (0.27)

[a]:Unstandardized Coefficients;[b]:Standardized Coefficients;CTD: Cumulative time on dialysis. †P < 0.05,‡P < 0.01

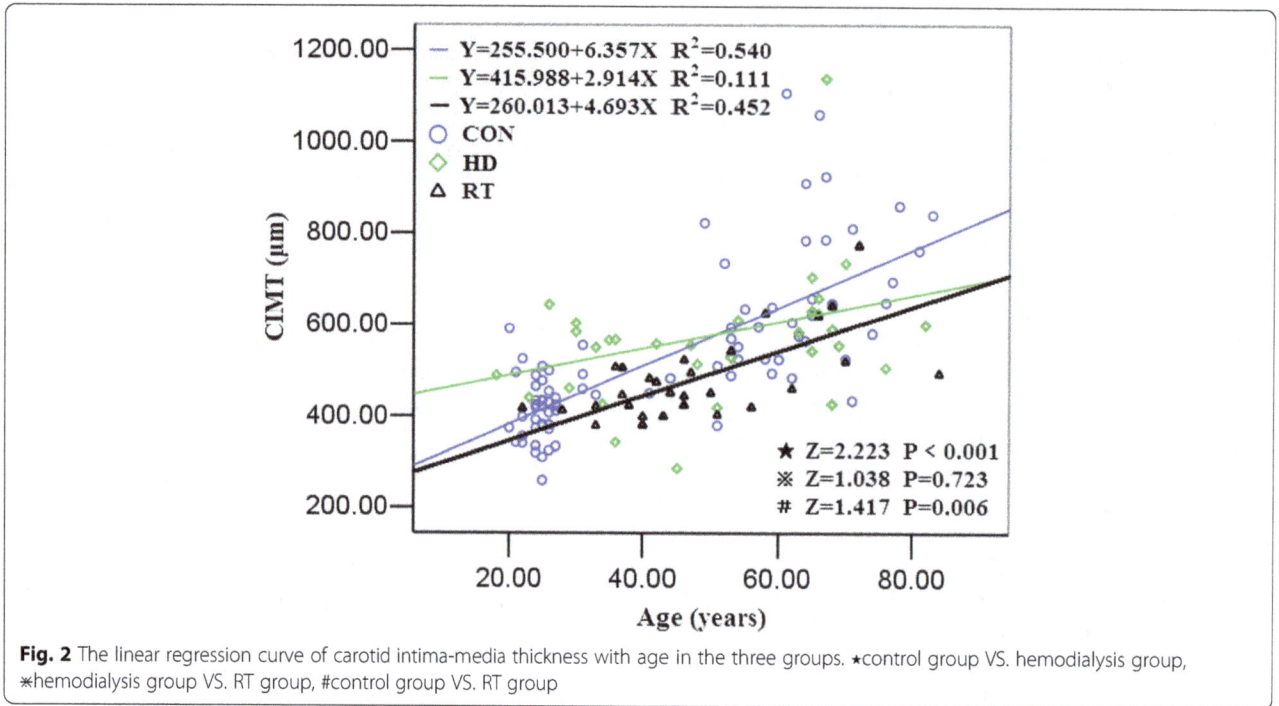

Fig. 2 The linear regression curve of carotid intima-media thickness with age in the three groups. ★control group VS. hemodialysis group, ✱hemodialysis group VS. RT group, #control group VS. RT group

decrease of HbA1c, suggesting CIMT could improve after the major risk factors of artery stiffness were removed. Our study showed the similar phenomena that renal transplantation may offer the benefit of removing the risk factors of atherosclerosis in the patients with ESRD, which was manifested as the decrease of CIMT in renal transplant recipients. Our study found that CIMT was positively correlated with the ages of patients.

Age is an important risk factor for the development of arteriosclerosis in the elastic arteries (e.g. aorta and carotid artery) [14]. Age-related arterial remodeling was significantly accelerated by hemodialysis therapy [15]. In this study, the slopes of CIMT-to-age were lower in renal transplant recipients than that in hemodialysis patients. Domingo et al. reported the similar results that the CIMT increased in the trend of age increase [16].

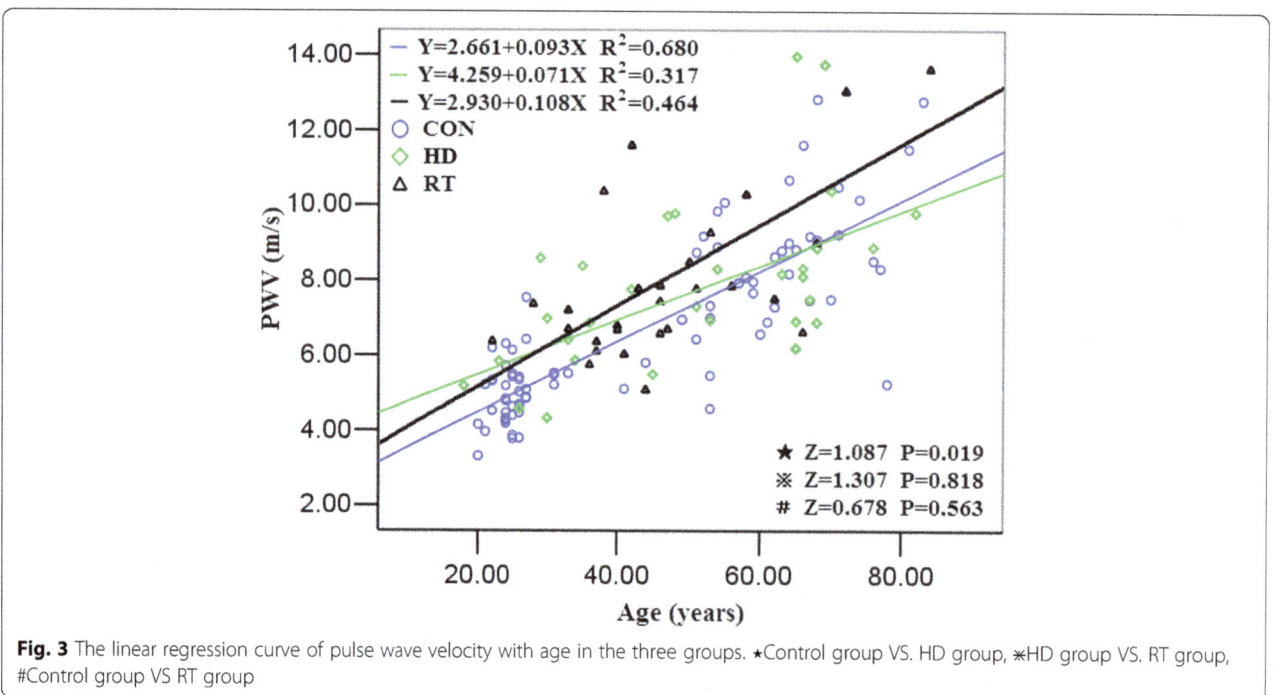

Fig. 3 The linear regression curve of pulse wave velocity with age in the three groups. ★Control group VS. HD group, ✱HD group VS. RT group, #Control group VS RT group

This result suggested that the primary risk factors (e.g. chronic renal insufficiency, arteriovenous fistula, etc.) were removed, and arterial remodeling was improved after renal transplantation.

PWV is another major parameter being used to assess the development of arteriosclerosis [17–19]. In this study, PWV in the hemodialysis patients was higher than that in the control group, but no significant increase was found compare with that of the transplant recipients. A few studies presented the similar results. The study by Birdwell et al. showed that no PWV increase (median: baseline 9.25 to 12-month 8.97 m/s) was detected in the group of 66 new renal transplant recipients within a follow-up period of 12 months [20]. In Bachelet-Rousseau's et al. study, in 88 patients, including 39 transplanted patients and 49 transplantation-pending patients, no significant difference of PWV between transplanted patients and transplantation-pending patients was observed, with the PWV of 9.2 (7.9–11.9) m/s and 9.8 (7.7–12.1) m/s, respectively [21], which can be explained that the restoration of renal function after transplantation had a positive effect on slowing the progression of arterial stiffness. Arterial stiffness was associated with many risk factors. Age was recognized to be an independent risk factor of arterial elasticity. Our study showed that the higher regression coefficients between age and PWV were shown in hemodialysis patients than transplant recipients ($\beta = 0.071$ and 0.108, respectively), which indicates that the progression of vascular stiffness was improved in the transplant recipients. After renal transplantation, the cardiovascular risk factors of kidney disease, including disorders of calcium and phosphorus metabolism and the hemodynamics factors are improved, which bring the improvement on the development of arterial stiffness [22]. In addition, immunosuppressant drugs can reduce vascular inflammatory reaction and improve the progression of arteriosclerosis. Therefore, the effect of age background on RT patients was increased and the weights of other risk factors was decreased,with a different set of that in hemodialysis patients. Covic et al. showed that PWV was decreased in transplant recipients ([6.59 ± 1.62] m/s), while it was increased when patients ([7.19 ± 1.88] m/s) were receiving dialysis treatment [23].

There were some limitations in this study. This is an observational single-center study with relatively small sample size. A longitudinal study with large sample size are needed to evaluate the morphologic changes of carotid arteries and their association with cardiovascular factors (e.g., anemia, transplant time, etc.).

Conclusions

In conclusion, our study demonstrated that the significantly lower PWV and CIMT in transplant recipients than that in the patients with hemodialysis, which indicate that PWV and CIMT may be used as the predictive factor for the improvement of atherosclerosis progression.

Abbreviations
CI: Confidence interval; CIMT: Carotid intima-media thickness; ESRD: End-stage renal disease; FBG: Fasting blood glucose; HbA1c: Hemoglobin A1c; HD: Hemodialysis; HDL-C: High-density lipoprotein cholesterol; ICC: Intraclass correlation coefficient; IQR: Interquartile range; LDL-C: Low-density lipoprotein cholesterol; PWV: Pulse wave velocity; RT: Renal transplant; SD: Standard deviation; TC: Total cholesterol; TG: Triglyceride

Acknowledgments
Thanks to Professor Feng Zhang at department of radiology, University of Washington School of Medicine for revising the article.

Funding
The research was is financially supported by the Shanghai Health and Family Planning Commission Fund (grand number 201440290 and 201640043), Shanghai Science and Technology Committee Fund (grand number 15411969100 and 16411969300), Interdisciplinary Program of Shanghai Jiao Tong University (project number YG2015MS28), Three - year Plan for Clinical Skills and Innovation in Municipal Hospitals (project number 16CR3105B) and Technology Transfer Project of Sience & Technogy Dept., Shanghai Jiao Tong University School of Medicine (grand number ZT201710 and ZT201711). The funding source has estimated the feasibility of the study, but has no role in the collection, analysis, or interpretation of the data or in the decision to submit the manuscript for publication.

Authors' contributions
ZJL, LFD, and XHL designed this study, and they all performed statistical analyses. ZJL, YQ, and LFD conducted the study and collected important background data. ZJL and XHL drafted the manuscript. All authors read and approved the final manuscript.

Competing interests
The authors declare that they have no competing interests.

Author details
[1]Department of Ultrasound, Shanghai General Hospital, Shanghai Jiaotong University School of Medicine, No.100 Hai Ning Road, Hongkou District, Shanghai 200080, China. [2]Department of Urology, Shanghai General Hospital, Shanghai Jiaotong University School of Medicine, No.100 Hai Ning Road, Hongkou District, Shanghai 200080, China. [3]Department of Echocardiography, Shanghai General Hospital, Shanghai Jiaotong University School of Medicine, No.100 Hai Ning Road, Hongkou District, Shanghai 200080, China.

References
1. Liefeldt L, Budde K. Risk factors for cardiovascular disease in renal transplant recipients and strategies to minimize risk. Transpl Int. 2010;23(12):1191–204.
2. JG OL, Samaniego M, Barrio MC, Potena L, Zeevi A, Djamali A, et al. The influence of immunosuppressive agents on the risk of De novo donor-specific HLA antibody production in solid organ transplant recipients. Transplantation. 2016;100(1):39–53.
3. Wiseman AC. Immunosuppressive Medications. Clin J Am Soc Nephrol. 2016;11(2):332–43.

4. Patzer RE, Plantinga LC, Paul S, Gander J, Krisher J, Sauls L, et al. Variation in Dialysis facility referral for kidney transplantation among patients with end-stage renal disease in Georgia. JAMA. 2015;314(6):582–94.

5. Gibson AO, Blaha MJ, Arnan MK, Sacco RL, Szklo M, Herrington DM, et al. Coronary artery calcium and incident cerebrovascular events in an asymptomatic cohort. The MESA Study. JACC Cardiovasc Imaging. 2014; 7(11):1108–15.

6. Reference Values for Arterial Stiffness' Collaboration. Determinants of pulse wave velocity in healthy people and in the presence of cardiovascular risk factors: 'establishing normal and reference values'. Eur Heart J. 2010;31(19): 2338–50.

7. Wolf M, Weir MR, Kopyt N, Mannon RB, Von Visger J, Deng H, et al. A prospective cohort study of mineral metabolism after kidney transplantation. Transplantation. 2016;100(1):184–93.

8. Li ZJ, Liu Y, Du LF, Luo XH. Evaluating arterial stiffness in type 2 diabetes patients using ultrasonic radiofrequency. J Huazhong Univ Sci Technolog Med Sci. 2016;36(3):442–8.

9. Yuan LJ, Xue D, Duan YY, Cao TS, Zhou N. Maternal carotid remodeling and increased carotid arterial stiffness in normal late-gestational pregnancy as assessed by radio-frequency ultrasound technique. BMC Pregnancy Childbirth. 2013;13:122.

10. Kim HS, Seung J, Lee JH, Chung BH, Yang CW. Clinical significance of pre-transplant arterial stiffness and the impact of kidney transplantation on arterial stiffness. PLoS One. 2015;10(9):e0139138.

11. Nafar M, Khatami F, Kardavani B, Farjad R, Pour-Reza-Gholi F, Firoozan A. Atherosclerosis after kidney transplantation: changes of intima-media thickness of carotids during early posttransplant period. Urol J. 2007;4(2): 105–10.

12. Mitsnefes MM, Kimball TR, Witt SA, Glascock BJ, Khoury PR, Daniels SR. Abnormal carotid artery structure and function in children and adolescents with successful renal transplantation. Circulation. 2004;110(1):97–101.

13. Danielson KK, Hatipoglu B, Kinzer K, Kaplan B, Martellotto J, Qi M, et al. Reduction in carotid intima-media thickness after pancreatic islet transplantation in patients with type 1 diabetes. Diabetes Care. 2013;36(2): 450–6.

14. Wang M, Monticone RE, Lakatta EG. Arterial aging: a journey into subclinical arterial disease. Curr Opin Nephrol Hypertens. 2010;19(2):201–7.

15. Avramovski P, Janakievska P, Sotiroski K, Sikole A. Accelerated progression of arterial stiffness in dialysis patients compared with the general population. Korean J Intern Med. 2013;28(4):464–74.

16. Hernández D, Triñanes J, Salido E, Pitti S, Rufino M, González-Posada JM, et al. Artery Wall assessment helps predict kidney transplant outcome. PLoS One. 2015;10(6):e0129083.

17. Townsend RR, Wilkinson IB, Schiffrin EL, Avolio AP, Chirinos JA, Cockcroft JR, et al. Recommendations for improving and standardizing vascular research on arterial stiffness: a scientific statement from the American Heart Association. Hypertension. 2015;66(3):698–722.

18. Myers OB, Adams C, Rohrscheib MR, Servilla KS, Miskulin D, Bedrick EJ, et al. Age, race, diabetes, blood pressure, and mortality among hemodialysis patients. J Am Soc Nephrol. 2010;21(11):1970–8.

19. Utescu MS, Couture V, Mac-Way F, De Serres SA, Marquis K, Larivière R, et al. Determinants of progression of aortic stiffness in hemodialysis patients: a prospective longitudinal study. Hypertension. 2013;62(1):154–60.

20. Birdwell KA, Jaffe G, Bian A, Wu P, Ikizler TA. Assessment of arterial stiffness using pulse wave velocity in tacrolimus users the first year post kidney transplantation: a prospective cohort study. BMC Nephrol. 2015;16:93.

21. Bachelet-Rousseau C, Kearney-Schwartz A, Frimat L, Fay R, Kessler M, Benetos A. Evolution of arterial stiffness after kidney transplantation. Nephrol Dial Transplant. 2011;26(10):3386–91.

22. Molnar MZ, Foster CE 3rd, Sim JJ, Remport A, Krishnan M, Kovesdy CP, et al. Association of pre-Transplant Blood Pressure with post-transplant outcomes. Clin Transpl. 2014;28(2):166–76.

23. Covic A, Goldsmith DJ, Gusbeth-Tatomir P, Buhaescu I, Covic M. Successful renal transplantation decreases aortic stiffness and increases vascular reactivity in dialysis patients. Transplantation. 2003;76(11):1573–7.

Assessment of thoracic ultrasound in complementary diagnosis and in follow up of community-acquired pneumonia (cap)

Maria D'Amato[1]*[iD], Gaetano Rea[2], Vincenzo Carnevale[3], Maria Arcangela Grimaldi[4], Anna Rita Saponara[5], Eric Rosenthal[6], Michele Maria Maggi[7], Lucia Dimitri[8] and Marco Sperandeo[9]

Abstract

Background: Chest X-ray (CXR) is the primary diagnostic tool for community-acquired pneumonia (CAP). Some authors recently proposed that thoracic ultrasound (TUS) could valuably flank or even reliably substitute CXR in the diagnosis and follow-up of CAP. We investigated the clinical utility of TUS in a large sample of patients with CAP, to challenge the hypothesis that it may be a substitute for CXR.

Methods: Out of 645 consecutive patients with a CXR-confirmed CAP diagnosed in the emergency room of our hospital over a three-years period, 510 were subsequently admitted to our department of Internal Medicine. These patients were evaluated by TUS by a well-trained operator who was blinded of the initial diagnosis. TUS scans were performed both at admission and repeated at day 4-6th and 9-14th during stay.

Results: TUS identified 375/510 (73.5%) of CXR-confirmed lesions, mostly located in posterior-basal or mid-thoracic areas of the lungs. Pleural effusion was detected in 26.9% of patients by CXR and in 30.4% by TUS. TUS documented the change in size of the consolidated areas as follows: 6.3 ± 3.4 cm at time 0, 2.5 ± 1.8 at 4-6 d, 0.9 ± 1.4 at 9-14 d. Out of the 12 patients with delayed CAP healing, 7 of them turned out to have lung cancer.

Conclusions: TUS allowed to detect lung consolidations in over 70% of patients with CXR-confirmed CAP, but it gave false negative results in 26.5% of cases. Our longitudinal results confirm the role of TUS in the follow-up of detectable lesions. Thus, TUS should be regarded as a complementary and monitoring tool in pneumonia, instead of a primary imaging modality.

Keywords: Community acquired pneumonia (CAP), Thoracic ultrasound (TUS), Complementary diagnostic tool, Follow-up

Background

Community-acquired pneumonia (CAP) is one of the most common infectious diseases contributing to mortality and morbidity worldwide [1]. Pneumonia exhibits a broad range of severity and induces many diagnostic and therapeutic challenges [2]. According to the American College of Radiology Appropriateness Criteria Expert Panel on Thoracic Radiology, a chest X-ray (CXR) is usually appropriate in patients with positive physical examination or risk factors for pneumonia [2, 3]. Standard CXR can identify pneumonia in almost all areas of the lung, and also helps to define its severity (multilobar or not) and the presence of complications, such as cavitations [4], and co-morbidity (intrathoracic diseases of the mediastinum and the heart). Computed Tomography (CT) is the golden standard for CAP diagnosis. However, it has a more limited role in daily clinical practice and is mostly used in dubious cases or in the assessment of complicated pneumonia, due to its higher cost and radiation exposure [2].

Besides these traditional diagnostic tools, thoracic ultrasound (TUS) is gaining growing popularity as a possible complementary tool for the diagnosis of pulmonary diseases. Some authors even went so far to say that TUS could represent an alternative tool for the diagnosis of pulmonary diseases, due to its intrinsic characteristics. TUS is a non-invasive and radiation free method, readily

* Correspondence: marielladam@hotmail.it
[1]Department of Pneumology, "Federico II University", AO "Dei Colli" Monaldi Hospital, Via Domenico Fontana,134, Naples, Italy
Full list of author information is available at the end of the article

available in many clinical departments and are also suitable for bedside exam in critical care settings. Moreover, several studies by our and other groups showed that TUS may provide useful information in different pleural-pulmonary diseases [5, 6] and particularly in CAP [7]. Some authors even proposed TUS a possible substitute for CXR for the diagnosis of CAP [8], at least in selected groups of patients as pregnant women, children, or whenever radiation exposure should be limited. However, TUS cannot visualize foci of pneumonia which are not adherent to the pleural surface or positioned where ultrasound cannot penetrate. It should also be stressed that until now the current evidence-based guidelines on pneumonia diagnosis and management do not include TUS [9]. On the other hand, the TUS method could have a relevant complementary role in CAP diagnosis and management. Considering that the roles of several putative biomarkers in the management of patients with pneumonia are not definite, and can not provide clues for the occurrence of supervening complications [3, 4, 9–11]. In this sense, TUS could be an option to monitor the evolution of pneumonia foci following a CXR-confirmed diagnosis [12]. Despite the mentioned results and the growing number of studies on this matter, the debate on the role of TUS in the diagnosis and management of CAP is still ongoing.

Our study was aimed to investigate the clinical performance of TUS in the primary diagnosis and in the management of CAP, as compared to standard CXR. We evaluated the following aspects: a) how many cases of CAP were confirmed by TUS after clinical and CXR diagnosis, and b) how changes in TUS imaging appearances, from onset to recovery of CAP, could help identifying therapy failure or the need to investigate an alternative diagnosis.

Methods

Patients

We investigated all patients consecutively admitted to our department of Internal Medicine between September 2013 and November 2016 with a CXR-confirmed diagnosis of CAP. In the Emergency Room (ER) all patients had undergone a conventional diagnostic work-up, including anamnesis, physical examination, laboratory tests and chest radiography. The diagnosis of CAP was posed according to the American Thoracic Society (ATS) guidelines [13]. The CURB65 score [14] was used to drive the allocation of patients as follows: severe cases, with 3 or 4 criteria were referred to the intensive care unit –ICU– or to our Internal Medicine department; non-severe cases, at moderate risk, with 1 or 2 criteria were referred to ward or management as outpatients; non-severe cases, at low risk and with 0 criteria, were not hospitalized [15]. All patients timely received empirical therapy, according to guidelines for the evaluation and treatment of CAP. Patients with either contingent

constraints or clinical conditions averting a complete TUS scan were conservatively excluded.

All participants gave witnessed informed consent and the study was approved by the ethics committee of SUN-AO dei Colli- Naples-Italy.

Thoracic ultrasound examination

In all patients admitted to our department, TUS was performed by a blinded operator, who was not aware of CXR results, nor of the entire clinical-laboratory picture. In order to follow the evolution of CAP foci after therapy, TUS was performed in at least three repeated sittings: on day 0 (initial), between days 4 and 6 (intermediate), and between days 9 and 14 (final), according to a defined work-up [12] (see Table 1 for details. TUS was performed at the bedside by a physician with at least 10 years of ultrasound experience. An Esaote Technos MPX, Twice and My Lab30 Gold and Twice device (Genoa, Italy) using a multi-frequency (3.5–5 MHz and 3–8 MHz) convex probe and the pre-setting for thoracic ultrasound in B mode was used (depth of images penetration: 7–14 cm; gain control: 40-50%; use of harmonic imaging; electronic focus: pleural line). Each TUS was assessed for the number, location, shape, size, and breath-dependent changes of the consolidation area attributable to pneumonia. Two main sonographic patterns of lung consolidation were defined: hypoechoic consolidation and mixed consolidation (hypoechoic and hyperechoic). The dimensions of the consolidated areas are reported as the average between longitudinal and transversal axes. Local and basal pleural effusions were also recorded. In addition, the presence of spot and/or linear/arborescent hyperechoic images on TUS, improperly referred to as an air bronchogram, were also recorded. The presence of artefacts (increased TUS B-line counts in the hemithorax with consolidation) was not considered in this study, because such artefacts are at best a sensitive, but very non-specific sign of lung injury, common to many conditions [16, 17].

Table 1 TUS procedures

- Pulmonary thoracic assessment setting (including: tissue harmonics imaging activation, the time gain compensation (TGC) should not exceed 50%, electronic imaging focus on the pleural line) using mainly a 3.5-5 MHz convex probe EsaoteTechnosMpx, My Lab 30 and Twice (Genova, Italy).

- Patients' chests were examined posteriorly, lateral and anteriorly, while sitting. A few patients were examined in a semi-supine position, due to severe discomfort when sitting upright. Posteriorly, we opted for longitudinal and transversal interscapular and paravertebral line scans. Anteriorly, the longitudinal and transversal interclavicular, parasternal line and supraclavicular scans were used. Laterally, we used the longitudinal and transversal anterior, median and posterior line axillary views.

- The duration of ultrasound probe application in each site (posterior, lateral and anterior) was 4–5 min and overall time needed to complete the entire lung examination was 12–15 min.

The positive clinical evolution of CAP was detected by clinical assessment and CXR, and faced to the changes of TUS findings during stay and/or within 30 days on an outpatient basis after discharge.

Assessment of inter-reader agreement
Video-clips recorded during TUS examinations (each lasting a minimum of 3 min) were later reviewed by a second examiner, who was blinded of all previous TUS findings; clips for control assessment were randomly assigned to one of two examiners with 20 years of experience in transthoracic ultrasound.

Statistical analysis
The results concerning the dimensions of TUS-detectable lesions are presented both as range and as mean ± SD. Inter-reader agreement was assessed using Spearman's coefficient for all parameters. The significance of changes in size of US-detectable lesions over time was tested by Repeated Measures ANOVA. A p value of <0.05 was considered significant.

In the clinical application phase of the study, a repeated measurements ANOVA model (on basal, 4th day, and 8–10th day) was used to assess dimensional changes over time in lung consolidation areas and was carried out via linear mixed models. Within-patients correlation was accounted for by an unstructured correlation type matrix [18]. Hochberg's method was followed to obtain p-values corrected for multiple comparisons. P-values <0.05 were considered significant. All analyses were performed using SAS Release 9.1 (SAS Institute, Cary, NC, USA). Inter-reader agreement was assessed using Spearman's coefficient for all parameters.

Results
Patients
Seven hundred ninety-six consecutive adult patients presented to the emergency room of the "Casa Sollievo della Sofferenza" Hospital (San Giovanni Rotondo - Italy) with symptoms and clinical/laboratory signs consistent with the diagnosis of CAP. Following the conventional diagnostic work-up, in 736 of them the diagnosis was confirmed by chest X-ray (CXR), and 91 patients were discharged and managed as outpatients after the ER workup. Among the 645 patients admitted to the hospital, 32 were referred to the intensive care unit, and 613 to our department. Among the latter, 103 patients were excluded (see methods). Five hundred ten patients admitted to our department were finally studied (see Fig. 1). The demographic and clinical characteristics of investigated patients are reported in Table 2.

Initial TUS findings
The topographic distribution of lung consolidation detected by TUS is indicated in Table 3. TUS imaging was negative for consolidation attributable to pneumonia in 135 adults with CXR-recorded pneumonia, which implies a false negative rate of 26.5%. This was due in 72/135 patients to single consolidations that were neither sub-pleural nor retro-scapular, and in 63/135 patients to multiple, even bilateral, and mostly not strictly sub-pleural, consolidations, which were visible only minimally using TUS (Fig. 2). Of the latter group, 39 patients were subsequently found to be immuno-compromised (Fig. 3).

Among US-detectable lesions (found in 375/510 pts. = 73.5%), most were posterior basal o midthoracic (see Table 3). Maximal length of the consolidation area ranged from 3.5 to 9.5 cm (mean ± SD: 6.3 ± 3.4 cm). The CXR features varied from complete lobar consolidation to patchy or less severe opacity, whereas TUS imaging showed two main patterns: hypoechoic in 135/375 (36%) and mixed in 240/375 (64%).

Pleural effusion associated to detectable consolidation was detected by TUS in 114/375 (30.4%) patients and in 137/510 (26.9%) patients by CXR. Spots, stripes and/or linear/arborescent hyperechoic images were present in 54.9% of all patients (206/375), and no difference was observed in prevalence between genders, or specific association with disease severity or greater dimension of consolidation.

Treatment-induced changes of TUS findings
By monitoring lung consolidations in subjects with moderate risk CAP using a convex probe (3.5-5 MHz), TUS modifications were: initial dimensions 3.5 to 9.5 cm (6.3 ± 3.4), intermediate dimensions 2.1 to 4.3 cm (2.5 ± 1.8 cm); final dimensions 0.3 to 1.0 cm (0.9 ± 1.4 cm) ($p < 0.001$ by ANOVA). A favourable outcome was confirmed in all except 12 patients by a final normal CXR and/or a subsequent clinical assessment including normal CXR and TUS within the first month, together with complete disappearance of fever and of the most relevant symptoms and physical signs. A persistent localized pleural line thickening (> 3.0 mm with 3.5 MHz convex transducer) after resolution was observed in all pneumonia patients. In 12/375 (3.2%) patients (three women and nine men) pulmonary consolidation, diameter 4.5 to 5.5 cm, did not significantly improve despite intensive antibacterial therapy, with no satisfactory clinical improvement or resolution of fever. In all 12, a chest CT was performed: in five patients the diagnosis of pneumonia was confirmed, and all recovered, although with delay. In the other seven patients, the diagnosis of lung cancer suggested by chest CT was subsequently confirmed at histology on US-guided fine needle aspiration biopsy (FNAB) of the lung nodules. In these cases, previous bronchoscopy did not provide any diagnostic yield, conceivably because of the peripheral site of the lesions. The spot and linear

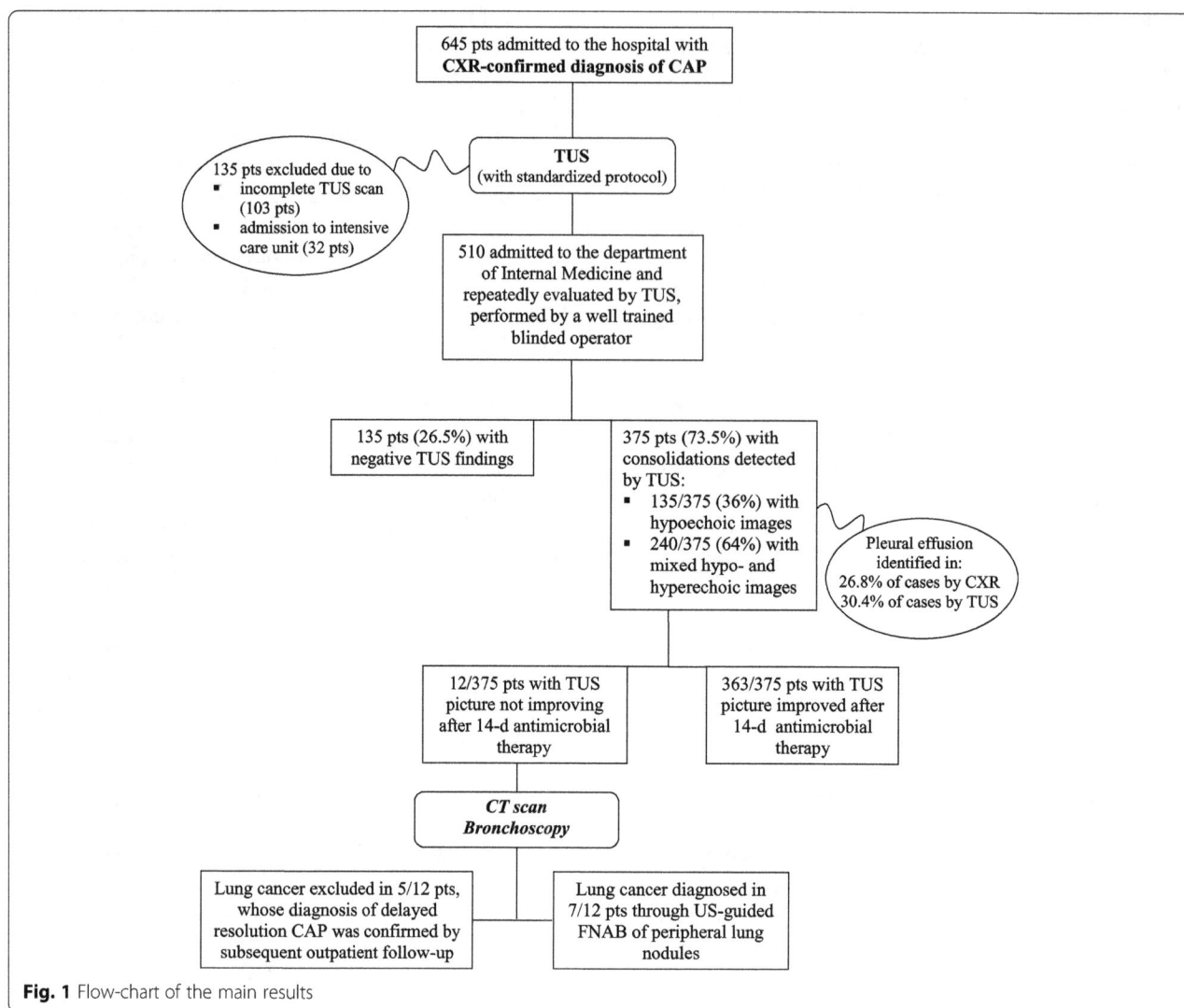

Fig. 1 Flow-chart of the main results

Table 2 Characteristics of the included patients ($n = 510$)

Age (years), (mean ± SD)	Range 32-78 (58.4 ± 14.7)
Gender (M/F)	281/229
CURB 65	2.4 ± 0.6
Mean hospital stay	8.9 ± 2.5 days
Consolidated areas identified by TUS	375/510
Size of Consolidated areas (cm)	6.3 ± 3.4
Comorbidity(more than one in 60 pts)	455/510 pts.(89.2%)
Diabetes mellitus	96 (18.8%)
COPD	107 (21%)
Pulmonary fibrosis	28 (5.5%)
Heart failure (III-IV NYA)	80 (15.7%)
Chronic kidney diseases	12(2.3%)
Oncological diseases	68 (13.3%)
Coronary disease	56(11%)

Table 3 Topographic distribution detected at lung ultrasound examination of pneumonia patients ($n = 375$)

Localization of pulmonary focus	Number of patients ($n = 375$)
Posterior-basal	202 (54%)
Posterior mid-thoracic	60 (16%)
Posterior-lateral mid-thoracic	75 (20%)
Anterior mid-thoracic	15 (4%)
Para-cardiac	12 (3.2%)
Anterior apical	6 (1.6%)
Posterior apical	3 (0.8%)
Multiple consolidation	31 (8.3%)

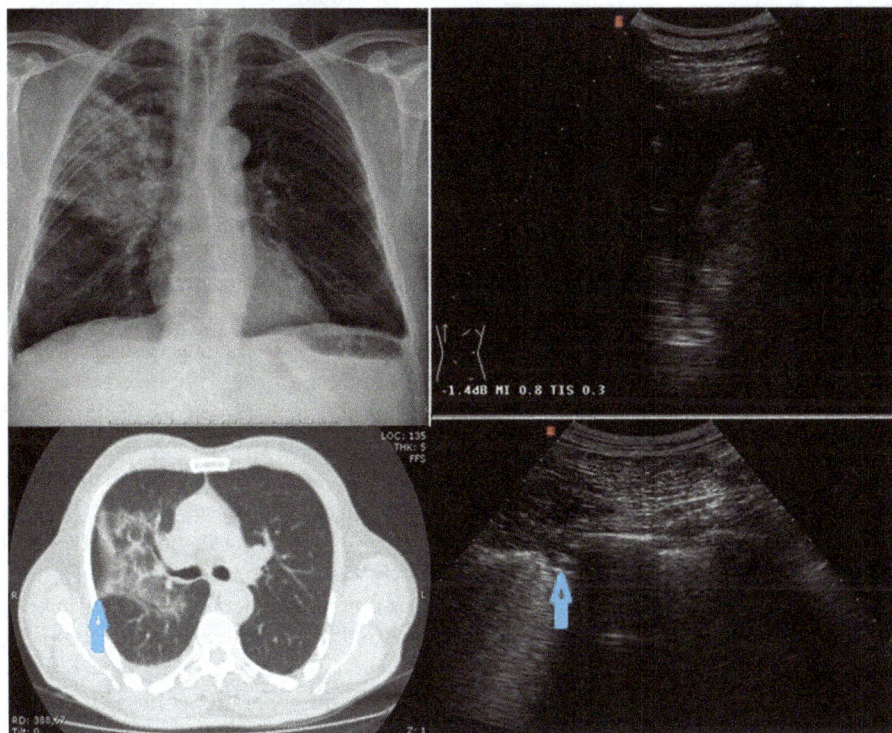

Fig. 2 Right lobar pneumonia. Lung consolidation is well defined by CXR (top left) and CT (bottom left); by TUS, pleural effusion is easily identified (top right) but only a very small density and adherent to pleura pneumonia is visible (blue arrows) (bottom right)

hyperechoic images were observed in 5/7 of the patients with a subsequent diagnosis of lung cancer.

Inter-reader agreement

Inter-reader agreement was excellent (Spearman's coefficient ≥ 0.90 for all parameters).

Positive TUS findings in patients with negative CXR imaging

Pneumonia that was not preliminarily CXR-proven but was suggested by the clinical picture and by the finding of TUS areas attributable to consolidation was identified in ten patients. They showed small sub-pleural consolidation areas of 1.0 to 1.5 cm; these cases did not progress toward greater extension of consolidation, and those considered doubtful for pneumonia were excluded from the subsequent data analysis of TUS imaging distribution.

Discussion

Our current results, obtained from the largest ever investigated series, substantially confirm the previous ones we obtained from an independent series of inpatients [12]. In most cases of CAP, TUS examination detects the sites of inflammation, which have typical although not specific patterns. TUS allows the measurement of dimensions of the pulmonary focus before and after medical therapy, which implies the possible use of this tool to monitor treatment efficacy. The present data also confirm the higher sensibility of TUS in identifying pleural effusion and its role to facilitate fluid drainage. Accordingly, in US-detectable cases TUS appears to valuably integrate the diagnostic information obtained from a CXR alone [19]. Due to these and other reasons, several authors went so far to even suggest that CXR can be replaced by TUS in the clinic to identify CAP [20, 21]. However, our current results mandate extreme caution on this matter.

Actually, most cases of CAP (around 80% of cases) are subpleural (that is adherent to the 70% of pleura visualized by TUS) and begin peripherally. This explains why CAP is also most often visible by TUS [13, 22]. In our series, 73.5% of CXR-positive lung consolidations due to CAP were also visible with TUS, being localized in sub-pleural areas (see details on location in Table 3). In these sites, hypoechoic and mixed (hypoechoic and hyperechoic) lesions corresponded to the foci of pneumonia identified by CXR. This result confirms in a large cohort of patients the reliability of TUS imaging to corroborate the diagnosis of CAP obtained from CXR. However, it should also be stressed as more than one out of four cases of CAP (26.5%) were not detectable by TUS, even if performed with the highest methodological accuracy (standardized complete scan, technical accuracy, involvement of only highly experienced operators, and so on)

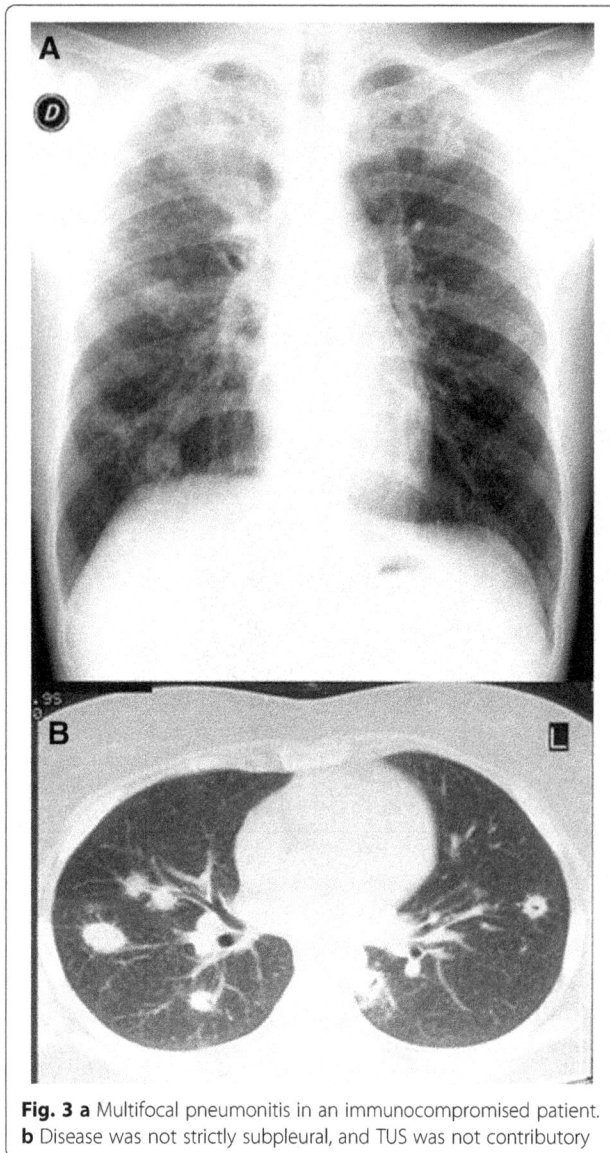

Fig. 3 a Multifocal pneumonitis in an immunocompromised patient. **b** Disease was not strictly subpleural, and TUS was not contributory

which would have been detected by CXR, can remain undiagnosed. Indeed, TUS and CXR examine lungs in different ways, with only a partial overlap.

In adjunct, it should be stressed as, even in US-amenable areas, TUS findings as spots, stripes and/or linear/arborescent hyperechoic images (improperly called air bronchograms) are not disease-specific. Therefore, TUS imaging is not helpful to differentiate between pneumonia and other lung diseases [17], including cancer [17, 25]. In particular, no study or meta-analysis so far demonstrated that linear/arborescent hyperechoic images on TUS do really correspond to the CT imaging finding of air bronchogram [22]. As a matter of fact, noteworthy, we also found this US feature also in 5/7 patients finally diagnosed to have lung cancer. This latter finding definitely confirms as certain optimistic statements on this matter are not realistic at all, CT remains the gold standard for imaging diagnosis. Moreover, according to our previous experience, we deliberately chose not to include the evaluation of B-line or "ring-down" artefacts among the investigated parameters. Despite their wide popularity, these TUS signs may be found in patients with different conditions, because these artefacts are generated behind the pleural line because of the high difference of acoustic impedance between soft tissue and air, or between fluid and air. Such a difference is enhanced in a number of pleuro-pulmonary diseases [18]. As a consequence, the attention to this acoustic phenomenon could be highly misleading in patients with co-morbidities, as were most patients from our series and in the common clinical practice.

On the other hand, our results stressed as TUS monitoring allows for follow-up care after the preliminary clinical-radiological diagnosis of pneumonia [4, 11–13], being capable to demonstrate the decrease in size of consolidation. This could be a precious clinical information, since the management of patients with CAP who fail to improve constitutes a relevant challenge for clinicians. Changes in CRP levels for CAP patients are sufficiently useful to discriminate between true treatment failure and slow response to treatment and can help clinicians in management decisions when patients fail to improve [28, 29]. CT should be performed to help rule out lung cancer when there is a lack of dimensional reduction of consolidations, and/or failure of symptom regression. Under these conditions and according to our results, TUS can be used to provide bedside information on the persistence of lung consolidation and can be a useful adjunctive tool to check the response to treatment [29–32]. The late observation of persistent localized pleural-line thickening after resolution is seemingly only the signature of the recent pneumonia. Our data suggest a wider use of TUS in the follow-up after the initial CXR diagnosis of sub-pleural pneumonia, whose progressive reduction in size is reliably assessed. Accordingly, TUS

[23]. Several reasons underpin this high false positive rate. As a fact, TUS cannot visualize foci of pneumonia which are not adherent to the pleural surface or are positioned where ultrasound cannot penetrate (e.g. adjacent to the mediastinum) [24–26]. Moreover, TUS is not a valid aid in immunocompromised patients of intensive care units [27] who commonly suffer from severe *Staphylococcus*, *Aspergillus*, *Candida*, *Mycoplasma* and viral pneumonia. Such pneumonia foci are often intra-parenchymal, multiple, and/or outside the TUS-visible pleura. This is also indirectly supported by our current findings, since most cases of CXR-confirmed CAP we did not detect by TUS had insufficient pleural contact and were also clinically more severe, as is usually observed in immunocompromised patients [24]. As a consequence, performing TUS alone, many pneumonias

Assessment of thoracic ultrasound in complementary diagnosis and in follow up of community-acquired...

161

could also decrease the need to repeat radiological procedures, particularly in the follow-up of pregnant patients or in the follow-up of patients not requiring hospital admission. When scheduling follow-up on an outpatient basis, TUS is seemingly a less expensive procedure and it is already successfully used to monitor other conditions and diseases [33].

Discordant results have been reported on TUS-positive and CXR–negative by other authors [2, 3, 13, 22]. Such discrepancies may result from Rx–negative small lung consolidations detected exclusively on TUS. Alternatively, they may stem from the different relationship between lung consolidations and the pleura, or from an alternative diagnosis (not CAP), or from the presence of sub-segmental lung focal areas of atelectasis beyond terminal bronchioles [23].

Our study has several strengths. Firstly, we prospectively validated our previous results by studying an independent large series of unselected patients. All patients of our series were managed in a substantially coherent way, at variance with previous studies suffering from a wide variability in criteria of admission [31], management, and discharge of pneumonia patients without follow up.

Our study has some limits, too. In fact, we tried to mimic the common practice through the unselective inclusion of all patients coming to the emergency room of our hospital and being suitable for subsequent (repeated) observation in our Internal Medicine department. Such a design was aimed to reduce possible observational bias, but this way we excluded patients with an insufficient number of TUS assessments, which implied the exclusion of patients admitted to other units, including ICU. Accordingly, the number of recruited patients with more severe disease and with likely more significant co-morbidities and further complications was lower. On the other hand, the exclusion of those managed as outpatients also excluded less severe cases. In addition, all TUS were performed by a highly trained staff and this could undermine the generalizability of our results. Actually, TUS requires a technically experienced operator and appropriate machine settings [11, 12, 30]. The clinical assessment of TUS consolidation mostly depends on the subjective expertise of the ultrasound operator, as in most sonographic diagnoses. Interpretation of TUS is not the easiest component of any ultrasound course and has many pitfalls, mostly for false-negative results. This is a risk increased by over-confidence [21]. As a fact, the negative ethical and potential medico-legal implications of omitting a CXR (co-morbidity associated, intraparenchimal not subpleural consolidation and therefore incorrect or incomplete diagnosis), particularly when addressing the therapeutic choices, are evident [34].

Conclusion

In conclusion, we exclude that TUS could reliably replace CXR, and we confirm that the assessment of physical signs, CXR, and biomarkers such as procalcitonin and CRP, remain the pillars for the diagnosis of pneumonia. On the other hand, TUS represents a highly valuable complementary imaging procedure, which can be performed at bedside, and easily repeated after the initial assessment. Therefore we recommend its use as a complementary and monitoring tool.

Acknowledgments
Not applicable.

Funding
Not applicable.

Authors' contributions
All authors contributed to the conception and design of the study, as to the acquisition, analysis and interpretation of data. They also contributed in drafting and critically revising the manuscript, and read and approved the final manuscript, so take public responsibility of its content. All authors are responsible for accuracy or integrity any part of the work. In particular the prominent contribution was as follows: MD and MS: wrote the manuscript. VC: made substantial contributions to conception and design. MS, MAG, GR made substantial contribution in acquisition of data, and data analysis and interpretation. ER, MMM: made substantial contributions to data analysis and interpretation. AS and LD: was involved in critically revising the manuscript for intellectual content. MD, GR e MS: were involved in data acquisition and database synthesis and cleaning. All authors read and approved the final manuscript.

Competing interests
The authors declare that they have no competing interests.

Author details
[1]Department of Pneumology, "Federico II University", AO "Dei Colli" Monaldi Hospital, Via Domenico Fontana,134, Naples, Italy. [2]Department of Radiology, AO "Dei Colli" Monaldi Hospital, Naples, Italy. [3]Unit of Internal Medicine, "Casa Sollievo della Sofferenza" Hospital, IRCCS, San Giovanni Rotondo (FG), Italy. [4]Unit of Internal Medicine and Pneumology, "Casa Sollievo della Sofferenza" Hospital, IRCCS, San Giovanni Rotondo (FG), Italy. [5]Unit of Internal Medicine, Local Health Service, Potenza, Italy. [6]Department of Internal Medicine, Hospital Archet 1, Nice, France. [7]Unit of Emergency Medicine, "Casa Sollievo della Sofferenza" Hospital, IRCCS, San Giovanni Rotondo (FG), Italy. [8]Unit of Pathology, "Casa Sollievo della Sofferenza" Hospital, IRCCS, San Giovanni Rotondo (FG), Italy. [9]Unit of Interventional and Diagnostic Ultrasound of Internal Medicine, "Casa Sollievo della Sofferenza" Hospital, IRCCS, San Giovanni Rotondo (FG), Italy.

References
1. Spellberg B. Community-acquired pneumonia. N Engl J Med. 2014;370:1861–2.
2. Dean NC, Jones JP, Aronsky D, Brown S, Vines CG, Jones BE, Allen T. Hospital admission decision for patients with community-acquired pneumonia: variability among physicians in an emergency department. Ann Emerg Med. 2012;59:35–41.
3. Gibot S, Béné MC, Noel R, Massin F, Guy J, Cravoisy A, et al. Combination biomarkers to diagnose sepsis in the critically ill patient. Am J Respir Crit Care Med. 2012;186:65–71.
4. Kirsch J, Ramirez J, Mohammed TL, Amorosa JK, Brown K, Dyer DS, et al. ACR appropriateness criteria® acute respiratory illness in immunocompetent patients. J Thorac Imaging. 2011;26:W42–4.
5. Reissig A, Gorg C, Mathis G. Transthoracic sonography in the diagnosis of pulmonary diseases: a systematic approach. Ultraschall Med. 2009;30:438–54.

6. Sartori S, Tombesi P. Emerging roles for transthoracic ultrasonography in pulmonary diseases. World J Radiol. 2010;2:203–14.

7. Gehmacher O, Mathis G, Kopf A, Scheier M. Ultrasound imaging of pneumonia. Ultrasound Med Biol. 1995;21:1119–22.

8. Thomas Berlet Thoracic ultrasound for the diagnosis of pneumonia in adults: a meta-analysis. Respir Res. 2015;16:89.

9. Rothrock SG, Green SM, Fanelli JM, Cruzen E, Costanzo KA, Pagane J. Do published guidelines predict pneumonia in children presenting to an urban ED? Pediatr Emerg Care. 2001;17:240–3.

10. Wunderink RG, Waterer GW. Update in pulmonary infections 2010. Am J Respir Crit Care Med. 2011;184:186–90.

11. Sperandeo M, Filabozzi P, Varriale A, Carnevale V, Piattelli ML, Sperandeo G, Brunetti E, Decuzzi M. Role of thoracic ultrasound in the assessment of pleural and pulmonary diseases. J Ultrasound. 2008;11:39–46.

12. Sperandeo M, Carnevale V, Muscarella S, Sperandeo G, Varriale A, Filabozzi P, Piattelli ML, D'Alessandro V, Copetti M, Pellegrini F, Dimitri L, Vendemiale G. Clinical application of transthoracic ultrasonography in inpatients with pneumonia. Eur J Clin Invest. 2011;41:1–7.

13. American Thoracic Society; Infectious Diseases Society of America. Guidelines for the management of adults with hospital-acquired, ventilator-associated, and healthcare-associated pneumonia. Am J Respir Crit Care Med. 2005;171:388–416.

14. Liu B, Yin Q, Chen YX, Zhao YZ, Li CS. Role of Presepsin (sCD14-ST) and the CURB65 scoring system in predicting severity and outcome of community-acquired pneumonia in an emergency department. Respir Med. 2014;108:1204–13.

15. Lim WS, van der Eerden MM, Laing R, Boersma WG, Karalus N, Town GI, et al. Defining community acquired pneumonia severity on presentation to hospital: an international derivation and validation study. Thorax. 2003;58:377–82.

16. Zanforlin A, Smargiassi A, Inchingolo R, Sher S, Ramazzina E, Corbo GM, et al. B-lines: to count or not to count? JACC Cardiovasc Imaging. 2014;7:635–6.

17. Trovato GM, Sperandeo M. Sounds, ultrasounds, and artifacts: which clinical role for lung imaging? Am J Respir Crit Care Med. 2013;187:780–1.

18. Sperandeo M, Varriale A, Sperandeo G, et al. Assessment of ultrasound acoustic artifacts in patients with acute dyspnea: a multicenter study. Acta Radiol. 2012;53:885–92.

19. Miyashita N, Akaike H, Teranishi H, Nakano T, Ouchi K, Okimoto N. Chest computed tomography for the diagnosis of mycoplasma pneumoniae infection. Respirology. 2014;19:144–5.

20. Ye X, Xiao H, Chen B, Zhang S. Accuracy of lung ultrasonography versus chest radiography for the diagnosis of adult community-acquired pneumonia: review of the literature and meta-analysis. PLoSOne. 2015;24:10.

21. Jones BP, Tay ET, Elikashvili I, Sanders JE, Paul AZ, Nelson BP, et al. Feasibility and safety of substituting lung ultrasonography for chest radiography when diagnosing pneumonia in children: a randomized controlled trial. Chest. 2016;150:131–8.

22. Sperandeo M, Filabozzi P, Carnevale V. Ultrasound diagnosis of ventilator-associated pneumonia: a not-so-easy issue. Chest. 2016;149:1350–1.

23. Sperandeo M, Rea G, Santantonio A, Carnevale V. Lung ultrasound in diagnosis of transient tachypnea of the newborn: limitations and pitfalls. Chest. 2016;150:977–8.

24. Craven DE, Palladino R, McQuillen DP. Healthcare-associated pneumonia in adults: management principles to improve outcomes. Infect Dis Clin North Am. 2004;18:939–62.

25. Jeon KN, Bae K, Park MJ, Choi HC, Shin HS, Shin S, et al. US-guided transthoracic biopsy of peripheral lung lesions: pleural contact length influences diagnostic yield. Acta Radiol. 2014;55:295–301.

26. Zhang Y, Qiang JW, Shen Y, Ye JD, Zhang J, Zhu L. Using air bronchograms on multi-detector CT to predict the invasiveness of small lung adenocarcinoma. Eur J Radiol. 2016;85:571–7.

27. Piccoli M, Trambaiolo P, Salustri A, Cerquetani E, Posteraro A, Pastena G, et al. Bedside diagnosis and follow-up of patients with pleural effusion by a hand-carried ultrasound device early after cardiac surgery. Chest. 2005;128:3413–20.

28. Liapikou A, Ferrer M, Polverino E, Balasso V, Esperatti M, Piñer R, et al. Severe community-acquired pneumonia: validation of the Infectious Diseases Society of America/American Thoracic Society guidelines to predict an intensive care unit admission. Clin Infect Dis. 2009;48:377–85.

29. Catalano D, Trovato G, Sperandeo M, Sacco MC. Lung ultrasound in pediatric pneumonia. The persistent need of chest X-rays. Pediatr Pulmonol. 2014;49:617–8.

30. Catalano D, Trovato FM, Pirri C, Trovato GM. Outpatient diagnosis and therapeutic units linked with ED referrals: a sustainable quality-centered approach. Am J Emerg Med. 2013;31:1612.

31. Sperandeo M, Rotondo A, Guglielmi G, Catalano D, Feragalli B, Trovato GM. Transthoracic ultrasound in the assessment of pleural and pulmonary diseases: use and limitations. Radiol Med. 2014;119:729–40.

32. Ruiz-González A, Falguera M, Porcel JM, Martínez-Alonso M, Cabezas P, Geijo P, et al. C-reactive protein for discriminating treatment failure from slow responding pneumonia. Eur J Intern Med. 2010;21:548–52.

33. Medford AR. Chest ultrasonography as a replacement for chest radiography for community-acquired pneumonia. Chest. 2013;143:877–8.

34. Goss CH, Rubenfeld GD, Park DR, Sherbin VL, Goodman MS, Root RK. Cost and incidence of social comorbidities in low-risk patients with community-acquired pneumonia admitted to a public hospital. Chest. 2003;124:2148–55.

20

Superb microvascular imaging (SMI) compared with conventional ultrasound for evaluating thyroid nodules

Ruigang Lu[1†], Yuxin Meng[2†], Yan Zhang[1], Wei Zhao[1], Xun Wang[3], Mulan Jin[4] and Ruijun Guo[1*]

Abstract

Background: Superb microvascular imaging (SMI) for depiction of microvascular flow in thyroid nodules was compared with color/power Doppler imaging (CDI/PDI) and contrast-enhanced ultrasonography (CEUS). In addition, the diagnostic performance of conventional ultrasound combined with SMI for differentiating benign and malignant thyroid nodules was evaluated.

Methods: Preoperative conventional ultrasound consisting of gray-scale ultrasonography and CDI/PDI, followed by SMI and CEUS, was used to record 52 thyroid nodules. Two radiologists analyzed the gray-scale ultrasound signs and nodules' microvascular flow patterns to differentiate between benign ($n = 13$) and malignant nodules ($n = 39$).

Results: SMI was significantly more effective in the detection of microvascular flow signals than CDI/PDI. In malignant nodules, SMI depicted the presence of incomplete surrounding periphery microvasculature and of disordered heterogeneous internal microvasculature. Benign nodules showed complete surrounding periphery microvasculature (ring sign) and homogeneity internal branching. The accuracies of conventional ultrasound combined with CDI/ PDI, SMI, or CEUS for predicting malignancy were 67.31, 86.54, and 92.31%, respectively. The accuracy of SMI differed significantly from CDI/PDI ($P = 0.012$), but not from CEUS ($P = 0.339$).

Conclusions: Microvascular flow and vessel branching in the peripheral and internal microvasculature of thyroid nodules is depicted with greater detail and clarity with SMI compared with conventional ultrasound. SMI offers a safe and low-cost alternative to CEUS for differentiating between benign and malignant thyroid nodules.

Keywords: Superb microvascular imaging, Thyroid nodule, CEUS, Microvascular, CDI/PDI, Microvessel density

Background

Thyroid nodules are a common finding. With development of ultrasonic technology and improvement in resolution, the rate of detection of thyroid nodules has risen, especially in younger persons [1]. In clinical practice, ultrasound is the primary imaging method for evaluating thyroid nodules. However, some of the typical characteristics of malignant nodules have a diagnostic accuracy of only 74 to 82%, including hypoechogenicity, irregular margins, being taller than wide, microcalcifications, absence of halo, and presence of perforator vessel(s) [2, 3]. None of these features is specific enough to classify a

lesion as malignant, and sensitivity is also significantly lower for any single feature [4]. It is therefore important to explore a complementary method which could improve the identification of benign and malignant nodules.

It is well known that blood vessels are important to the growth of a nodule, but conventional color or power Doppler imaging (CDI and PDI, respectively) are not very sensitive to microvascularity patterns and low blood flow velocity [5]. Vessel extraction methods, such as minimal path techniques to effectively locate tiny vessels, might be of help to extract vessel-related information for further diagnosis [6], although they are limited by some inherent problems like endpoint, shortcut and accumulation issues [7]. A recent improved means of visualizing low flow in microvessels is superb microvascular imaging (SMI) ultrasound technology, implemented with the Aplio 500 US

* Correspondence: Ruijunguo2016@sina.com

†Equal contributors

[1]Department of Ultrasonography, Beijing Chao-Yang Hospital, Capital Medical University, Beijing 100020, China

Full list of author information is available at the end of the article

system by Toshiba (Toshiba Medical Systems, Tokyo, Japan). SMI uses advanced clutter suppression to extract flow signals from large to small vessels, and depicts this information at high frame rates as a color overlay image or as a grayscale map of flow (color or monochrome SMI, respectively).

The present study compares the flow imaging abilities of SMI, CDI/PDI, and CEUS for depicting microvascular flow in thyroid nodules, and evaluates the efficacy of these methods for identifying benign and malignant thyroid nodules.

Methods

The study was conducted from March to November 2016. Fifty prospective patients (45 women and 5 men; 52 tumors) who were referred for surgery due to suspicion of malignancy after gray-scale ultrasound or palpation, were enrolled. The mean age of these patients was 47 years (range: 20-65 years).

All patients enrolled underwent ultrasound examination of the thyroid consisting of the following modalities: gray-scale ultrasound; CDI; PDI; color and monochrome SMI; and CEUS using an Aplio 500 ultrasound system with a broad bandwidth linear array transducer (imaging frequency, 14 MHz). The nodules studied were solid or cystic solid with a solid component greater than 50% and a maximum diameter of 0.5-3.0 cm. For all subjects, the settings for cross section, constant color sampling frame size, and moderation scale were identical throughout the imaging portion of the study. In selected patients, pulsed Doppler was also used during monochrome SMI to examine a few specific microvessels inside the nodule, to verify that the observed vessels were real microvasculature.

Two senior radiologists read all the fixed and dynamic pictures independently. Nodules were scored by analyzing microvasculature and branching using a visual-analog scale of 0 (worst) to 10 (best), based on the semiquantitative percentage of nodule volume occupied by vessel signals. For each patient, the following characteristics were recorded: vessel branching detail, peripheral vascularization surrounding the nodule, and homogeneous or heterogeneous disordered distribution of internal small branching microvasculature.

Images and cine loops of the thyroid nodules from all 5 modalities, acquired during the ultrasound examinations, were independently analyzed by 2 radiologists (blinded to the histology pathology results). The observers independently scored the digital clips from each of the 5 flow modes, and each nodule with regard to overall flow detection and vessel branching details, scoring them as 0 (worst) to 10 (best). The qualitative scores (i.e., for overall flow detection and vessel branching details) were compared on a per nodule basis using a nonparametric Wilcoxon signed rank test.

All tests were performed using Stata 12.0 software (Stata Corp, College Station, TX), with $P < 0.05$ indicating statistical significance. To assess the consistency of the vascularity scores determined by the 2 observers, k-coefficients were calculated.

Results

For the 52 solid nodules, the results of histology yielded 39 malignant (papillary thyroid carcinoma) and 13 benign nodules. The latter consisted of 5 follicular adenomas, 6 nodular goiters, 1 parathyroid adenoma, and 1 shrinking cyst. The details of microvasculature within the nodules were recorded semi-quantitatively (Fig. 1).

Both color and monochrome SMI delivered clearer and more cohesive vessel branching detail in the nodules compared with CDI/PDI. In malignant nodules, SMI revealed disordered heterogeneous internal microvessel distribution, scarce vascularity in hypoechoic nodules or interrupted surrounding peripheral microvasculature (Figs. 2 and 4). In benign nodules, SMI showed complete surrounding periphery microvasculature and homogeneous internal microvessel distributions (Figs. 3 and 4). The characteristics of the nodules according to microvascular flow of CDI/PDI, SMI, and CEUS were evaluated and the accuracy of the 3 imaging microvascular flow patterns was assessed.

Pulsed Doppler guided by monochrome SMI established that the small branching microvessels detected by monochrome SMI are real and can be measured (Figs. 2e, 3e and 4e). CEUS features of the nodule (Figs. 2f, 3f and 4f). Observations included heterogeneous hypoechoic enhancement of the middle nodule, and homogeneous hyperechoic enhancement in the right nodule (Figs. 4f). The results for the various ultrasound modalities in the depiction of microvascular flow in thyroid nodules are summarized in Table 1.

The consistency of scores for a subset of 52 nodules among the CDI/PDI, SMI, and CEUS images acquired by 2 independent operators was assessed. The k-coefficients of CDI/PDI, SMI, and CEUS were 0.949, 0.871, and 0.918, respectively. The diagnostic accuracies of the 3 methods are presented in Table 2. The accuracies of conventional ultrasound combined with CDI/ PDI, SMI, or CEUS for predicting malignancy were 67.31, 86.54, and 92.31%, respectively. SMI differed significantly from CDI/PDI ($\chi2 = 6.372$, $P = 0.012$), but not from CEUS ($\chi2 = 0.915$, $P = 0.339$).

Discussion

Ultrasound is the primary imaging method for the evaluation of thyroid nodules [4]. Flow imaging of thyroid nodules can differentiate between benign and malignant

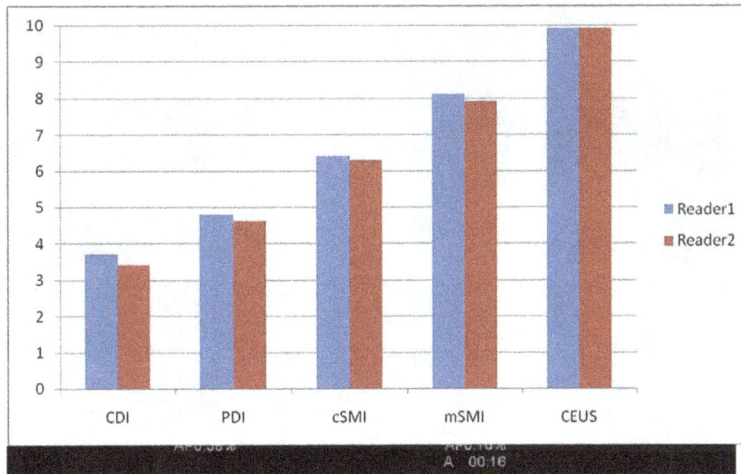

Fig. 1 Overall flow detection scored on a subjective scale of 0 to 10 for CDI, PDI, color SMI (cSMI), monochrome SMI (mSMI), and CEUS of average distribution for all nodules

nodules. However, there are technical limitations in using CDI/PDI for detecting small blood vessels and low blood flow. Currently, microvessel density is the gold standard for determining tumor angiogenesis [8, 9]. The radiological evaluation of tumor angiogenesis includes morphological abnormalities of the microvessels, and differences in neonatal microvascular density and function [10, 11]. However, microvessel density can only be measured postoperatively, and therefore cannot be used to prevent unneeded invasive procedures, that is, for identifying benign lesions that should not be operated on.

SMI is a relatively new imaging modality that is implemented on the Toshiba Aplio 500 ultrasound system. It enables better depiction of microvascularity and low-velocity blood flow compared with conventional ultrasound methods. Low-level echoes that are near the noise level of the equipment, are detected by the SMI procedure for maximum information with minimum noise, but improper adjustment of the system gain may cause SMI imaging information distortion. In the present study, SMI did indeed reveal more small branches of microvasculature compared with CDI/PDI, and show the distribution

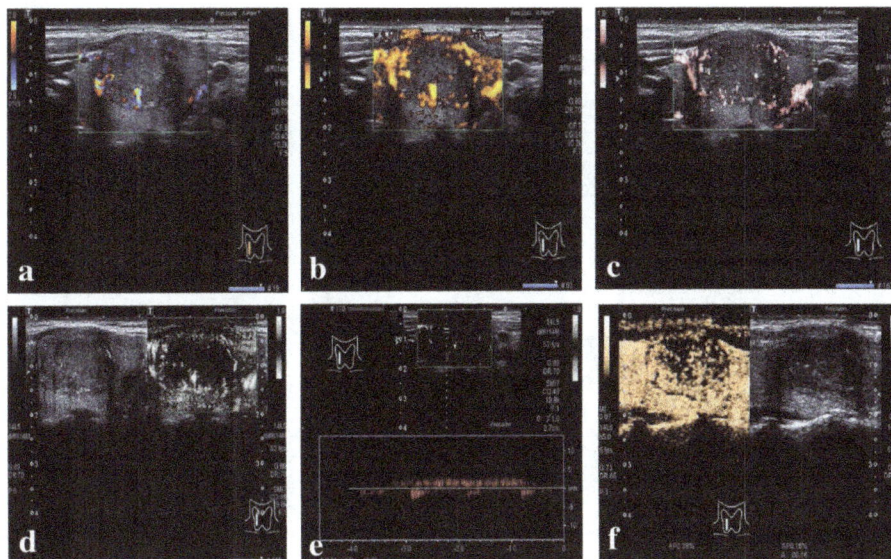

Fig. 2 A papillary thyroid carcinoma located in the right lobe. **a** CDI and **b** PDI show peripheral and internal vascularity of the nodule, with **c** color SMI and **d** monochrome SMI depicting more detailed peripheral vascularity surrounding the nodule as well as internal disordered small branching microvessels. **e** Pulsed Doppler (guided by monochrome SMI) established that the small branching microvasculature was real and measurable. **f** CEUS features of the nodule. The nodule enhances later compared with normal thyroid parenchyma, with disordered heterogeneous hypoechoic enhancement and incomplete peripheral enhancement

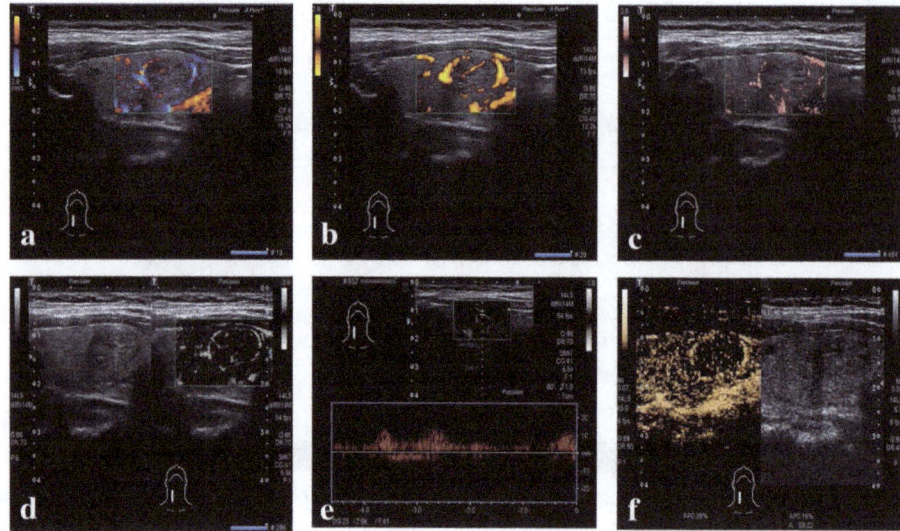

Fig. 3 An isoechoic thyroid nodule located in the right lobe. **a** CDI and **b** PDI show some peripheral vascularization around the nodule. **c** Color SMI and **d** monochrome SMI show complete peripheral vascularization surrounding the nodule, with internal microvascularization and small branching details. **e** Pulsed Doppler (guided by monochrome SMI) established that the small branching microvasculature was real and measurable. **f** CEUS shows ring enhancement around the nodule and homogeneous internal enhancement. Histology: adenoma

inside nodules and adjacent thyroid parenchyma in better detail. Judged by the detail in its images, SMI is highly accurate.

According to several reports, CEUS is able to depict microperfusion in thyroid nodules. Zhang et al. [3] demonstrated that ring enhancement was closely associated with the benign character of lesions, whereas heterogeneous enhancement was helpful for detecting malignant lesions. Jiang reported that lower contrast enhancement levels are an important diagnostic indication of tiny papillary thyroid carcinoma [12]. This study compared SMI with CEUS and found that SMI provides better display of the network of small microvascular branches and their distribution in nodules, although

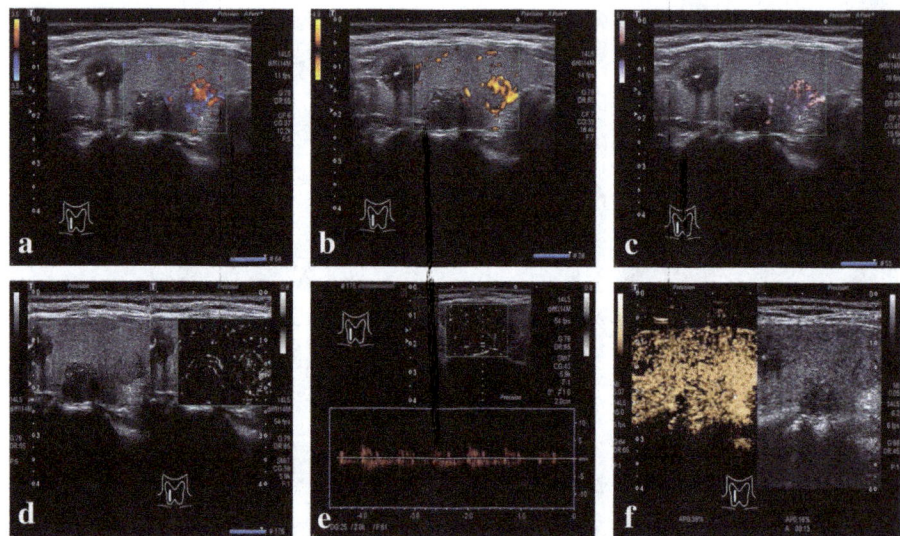

Fig. 4 A papillary thyroid carcinoma (➜) and an adenoma (⇑) coexist in the right lobe. **a** CDI and **b** PDI show peripheral vascularization and peripheral interrupted vascularization of the nodule and internal microvascularization. **c** Color SMI and **d** monochrome SMI show more vascularization, in particular curved and ring peripheral vascularization surrounding the nodule as well as internal microvascularization with small branching details. **e** Pulsed Doppler (guided by monochrome SMI) established that the small branching microvasculature was real and measurable. **f** CEUS shows disordered heterogeneous hypoechoic enhancement with incomplete peripheral enhancement (➜) and ring enhancement around the nodule and homogeneous hyperechoic internal enhancement (⇑).

Table 1 CDI/PDI, SMI, and CEUS for depiction of microvascular flow distribution in thyroid nodules

	Disordered heterogeneous	Homogeneous	Ring	None	Sum
CDI/PDI	40	3	3	6	52
SMI	38	5	7	2	52
CEUS	37	6	8	1	52

CEUS blood pool imaging can show thicker blood branches and vascular perfusion clearly. CEUS is believed by some researchers to have a high sensitivity to blood flow, resulting in coverage of real blood vessels [13]. However, another characteristic of CEUS is harmonic imaging, coupled with low mechanical index, low frequency, and a low frame rate (6-13 fps), which unfortunately affects the 2-dimensional display of the image. Another drawback of CEUS is variation in the contrast agent in-out time and patients' swallowing, resulting in an unsatisfactory 3-dimensional display of microvasculature.

In the present study, SMI and CEUS were similar in the high consistency of differentiation between benign and malignant nodules. The results of conventional ultrasound combined with CEUS tended to be better than those combined with SMI, but SMI is also the more economical method and avoids the hazards associated with the contrast agent used in CEUS. Furthermore, SMI has already shown potential in the characterization of brain tumors prior to surgery [14] and in the early diagnosis of breast cancer [15, 16]. Zhan et al. [14] considered the value of SMI when combined with conventional ultrasound without contrast administration and determined that SMI was helpful in the differential diagnosis of benign and malignant avascular breast lesions, especially those in BI-RADS category 4.

To the best of our knowledge there is only one previous comparison in the literature of the diagnostic value of SMI and CEUS for the differentiation of tumors. This is a retrospective study by Xiao et al., [16] who compared the diagnostic utility of SMI and CEUS for breast lesions, using root hair-like and crab claw-like patterns as criteria for malignant lesions. Based on the microvascular architecture patterns, the sensitivity, specificity, and accuracy of monochromatic SMI for differentiation

were 78, 91, and 85%, respectively, and the corresponding rates using CEUS were 90, 88, and 89%. Areas under the curve for monochromatic SMI and CEUS were not significantly different ($P = 0.013$) [15]. These breast cancer data are closely similar to the thyroid cancer data obtained in the present prospective study comparing SMI and CEUS for differentiating malignant from benign thyroid nodules. That is, we report an ~87% accuracy for SMI combined with conventional ultrasound, and a ~92% accuracy for CEUS with conventional ultrasound ($P = 0.339$). The main limitation in this study, is formed by the homogeneous background of the patients with none of the nodules being follicular carcinoma. Those typically require hemi-thyroidectomy or lobectomy for definitive diagnosis.

Our results indicate that SMI has the potential to become the method of choice for detecting microvasculature in thyroid nodules. This conclusion is in accord with previous studies showing the use of SMI for better characterization of the vascularity of breast tumors [14, 15]. Blood flow detection and depiction of microvessel architecture are superior with this new noninvasive ultrasound imaging method. SMI combined with conventional ultrasound may become the tool of choice for differentiating benign from malignant thyroid nodules. Furthermore, because SMI does not require a contrast agent, it is more economical than CEUS and avoids the adverse reactions associated with the contrast agent.

Conclusion

SMI detects more small branches of microvasculature compared with CDI/PDI, and also shows the distribution inside nodules and adjacent thyroid parenchyma in better detail. SMI and CEUS are similar in the high consistency of differentiation between benign and malignant nodules, but SMI is also the more economical method and avoids the hazards associated with the contrast agent used in CEUS. Compared with conventional ultrasound, SMI therefore offers a superior alternative for the differentiation of benign and malignant thyroid nodules.

Table 2 Diagnostic accuracy of conventional ultrasound combined with CDI/PDI, SMI and CEUS in predicting benign and malignant thyroid nodules

	Benign or malignant		
	Conform	Not conform	Sum
CDI/PDI	35	17	52
SMI	45	7	52
CEUS	48	4	52

Abbreviations

CDI/PDI: Color/Power Doppler imaging; CEUS: Contrast-enhanced ultrasonography; SMI: Superb microvascular imaging

Acknowledgements

Not applicable

Funding

None

Authors' contributions

RG and RJ designed the study. YZ and WZ collected and analysed the data. YX advised on histological staining and analysis. XW and ML contributed samples collection and intellectual input. RG and WZ drafted and wrote the manuscript. RJ revised the manuscript critically for intellectual content. All authors gave intellectual input to the study and approved the final version of the manuscript. RJ conceived the study, finalized the manuscript and acts as guarantor. All authors approved submission.

Competing interests

The authors declare that they have no competing interests.

Author details

[1]Department of Ultrasonography, Beijing Chao-Yang Hospital, Capital Medical University, Beijing 100020, China. [2]Department of Endocrinology, Beijing No. 6 Hospital, Beijing 100007, China. [3]Department of Otorhinolaryngology Head and Neck Surgery, Beijing Chao-Yang Hospital, Capital Medical University, Beijing 100020, China. [4]Department of Pathology, Beijing Chao-Yang Hospital, Capital Medical University, Beijing 100020, China.

References

1. Colonna M, Uhry Z, Guizard AV, Delafosse P, Schvartz C, Belot A, et al. Recent trends in incidence, geographical distribution, and survival of papillary thyroid cancer in France. Cancer Epidemiol. 2015;39:511–8.
2. Smith-Bindman R, Lebda P, Feldstein VA, Sellami D, Goldstein RB, Brasic N, et al. Risk of thyroid cancer based on thyroid ultrasound imaging characteristics: results of a population-based study. JAMA Intern Med. 2013;173:1788–96.
3. Zhang B, Jiang YX, Liu JB, Yang M, Dai Q, Zhu QL, et al. Utility of contrast-enhanced ultrasound for evaluation of thyroid nodules. Thyroid. 2010;20:51–7.
4. Haugen BR, Alexander EK, Bible KC, Doherty GM, Mandel SJ, Nikiforov YE, et al. 2015 American Thyroid Association management guidelines for adult patients with thyroid nodules and differentiated thyroid cancer: the American Thyroid Association guidelines task force on thyroid nodules and differentiated thyroid cancer. Thyroid. 2016;26:1–133.
5. Niu LJ, Hao YZ, Zhou CW. Diagnostic value of ultrasonography in thyroid lesions. Zhonghua Er Bi Yan Hou Tou Jing Wai Ke Za Zhi. 2006;41:415–8.
6. Wink O, Niessen WJ, Viergever MA. Multiscale vessel tracking. IEEE Trans Med Imaging. 2004;23:130–3.
7. Chen Y, Zhang Y, Yang J, Cao Q, Yang G, Chen J, et al. Curve-like structure extraction using minimal path propagation with backtracking. IEEE Trans Image Process. 2016;25:988–1003.
8. Weidner N. Current pathologic methods for measuring intratumoral microvessel density within breast carcinoma and other solid tumors. Breast Cancer Res Treat. 1995;36:169–80.
9. Elston CW, Ellis IO. Pathological prognostic factors in breast cancer. I. The value of histological grade in breast cancer: experience from a large study with long-term follow-up. Histopathology. 2002;41:154–61.
10. Shaked Y, Bertolini F, Man S, Rogers MS, Cervi D, Foutz T, et al. Genetic heterogeneity of the vasculogenic phenotype parallels angiogenesis; implications for cellular surrogate marker analysis of antiangiogenesis. Cancer Cell. 2005;7:101–11.
11. Testa AC, Ferrandina G, Fruscella E, Van Holsbeke C, Ferrazzi E, Leone FP, et al. The use of contrasted transvaginal sonography in the diagnosis of gynecologic diseases: a preliminary study. J Ultrasound Med. 2005;24:1267–78.
12. Jiang J, Liu N, Zhou Q. Diagnosis of thyroid microcarcinoma using contrast-enhanced ultrasound. Chin J Ultrasonogr. 2012;21:595–7.
13. Chen HY, Chen Y, Zhu H. Comparative study of superb microvascular imaging and contrast-enhanced ultrasound in differentiating thyroid micronodules. Chin J Ultrasonogr. 2016;25:44–7.
14. Ishikawa M, Ota Y, Nagai M, Kusaka G, Tanaka Y, Naritaka H. Ultrasonography monitoring with superb microvascular imaging technique in brain tumor surgery. World Neurosurg. 2017;97:749.e11–.e20.
15. Zhan J, Diao XH, Jin JM, Chen L, Chen Y. Superb microvascular imaging-a new vascular detecting ultrasonographic technique for avascular breast masses: a preliminary study. Eur J Radiol. 2016;85:915–21.
16. Xiao XY, Chen X, Guan XF, Wu H, Qin W, Luo BM. Superb microvascular imaging in diagnosis of breast lesions: a comparative study with contrast-enhanced ultrasonographic microvascular imaging. Br J Radiol. 2016;89: 20160546.

21

Quantification of FDG-PET/CT with delayed imaging in patients with newly diagnosed recurrent breast cancer

Christina Baun[1]*[iD], Kirsten Falch[1], Oke Gerke[1,2], Jeanette Hansen[1], Tram Nguyen[1], Abass Alavi[3], Poul-Flemming Høilund-Carlsen[1] and Malene G. Hildebrandt[1]

Abstract

Background: Several studies have shown the advantage of delayed-time-point imaging with 18F-FDG-PET/CT to distinguish malignant from benign uptake. This may be relevant in cancer diseases with low metabolism, such as breast cancer. We aimed at examining the change in SUV from 1 h (1h) to 3 h (3h) time-point imaging in local and distant lesions in patients with recurrent breast cancer. Furthermore, we investigated the effect of partial volume correction in the different types of metastases, using semi-automatic quantitative software (ROVER™).

Methods: One-hundred and two patients with suspected breast cancer recurrence underwent whole-body PET/CT scans 1h and 3h after FDG injection. Semi-quantitative standardised uptake values (SUVmax, SUVmean) and partial volume corrected SUVmean (cSUVmean), were estimated in malignant lesions, and as reference in healthy liver tissue. The change in quantitative measures from 1h to 3h was calculated, and SUVmean was compared to cSUVmean. Metastases were verified by biopsy.

Results: Of the 102 included patients, 41 had verified recurrent disease with in median 15 lesions (range 1-70) amounting to a total of 337 malignant lesions included in the analysis. SUVmax of malignant lesions increased from 6.4 ± 3.4 [0.9-19.7] (mean $\pm$ SD, min and max) at 1h to 8.1 ± 4.4 [0.7-29.7] at 3h. SUVmax in breast, lung, lymph node and bone lesions increased significantly ($p < 0.0001$) between 1h and 3h by on average 25, 40, 33, and 27%, respectively. A similar pattern was observed with (uncorrected) SUVmean. Partial volume correction increased SUVmean significantly, by 63 and 71% at 1h and 3h imaging, respectively. The highest impact was in breast lesions at 3h, where cSUVmean increased by 87% compared to SUVmean.

Conclusion: SUVs increased from 1h to 3h in malignant lesions, SUVs of distant recurrence were in general about twice as high as those of local recurrence. Partial volume correction caused significant increases in these values. However, it is questionable, if these relatively modest quantitative advances of 3h imaging are sufficient to warrant delayed imaging in this patient group.

Keywords: FDG-PET/CT, Breast cancer, Delayed-time-point, Standardised uptake values, Partial volume correction

* Correspondence: Christina.baun@rsyd.dk
[1]Department of Nuclear Medicine, University Hospital, Sdr. Boulevard 29, 5000 Odense C, Denmark
Full list of author information is available at the end of the article

Background

Breast cancer is the most frequent cancer among women in western countries, and up to 30% of patients are likely to develop recurrence [1, 2]. 18F-fluoro-deoxy-glucose positron emission tomography/computed tomography (FDG-PET/CT) is useful in the diagnosis, staging and therapeutic follow-up of patients with recurrent breast cancer, and is especially better than conventional imaging at detecting distant metastases [3–5].

FDG is not specific for malignancy; however, recent studies have shown the advantage of delayed or dual-time imaging with FDG-PET to distinguish malignant from benign uptake [6–8]. The underlying rationale is that malignant cells have more glucose transporters and hexokinases and less glucose-6-phosphatase (G6Pase), which leads to FDG accumulation over time compared to benign cells [9, 10]. Delayed scan time-points may thus improve the image quality due the greater difference between tumour and background levels [11–14]. This may be relevant in cancer diseases with low metabolism, such as breast cancer.

Only a few studies have examined the use of delayed time-point imaging (DTPI) in whole-body FDG-PET/CT to show the FDG accumulation over time associated with distant metastases [15–17]. The literature suggests that more prospective studies are needed to provide a better understanding of the use of DTPI in detecting recurrent breast cancer [6, 18, 19]. Analysis of PET data is often performed semi-quantitatively by measuring standardised uptake values (SUV) in lesions suspected of malignancy [20–22]. SUV has been referred to correlate well with histological and biological tumour characteristics, and can be an important tool in the diagnostic report for breast cancer patients [23–25]. SUV is strongly affected by the partial volume effect (PVE), however, which can cause a significant underestimation of the lesion uptake level [26–28]. Although methods for partial volume correction (PVC) have been developed to overcome this limitation, no method has yet found its place in daily clinical practice. Further evidence is needed to state the usefulness and feasibility of these software methods [29–32].

We aimed at examining the value of whole-body FDG-PET/CT performed at 3 h (3h) compared to the standard imaging time-point at 1 h (1h), in patients suspected of recurrent breast cancer, using quantitative software that included PVC.

Our objectives were to investigate i) the change in standardised uptake values from early (1h) to delayed (3h) time-point imaging in local and distant lesions, by measuring SUVmax, SUVmean and correcting SUVmean for PVE (cSUVmean), and ii) the effect of PVC by comparing SUVmean and cSUVmean at both time-points.

Methods

One-hundred and two women with suspected breast cancer recurrence or with verified local recurrence and potential distant disease were enrolled in the study. The patients were part of a larger prospective accuracy study comparing FDG-PET/CT to conventional imaging in detecting recurrent breast cancer [33]. The prospective study was conducted at the PET centre, Odense University Hospital, Denmark, from December 2011 to September 2014. Exclusion criteria were history of other malignancies, age < 18 years, pregnancy or breastfeeding, diabetes mellitus, or considered unable to cooperate. For further methodological details we refer to our recent publication [33].

FDG-pet/CT

Patients were required to fast for at least 6 h before the FDG-PET/CT scan. A maximum blood glucose level of 144 mg/dL was allowed prior to intravenous injection of 4 MBq/kg FDG. Whole-body FDG-PET/CT scans were performed 1h and 3h after FDG injection on a General Electric Discovery STE or Discovery RX system (GE Healthcare, Milwaukee, USA). A low-dose CT scan (140 kV, 30-110 mA; Auto- and Smart mA) was performed followed by a 3D PET scan. Acquisition time was of 2.5 min/frame for the 1h scan and 3.5 min/frame for the 3h scan, for patients with a normal body mass index (BMI) between 18.5 kg/m^2 and 24.9 kg/m^2. If BMI was lower or higher, the scan time was adjusted according to BMI and either decreased or increased by ½ min/frame, respectively. Images were reconstructed iteratively using an ordered subset expectation maximization (OSEM) algorithm, with 2 iterations, and 21 or 28 subsets, a slice thickness of 3.3 mm and matrix size of 128 × 128 (pixel size of 5.47mm^2) with CT-based attenuation correction and 5 mm Gaussian post-filtering.

Reference standard

Suspected recurrence was verified by biopsy. If biopsy was not possible, a composite reference standard comprising all available imaging procedures (MRI, CT, PET/CT, bone scan, ultrasound, x-ray and mammography) and/or clinical follow-up data over 6 months was used as gold standard, using the patients' medical files as necessary. In patients with multiple lesions, it was not possible to obtain a biopsy from all lesions for ethical reasons. The patients were categorised into groups of 'local recurrence' or 'distant recurrence' based on reference standard and in accordance with treatment decision.

Image interpretation

The scans were visually interpreted by an experienced nuclear medicine physician using the General Electric acquisition workstation. The 1h and 3h images were read independently. Each lesion was described with anatomic site and exact image number for further semi-quantitative analysis. The lesions were divided into seven subgroups according to lesion site: cerebrum, lung, liver, breast, lymph node, bone and 'other' (subcutaneous and muscle metastasis).

Semi-quantitative analysis

Semi-quantitative analysis of the malignant lesions was retrospectively performed using dedicated image analysis software (ROVER™, ABX, Radeberg, Germany). This software provides semi-automatic image segmentation with a model-free method for PVE correction of SUV-mean values. The software performs lesion delineation within a user-defined 3D mask using fixed, peak-based thresholding to delineate the lesion region-of-interest (ROI), which represents the metabolic active tumour volume (MTV). In the following step, ROVER performs PVC using an algorithm that defines a spill-out region of the lesion ROI from which a background corrected estimate of the spill-out region is calculated and used to perform PVC of SUVmean resulting in cSUVmean. Further details regarding software algorithms are explained by Hofheinz et al. [32, 34]. The ROVER software was used in standard mode with a threshold setting of 40% of maximum 3D mask value, including a minimum ROI volume of 1cm^3 and excluding ROI intersection. SUV values were normalised to body weight. Manually placement of 3D masks was performed after visual identification of the lesion by the interpreting physician. Masks were placed 2-4 pixels beyond the visual margin of each lesion, and ROVER automatically delineated the lesion ROI and performed PVC. It automatically calculated ROI values of SUVmax, SUVmean, cSUVmean and MTV. Separate 3D masks were used for the same lesions in the 1h and 3h scans. If a lesion had no discernible FDG uptake in the early images, the 3D mask was placed as close as possible to the assumed origin based on anatomic orientation. A reference measurement in healthy liver tissue was obtained in all patients at both time-points. This was performed by drawing a mask of approximately 36 cm^3 in the upper right lobe of healthy liver tissue, avoiding malignancies and organ boundaries. Potential metastatic lesions without FDG-uptake would not be registered for analysis. The difference in SUV-max, SUVmean, cSUVmean, and MTV between the two time-points were calculated as $\Delta SUV = SUV3h - SUV1h$, and $\Delta MTV = MTV3h - MTV1h$.

Statistical analysis

Descriptive statistics were performed for demographic variables and scanning parameters. The semi-quantitative analysis parameters from the 1h and 3h scans were expressed as mean ± standard deviation (SD) and range. Boxplots were used for graphical display of the data. The differences in SUVs between the two time-points as well as the difference between SUVmean and cSUVmean measurements at each time-point were estimated together with 95% confidence intervals (CI) and p-values that were derived from univariate linear regression models using robust standard errors to allow for intragroup correlation (i.e. multiple lesions in the same patient). Subgroup analyses were conducted by recurrence category (distant versus local recurrence) and lesion site, where healthy liver tissue was used as the reference category. Analyses were supplemented by relative changes of mean values in groups, e.g. (mean value of 3h measurements − mean value of 1h measurements)/ (mean value of 1h measurements)*100%.

Statistical tests were two-sided with a significance level of 5%. Analyses were conducted with Stata/MP 14.0 (StataCorp LP, College Station, Texas 77845, USA).

Results

Of the 102 patients who initially agreed to participate in the study one patient changed her mind before FDG-PET/CT, another was excluded due to a previous biopsy-verified bone metastasis, and a third patient did not complete the 3h scan, leaving 99 women available for analysis. Forty-one of these (41.4%) were diagnosed with recurrent breast cancer, with a total of 337 malignant lesions (mean 15, range 1-70) available for analysis. The patient and scanning characteristics are given in Table 1.

Nineteen patients had local recurrence comprising 21 lesions, and 22 patients had distant disease with 316 lesions. All patients had at least one biopsy to verify recurrence. Biopsies were primarily taken from breast lesions. For patients with recurrent disease and multiple distant metastases, only one distant lesion was verified by biopsy due to ethical aspect. All remaining metastatic lesions were verified by the composite reference standard, as

Table 1 Patient and scanning characteristics of 1h and 3h FDG-PET/CT, performed in the 41 patients with recurrent breast cancer

Patient characteristics	Mean ± SD, range
Patient age (years)	62 ± 4.2 [57;74]
Body mass index	27 ± 7.1 [22;32]
Blood glucose level (mmol/L)	5.4 ± 1.0 [3.8;7.7]
Years since treatment of primary breast cancer	6 ± 8.2 [0;30]
Scanning characteristics	
Dose (MBq)	281 ± 56.0 [208;401]
Time (min) between injection and early scan (1h)	62 ± 6.0 [53;80]
Time (min) between injection and late scan (3h)	180 ± 6.0 [170;200]

described in the method section. Distribution of lesions and biopsies are shown in Table 2.

Local vs. distant recurrence

The overall SUV measurements for all 41 patients increased, on average, significantly between 1h and 3h, i.e., SUVmax by 1.8 (+ 28% increase), SUVmean by 1.1 (+ 28%), and cSUVmean by 2.3 (+ 35%). Overall, MTV decreased significantly over time, particularly for patients with distant recurrence in whom it decreased by 16%, shown in Table 3.

The values of distant recurrence were in general about twice as high as those of local recurrence, but the relative average increase was the same for the two groups. In both groups, the relative increase in cSUVmean (35-36%) was greater than the increase in SUVmean and SUVmax (25-28%). Despite these average tendencies, some lesions showed reduced SUVmax values at 3h, i.e., 8 lesions (38%) in patients with local recurrence and 31 lesions (10%) in patients with distant recurrence.

Changes by lesion subgroup

Except for and the lesion group 'other', all subgroups showed a significant increase in SUVmax and SUV-mean over time, compared to the reference measurements in healthy liver tissue (Fig. 1). Lymph node metastases showed the highest absolute increase in SUVmax by 2.1 [1.4-2.8] (mean, 95% CI) (+ 33%), SUVmean by 1.5 [0.1-0.7] (+ 36%) and cSUVmean by 3.2 [2.6-3.2] (+ 47%). The highest relative increase in SUVmax, SUVmean and cSUVmean over time was seen for lung metastases at 40, 44 and 52%, respectively. Breast lesions showed the smallest absolute increase from 1h to 3h in SUVmax, SUVmean and cSUVmean at 0.7 [0.2-1.1] (+ 25%), 0.4 [0.1-0.7] (+ 24%) and 1.2 [0.4-1.9] (+ 42%). Liver lesions showed the lowest relative increase in SUVmax, SUVmean and, cSUVmean of 18, 16 and 18% respectively. Reference tissue in healthy liver showed a significant average decrease in SUVmax by 11 and 20%, respectively.

Despite the overall increase in SUV for lesion subgroups, some lesions showed reduced SUV over time, i. e., 1 (4%) in the lung, 1 (14%) in liver, 11 (41%) in breast, 3 (6%) in lymph nodes, 22 (7%) in bone and 1 (10%) of the 'other' lesions. The percentages of lesions with decreased values between the two time-points were the same for SUVmax, SUVmean and cSUVmean. Due to only one cerebral metastasis, this lesion group was not considered representative and is not commented upon in the results or discussion sections. MTV decreased, on average, significantly for all lesion subgroups between 1h and 3h; however, for liver lesions and 'other' lesions the decrease was not significant. The greatest decrease (of 43%) in MTV was seen in breast lesions. For details regarding lesion subgroups, see supplementary data given in Additional file 1.

Partial volume correction

For all lesions as a whole, cSUVmean was significantly higher than SUVmean at both 1h (mean difference of 2.5 equal to 63%) and 3h (3.6 equal to 71%) except lesions 'other' and liver metastases at 1h, which was insignificantly higher (Table 4). For patients with local recurrence cSUVmean was 70% higher than SUVmean at 1h and 84% at 3h and for distant recurrence 63% higher at 1h and 71% at 3h, see Table 4.

At lesion site the largest difference was at 3h for breast lesions, where cSUVmean was 87% higher than SUV-mean. The smallest difference was at 1h for liver lesions, in which cSUVmean was 39% higher than SUVmean (Table 4). Generally, cSUVmean varied more than SUV-mean in all lesion sites (Fig. 2). Further details regarding lesion subgroups, see supplementary data given in Additional file 1.

Discussion

This study of malignant lesions in 41 out of 99 analysed patients with breast cancer recurrence showed significant overall increase in uptake of FDG between 1h and 3h scans. The values of distant recurrence were in general about twice as high as those of local recurrence, but the relative increase was the same for the two groups (Table 3). Lymph node metastases showed the highest absolute increase in SUV between the two time-points, whereas lung metastases displayed the highest relative increase. PVC led to higher uptake estimates, especially for patients with local recurrence and for breast lesions at the 3h scan (Table 4 and Fig. 2). We found decreased SUV over time in reference tissue (healthy liver) as expected and hence an increased tumour-to-background ratio for delayed imaging.

Table 2 Distribution of 337 malignant lesions in 41 recurrent breast cancer patients, according to recurrence status and lesion site. Lesion group 'other' consisted of subcutaneous and muscle metastases

Sites of recurrence	Number of patients	Number of lesions	Number of biopsies
Local recurrence	19	21	19
Distant recurrence	22	316	22
Cerebrum	1	1 (0.3%)	1
Lung	6	25 (7.4%)	1
Liver	4	7 (2.1%)	3
Breast	23	27 (8.0%)	21
Lymph node	13	54 (16.0%)	8
Bone	18	213 (63.2%)	7
Other	2	10 (3.0%)	5

Table 3 Standard uptake values (SUVmax, SUVmean, partial volume corrected SUVmean (cSUVmean) and MTV of malignant lesions at 1h and 3h (mean ± SD, min and max), and the change over time (ΔSUV with 95% CI) by patient recurrence status. **Δ**SUV% and ΔMTV% were calculated by using mean values of 1h and 3h groups. *P*-values refer to the hypothesis test that the mean difference of the paired observations at 1h and 3h is equal to 0

	1h	3h	ΔSUV (3h-1h)	p-value	ΔSUV%
All 41 patients with recurrence (337 lesions)					
SUVmax	6.4 ± 3.4 [0.9-19.7]	8.1 ± 4.4 [0.7-29.7]	1.8 [1.5 to 2.1]	< 0.0001	28
SUVmean	4.0 ± 2.0 [0.5-11.3]	5.1 ± 2.6 [0.4-16.5]	1.1 [1.0 to 1.3]	< 0.0001	28
cSUVmean	6.5 ± 3.5 [0.7-20.8]	8.8 ± 4.7 [0.5-30.9]	2.3 [1.9 to 2.6]	< 0.0001	35
MTV (cc)	12.5 ± 42.4 [0.3-562]	10.4 ± 39.9 [0.2-565.5]	−2.1 [− 3.1 to − 1.0]	< 0.0001	− 17
19 patients with local recurrence (21 lesions)					
SUVmax	3.0 ± 1.9 [0.9-8.7]	3.8 ± 3.0 [0.7-12.3]	0.8 [0.2 to 1.4]	0.006	27
SUVmean	1.9 ± 1.3 [0.5-5.9]	2.4 ± 2.0 [0.4-8.6]	0.5 [0.08 to 0.9]	0.022	25
cSUVmean	3.2 ± 2.4 [0.7-8.9]	4.4 ± 3.9 [0.5-14.4]	1.2 [0.3 to 2.1]	0.014	36
MTV (cc)	8.4 ± 10.3 [0.3-33.3]	5.7 ± 5.5 [0.2-22.3]	−2.8 [−6.2 to 0.7]	0.11	−33
22 patients with distant recurrence (316 lesions)					
SUVmax	6.6 ± 3.3 [1.2-19.7]	8.4 ± 4.4 [1.2-29.7]	1.8 [1.5 to 2.2]	< 0.0001	28
SUVmean	4.1 ± 2.0 [0.8-11.3]	5.3 ± 2.6 [0.6-16.5]	1.2 [1.0 to 1.4]	< 0.0001	28
cSUVmean	6.7 ± 3.5 [0.8-20.8]	9.1 ± 4.6 [0.8-30.9]	2.3 [2.0 to 2.7]	< 0.0001	35
MTV (cc)	12.8 ± 43.7 [0.4-562.0]	10.7 ± 41.1 [0.2-565.5]	−2.1 [−3.2 to −0.9]	0.001	−16

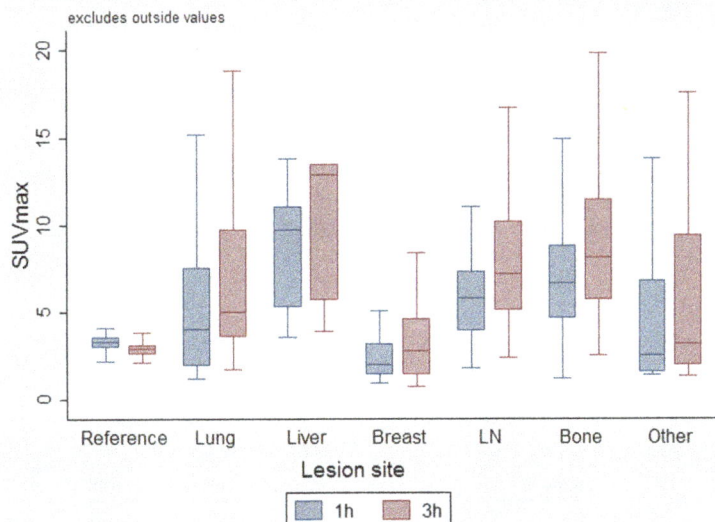

Fig. 1 Boxplots of SUVmax, at 1h and 3h imaging time-point, for the 337 malignant lesions according to the different subgroups and reference tissue (healthy liver) in 41 patients with recurrent breast cancer. Due to only one cerebral lesion, data are not shown for this group

Table 4 Difference between SUVmean and cSUVmean for 1h and 3h measurements for all lesions according to recurrent status and lesion subgroups (mean and 95% CI). Percentage difference was calculated by using mean values of cSUVmean and SUVmean groups for 1h and 3h. P-values refer to the hypothesis test that the mean difference of the paired observations at each time-point for SUVmean and cSUVmean is equal to 0

Group	Difference 1h (cSUVmean-SUVmean)	p-value	% diff	Difference 3h (cSUVmean-SUVmean)	p-value	% diff
All lesions (337 lesions)	2.51 [2.14 – 2.88]	< 0.0001	63	3.64 [3.22 – 4.06]	< 0.0001	71
Local recurrence (21 lesions)	1.32 [0.74 – 1.91]	< 0.0001	70	2.02 [1.07 - 2.98]	< 0.0001	84
Distant recurrence (316 lesions)	2.59 [2.21 - 2.98]	< 0.0001	63	3.75 [3.32 - 4.18]	< 0.0001	71
Lung (25 lesions)	1.88 [0.48 – 3.27]	0.018	60	3.09 [1.28 - 4.91]	0.007	68
Liver (7 lesions)	2.17 [−0.80 – 5.14]	0.103	39	2.67 [0.91 - 4.44]	0.017	41
Breast (27 lesions)	1.09 [0.59 - 1.60]	< 0.0001	63	1.86 [1.06 - 2.66]	< 0.0001	87
Lymph node (54 lesions)	2.77 [1.62 - 3.92]	< 0.0001	69	4.49 [3.16 - 5.82]	< 0.0001	82
Bone (213 lesions)	2.73 [2.43 - 2.92]	< 0.0001	63	3.80 [3.45 - 4.14]	< 0.0001	69
Other (10 lesions)	2.32 [−21.82 – 26.46]	0.437	78	2.73 [−21.54 – 27.00]	0.389	73

Although our study, in line with previous literature, demonstrated an increased tumour-to-background ratio in delayed images, the diagnostic accuracy at patient level did not improve in our overall prospective accuracy study [33]. The clinical usefulness of delayed imaging in this category of patients may thus be limited. Furthermore, it is our experience that DTPI caused planning challenges in daily workflow and patient discomfort due to a longer fasting period.

Change in SUV from early to late time-point imaging
Patients with local recurrence had in general lower SUV-max and SUVmean measurements compared to the group with distant recurrence at both time-points. This

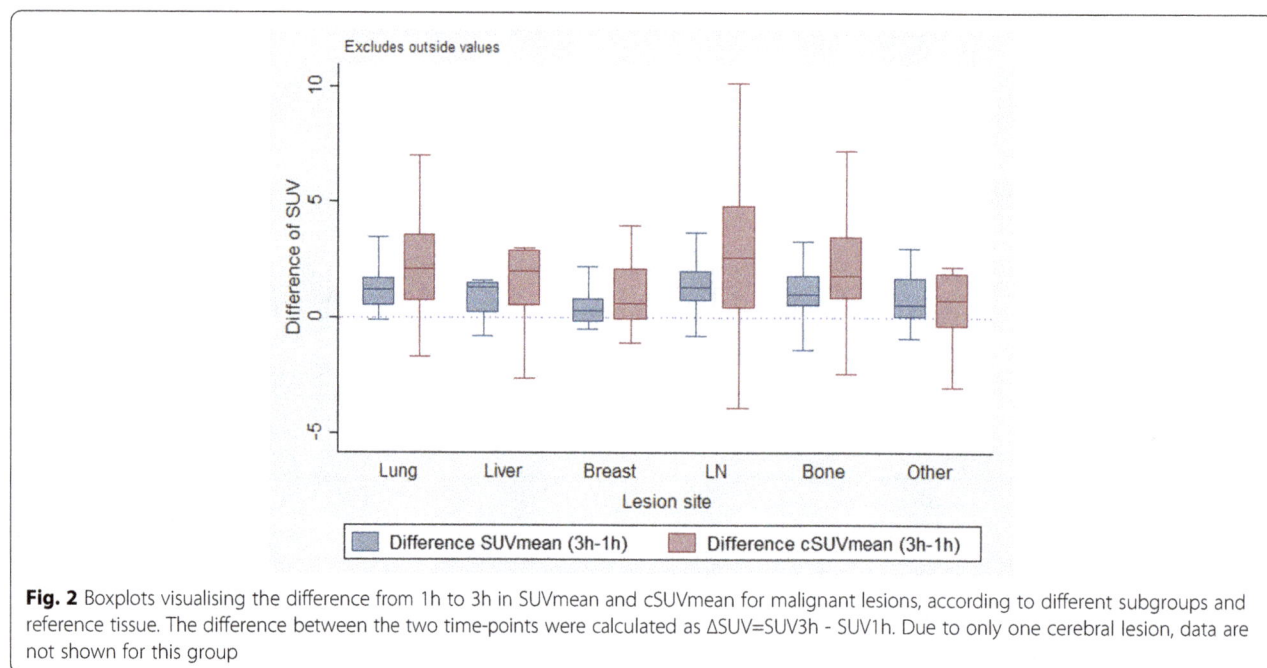

Fig. 2 Boxplots visualising the difference from 1h to 3h in SUVmean and cSUVmean for malignant lesions, according to different subgroups and reference tissue. The difference between the two time-points were calculated as ΔSUV=SUV3h - SUV1h. Due to only one cerebral lesion, data are not shown for this group

could partly be due to the finding that 8 of the 21 lesions (38%) in the group with local recurrence showed decreased SUV from 1h to 3h compared to only 10% in patients with distant recurrence. Suga et al. reported similar results from 52 patients with suspected local recurrence of breast cancer, where SUVmax increased in 84% of the lesions and decreased in 16% of the lesions between 1h and 2h scans, while overall SUVmax increased by 18% [35]. The higher increase in SUVmax in our study could be due to the later imaging point at 3h. Several studies have performed delayed or dual-time imaging in breast cancer but have only shown a small improvement in detecting local recurrence, despite an increased tumour-to-background ratio [11, 12, 36, 37].

Distant metastases in lung, lymph node, liver and bone all increased in SUVmax, SUVmean, and cSUVmean from 1h to 3h, and especially for lymph node metastases. These findings are supported by the literature, where several publications have stated the increased FDG accumulation over time in different malignant lesions [7, 16, 17, 35].

In our study, we used healthy liver tissue for reference measurement, which has previously been demonstrated useful by Chirindel et al. [38]. For bone metastases, we found a significant increase for SUVmax, SUVmean, and cSUVmean between 1h and 3h. These findings are supported by a study of bone metastases in breast cancer patients from Tian et al. [39]. Other diagnostic studies of bone metastases and FDG-PET/CT have found that FDG has a high sensitivity for detecting osteolytic and mixed bone lesions compared to osteoblastic lesions, which can be false-negative due to low metabolic activity [40, 41].

SUV can be influenced by a range of physiological and technical parameters, which should be taken in consideration by quantitative image analysis, to minimize bias [42–44]. SUVmax demonstrates a high inter-observer reproducibility and is often used as a semi-quantitative measure of FDG-uptake. However, SUVmax is more sensitive to image noise, and has been shown to have a lower inter-study repeatability than SUVmean [45, 46]. While SUVmean may be a more reliable measure in heterogeneous tumours, it can be observer-dependent due to lesion delineation dependency with variability in mask placement and sensitivity to PVE, especially in smaller lesions [26, 27, 47].

Impact of PVC performed with ROVER software
PVC of SUVmean had as expected a significant impact in our study, in both the overall lesion group and the various subgroups. However, PVC increased the standard deviation of cSUVmean compared to uncorrected SUVmean, probably due to incorrect lesion delineation caused by segmentation challenges (Fig. 2). The highest impact of PVC was seen for breast lesions which also

had the smallest MTV according to ROVER. Our results agree with the literature, showing that partial volume effects influence measured uptake in all lesions, especially those smaller or of a size close to the limited spatial resolution of the PET scanner, for which it causes a significant underestimation of lesion extent and activity level [26, 27, 47].

Several studies have demonstrated observer-related variability associated with manual delineation of ROI, which can be reduced by the use of automatic or semi-automatic contour drawing [48–50]. Prevalently employed automatic delineation methods employing different threshold and cut-offs, however, are also known to be suboptimal in many cases, leading to segmentation bias [20, 49]. We used ROVER software for PVC, which has previously been shown to be feasibly and clinically useful [31, 34]. ROVER software included background subtraction for each lesion, but despite this we discovered practical challenges due to non-uniformity of lesions and background activity. We experienced against expectation a decrease in MTV defined by ROVER from 1h to 3h, despite the general known tendency of increased FDG accumulation over time in malignant lesions. This issue was probably caused by crucial segmentation challenges associated with the semi-automatic lesion delineation. Thus, by visual inspection of the automatic lesion delineation in our study, the lesion ROI in the 1h image often included background voxels and thereby overestimated lesion size, compared to the same lesion in the 3h image, where the lesion delineation appeared more well-defined (Fig. 3). This indicates that the threshold-based segmentation in ROVER led to overestimated volumes of small lesions, particularly in the early scan, where the lesion-to-background ratio was low, and through that an underestimation of SUVmean. We used a fixed 40% threshold setting to semi-automatically delineate lesions. This approach was based on the current use in the literature and similar to the threshold of 41% recommended by updated European guidelines [48, 51]. A more systematic search of other threshold levels or rather alternative segmentation methods that can provide more accurate lesion delineation could be beneficial [32, 42, 49], but lies outside the scope of this article.

Strengths and limitations of the study
The main strengths of our study are its prospective design and clinically representative patient group with newly diagnosed recurrence – verified by biopsy in all patients – and, hence, yet untreated metastases. The scanning protocol consisted of whole-body scans at both 1h and 3h allowing us to compare SUV measurements over time in all recurrent lesions. A major limitation was that histological proof was not available for all lesions due to ethical and practical reasons, and therefore a composite reference

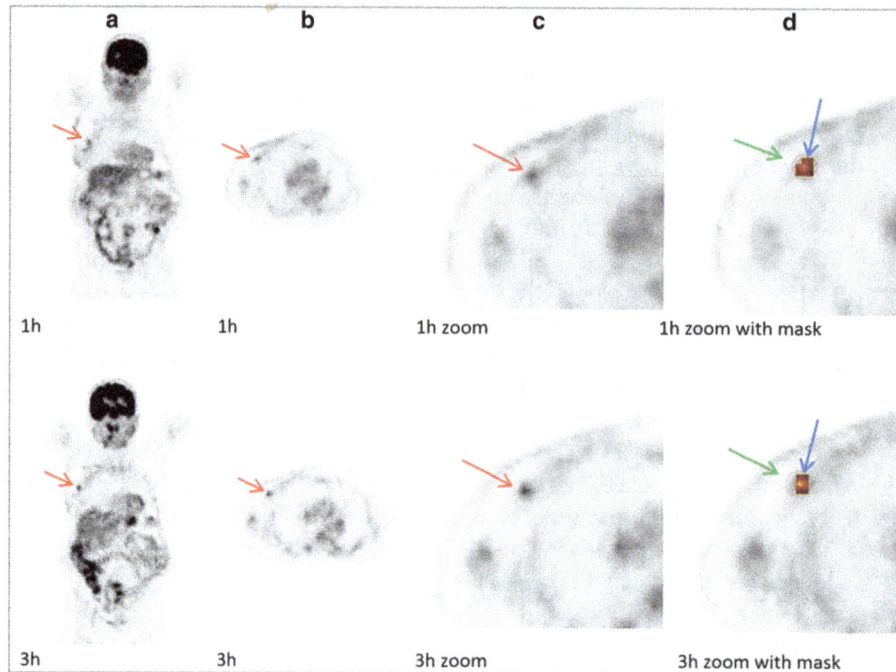

Fig. 3 FDG-PET/CT images of a 73 years old woman with local recurrence in her right breast (red arrow) displayed in ROVER. **a** Maximum intensity projection images 1 h (1h) and 3 h (3h) after injection, **b** Transaxial images of thorax at 1h and 3h, **c** Zoomed transaxial images of the left side of thorax at 1h and 3h, and **d** Zoomed transaxial images with masks at 1h and 3h, where the green arrow shows the user defined 3D mask (equal mask size at 1h and 3h images), and the blue arrow shows the lesion ROI delineated by the ROVER software, which yielded the following values after 1h and 3h, respectively: MTV (cc) 3.8 and 2.1; SUVmax 3.2 and 3.7; SUVmean 1.8 and 2.6; cSUVmean 2.3 and 5.1

standard was the best option. Another limitation was the observed suboptimal segmentation with a fixed 40% of maximum value threshold. Segmentation methods using separate masks for 1h and 3h images in each patient were associated with challenges such as spatial mismatch between 1h and 3h acquisitions. This could contribute to segmentation variability and potentially incorrect comparison of quantitative results from the two time-points. Being the outcome of a single institution study, the generalizability of our results is uncertain.

The overall intention with this study was to consider whether a 3h scan should replace the 1h standard imaging in patients with metastatic breast cancer. Although we found an increased tumour-to-background ratio in 3h compared to 1h scans, this was not associated with improved diagnostic accuracy on a per-patient level as shown in our previous publication [33]. Furthermore, 3h protocols cause challenges regarding planning, patient discomfort and healthcare costs. Based on these experiences, it may not be justified to replace the standard 1h by a delayed imaging protocol.

Conclusion

SUVs of FDG increased significantly from 1h to 3h in malignant lesions of recurrent breast cancer and in all

types of lesions, while reference measurements in healthy liver tissue decreased. PVC increased these values significantly as expected, especially in breast metastases. However, the demonstrated modest quantitative advances of 3h imaging can hardly justify delayed PET imaging on a routine basis in this patient group.

Abbreviations

1h: 1 h; 3h: 3 h; BMI: Body mass index; CI: Confidence interval; cSUVmean: Partial volume corrected SUVmean; CT: Computed tomography; DTPI: Delayed time-point imaging; FDG-PET/CT: ^{18}F-fluoro-deoxy-glucose positron emission tomography/computed tomography G6PaseGlucose-6-phosphatase; MBq: Mega Becquerel; MRI: Magnetic resonance imaging; MTV: Metabolic active tumour volume; OSEM: Ordered subset expectation maximization; PVC: Partial volume correction; PVE: Partial volume effect; ROI: Region-of-interest; SD: Standard deviation; SUV: Standard uptake values; SUVmax: Maximum standard uptake value; SUVmean: Mean standard uptake value

Acknowledgements

The authors would like to express their gratitude towards two reviewers whose comments significantly improved former versions of the manuscript. Moreover, the authors acknowledge the support of the staff at the Department of Nuclear Medicine, Odense University Hospital, Denmark. Special thanks to the PET/CT technologists for technical assistance with the imaging studies and to Birgitte B. Olsen for ongoing constructive feedback on the project.

Funding

The project was implemented without the involvement of private organizations or companies.

Authors' contributions

CB, MGH, KF AA and PFC conceptualised and designed the study CB and MGH acquired and analysed data and drafted the manuscript. KF acquired and analysed data. JH and OG analysed and interpreted data. PFHC, AA, OG and TQN enhanced the intellectual content of and reviewed the manuscript. All authors have read and approved the final version of the manuscript.

Competing interests

The authors declare that they have no competing interests.

Author details

[1]Department of Nuclear Medicine, University Hospital, Sdr. Boulevard 29, 5000 Odense C, Denmark. [2]Centre of Health Economics Research, University of Southern Denmark, Odense, Denmark. [3]University of Pennsylvania, Philadelphia, USA.

References

1. Jemal A, Bray F, Center MM, Ferlay J, Ward E, Forman D. Global cancer statistics. CA Cancer J Clin. 2011;61(2):69–90.
2. International Agency for Research on Cancer, Globocan 2012. http://globocan.iarc.fr/Pages/fact_sheets_cancer.aspx. Accessed 11 May 2016.
3. Groheux D, Espie M, Giacchetti S, Hindie E. Performance of FDG PET/CT in the clinical management of breast cancer. Radiology. 2013;266(2):388–405.
4. Pennant M, Takwoingi Y, Pennant L, Davenport C, Fry-Smith A, Eisinga A, Andronis L, Arvanitis T, Deeks J, Hyde C. A systematic review of positron emission tomography (PET) and positron emission tomography/computed tomography (PET/CT) for the diagnosis of breast cancer recurrence. Health Technol Asses. 2010;14(50):1–103.
5. Eubank WB, Mankoff DA, Vesselle HJ, Eary JF, Schubert EK, Dunnwald LK, Lindsley SK, Gralow JR, Austin-Seymour MM, Ellis GK, et al. Detection of locoregional and distant recurrences in breast cancer patients by using FDG PET. Radiographics. 2002;22(1):5–17.
6. Cheng G, Torigian DA, Zhuang H, Alavi A. When should we recommend use of dual time-point and delayed time-point imaging techniques in FDG PET? Eur J Nucl Med Mol I. 2013;40(5):779–87.
7. Matthies A, Hickeson M, Cuchiara A, Alavi A. Dual time point 18F-FDG PET for the evaluation of pulmonary nodules. J Nucl Med. 2002;43(7):871–5.
8. Houshmand S, Salavati A, Segtnan EA, Grupe P, Hoilund-Carlsen PF, Alavi A. Dual-time-point imaging and delayed-time-point Fluorodeoxyglucose-PET/computed tomography imaging in various clinical settings. PET Clin. 2016;11(1):65–84.
9. Cheng G, Alavi A, Lim E, Werner TJ, Del Bello CV, Akers SR. Dynamic changes of FDG uptake and clearance in normal tissues. Mol Imaging Biol. 2013;15(3):345–52.
10. Gillies RJ, Robey I, Gatenby RA. Causes and consequences of increased glucose metabolism of cancers. J Nucl Med. 2008;49(Suppl 2):24s–42s.
11. Boerner AR, Weckesser M, Herzog H, Schmitz T, Audretsch W, Nitz U, Bender HG, Mueller-Gaertner HW. Optimal scan time for fluorine-18 fluorodeoxyglucose positron emission tomography in breast cancer. Eur J Nucl Med. 1999;26(3):226–30.
12. Kumar R, Loving VA, Chauhan A, Zhuang H, Mitchell S, Alavi A. Potential of dual-time-point imaging to improve breast cancer diagnosis with (18)F-FDG PET. J Nucl Med. 2005;46(11):1819–24.
13. Mavi A, Urhan M, Yu JQ, Zhuang H, Houseni M, Cermik TF, Thiruvenkatasamy D, Czerniecki B, Schnall M, Alavi A. Dual time point 18F-FDG PET imaging detects breast cancer with high sensitivity and correlates well with histologic subtypes. J Nucl Med. 2006;47(9):1440–6.
14. Beaulieu S, Kinahan P, Tseng J, Dunnwald LK, Schubert EK, Pham P, Lewellen B, Mankoff DA. SUV varies with time after injection in (18)F-FDG PET of breast cancer: characterization and method to adjust for time differences. J Nucl Med. 2003;44(7):1044–50.
15. Basu S, Mavi A, Cermik T, Houseni M, Alavi A. Implications of standardized uptake value measurements of the primary lesions in proven cases of breast carcinoma with different degree of disease burden at diagnosis: does 2-deoxy-2-[F-18]fluoro-D-glucose-positron emission tomography predict tumor biology? Mol Imaging Biol. 2008;10(1):62–6.
16. Chan WL, Ramsay SC, Szeto ER, Freund J, Pohlen JM, Tarlinton LC, Young A, Hickey A, Dura R. Dual-time-point (18)F-FDG-PET/CT imaging in the assessment of suspected malignancy. J Med Imag Radiat On. 2011;55(4):379–90.
17. Lee JW, Kim SK, Lee SM, Moon SH, Kim TS. Detection of hepatic metastases using dual-time-point FDG PET/CT scans in patients with colorectal cancer. Mol Imaging Biol. 2011;13(3):565–72.
18. Basu S, Alavi A. Partial volume correction of standardized uptake values and the dual time point in FDG-PET imaging: should these be routinely employed in assessing patients with cancer? Eur J Nucl Med Mol I. 2007;34(10):1527–9.
19. Kadoya T, Aogi K, Kiyoto S, Masumoto N, Sugawara Y, Okada M. Role of maximum standardized uptake value in fluorodeoxyglucose positron emission tomography/computed tomography predicts malignancy grade and prognosis of operable breast cancer: a multi-institute study. Breast Cancer Res Tr. 2013;141(2):269–75.
20. Vriens D, Visser EP, de Geus-Oei LF, Oyen WJ. Methodological considerations in quantification of oncological FDG PET studies. Eur J Nucl Med Mol I. 2010;37(7):1408–25.
21. Gamez-Cenzano C, Pino-Sorroche F. Standardization and quantification in FDG-PET/CT imaging for staging and restaging of malignant disease. PET Clin. 2014;9(2):117–27.
22. Basu S, Zaidi H, Houseni M, Bural G, Udupa J, Acton P, Torigian DA, Alavi A. Novel quantitative techniques for assessing regional and global function and structure based on modern imaging modalities: implications for normal variation, aging and diseased states. Semin Nucl Med. 2007;37(3):223–39.
23. Groheux D, Giacchetti S, Moretti JL, Porcher R, Espie M, Lehmann-Che J, de Roquancourt A, Hamy AS, Cuvier C, Vercellino L, et al. Correlation of high 18F-FDG uptake to clinical, pathological and biological prognostic factors in breast cancer. Eur J Nucl Med Mol I. 2011;38(3):426–35.
24. Morris PG, Ulaner GA, Eaton A, Fazio M, Jhaveri K, Patil S, Evangelista L, Park JY, Serna-Tamayo C, Howard J, et al. Standardized uptake value by positron emission tomography/computed tomography as a prognostic variable in metastatic breast cancer. Cancer. 2012;118(22):5454–62.
25. Garcia Vicente AM, Soriano Castrejon A, Leon Martin A, Chacon Lopez-Muniz I, Munoz Madero V. Munoz Sanchez Mdel M, Palomar Munoz a, Espinosa Aunion R, Gonzalez Ageitos a: molecular subtypes of breast cancer: metabolic correlation with (1)(8)F-FDG PET/CT. Eur J Nucl Med Mol I. 2013;40(9):1304–11.
26. Soret M, Bacharach SL, Buvat I. Partial-volume effect in PET tumor imaging. J Nucl Med. 2007;48(6):932–45.
27. Hoetjes NJ, van Velden FH, Hoekstra OS, Hoekstra CJ, Krak NC, Lammertsma AA, Boellaard R. Partial volume correction strategies for quantitative FDG PET in oncology. Eur J Nucl Med Mol I. 2010;37(9):1679–87.
28. Gallivanone F, Canevari C, Sassi I, Zuber V, Marassi A, Gianolli L, Picchio M, Messa C, Gilardi MC, Castiglioni I. Partial volume corrected 18F-FDG PET mean standardized uptake value correlates with prognostic factors in breast cancer. Q J Nucl Med. 2014;58(4):424–39.
29. Aston JA, Cunningham VJ, Asselin MC, Hammers A, Evans AC, Gunn RN. Positron emission tomography partial volume correction: estimation and algorithms. J Cerebr Blood F Met. 2002;22(8):1019–34.
30. Boussion N, Hatt M, Lamare F, Bizais Y, Turzo A, Cheze-Le Rest C, Visvikis D. A multiresolution image based approach for correction of partial volume effects in emission tomography. Phys Med Biol. 2006; 51(7):1857–76.
31. Torigian DA, Lopez RF, Alapati S, Bodapati G, Hofheinz F, van den Hoff J, Saboury B, Alavi A. Feasibility and performance of novel software to quantify metabolically active volumes and 3D partial volume corrected SUV and metabolic volumetric products of spinal bone marrow metastases on 18F-FDG-PET/CT. Hell J Nuc Med. 2011;14(1):8–14.
32. Hofheinz F, Langner J, Petr J, Beuthien-Baumann B, Oehme L, Steinbach J, Kotzerke J, van den Hoff J. A method for model-free partial volume correction in oncological PET. Eur J Nucl Med Mol I Research. 2012;2(1):16.
33. Hildebrandt MG, Gerke O, Baun C, Falch K, Hansen JA, Farahani ZA, Petersen H, Larsen LB, Duvnjak S, Buskevica I, et al. [18F]Fluorodeoxyglucose-positron emission tomography (PET)/computed tomography (CT) in suspected recurrent breast Cancer: a prospective comparative study of dual-time-point FDG-PET/CT, contrast-enhanced CT, and bone scintigraphy. J Clin Oncol. 2016;34:1889–97.
34. Hofheinz F, Potzsch C, Oehme L, Beuthien-Baumann B, Steinbach J, Kotzerke J, van den Hoff J. Automatic volume delineation in oncological PET. Evaluation of a dedicated software tool and comparison with manual delineation in clinical data sets. Nuklearmedizin. 2012;51(1):9–16.
35. Suga K, Kawakami Y, Hiyama A, Matsunaga N. Differentiation of FDG-avid loco-regional recurrent and compromised benign lesions after surgery for breast cancer with dual-time point F-18-fluorodeoxy-glucose PET/CT scan. Ann Nucl Med. 2009;23(4):399–407.

36. Caprio MG, Cangiano A, Imbriaco M, Soscia F, Di Martino G, Farina A, Avitabile G, Pace L, Forestieri P, Salvatore M. Dual-time-point [18F]-FDG PET/CT in the diagnostic evaluation of suspicious breast lesions. Radiol Med. 2010;115:215–24.
37. Choi WH, Yoo IR, JH O, Kim SH, Chung SK. The value of dual-time-point 18F-FDG PET/CT for identifying axillary lymph node metastasis in breast cancer patients. Brit J Rad. 2011;84(1003):593–9.
38. Chirindel A, Alluri KC, Tahari AK, Chaudhry M, Wahl RL, Lodge MA, Subramaniam RM. Liver standardized uptake value corrected for lean body mass at FDG PET/CT: effect of FDG uptake time. Clin Nucl Med. 2015;40(1):e17–22.
39. Tian R, Su M, Tian Y, Li F, Li L, Kuang A, Zeng J. Dual-time point PET/CT with F-18 FDG for the differentiation of malignant and benign bone lesions. Skelet Radiol. 2009;38(5):451–8.
40. Hamaoka T, Madewell JE, Podoloff DA, Hortobagyi GN, Ueno NT. Bone imaging in metastatic breast cancer. J Clin Oncol. 2004;22(14):2942–53.
41. Cook GJ, Houston S, Rubens R, Maisey MN, Fogelman I. Detection of bone metastases in breast cancer by 18FDG PET: differing metabolic activity in osteoblastic and osteolytic lesions. J Clin Oncol. 1998;16(10):3375–9.
42. Boellaard R, Krak NC, Hoekstra OS, Lammertsma AA. Effects of noise, image resolution, and ROI definition on the accuracy of standard uptake values: a simulation study. J Nucl Med. 2004;45(9):1519–27.
43. Huang SC. Anatomy of SUV. Standardized uptake value. Nucl Med Biol. 2000;27(7):643–6.
44. Keyes JW Jr. SUV: standard uptake or silly useless value? J Nucl Med. 1995; 36(10):1836–9.
45. Krak NC, Boellaard R, Hoekstra OS, Twisk JW, Hoekstra CJ, Lammertsma AA. Effects of ROI definition and reconstruction method on quantitative outcome and applicability in a response monitoring trial. Eur J Nucl Med Mol I. 2005;32(3):294–301.
46. Nahmias C, Wahl LM. Reproducibility of standardized uptake value measurements determined by 18F-FDG PET in malignant tumors. J Nucl Med. 2008;49(11):1804–8.
47. Bai B, Bading J, Conti PS. Tumor quantification in clinical positron emission tomography. Theranostics. 2013;3(10):787–801.
48. Boellaard R. Standards for PET image acquisition and quantitative data analysis. J Nucl Med. 2009;50(Suppl 1):11s–20s.
49. Tomasi G, Turkheimer F, Aboagye E. Importance of quantification for the analysis of PET data in oncology: review of current methods and trends for the future. Mol Imaging Biol. 2012;14(2):131–46.
50. Houshmand S, Salavati A, Hess S, Werner TJ, Alavi A, Zaidi H. An update on novel quantitative techniques in the context of evolving whole-body PET imaging. PET Clin. 2015;10(1):45–58.
51. Boellaard R, Delgado-Bolton R, Oyen WJ, Giammarile F, Tatsch K, Eschner W, Verzijlbergen FJ, Barrington SF, Pike LC, Weber WA, et al. FDG PET/CT: EANM procedure guidelines for tumour imaging: version 2.0. Eur J Nucl Med Mol I. 2015;42(2):328–54.

22

Evaluation of left atrial volume and function using single-beat real-time three-dimensional echocardiography in atrial fibrillation patients

Qian Zhang, Ju-fang Wang, Qing-qing Dong, Qing Yan, Xiang-hong Luo, Xue-ying Wu, Jian Liu and Ya-ping Sun[*]

Abstract

Background: This study was aimed to evaluate the feasibility and accuracy of real-time three-dimensional echocardiography (RT-3DE) measurement of left atrial (LA) volume and function in comparison with two-dimensional echocardiography (2DE) measurements in atrial fibrillation (AF) patients.

Methods: A total of 50 pairs of AF patients and healthy controls were enrolled in this study. Indexed LA end-diastole volume (ILAEDV) and indexed LA end-systolic volume (ILAESV), as well as LA function indices such as segmental LA ejection fraction (LAEF), were assessed using 2DE Simpson's method and the RT-3DE method.

Results: The images showed that regional LA volume–time curves and LAEF were disordered in AF patients. ILAEDV and ILAESV were markedly increased and global LAEF was significantly decreased in AF patients compared with those in healthy controls ($P < 0.01$). No significant differences were found in ILAEDV, ILAESV, and LAEF levels as determined by the RT-3DE method or 2DE Simpson's method. Bland–Altman analysis showed that the two methods agreed well for measuring ILAEDV, ILAESV, and segmental LAEF.

Conclusion: The RT-3DE method may be a feasible and accurate method for evaluating LA volume and function of AF patients in clinical practice.

Keywords: Real-time three-dimensional echocardiography, Atrial fibrillation, Left atrial volume, Left atrial function

Background

Atrial fibrillation (AF) is one of the most common sustained cardiac arrhythmias and is associated with increased morbidity and mortality, with its incidence ranging from 2.73% in 1993 to 2.83% in 2007 [1, 2]. There is strong evidence that left atrial (LA) volume and ejection fraction (EF) are important factors that influence AF development [3, 4]. Previous studies indicated that measuring LA volume is valuable for predicting AF recurrence [5, 6]. Segmental EF is a more sensitive index of segmental LV function than global EF in AF patients [7].

Two-dimensional echocardiography (2DE) using Simpson's method has been widely used for assessing LA

volume and segmental LAEF in previous studies [8, 9]. However, this method not only requires the acquisition of a series of contiguous images that cover the entire LA but also requires manual tracking, making it time consuming. Moreover, geometric assumptions that have a risk for underestimating volumes are required for the 2DE method [10, 11]. Three-dimensional echocardiography (3DE) is a recently developed technology that has an advantage in overcoming the geometric limitations of 2DE [12]. The single-beat real-time 3DE (RT-3DE) method has been widely used to produce integrated, instantaneous, and large volumes at high volume rates of 3D cardiac images in a single cardiac cycle and to automatically measure the LA volume [13]. RT-3DE may be feasible for clinical application, superior to 2DE for patients with severe mitral regurgitation [14] and aortic regurgitation [15]. However, few studies have focused on

* Correspondence: sunyanhsh@hotmail.com
Department of Echocardiography, Shanghai General Hospital, Shanghai Jiao Tong University School of Medicine, No.100 Hai Ning Road, Shanghai 200080, China

the clinical use of RT-3DE for detecting the LA volume and EF, compared with 2DE.

In this study, segmental LAEF and LA volume in AF patients and healthy controls were measured using the single-beat RT-3DE method and 2DE Simpson's method. The study assessed the accuracy and feasibility of RT-3DE measurements of LA volume and function compared with standard 2DE measurements in AF patients.

Methods

Subjects

Between June and September 2014, a total of 50 consecutive AF patients who visited the hospital for radiofrequency ablation were enrolled. AF was diagnosed by combined conventional electrocardiography (ECG) and dynamic electrocardiography (DCG). The conventional 12-lead ECG was used for recording the rate and rhythm of heartbeats in the patients in a resting condition, and DCG monitored the electrical activity in the states of resting, activity, working, studying and sleeping for consecutive 24 h. If AF could not be confirmed by ECG, patients were subjected to DCG monitor from 9 o'clock to 9 o'clock on the next day. Patients with other cardiovascular diseases, metabolic disorders, anemia, liver and renal failures, and lung diseases that could affect cardiac morphology and function were excluded. A total of 50 age- and sex-matched healthy volunteers who underwent a routine physical examination at our hospital were included as the control group.

2DE Simpson's measurement

Participants were placed in the left lateral position and connected to an electrocardiogram monitor. The apical four-chamber view was obtained using a 4V1c transducer (1–4 MHz). The frame rate was 51 ± 5 frames/s. Segmental LAEF, LA end-diastolic volume (LAEDV), and LA end-systolic volume (LAESV) were measured using a Simpson's method from the apical four-chamber view [16, 17]. The measurement was performed using an echocardiographic system (Siemens Acuson SC2000 diasonograph, Siemens Medical Solutions USA). LAEDV and LAESV were adjusted for body surface area (BSA) and were defined as indexed LA end-diastolic volume (ILAEDV) and indexed LA end-systolic volume (ILAESV).

RT-3DE measurement

To conduct the apical four-chamber view, the 4Z1c probe (1–4 MHz) was used to collect LA images during a breath-hold over 5 s. The detectable depth was 16 cm, and the 3D pyramid scanning was $90° \times 90°$ with temporal resolution of ≥ 40 frames/s. Meanwhile, the plane images of the apical four-chamber, three-chamber, and short-axis views were synchronously displayed (Additional file 1: Fig. S1). The full image for LA volume (Additional file 2: Fig.

S2) was analyzed by manual tracking of LAED and LAES endocardium (Additional file 3: Fig. S3). Data of segmental LAEF, LAEDV, and LAESV were obtained. LAEDV and LAESV were corrected for BSA and recorded as ILAEDV and ILAESV. Regional LA volume–time curves and segmental LAEF were constructed using segmental values representing a whole cardiac cycle.

Interobserver variability

All the above analyses were performed by an experienced physician who was blinded to the group assignment and subjects' clinical status. To determine the interobserver variability, all measurements were repeated by a second physician blinded to the values obtained by the first physician, after an average of 1 week. The 2DE Simpson's measurement and RT-3DE measurement were completed within 2 h of each other in one patient. Patients and healthy controls were evaluated in the same examination room. AF patients were examined and evaluated before radiofrequency ablation.

Statistical analysis

All data are presented as mean $\pm$ standard deviation (SD). Paired t test was used to compare continuous variables between the control and case groups. Bland–Altman analysis was used to assess the agreement between 2DE Simpson's measurement and RT-3DE measurement. The agreement between the two methods (2DE Simpson's and RT-3DE) was expressed as 95% limits of agreement, as recommended by Bland and Altman [18]. All analyses were performed using the Stata software (version 11.2; StataCorp, TX, USA). P values of <0.05 were considered to be significant.

Results

Characteristics of the subjects

There were 29 male and 21 female subjects in the control group (mean age, 60.36 ± 1.30 years) and 32 males and 18 females in the case group (mean age, 60.06 ± 1.12 years). BSA was 1.61 ± 0.016 m^2 and 1.63 ± 0.017 m^2 for the control and case groups, respectively. No significant differences were observed with regard to age ($P = 0.22$), sex ($P = 0.54$), and BSA ($P = 0.11$) of the subjects in the two groups.

RT-3DE images of LA volume, volume variations, and segmental LAEF during a single heartbeat

Compared with healthy controls, BSA-adjusted LA volume was greater in age-, sex- and BSA-matched AF patients (Fig. 1). Regional LA volume–time curves (Fig. 2a) and segmental LAEF during the cardiac cycle (Fig. 3a) of the control group were orderly arranged; in contrast, the curves in the case group were unordered (Fig. 2b and Fig. 3b).

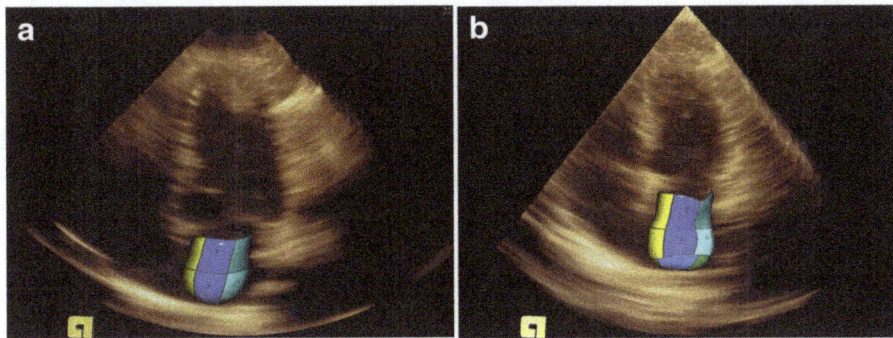

Fig. 1 Real-time three-dimensional echocardiography (RT-3DE) images of left atrial volume of healthy controls (**a**) and patient cases (**b**)

Comparison of LA volume and segmental LAEF between 2DE biplane Simpson's measurement and RT-3DE measurement

The RT-3DE measurement showed that ILAEDV and ILAESV levels were significantly increased in the case group compared with the control group, but LAEF levels significantly decreased (all $P < 0.01$) (Table 1).

Similarly, the results of 2DE Simpson's measurement showed that ILAEDV and ILAESV levels were markedly increased in the case group compared with the control group (all $P < 0.01$). Moreover, the case group had lower global LAEF than the control group ($P < 0.01$) (Table 1).

However, no significant differences were found in ILAEDV ($P = 0.57$ in control, $P = 0.066$ in case), ILAESV ($P = 0.84$ in control, $P = 0.93$ in case), and LAEF ($P = 0.062$ in control, $P = 0.17$ in case) levels between the RT-3DE measurement and 2DE Simpson's measurement.

Bias between 2DE Simpson's measurement and RT-3DE measurement of LA volume and segmental LAEF

The Bland–Altman plots (Fig. 4) showed a good agreement between 2DE biplane Simpson's measurement and RT-3DE measurement. The Bland–Altman plots graphically showed that the mean differences (between 0.02

and 0.04) were nearly 0 for all tests. No systematic differences in SD (between 0.03 and 0.56) and random error (95% limits of agreement) were found.

Discussion

There were no significant differences in LAEDV, LAESV, and segmental LAEF between the results of RT-3DE measurement and 2DE Simpson's measurement. Furthermore, the two methods agreed well for measuring segmental LAEF. The study results suggested that single-beat RT-3DE measurement is as accurate and feasible as 2DE Simpson's measurement of LA volume and function in AF patients.

Evidence has proved that 2DE Simpson's measurement is reliable for assessing LA volume and function [10]. The 2DE method requires the measurement of the apical four-chamber view and apical two-chamber view to evaluate LA volume and function, whereas the RT-3DE method only requires the measurement of the apical four-chamber view for the acquisition of related data. The 2DE Simpson's method is more complicated and could be more time consuming than the RT-3DE method. The single-beat RT-3DE method has overcome the drawbacks of 2DE in geometric assumption and offers 3D pyramid scanning of 90° × 90° and a 16-cm

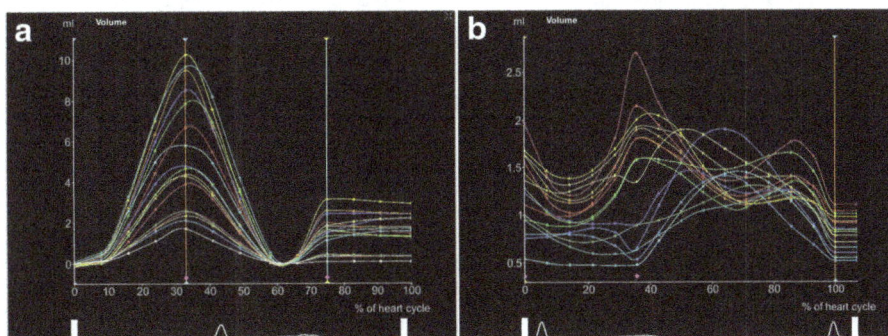

Fig. 2 The regional left ventricular volume–time curve of healthy controls (**a**) and patient cases (**b**) by real-time three-dimensional echocardiography (RT-3DE)

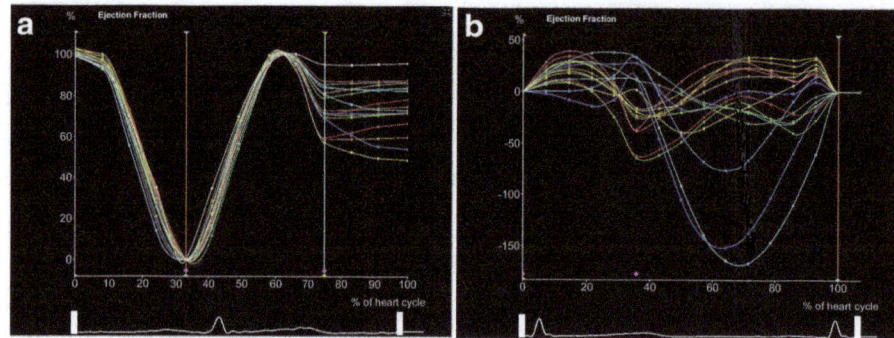

Fig. 3 Segmental ejection fraction (EF) (%) of healthy controls (**a**) and patient cases (**b**) by real-time three-dimensional echocardiography (RT-3DE)

depth, which covers the entire LA volume with acceptable image quality and eliminates the stitch artifact of previous RT-3DE [19]. The single-beat RT-3DE method can accurately and rapidly calculate the LA volume and function index and provide a visual observation of LA volume and function at each stage of every cardiac cycle. These superior features will be beneficial for AF patients with arrhythmia.

Previous studies have validated the feasibility of RT-3DE in clinical assessment. RT-3DE was used by Cong et al. to determine LA volume and function during normotensive and preeclamptic pregnancy [20]. Although Marsan et al. [21] measured LA volumes and segmental LAEF using RT-3DE in AF patients, LA volume variations in a cardiac cycle were not visually presented as images, and the comparison between new RT-3DE and conventional 2DE was not performed. Furthermore, there were no significant differences in ILAEDV, ILAESV, and segmental LAEF levels that were determined using the single-beat RT-3DE method and 2DE Simpson's method. Moreover, the two methods had good agreement for measuring segmental LAEF. Although the high correlation between LA volumes and LAEF using 2DE and RT-3DE may have been because of the single physician performing the measurements to some extent, these findings still suggested that the RT-3DE method was as feasible as the 2DE method for assessing LA volume and function.

In addition, LA volume and segmental LAEF are suggested to be robust markers of adverse cardiovascular events [22] and are found to reflect LA dysfunction [23, 24] and are associated with the risk for incident AF [4, 25, 26]. LA volume has a predictive role for congestive heart failure in AF patients [24]. In our study, regional LA volume–time curves of AF patients were discordant with those of healthy controls, and LA volume-related ILAEDV and ILAESV levels were remarkably increased. In addition, segmental LAEF was clearly reduced in AF patients compared with that in healthy controls. These results suggested LA dysfunction and unsynchronized LA volume enlargement in a cardiac cycle in AF patients, which were largely consistent with previous studies [27–29].

This study is limited by the fact that the population size is relatively small. In addition, LA function of AF patients was preliminarily evaluated without long-term follow-up data after radiofrequency ablation. Therefore, an investigation of a large number of AF patients with a long-term follow-up is required for confirming the results of this study. Moreover, the effects of 2DE and RT-3DE measurements were not compared with a gold standard such as magnetic

Table 1 Comparison of ILAEDV, ILAESV and segmental LAEF between two groups

Parameter	Method	Control	Case	P value
ILAEDV (ml)	Simpson's	12.60 ± 0.35 (0.20)	27.40 ± 1.50[a](0.39)	<0.01
	RT-3DE	12.56 ± 0.35 (0.20)	27.38 ± 1.51[a](0.39)	<0.01
ILAESV (ml)	Simpson's	8.40 ± 0.25 (0.21)	22.26 ± 1.17[a](0.37)	<0.01
	RT-3DE	8.41 ± 0.25 (0.21)	22.28 ± 1.17[a](0.37)	<0.01
Segmental LAEF (%)	Simpson's	46.94 ± 0.92 (0.14)	21.87 ± 1.20[a](0.40)	<0.01
	RT-3DE	47.49 ± 0.76 (0.11)	21.52 ± 1.30[a](0.43)	<0.01

Data were presented as mean ± standard error of mean (coefficient of variation). *ILAEDV* indexed left atrial end-diastolic volume, *ILAESV* indexed left atrial end-systolic volume, *LAEF* left atrial ejection fraction. [a], significant difference between the case group and control group

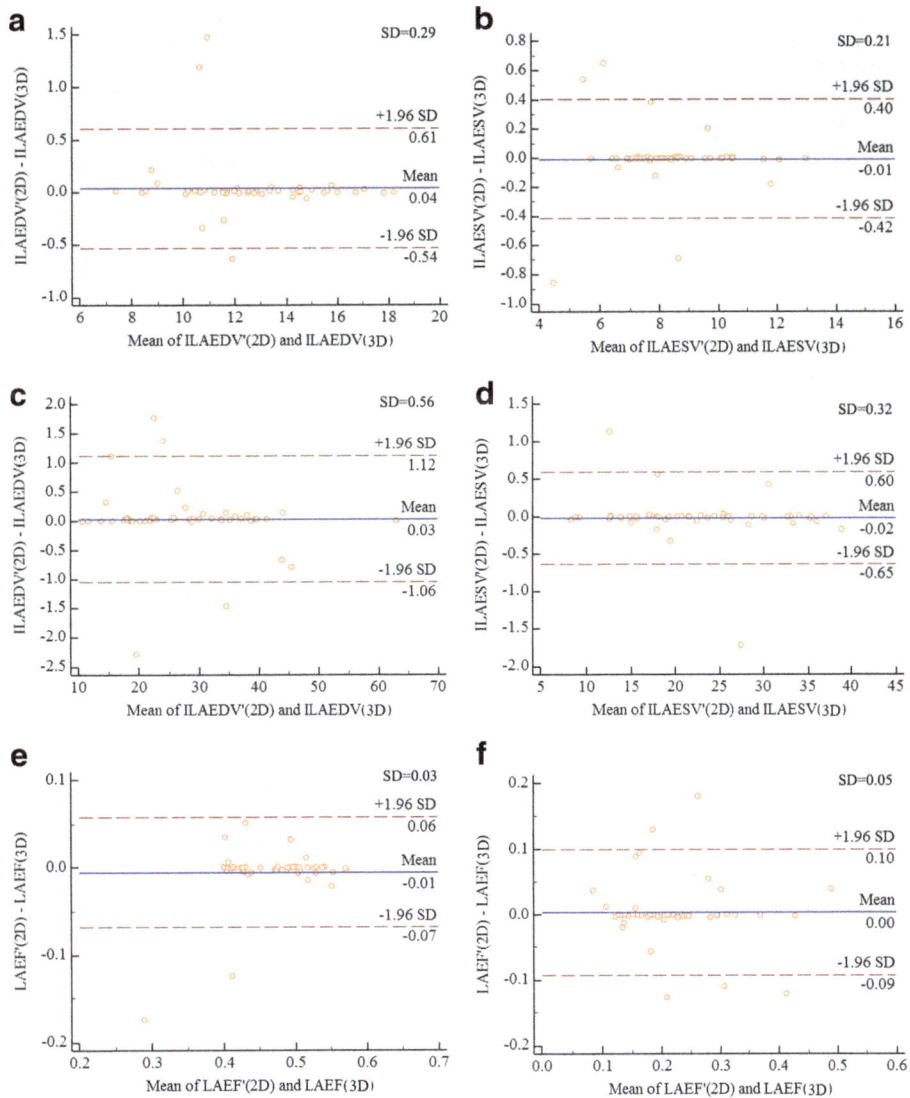

Fig. 4 a The correlation of 2DE and RT-3DE measurement of ILAEDV in control group; **b** the correlation of 2DE and RT-3DE measurement of ILAESV in control group; **c** the correlation of 2DE and RT-3DE measurement of ILAEDV in case group; **d** the correlation of 2DE and RT-3DE measurement of ILAESV in case group; **e** the correlation of 2DE and RT-3DE measurement of IAEF in control group; **f** the correlation of 2DE and RT-3DE measurement of IAEF in case group

resonance imaging; we will focus on this point in subsequent analyses and investigate the effect factors of image quality or heart size.

Conclusion

In conclusion, this study showed that semiautomated measurements by the single-beat RT-3DE method had low bias compared with the 2DE Simpson's method for assessing LA volume and function in AF patients. Compared with 2DE, RT-3DE had the advantage of displaying the 3D anatomy directly. With more experience, RT-3DE may be more acceptable and feasible in clinical practice for AF patients than conventional 2DE.

Abbreviations

2DE: Two-dimensional echocardiography; AF: Atrial fibrillation; BSA: Body surface area; DCG: Dynamic electrocardiography; ECG: Electrocardiography; EF: Ejection fraction; ILAEDV: Indexed LA end-diastole volume; ILAESV: Indexed LA end- systolic volume; LA: Left atrial; LAEF: LA ejection fraction; RT-3DE: real-time three-dimensional echocardiography; SD: Standard deviation

Acknowledgments

None.

Funding

None.

Authors' contributions

QZ, JFW, and QQD designed this study, and they all performed statistical analyses. XHL, XYW, and JL conducted the study and collected important background data. QY and YPS drafted the manuscript. All authors read and approved the final manuscript.

Competing interests

The authors declare that they have no competing interests.

References

1. Vidaillet H, Granada JF, Chyou P-H, Maassen K, Ortiz M, Pulido JN, Sharma P, Smith PN, Hayes J. A population-based study of mortality among patients with atrial fibrillation or flutter. Am J Med. 2002;113(5):365–70.
2. Piccini JP, Hammill BG, Sinner MF, Jensen PN, Hernandez AF, Heckbert SR, Benjamin EJ, Curtis LH. Incidence and prevalence of atrial fibrillation and associated mortality among Medicare beneficiaries: 1993–2007. Circulation. 2012;5(1):85–93.
3. Vaziri SM, Larson MG, Benjamin EJ, Levy D. Echocardiographic predictors of nonrheumatic atrial fibrillation. The Framingham heart study. Circulation. 1994;89(2):724–30.
4. Tsang TSM, Barnes ME, Bailey KR, Leibson CL, Montgomery SC, Takemoto Y, Diamond PM, Marra MA, Gersh BJ, Wiebers DO. Left atrial volume: important risk marker of incident atrial fibrillation in 1655 older men and women. Mayo Clin Proc. 2001;76(5):467–75.
5. Marchese P, Bursi F, Delle Donne G, Malavasi V, Casali E, Barbieri A, Melandri F, Modena M. Indexed left atrial volume predicts the recurrence of non-valvular atrial fibrillation after successful cardioversion. Eur Heart J Cardiovasc Imaging. 2011;12(3):214–21.
6. Procolo M, Vincenzo M, Luca R, Natalia N, Delle DG, Mirza B, Alessra C, Antonio L, Grazia MM. Indexed left Atrial volume is superior to left Atrial diameter in predicting Nonvalvular Atrial fibrillation recurrence after successful Cardioversion: a prospective study. Echocardiogr J Card. 2012; 29(3):276–284(279).
7. Llerena LR, Toruncha A, Llerena L, Pereiras R, Dopico A, Cruz-Hernández A, Hernández-Cañero A. Comparison of segmental and global ejection fraction in ischaemic heart disease. Cor Et Vasa. 1985;27(4):259–65.
8. Folland ED, Parisi AF, Moynihan PF, Jones DR, Feldman CL, Tow DE. Assessment of left ventricular ejection fraction and volumes by real-time, two-dimensional echocardiography. A comparison of cineangiographic and radionuclide techniques. Circulation. 1979;60(4):760–6.
9. Schiller NB, Shah PM, Crawford M, Demaria A, Devereux R, Feigenbaum H, Gutgesell H, Reichek N, Sahn D, Schnittger I. Recommendations for Quantitation of the left ventricle by two-dimensional echocardiography. J Am Soc Echocardiogr. 1989;2(5):358.
10. Bellenger N, Burgess M, Ray S, Lahiri A, Coats A, Cleland J, Pennell D. Comparison of left ventricular ejection fraction and volumes in heart failure by echocardiography, radionuclide ventriculography and cardiovascular magnetic resonance. Are they interchangeable? Eur Heart J. 2000;21(16): 1387–96.
11. Jenkins C, Bricknell K, Chan J, Hanekom L, Marwick TH. Comparison of two- and three-dimensional echocardiography with sequential magnetic resonance imaging for evaluating left ventricular volume and ejection fraction over time in patients with healed myocardial infarction. Am J Cardiol. 2007;99(3):300–6.
12. Jenkins C, Bricknell K, Hanekom L, Marwick TH. Reproducibility and accuracy of echocardiographic measurements of left ventricular parameters using real-time three-dimensional echocardiography. J Am Coll Cardiol. 2004;44(4):878.
13. Marsan NA, Tops LF, Nihoyannopoulos P, Holman ER, Bax JJ. Real-time three dimensional echocardiography: current and future clinical applications. Heart. 2009;95(22):1881–90.

14. Izumo M, Shiota M, Kar S, Gurudevan SV, Tolstrup K, Siegel RJ, Shiota T. Comparison of real-time three-dimensional transesophageal echocardiography to two-dimensional transesophageal echocardiography for quantification of mitral valve prolapse in patients with severe mitral regurgitation. Am J Cardiol. 2013;111(4):588–94.
15. Ewe SH, Delgado V, van der Geest R, Westenberg JJ, Haeck ML, Witkowski TG, Auger D, Marsan NA, Holman ER, de Roos A. Accuracy of three-dimensional versus two-dimensional echocardiography for quantification of aortic regurgitation and validation by three-dimensional three-directional velocity-encoded magnetic resonance imaging. Am J Cardiol. 2013;112(4):560–6.
16. Feigenbaum H, Armstrong WF, Ryan T: Feigenbaum's echocardiography. © Copyright 2010. In. Philadelphia: Lippincott Williams & Wilkins.
17. Armstrong WF, Ryan T. Feigenbaum's echocardiography. Philadelphia: Lippincott Williams & Wilkins; 2012.
18. Bland MJ, Altman DG. Statistical methods for assessing agreement between two methods of clinical measurement. Lancet. 1986;1(8476):931–6.
19. Nemes A, Geleijnse ML, Soliman OI, Anwar AM, Vletter WB, McGhie JS, Csanády M, Forster T, Ten Cate FJ. The role of real-time three-dimensional echocardiography in the evaluation of hypertrophic cardiomyopathy. Orv Hetil. 2009;150(42):1925–31.
20. Cong J, Yang X, Zhang N, Shen J, Fan T, Zhan Z. Quantitative analysis of left atrial volume and function during normotensive and preeclamptic pregnancy: a real-time three-dimensional echocardiography study. Int J Cardiovasc Imaging. 2015;31:1–8.
21. Marsan NA, Tops LF, Holman ER, Veire NRVD, Zeppenfeld K, Boersma E, Wall EEVD, Schalij MJ, Bax JJ. Comparison of left atrial volumes and function by real-time three-dimensional echocardiography in patients having catheter ablation for atrial fibrillation with persistence of sinus rhythm versus recurrent atrial fibrillation three months later. Am J Cardiol. 2008;102(7):847–53.
22. Hoit BD. Left atrial size and function: role in prognosis. J Am Coll Cardiol. 2014;63(6):493–505.
23. Sasaki S, Tamura H, Watanabe T, Wanezaki M, Nishiyama S, Ishino M, Sato C, Arimoto T, Takahashi H, Shishido T. Abstract 16303: left Atrial ejection fraction is a feasible parameter to predict poor prognosis in patients with heart failure and sinus rhythm. Circulation. 2012;21:A16303.
24. Suwa Y, Miyasaka Y, Tsujimoto S, Maeba H, Shiojima I. Left Atrial volume as an independent predictor of congestive heart failure in patients with Atrial fibrillation. Circulation. 2015;132(Suppl 3):-A15191.
25. Kohari M, Zado E, Marchlinski FE, Callans DJ, Han Y. Left atrial volume best predicts recurrence after catheter ablation in patients with persistent and longstanding persistent atrial fibrillation. Pacing Clin Electrophysiol. 2014; 37(4):422–9.
26. Pellicori P, Lukaschuk E, Joseph A, Bourantas C, Sherwi N, Loh H, Rigby A, Zhang J, Clark AL, Cleland JGF. Clinical significance of left atrial ejection fraction measured by MRI in patients with suspected heart failure. Eur Heart J. 2013;34(12):287–8.
27. Jaïs P, Peng JT, Shah DC, Garrigue S, Hocini M, Yamane T, Haïssaguerre M, Barold SS, Roudaut R, Clémenty J. Left ventricular diastolic dysfunction in patients with so-called lone atrial fibrillation. J Cardiovasc Electrophysiol. 2000;11(6):623–5.
28. Grogan M, Smith HC, Gersh BJ, Wood DL. Left ventricular dysfunction due to atrial fibrillation in patients initially believed to have idiopathic dilated cardiomyopathy. Am J Cardiol. 1992;69(19):1570–3.
29. Tsang TSM, Gersh BJ, Appleton CP, Tajik AJ, Barnes ME, Bailey KR, Oh JK, Leibson C, Montgomery SC, Seward JB. Left ventricular diastolic dysfunction as a predictor of the first diagnosed nonvalvular atrial fibrillation in 840 elderly men and women. ACC Curr J Rev. 2002;40(9):1636–44.

The same modality medical image registration with large deformation and clinical application based on adaptive diffeomorphic multi-resolution demons

Chang Wang[1,2*], Qiongqiong Ren[1,2], Xin Qin[1] and Yi Yu[1,2]

Abstract

Background: Diffeomorphic demons can not only guarantee smooth and reversible deformation, but also avoid unreasonable deformation. However, the number of iterations which has great influence on the registration result needs to be set manually.

Methods: This study proposed a novel method to exploit the adaptive diffeomorphic multi-resolution demons algorithm to the non-rigid registration of the same modality medical images with large deformation. Firstly an optimized non-rigid registration framework and the diffeomorphism strategy were used, and then a similarity energy function based on the grey value was designed as registration metric, lastly termination condition was set based on the variation of this metric and iterations can be stopped adaptively. Quantitative analyses based on the registration evaluation indexes were conducted to prove the validity of this method.

Results: Registration result of synthetic image and the same modality MRI and CT image was compared with those obtained by other demons algorithms. Quantitative analyses demonstrated the proposed method's superiority. Medical image with large deformation was produced by rotational distortion and extrusion transform, and the same modality image registration with large deformation was performed successfully. Quantitative analyses showed that the registration evaluation indexes remained stable with an increase in transform strength. This method can be also applied to pulmonary medical image registration with large deformation successfully, and it showed the clinical application value. The influence of different driving forces and parameters on the registration result was analysed, and the result demonstrated that the proposed method is effective and robust.

Conclusions: This method can solve the non-rigid registration problem of the same modality medical image with large deformation showing promise for diagnostic pulmonary imaging applications.

Keywords: Diffeomorphic, Demons, Adaptive, Large deformation, Multi-resolution

Background

Non-rigid registration has been applied to inter-subjective registration to detect lesions and to establish a medical atlas. Comparisons of non-rigid registration algorithms have shown that those with demons based on the optical flow field theory provide superior results [1].

The demons algorithm was initially only applicable to image registration with small deformation. Therefore, many researchers have tried to improve it. In 2005, Wang and Pennec introduced the floating image gradient in the diffusion equation and proposed active demons [2, 3]. In 2006, Roglj et al. proposed symmetric demons method and demonstrated its high efficient [4]. In 2007, Vercauteren et al. applied the optimization framework of non-rigid registration to demons and proposed additive demons. In their method, non-rigid registration was equivalent to optimizing the similarity energy function, and iterations

* Correspondence: wangchang@xxmu.edu.cn
[1]School of Biomedical Engineering, Xinxiang Medical University, Xinxiang 453003, China
[2]Xinxiang City Engineering Technology Research Center of Neurosensor and Control, Xinxiang 453003, China

could be stopped adaptively [5]. In 2008, symmetric log-domain diffeomorphic demons algorithm was proposed, and Log Euclidean transformation was used to avoid time-consuming computations of Log spatial transformation [6]. In 2009, diffeomorphic demons was proposed, and it was shown that the final deformation is topologically invariant and that unreasonable deformations are not produced [7]. In 2010, Xu et al. introduced a regularization term and designed a new similarity energy function to ensure smooth and reversible deformations [8]. In 2012, Lei et al. proposed a new active gradient and curvature (G&C) demons algorithm using the curvature to control the deformation [9].

In recent years, some researchers have proposed non-rigid image registration methods with large deformation. In 2014, Lombaert et al. introduced the direct feature matching technique to find global correspondences between reference and moving images, and they proposed spectral log-demons method for diffeomorphic image registration with large deformation [10, 11]. In 2014, Kong et al. proposed a robust discriminative clustering method based on mutual information and used it to efficiently perform brain MRI segmentation [12]. In 2015, Zhao et al. used multilayer convolutional neural networks to determine scale and translation parameters and proposed the deep adaptive log-demons method for diffeomorphic image registration with large deformation [13]. In 2015, Yan et al. performed image registration with large deformation by combining manifold learning and diffeomorphic demons [14]. In 2016, Deng et al. proposed a data classification method based on fused fuzzy deep neural network and used it to efficiently discriminate WM, GM, and CSF [15].

Medical image registration plays an important role in diagnosing diseases and establishing a medical atlas. Large deformation may exist between reference image and moving image, and it could result in problems in non-rigid medical image registration with large deformation. This study proposes an adaptive diffeomorphic multi-resolution demons algorithm for medical image registration with large deformation. An optimized framework with non-rigid registration and the diffeomorphic deformation strategy were used, a similarity energy function based on the grey value was designed as a registration metric, and the termination condition was set based on the variation of this metric. Iterations could be stopped adaptively, and medical image registration with large deformation was performed. This method was tested using synthetic images and the same modality MRI and CT images, and the mean square error, normalized cross correlation, and structural similarity were used as evaluation indexes to verify the superiority of this method. Medical image registration with large deformation simulated by rotational distortion and extrusion

was performed successfully. Quantitative analyses of the influences of different driving forces and parameters on the registration result showed that our method is effective and robust. This method can be applied to the same modality medical image registration with large deformation, making it promising for diagnostic pulmonary imaging applications.

Methods

For the problems of the same modality medical image registration with large deformation, an adaptive diffeomorphic multi-resolution demons algorithm was proposed. An optimized framework with non-rigid registration and the diffeomorphic deformation strategy were used, a similarity energy function based on the grey value was designed, and termination conditions were set to stop iterations adaptively. We applied this method to the same modality medical image registration with large deformation and found that it shows promise for pulmonary medical image registration in clinical application.

Additive demons

Non-rigid image registration is essentially a multi-parameter optimization problem involving mapping a moving image to a reference image. It defines an appropriate objective function as registration metric and then optimizes this metric. For reference image F and moving image M, the registration metric should be optimized to seek the best transform t^{opt}. $t{:}R^n \rightarrow R^n$, $p \rightarrow t(p)$ is the mapping of pixel p of the moving image to pixel $t(p)$ of the reference image. The definition of registration metric is the crucial step in the non-rigid registration process. The mean square deviation based on the grey value as a registration metric can be calculated using Eq. 1.

$$Sim(F, M \circ t) = \frac{1}{2} \| F - M \circ t \|^2 = \frac{1}{2|\Omega_P|} \sum_{P \in \Omega_P} |F(p) - M(t(p))|$$

(1)

In Eq. 1, Ω is the common region of F and M after registration, and o is the transform operator. Directly minimizing the registration metric using Eq. 1 will lead to an unstable solution, and therefore, a regularization term needs to be added to restrict the geometric transform. The revised energy function $E(t)$ is expressed using Eq. 2.

$$E(t) = \frac{1}{\sigma_i} Sim(F, M \circ t) + \frac{1}{\sigma_t} Reg(t)$$

(2)

In Eq. 2, σ_i is the local noise level, and σ_t is the regularization parameter. Cachier et al. [16] introduced the parameters c (not ruled spatial transform) and t (ruled spatial transform). Then, the new energy function is expressed using Eq. 3.

$$E(c,t) = \left\| \frac{1}{\sigma_i}(F-M \circ c) \right\|^2 + \frac{1}{\sigma_x^2} Dist(c,t)^2 + \frac{1}{\sigma_t}\ Reg(t) \quad (3)$$

In Eq. 3, $Dist(c,t) = \|c - t\|$, σ_x is the uncertainty degree between c and t. The displacement field u is produced using the space geometric transform, and two vectors are added directly to form a new vector. The energy function of additive demons algorithm comprised similarity measure term, deformation error term, and regularization term. The final energy function is expressed as follows:

$$E(u) = \frac{1}{\sigma_i^2} \| F-M \circ (t + u) \|^2 + \frac{1}{\sigma_x^2} \|u\|^2 \quad (4)$$

In Eq. 4, u is the updated displacement field, and $Dist(c,t) = \|c - t\| = \|u\|$. By minimizing the energy function with respect to the displacement field, the final displacement field is expressed using Eq. 5.

$$u(p) = - \frac{F(p)-M \circ t(p)}{J_P^2 + \frac{\sigma_i^2(p)}{\sigma_x^2}} J_P^T \quad (5)$$

In Eq. 5, $\sigma_i(p) = |F(p) - M \circ t(p)|$ and $J_P = -\nabla^T F(p)$.

Diffeomorphic deformation strategy

Diffeomorphic space was proposed in 2009, and it can make sure that the deformation is smooth, reversible, and topologically invariant. Diffeomorphic transform, which is based on the theory of Lie groups, is related to the exponential map of the velocity field v, that is, $\phi = \exp(v)$, and a practical and fast approximation method with a scaling-and-squaring strategy was described as follows.

Exponential $\phi = \exp(v)$

Input: Velocity field v.
Output: Diffeomorphic map $\phi = \exp(v)$
Choose N such that $2^{-N}v \to 0$
e.g., such that max $\|2^{-N}v\| \leq 0.5$ pixels
Scale velocity field $\phi \leftarrow 2^{-N}v$
for N times
do $\phi \leftarrow \phi \circ \phi$
end for

Algorithm implementation

The diffeomorphic deformation strategy was used for optimizing the energy function designed by additive demons. The deformation should always be topologically invariant. Rough deformation greatly influences the registration result; if it is calculated unsuitably, it is easy to fall into a local optimum. Therefore, a multi-resolution strategy was used, and rough deformation was calculated with low resolution. Then, the energy function was

minimised and the best registration result was obtained, and it can avoid the local optimum.

Iterations also have great influence on the registration result. If the number of iterations is not set properly, the best deformation field cannot be obtained. The consumed time will increase with the increasing of iterations. The mean square deviation based on the grey value was designed as a registration metric, and iterations could be stopped adaptively depending on the variation of energy function. It can eliminate the influence of iterations on registration result. The convergence condition was defined by Eq. 6.

$$\begin{cases} if & E(n)-E(n-1) < E(n-1) * stop\_criterium \quad break \\ else & continue \end{cases}$$

$$(6)$$

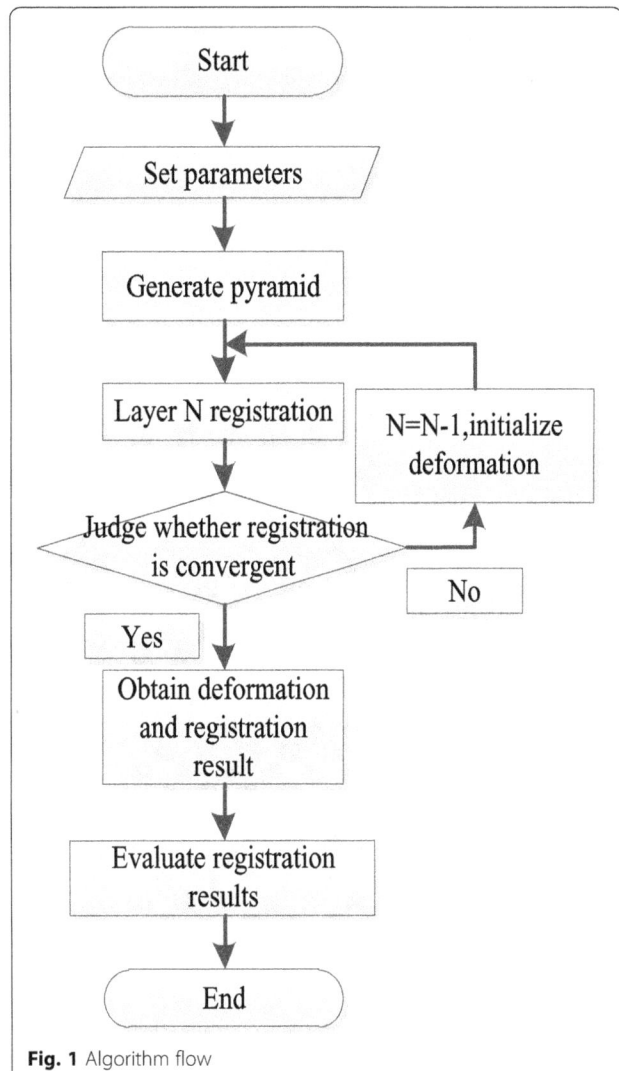

Fig. 1 Algorithm flow

When the displacement field was updated, three different demons driving forces were proposed as follows: Thirion's primitive driving force, $J_P = -\nabla^T F(p)$; Gauss–Newton-based advanced driving force, $J_P = -\nabla^T(M \cdot t(p))$; and symmetric driving force, $J_P = -(\nabla^T F + \nabla^T(M \cdot t(p)))/2$.

The steps for each registration layer can be described as follows:

Step 1: initialize displacement field.
Step 2: calculate demons driving force $u(p)$ and update velocity field v.
Step 3: regulate deformation field using Gauss filter.
Step 4: obtain exponential mapping of deformation field by diffeomorphic transform.
Step 5: calculate similarity measurement function $E(t)$ using Eq. 4.
Step 6: judge convergence condition.

Figure 1 shows the algorithm flow of proposed method.

Algorithm evaluation

The mean square error, normalized cross correlation, and structural similarity [17] were calculated as evaluation indexes. The mean square error is defined by Eq. 7.

$$MSE = \sqrt{\frac{\sum (S(x) - M(x))^2}{n}} \qquad (7)$$

The normalized cross-correlation coefficient is defined by Eq. 8.

$$CC = \frac{\sum (S(x) - \overline{S})(M(x) - \overline{M})}{\sqrt{\sum (S(x) - \overline{S})^2}\sqrt{\sum (M(x) - \overline{M})^2}} \qquad (8)$$

Here, n is the total pixel number, S is the reference image, M is the registration result, and $\overline{S}$ and $\overline{M}$ are the average grey values of each pixel point in the reference image and registration result, respectively.

Results

The superiority of our method was verified through comparisons with active demons, additive demons, and diffeomorphic demons. The experimental parameters were set as follows: Gaussian filter parameter G_σ, where $\sigma = 2$; deformation updating step-length $\sigma_x = 1.0$; multi-resolution layer number $N = 3$; and convergence condition $stop\_criterium = 0.005$.

Synthetic image registration

Figure 2 shows the synthetic checkerboard images that were processed to validate our method. This method can realize non-rigid image registration and estimate the deformation field effectively.

The same modality medical image registration

MRI images were selected from the Simulated Brain Database (http://www.bic.mni.mcgill.ca/brainweb/) provided by the Montreal Neurology Institute of McGill University. Their size is $217 \times 181 \times 181$, and T1-weighted MRI images were selected as reference and moving images. Figure 3(a–c) show the reference image, moving images and initial difference. Figure 3(d–e) show that our method

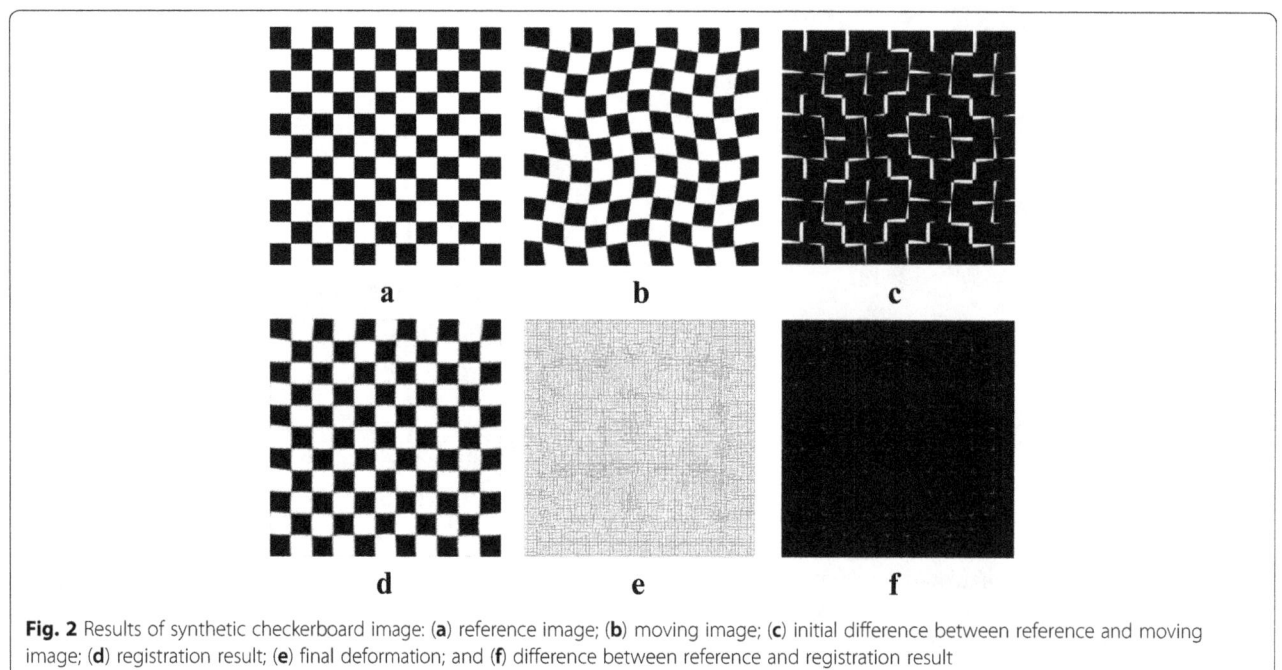

Fig. 2 Results of synthetic checkerboard image: (**a**) reference image; (**b**) moving image; (**c**) initial difference between reference and moving image; (**d**) registration result; (**e**) final deformation; and (**f**) difference between reference and registration result

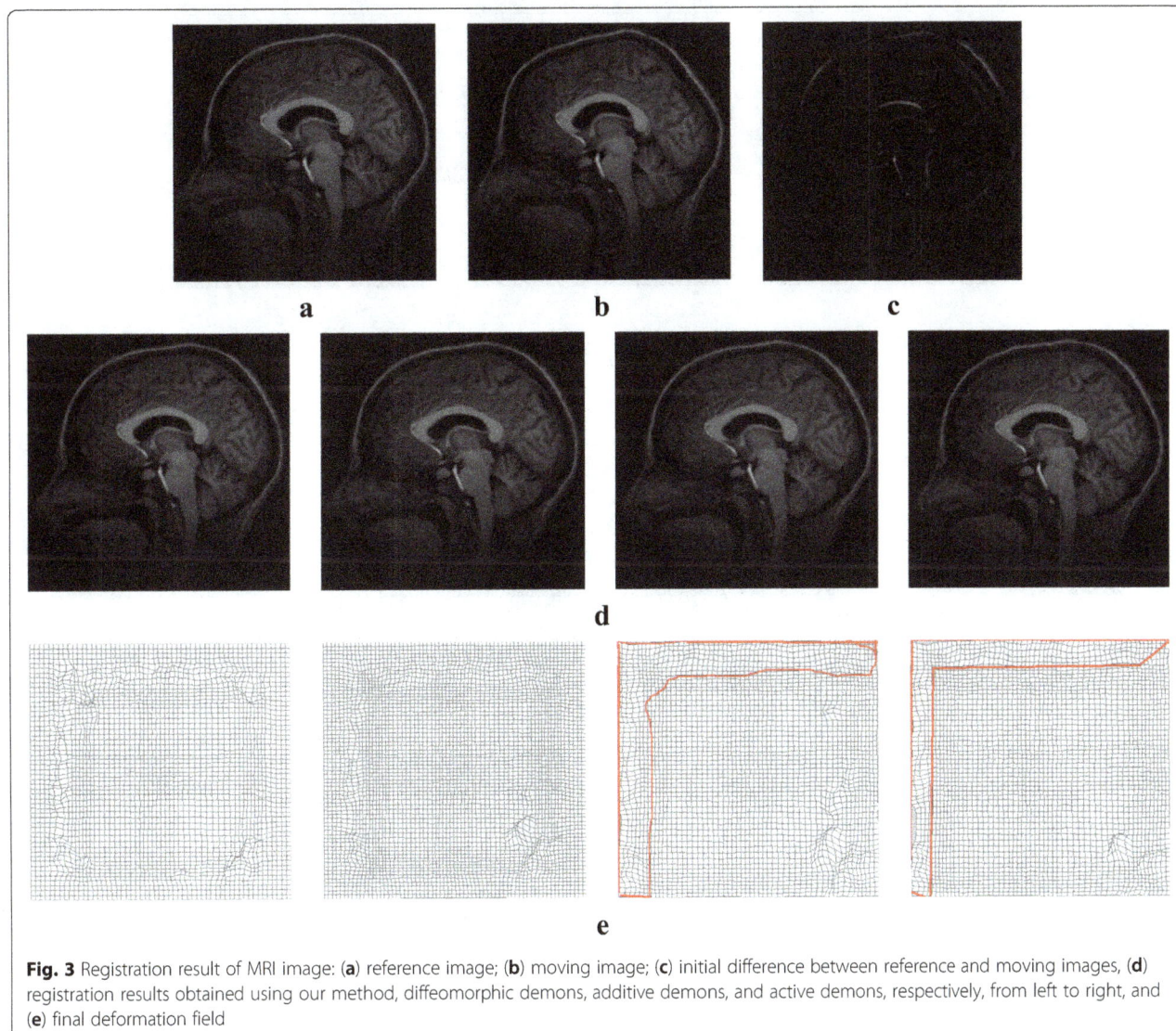

Fig. 3 Registration result of MRI image: (**a**) reference image; (**b**) moving image; (**c**) initial difference between reference and moving images, (**d**) registration results obtained using our method, diffeomorphic demons, additive demons, and active demons, respectively, from left to right, and (**e**) final deformation field

provides the best registration result and that the deformation field is smooth and reversible. The edge of deformation field is more reasonable than that in the case of active demons and additive demons. Table 1 shows the quantitative analysis of evaluation indexes for MRI image registration. It is seen that the normalized cross-correlation coefficient and structural similarity are the highest and the mean square error is the lowest; therefore, our method is superior to active demons, additive demons, and diffeomorphic demons.

CT images were selected from the Medical Image Database (http://www.med.harvard.edu/AANLIB) provided by Harvard Medical Center, and their size is 256×256. Figure 4 shows the registration result of CT images, and Table 2 shows the quantitative analysis of evaluation indexes for CT image registration. Comparative analysis showed that the registration and statistical results of CT image were the same as those of the MRI image, indicating that our method can be also applicable to CT image registration.

Table 1 Evaluation of registration result (MRI)

Experiment Method	MSE/(A.U.)	NCC/(A.U.)	Structural Similarity/(A.U.)
our method	514.7965	0.9993	0.9952
diffeomorphic demons	583.0147	0.9992	0.9937
additive demons	640.9294	0.9987	0.9906
active demons	1307.5	0.9944	0.9824

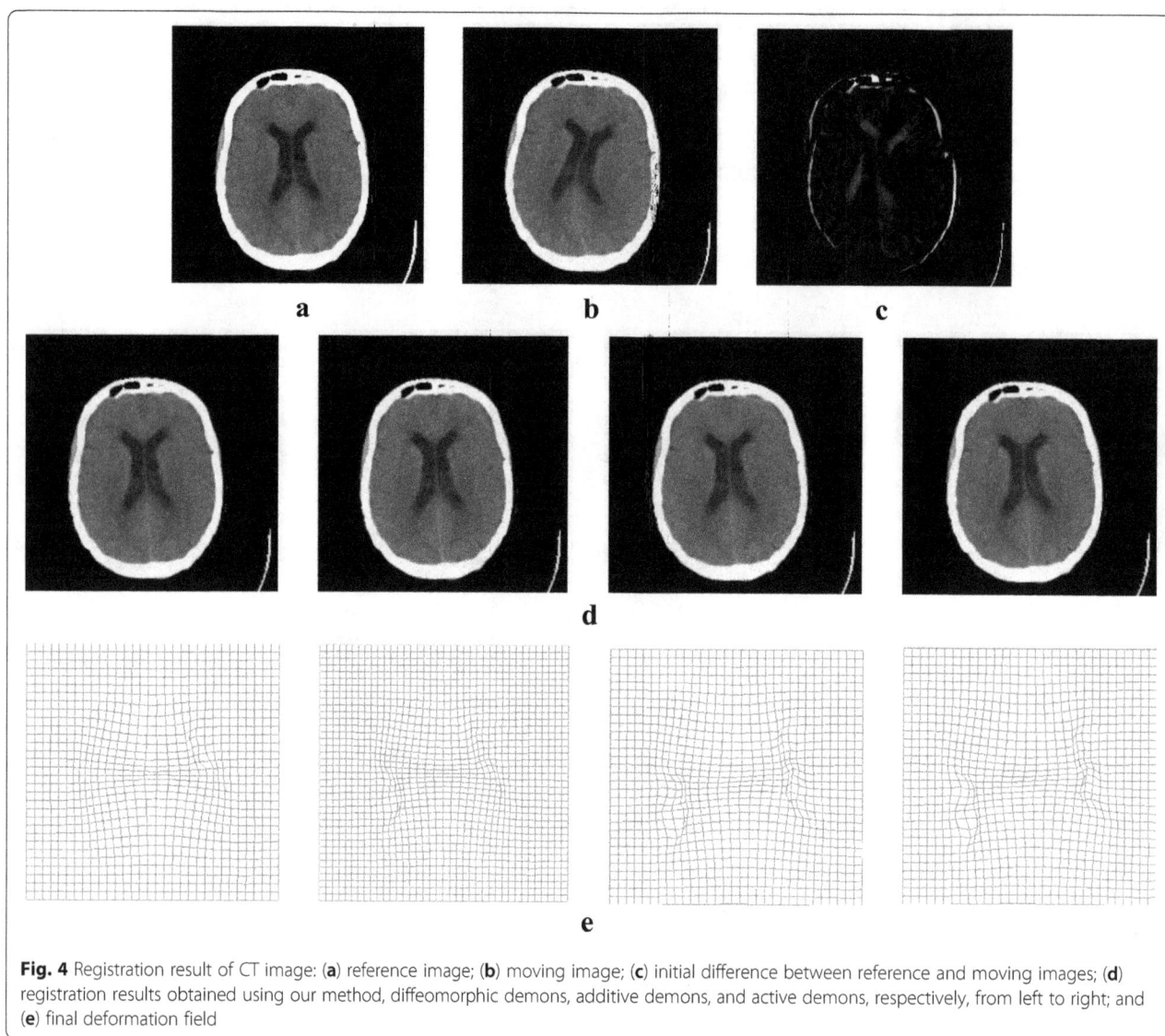

Fig. 4 Registration result of CT image: (**a**) reference image; (**b**) moving image; (**c**) initial difference between reference and moving images; (**d**) registration results obtained using our method, diffeomorphic demons, additive demons, and active demons, respectively, from left to right; and (**e**) final deformation field

Medical image registration with large deformation

Large deformation was produced by two types of free transforms: rotational distortion and extrusion. The deformation field was determined by the transform strength.

Medical image registration with large deformation produced by rotational distortion was performed using our proposed method, as shown in Fig. 5. Column 1 show moving images produced with rotational distortional strengths of 30–90%, column 2 shows the corresponding registration result, and column 3 shows the corresponding final deformation field. Table 3 shows the quantitative analysis result; the normalized cross-correlation coefficient and structural similarity decreased and the mean square error and the consumed time gradually increased with an increase in the deformation field strength.

Figure 6 shows the result for large deformation produced by extrusion. Column 1 show moving images produced for extrusion strengths of 10–70%, column 2 shows the corresponding registration result, and column

Table 2 Evaluation of registration result (CT)

Experiment Method	MSE/(A.U.)	NCC/(A.U.)	Structural Similarity/(A.U.)
our method	2257.2	0.9928	0.9762
diffeomorphic demons	2578.6	0.9905	0.9619
additive demons	2377.0	0.9920	0.9635
active demons	2332.2	0.9923	0.9644

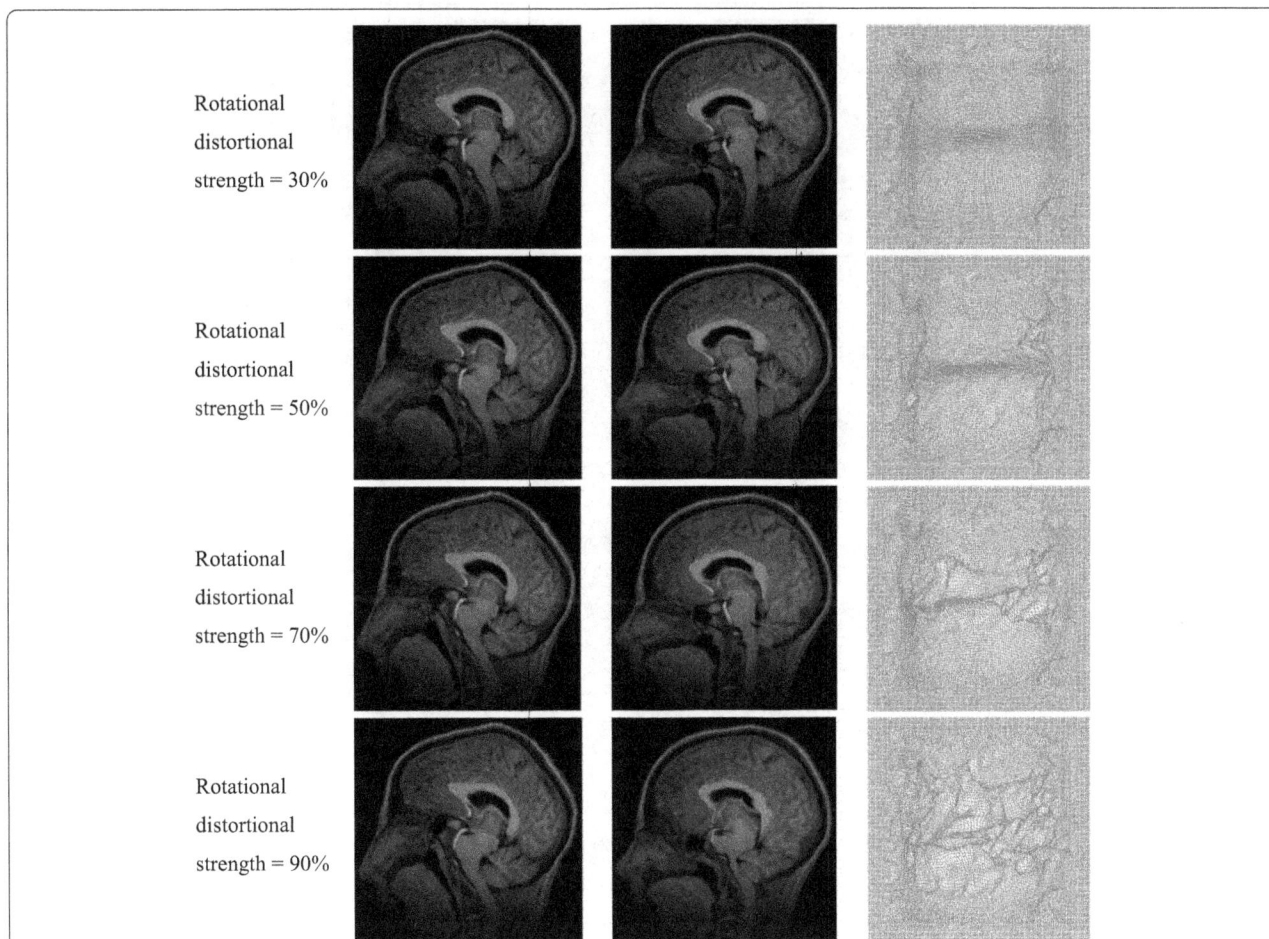

Fig. 5 Medical image registration with large deformation produced by rotational distortion. Column 1: moving images produced for rotational distortional strengths of 30–90%, column 2: corresponding registration results, and column 3: corresponding final deformation fields

3 shows the corresponding final deformation field. Table 4 shows the quantitative analysis result; the normalized cross-correlation coefficient, structural similarity, and mean square error basically remained stable and the consumed time gradually increased with an increase in the deformation field strength. Therefore, medical image registration with large deformation produced by both rotational distortion and extrusion can be performed efficiently.

Clinical application

Pulmonary medical images of the same individual show large deformations under different respiration states, and therefore, non-rigid registration of such images remains challenging. Thoracic images were selected from DIR-Lab (http://www.DIR-lab.com). DIR-Lab provides 12 cases, each of which contains a thoracic image with six phases. Slices with inhale and exhale phases were used as reference and moving images with large deformation. Figure 7 shows the registration result of pulmonary images. The deformation field obtained using our method was smooth and topologically invariant. Table 5 shows the quantitative analysis of the evaluation indexes for thoracic image registration with large deformation; the normalized cross-correlation coefficient and structural similarity are the highest and the mean square error is the lowest; and

Table 3 Evaluation of registration result (rotational distortion deformation)

Rotational Distortional Strength	MSE/(A.U.)	NCC/(A.U.)	Structural Similarity/(A.U.)
30%	531.6939	0.9991	0.9950
50%	1763.9	0.9898	0.9479
70%	2948.6	0.9717	0.9107
90%	5046.0	0.9169	0.8136

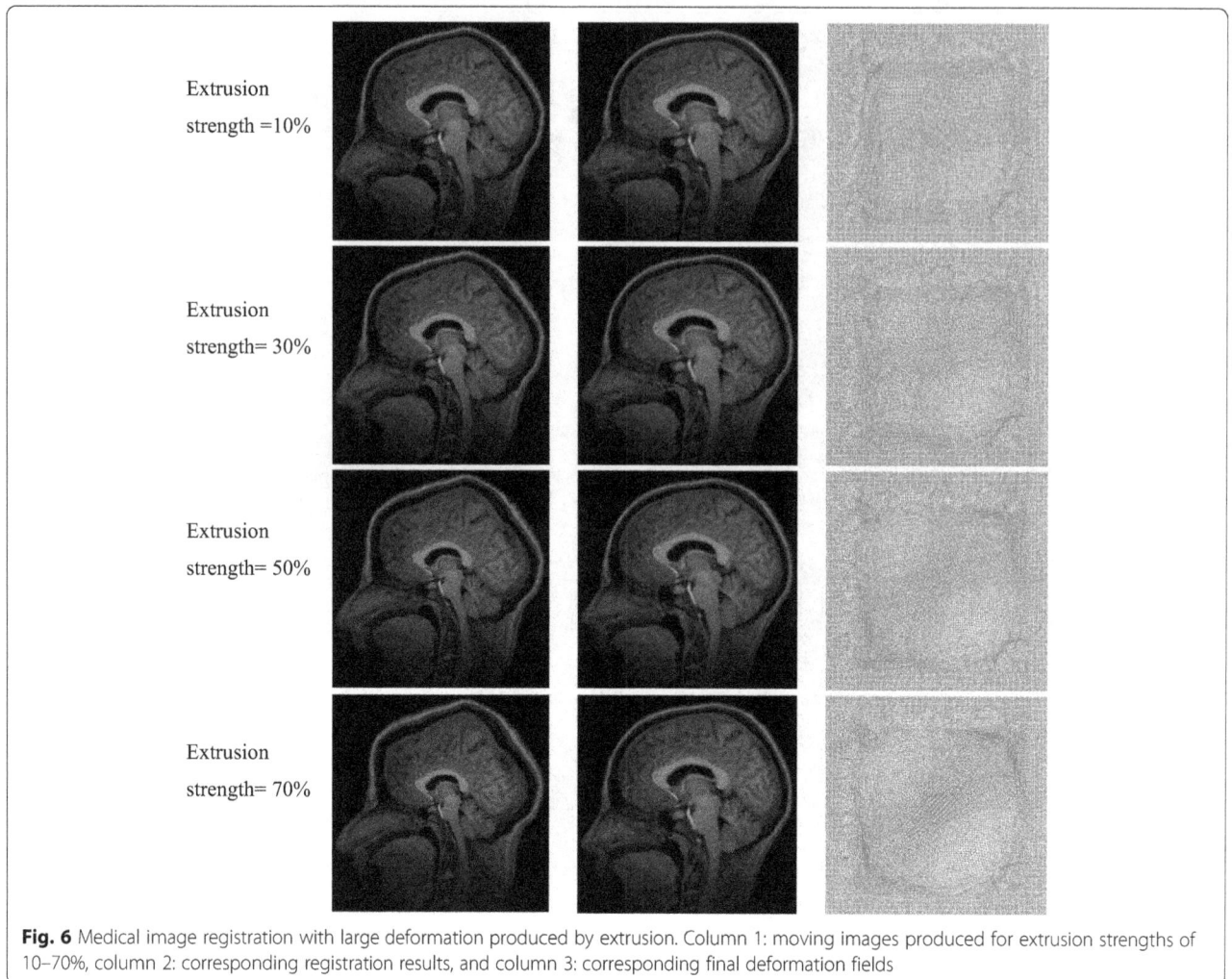

Fig. 6 Medical image registration with large deformation produced by extrusion. Column 1: moving images produced for extrusion strengths of 10–70%, column 2: corresponding registration results, and column 3: corresponding final deformation fields

the evaluation indexes obtained using our method were the closest to the standard value. The registration and statistical results indicate that our method can be clinically applied to the non-rigid registration of pulmonary images with large deformation.

Analysis of different driving forces

Thirion, Gauss-Newton, and symmetric driving forces were used, and the displacement field was defined differently. Figure 8 shows the variation of the energy function $E(t)$; the convergence is the fastest and the similarity measure based on energy function is the lowest with symmetric driving

Table 4 Evaluation of registration result (extrusion deformation)

Extrusion Strength	MSE/(A.U.)	NCC/(A.U.)	Structural Similarity/(A.U.)
10%	543.2	0.9991	0.9940
30%	545.1	0.9991	0.9944
50%	529.8	0.9991	0.9949
70%	559.4	0.9990	0.9946

forces. Table 6 shows the quantitative analysis; the symmetric driving force shows the best performance.

Influence of parameters on registration result

The Gaussian filter, deformation updating step-length, resolution layer, and convergence condition were used as experimental parameters. The resolution layer can only influence the registration speed, and the convergence condition can influence the registration accuracy. Table 7 shows details about the deformation updating step-length; the registration accuracy remained stable and the consumed time decreased with an increase in the step-length from 0.8 to 2.0.

Discussion

To verify the superiority of our method, synthetic images and the same modality MRI and CT images were used to perform non-rigid image registration with large deformation. Figures 3(e) and 4(e) show the obtained deformation fields for MRI and CT images. The edge and detail information of final deformation field obtained

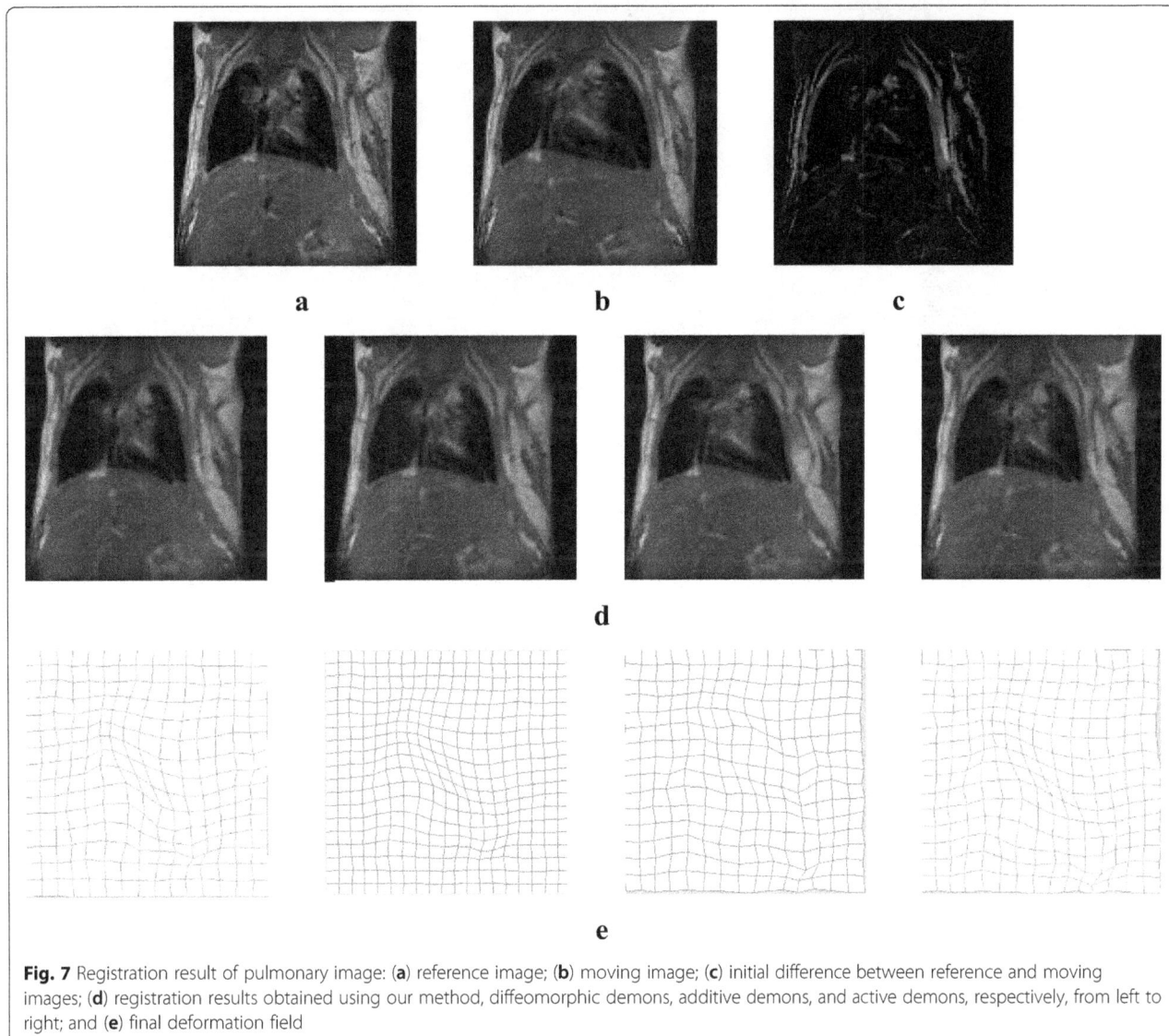

Fig. 7 Registration result of pulmonary image: (**a**) reference image; (**b**) moving image; (**c**) initial difference between reference and moving images; (**d**) registration results obtained using our method, diffeomorphic demons, additive demons, and active demons, respectively, from left to right; and (**e**) final deformation field

using our method are more accurate and reasonable than those obtained using active demons and additive demons. The diffeomorphism strategy was used to guarantee smooth and reversible deformation; by contrast, active demons and additive demons produce unreasonable deformation during registration. This conclusion agrees with that reported previously [7, 8]. Tables 1 and 2 show quantitative analysis results for the same modality MRI and CT image registration, respectively; it is seen that the mean square error is the lowest and normalized cross-correlation and structural similarity are the highest when using the proposed method. Therefore, the proposed method is superior to active demons, additive demons, and diffeomorphic demons. Large deformation was simulated by two types of free transform, rotational distortion and extrusion, and the

Table 5 Evaluation of registration result (lung)

Experiment Method	MSE/(A.U.)	NCC/(A.U.)	Structural Similarity/(A.U.)
our method	1371.9	0.9685	0.7911
diffeomorphic demons	1427.4	0.9678	0.7847
additive demons	1409.3	0.9385	0.7088
active demons	1401.8	0.9377	0.7043
standard result	1002.1	0.9874	0.8210

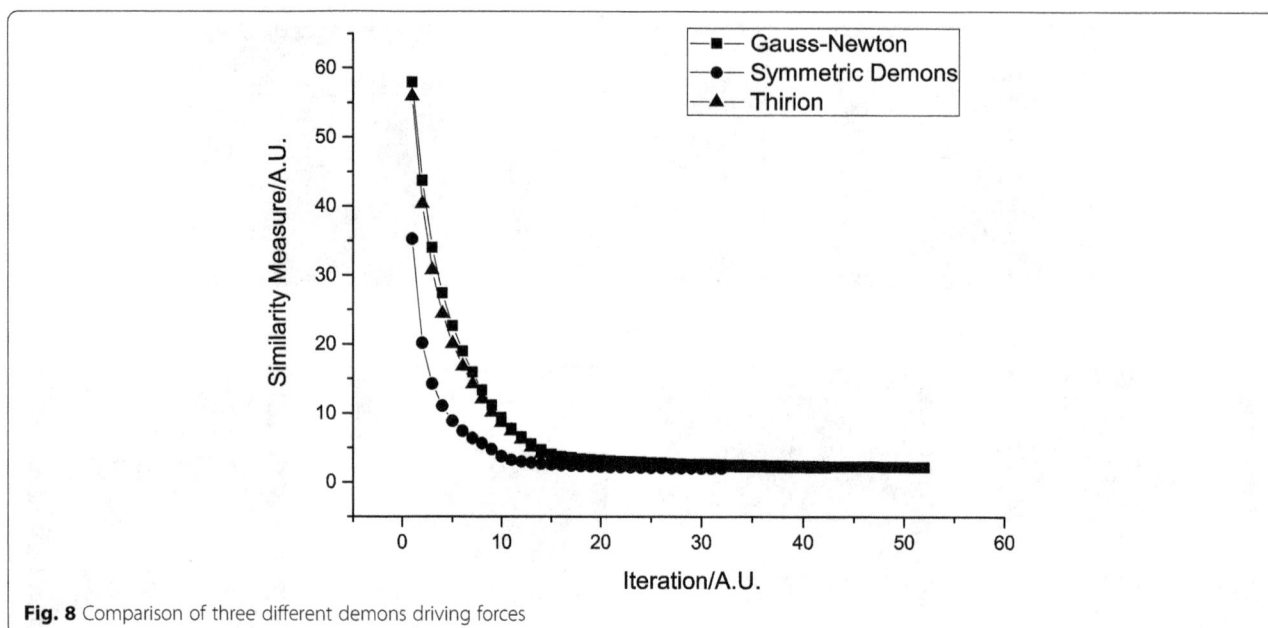

Fig. 8 Comparison of three different demons driving forces

deformation field was determined by the transform strength. The same modality medical image registration with large deformation was performed successfully, as seen from the registration results in Figs. 5 and 6 and the quantitative analysis results in Tables 3 and 4.

The influence of the deformation updating step-length on registration result was analysed. The result shows that non-rigid registration with large deformation can be performed successfully and that the evaluation indexes remain stable when the update is within a reasonable range. The registration speed accelerates with an increase in the step-length update, and the proposed algorithm is robust. The influence of driving forces on the registration result was also analysed; the result shows that the convergence of the proposed algorithm is the fastest and that the evaluation indexes are the most perfect with symmetric driving force. The finding for the driving force is consistent with those reported previously [5, 7]. A similarity energy function based on the grey value was designed, and the termination condition was set according to the variation of the energy function. Furthermore, iterations could be stopped adaptively, and therefore, the registration speed was accelerated. By contrast, when implementing active demons and diffeomorphic demons, the number of iterations needs to be set manually, and this greatly influences

the registration result. If the number of iterations is insufficient, the best registration result cannot be obtained. Diffeomorphic demons use the diffeomorphic deformation strategy to guarantee smooth and reversible deformation; however, they are time-consuming. By contrast, additive demons consume less time; however, they cannot guarantee smooth and topologically invariant deformation, and they are prone to producing unreasonable deformations. The proposed algorithm can stop iterations automatically, thus greatly accelerating the registration speed and ensuring a smooth and topologically invariant deformation field.

Pulmonary medical images of the same individual under different respiration states show large deformation, and registration of such images is crucial for planning the treatment of thoracic malignancies and quantitatively analysing pulmonary function. Quantitative analyses showed that pulmonary medical images with large deformation were successfully and efficiently registered using our proposed method, and the deformation was smooth and topologically invariant. Therefore, our proposed

Table 6 Evaluation of registration result based on different driving forces

Experiment Method	MSE/(A.U.)	NCC/(A.U.)	Structural Similarity/(A.U.)
Thirion	514.79	0.9993	0.9948
Gauss-Newton	476.1	0.9993	0.9948
Symmetric Demons	465.0	0.9994	0.9952

Table 7 Influence of deformation updating step-length σ_x on registration accuracy

Registration Accuracy	σ_x				
	2.0	1.5	1.2	1.0	0.8
MSE/(A.U.)	464.81	479.2040	485.8915	508.2908	522.31
NCC/(A.U.)	0.9993	0.9993	0.9992	0.9992	0.9991
Structural Similarity/(A.U.)	0.9953	0.9949	0.9949	0.9943	0.9939
Time Consuming/(s)	136.46	150.37	193.94	222.06	287.1

method is promising for applications in diagnostic pulmonary imaging and radiation oncology.

Conclusion

This study proposed an adaptive diffeomorphic multi-resolution demons algorithm and solved the problem of the same modality medical image non-rigid registration with large deformation. Synthetic images and the same modality MRI and CT image registration were tested by this method, and quantitative analyses demonstrated the proposed method's superiority. Medical images with large deformation were produced by rotational distortion and extrusion transform, registration result and quantitative analyses demonstrated that image registration with large deformation could be performed successfully and efficiently using our method. Quantitative analyses under different driving forces demonstrated that our method based on symmetric driving force is the most efficient. The influence of parameters on registration result was analysed indicating that our method is robust. This method can be also applied to pulmonary medical image registration with large deformation, and have an important clinical application value.

Abbreviations
CSF: Cerebrospinal fluid; CT: Computed tomography; GM: Grey matter; MRI: Magnetic resonance imaging; MSE: Mean square error; NCC: Normalized cross correlation; WM: White matter

Acknowledgements
The authors are thankful for the supports from the School of biomedical engineering and Key Lab of Neurosense and Control (Xinxiang Medical University, Xinxiang, China).

Funding
This work is supported by the Fundamental Research Funds for Key Scientific Research Project of Henan Higher Education Institutions under grant no. 17A310005; Scientific and Technological Project of Henan Province under grant nos. 182102310528, 182102310555, and 152102310357; Natural Science Foundation of Xinxiang City under grant no. CXGG17005; Open Project of Biomedical Engineering School under grant no. 2018-BME-KFKT-06; and Disciplinary Group of Psychology and Neuroscience under grant no. 2016PN-KFKT-19.
The funding sponsors have estimated the feasibility of the study, but have no role in the collection, analysis, or interpretation of the data or in the decision to submit the manuscript for publication.

Authors' contributions
CW proposed adaptive diffeomorphic multi-resolution demons, designed evaluation indexes for registration results, and performed medical image registration; QQR and XQ prepared the medial images with large deformation, and performed the same modality medical image registration with large deformation; YY performed the analysis and interpretation of the registration results. All authors have been involved in drafting and revising the manuscript and approved the final version to be published. All authors read and approved the final manuscript.

Competing interests
The authors declare that they have no competing interests.

References
1. Hellier P, Barillot C, Corouge I. Retrospective evaluation of inter-subject brain registration. IEEE Trans on Medical Imaging. 2003;22:1120–30.
2. Wang H, Dong L, O'Daniel J. Validation of an accelerated 'demons' algorithm for deformable image registration in radiation therapy. Phys Med Biol. 2005;50:2887–905.
3. Pennec X, Cachier P. Understanding the demons algorithm: 3D non-rigid registration by gradient descent. Med Image Comput Comput Assist Interv. 1999:597–605.
4. Rogelj P, Kovacic S. Symmetric image registration. Med Image Anal. 2006;10: 484–93.
5. Vercauteren T, Pennec X, Perchant A. Non-parametric diffeomorphic image registration with the demons algorithm. Med Image Comput Comput Assist Interv. 2007:319–26.
6. Vercauteren T, Pennec X, Perchant A, et al. Symmetric log-domain diffeomorphic registration: a demons-based approach. Med Image Comput Comput Assist Interv. 2008:754–61.
7. Vercauteren T, Pennec X, Perchant A. Diffeomorphic demons: efficient non-parametric image registration. NeuroImage. 2009;45:61–72.
8. Xu F, Liu W, Li CF. A non-rigid registration of the cerebral CT images with large deformations. Chin J Biomed Eng. 2010;29:172–7.
9. Lei WJ, Zhu X, Jia YT, et al. Image registration method by combination of gradient and curvature driven. Comput Eng Appl. 2012;48:204–6.
10. Lombaert H, Grady L, Pennec X, et al. Spectral log-demons: diffeomorphic image registration with very large deformations. Int J Comput Vis. 2014;107: 254–71.
11. Lombaert H, Grady L, Pennec X, et al. Spectral demons- image registration via global spectral correspondence. Eur Conference Comput Vision. 2012: 30–44.
12. Kong YY, Deng Y, Dai QH. Discriminative clustering and feature selection for brain MRI segmentation. IEEE Signal Processing Letters. 2014;22:573–7.
13. Zhao L, Jia K. Deep adaptive log-demons: diffeomorphic image registration with very large deformations. Comput Math Methods Med. 2015;15:1–16.
14. Yan DQ, Liu CF, Liu SL, et al. A fast image registration algorithm for diffeomorphic image with large deformation. Acta Automat Sin. 2015;41: 1461–70.
15. Deng Y, Ren ZQ, Kong YY, et al. A hierarchical fused fuzzy deep neural network for data classification. IEEE Trans Fuzzy Syst. 2017;25:1006–12.
16. Cachier P, Bardinet E, Dormont D, et al. Iconic feature based-nonrigid registration: the PASHA algorithm. Comput Vis Image Underst. 2003;89:272–98.
17. Wang Z, Bovik AC, Sheikh HR. Image quality assessment: from error visibility to structural similarity. IEEE Trans Image Process. 2004;13:600–12.

24

Automatic brain tissue segmentation based on graph filter

Youyong Kong[1,2]* (iD), Xiaopeng Chen[1,2], Jiasong Wu[1,2], Pinzheng Zhang[1,2], Yang Chen[1,2] and Huazhong Shu[1,2]

Abstract

Background: Accurate segmentation of brain tissues from magnetic resonance imaging (MRI) is of significant importance in clinical applications and neuroscience research. Accurate segmentation is challenging due to the tissue heterogeneity, which is caused by noise, bias filed and partial volume effects.

Methods: To overcome this limitation, this paper presents a novel algorithm for brain tissue segmentation based on supervoxel and graph filter. Firstly, an effective supervoxel method is employed to generate effective supervoxels for the 3D MRI image. Secondly, the supervoxels are classified into different types of tissues based on filtering of graph signals.

Results: The performance is evaluated on the BrainWeb 18 dataset and the Internet Brain Segmentation Repository (IBSR) 18 dataset. The proposed method achieves mean dice similarity coefficient (DSC) of 0.94, 0.92 and 0.90 for the segmentation of white matter (WM), grey matter (GM) and cerebrospinal fluid (CSF) for BrainWeb 18 dataset, and mean DSC of 0.85, 0.87 and 0.57 for the segmentation of WM, GM and CSF for IBSR18 dataset.

Conclusions: The proposed approach can well discriminate different types of brain tissues from the brain MRI image, which has high potential to be applied for clinical applications.

Keywords: Magnetic resonance imaging, Brain tissue segmentation, Supervoxel generation, Graph filter

Background

Magnetic resonance imaging (MRI) has been widely employed to examine the anatomical structures of the human brain in both clinical application and neuroscience research [1, 2]. Compared to other medical imaging modalities, MRI has the advantage of the high spatial resolution and well soft-tissue contrasts [3, 4]. This powerful technique can yield exquisite differentiation between different types of tissues, including white matter (WM), grey matter (GM) and cerebrospinal fluid (CSF). Accurate segmentation of these tissues is of significant importance in the several applications [5–7]. Manual segmentation is extremely time-consuming due to millions of voxels in the brain MRI image. Besides, the segmentation result is prone to substantial intra-observer and inter-observer variation. Therefore, it is

essential to propose an effective approach for automatic and accurate segmentation of brain tissues from the MRI image.

Accurate segmentation can be challenging due to the tissue heterogeneity, which is caused by noise, bias filed and partial volume effects in brain MRI [8, 9]. To overcome these issues, great deals of efforts have been made to propose a number of approaches for brain tissue segmentation in the past two decades. These methods can be mainly categorized into three main-streams, i.e. level set methods [10], classification approaches [11–13] and atlas based methods [14]. The level set methods in natural images are extent to the brain tissue segmentation, which are sensitive to user initialization and parameter settings [10]. Several clustering methods have been employed for brain tissue segmentation, such as the Gaussian mixture model [11] and fuzzy C-means [12]. Besides, the tissue atlases have been employed to propose effective segmentation methods to enable accurate segmentation of tissues [14].

* Correspondence: kongyouyong@seu.edu.cn
[1]Laboratory of Image Science and Technology, Key Laboratory of Computer Network and Information Integration, School of Computer Science and Engineering, Southeast University, Nanjing, People's Republic of China
[2]International Joint Laboratory of Information Display and Visualization, Nanjing, People's Republic of China

The existing voxel-vise segmentation approach for MRI have drawbacks in neglecting the spatial information among data. Fortunately, the promising supervoxel technique provides a possible solution to make use of the statistical information of the local regions. In the past decade, this technique has been increasingly employed for natural image processing and analysis in the fields of computer vision and machine learning [15–17]. This powerful technique can group similar voxels into a meaningful supervoxel. The brain MRI image consists of approximately piecewise constant regions, which is suitable for generating appropriate supervoxels. Therefore, the supervoxel technique has been recently utilized for several brain MRI analysis applications, such as segmentation, registration and functional parcellation [18–21]. However, with approach supervoxels, it is still challenging to enable robust segmentation due to the tissue heterogeneity [22, 23].

To cope with these issues, this paper proposes an effective algorithm for the brain tissue segmentation based on supervoxel and graph filter. A novel distance metric is proposed to develop an efficient and effective supervoxel generation method to suppress the noise in the MRI image. After computing features from each supervoxel, a graph filter algorithm is employed to classify these supervoxels into different types of brain tissues. Experiments on two widely utilized MRI dataset demonstrate the superior performance of the proposed approach compared to the state-of-art voxel-vise and supervoxel based brain MRI segmentation algorithms. The proposed method achieves mean dice similarity coefficient (DSC) of 0.94, 0.92 and 0.90 for the segmentation of white matter (WM), grey matter (GM) and cerebrospinal fluid (CSF) for BrainWeb 18 dataset, and mean DSC of 0.85, 0.87 and 0.57 for the segmentation of WM, GM and CSF for IBSR18 dataset.

Methods
Materials
The MRI datasets in this study includes the BrainWeb 18 MRI dataset [24] and the Internet Brain Segmentation Repository (IBSR) dataset [25]. The BrainWeb 18 dataset has 18 MRI images from the McConnell Brain Imaging Centre. The images are simulated with different level of noise ranging from 0 to 9% and with an intensity non-uniformity (INU) level of 0, 20% or 40%. Each image includes $181 \times 217 \times 60$ voxels with 1 mm × 1 mm × 1 mm. The IBSR dataset is consisting of 18 real MRI images derived from healthy subjects. Each MRI volume has a size of $256 \times 256 \times 128$ voxels with 1 mm × 1 mm × 2 mm. All the images in the two datasets are provided with the ground truth tissue segmentation of WM, GM and CSF.

Methods
The proposed method mainly includes two steps, i.e. supervoxel generation and supervoxel classification. An effective supervoxel algorithm is first employed to over segment the brain MRI volume into a number of small compact supervoxels with homogenous appearance. These supervoxels are then classified into different types of tissues based on graph filter.

Supervoxel generation for brain MRI
In the past decade, a number of algorithms have been proposed to generate meaningful supervoxels with homogeneous regions. The commonly used algorithms are normalized cuts, mean shift, turbo pixels and the simple linear iterative clustering (SLIC) method. Normalized cuts [26] recursively partitions a graph to globally minimize the cost function. Its high computational complexity limits its application for images with a large size. Mean shift [27] is a gradient based method, which generates supervoxels by recursively moving to the kernel smoothed centroid. This approach cannot control the size and the compactness of supervoxels, which may produce irregular supervoxels. The turbo pixel method [28] perform supervoxel generation by evolving the geometric flow from seeds sampled uniformly on the image plane. The SLIC method [29] employs the k-means clustering to classify neighborhood voxels into each seed for generating compact supervoxels. This efficient method can control the number and compactness of the supervoxels.

Among these methods, the SLIC method has been widely applied for the high dimensional MRI images due to its efficiency [30–32]. SLIC initially generates a number of cluster centers sampled at regular intervals of length at each dimension of the image plane or volume. The length L is calculated by the number of voxel N and the number of supervoxels q as $L = \sqrt[3]{N/q}$. The cluster centers are then perturbed to the lowest position in a neighborhood to avoid placing them at an edge. The voxel within a $2L \times 2L \times 2L$ area round the center on the xyz plane are clustered into each supervoxel based on their intensity and location similarity, which guarantees the homogeneity and compactness of supervoxels. After clustering all the voxels into the nearest cluster center, a new center is calculated as the average intensity and spatial positions of all the voxels belonging to this cluster. The process of clustering is iteratively repeated until that the distance between the new centers and the previous ones is smaller than a threshold.

In the SLIC algorithm, images are considered as approximately uniform for homogeneous regions. However, MRI images are always contaminated by the Rician noise in the imaging process. The voxel similarity measurements in the SLIC method may be unreliable on MRI images. To overcome this problem, a novel voxel similarity measurement is proposed to suppress the noise as

$$d_{int} = \|G^*I_{N_i} - I_c\|$$
$$d = d_{int} + \gamma d_{spa} \qquad (1)$$

where I_{N_i} represent the intensity matrices of the cubic image patches with central voxel N_i and I_c denotes the intensity of seed c. Function G represents the standard Gaussian kernel and $*$ denotes the convolution operator. The intensity distance between the voxel N_i and the seed c is denoted as d_{int}, and the spatial similarity between the voxels and seed is represented as d_{spa}. A regularization parameter γ is introduced to weigh the relative importance between voxel intensity and the spatial proximity. The regularization parameter is set 0.2 empirically in this study. The parameter of Gaussian kernel is adopted to the noise level estimated using the median absolute deviation method [33].

Figure 1 illustrates the supervoxels generated from a noisy brain MRI image using the SLIC, monoSLIC [34], regularity preserved supervoxel (RSV) method [35] and our proposed method. It can be easily seen that the original SLIC method is sensitive to the noise, and generate irregular supervoxels. MonoSLIC and RSV methods can generate regular supervoxels with a bad adherence of the tissue boundaries, especially at the cortex regions. Our approach can guarantee the boundaries of supervoxels to adhere well the brain tissue boundaries in image. Furthermore, our suepervoxel algorithm makes the size of supervoxel as regular as possible. The proposed supervoxel technique has high potential to be applied for the MRI images of other organs or other medical images, such as computed tomography and ultrasound imaging [36, 37].

Supervoxel classification based on graph filter
After generating supervoxels for the 3D brain MRI image, it is essential to develop an effective approach to classify these supervoxels into different types of tissues to enable an accurate segmentation. Here we propose to classify these supervoxels based on an effective graph filter

approach [38]. An undirected weighted graph $G = \{V, A\}$ is constructed for the MRI image. As there are huge number of voxels in the brain MRI volume, we construct a graph among the above generated supervoxels, which can highly reduce the computational complexity. The nodes $V = \{v_1, v_2, ..., v_N\}$ of the graph are supervoxels, and A is a $N \times N$ weighted adjacency matrix. Each node is represented by the intensity features derived from the corresponding supervoxel. The weight between each node is obtained by computing the similarity between the nodes using the radial basis function between the features

$$A(i, j) = \exp\left\{-\frac{(v_i - v_j)^2}{2\alpha}\right\} \qquad (2)$$

where v_i represents the value of feature in node i and α represents hyper parameter. As the supervoxels in the same class have similar features, each node is only connected to K nearest neighbors in the graph.

Similar to traditional digital signal processing, filters can be performed on the graph signal. It has been demonstrated that a graph filter H can be linear and shift invariant with the assumption of the equation between the characteristic and minimal polynomials of the adjacency matrix. The graph filter is defined as

$$H = h(A) = \sum_{l=0}^{L} h_l A^l \qquad (3)$$

where A is the adjacency matrix, and L represents the taps of filter.

This study proposes a semi-supervised segmentation approach with a few number of known labels. The segmentation is performed by classification of supervoxels using an adaptive graph filter. The graph filter propagates the nodes of known labels to predict the nodes of unknown labels, defined as

$$s^{predict} = h(A)s^{known} \qquad (4)$$

The optimal taps can be adaptively determined by adaptively constructing filter based on the initial labels. For the nodes V^{known} of the the initial known labels, the the label s^{known} is set to -1 or 1 and the unknown labels

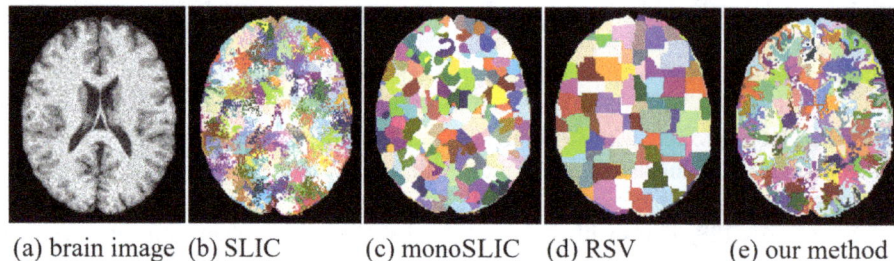

(a) brain image (b) SLIC   (c) monoSLIC   (d) RSV   (e) our method

Fig. 1 Supervoxels of a noisy brain MRI image using SLIC and our proposed method. **a** is the original brain MRI image, **b**, **c**, **d** and **e** are the supervoxel results from the SLIC, monoSLIC, RSV and the proposed method

are set to 0. A smaller subset of training nodes V^{train} is selected from the nodes with known labels V^{known}. A graph filter can be found from the training nodes that correctly classify the nodes in V^{known}. An adaptive filter can thus be estimated from the selected training nodes with a least square minimization problem

$$argmin \left\| Dh(A) \, s^{train} - 1_N \right\| \qquad (5)$$

where $D = diag(s^{known})$ is the diagonal matrix with initial known labels on its main diagonal. The binary classifier can be extent to the multi-class classification in brain tissue segmentation by the one-against-all strategy.

Results

The performance of the proposed method was evaluated on two widely used datasets, including the BrainWeb 18 MRI dataset [24] and the Internet Brain Segmentation Repository (IBSR) dataset [25]. The number of supervoxel was set to 4000 empirically for these two datasets in the experiments and the taps of filter L was set to 4 in the experiments.

The performance of the proposed approach is compared with other state-of-the-arts, including two voxel-wise methods and one promising supervoxel based methods. The two voxel-wise methods are the FMRIB Software Library v5.0 (FSL) [39] and Statistical Parametric Mapping (SPM8) [40], which are widely used in the neuroscience community. The FSL software employs expectation maximization algorithm with hidden Markov random field model for segmentation. The SPM8 tool utilizes atlas based approach with the probabilistic atlases of brain tissues. The supervoxel based method is a

recently developed approach especially for brain tissue segmentation [20].

Figure 2 illustrates the brain tissue segmentation results of the image volume with a noise level of 9% and an INU level of 40% from the BrainWeb dataset. In the figure, the 2D axial, sagittal and coronal views of 3D segmentation results are shown for visual inspections using the itk-snap tool [41]. The first and second columns are the image and the ground truth of the segmentation with red, green, blue voxels corresponding to CSF, GM and WM tissues, respectively. The third, fourth, fifth, sixth, seventh and eighth column illustrate the segmentation results of the FSL, FSL on denoised data, SPM8, SPM8 on denoised data, ITDS methods and our proposed algorithm. As the ground truth for reference, we can observe the advantage of our proposed segmentation over other three approaches. In particular, the proposed method shows apparently better delineations of the WM and GM tissues. With the results on the denoised data with FSL (the fifth column) and SPM8(the seventh column), the FSL and SPM method cannot obtain better results on denoised MRI volumes [33]. This may be because that these two segmentation models consider the noise in the MRI volume, and the denoised data corrupt the intrinsic features.

To further assess the performance objectively, quantitative evaluation is performed by calculating the dice similarity coefficient (DSC) and volume difference ratio (VDR) [42–44]. These metrics are commonly utilized benchmark evaluation strategies in the segmentation community. The DSC metric measures the similarity between automatic segmentation results and ground truth for each tissue, defined as

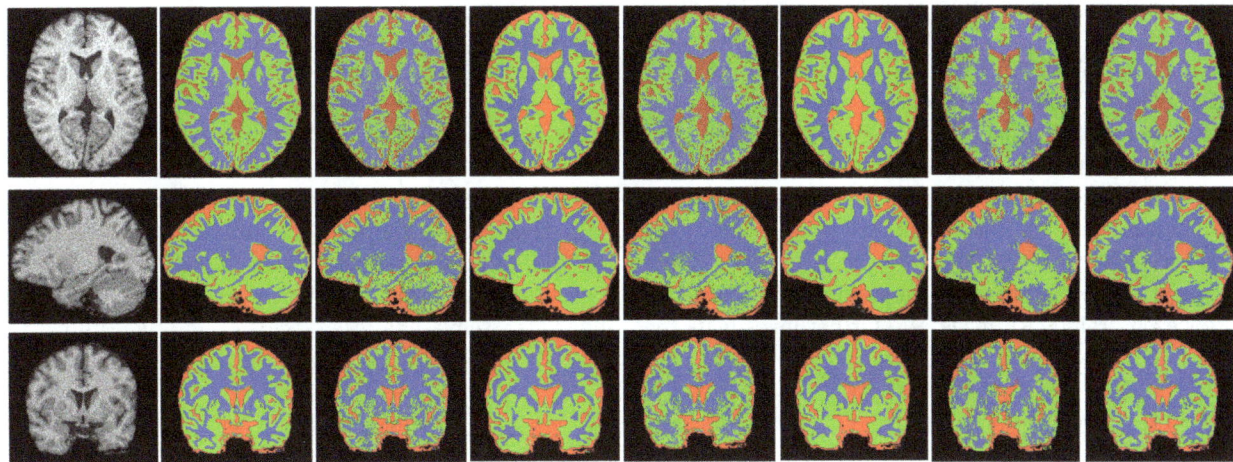

(a) Brain image (b) Truth　　　(c) FSL　　　(d) FSL(denoised)　　(e) SPM8　(f) SPM8(denoised) (g) ITDS　　　(h) Proposed

Fig. 2 Segmentation results using different methods for the brain image with 9% noise and INU level of 40% from the BrainWeb18 dataset. The colors of red, green and blue represents the labels of segmentation for cerebrospinal fluid (CSF), grey matter (GM) and white matter (WM). The three rows are the two dimensional axial, sagittal and coronal views of three dimensional segmentation results, respectively. Column (**a**) and (**b**) are the original image and the ground truth of the segmentation. Column (**c-g**) are the segmentation results of the FSL, FSL on denoised data, SPM8, SPM8 on denoised data, ITDS and the proposed method

Table 1 Performance of segmentation results on the BrainWeb18 dataset

	DSC			VDR		
	WM	GM	CSF	WM	GM	CSF
FSL	0.91 ± 0.04	0.88 ± 0.03	0.89 ± 0.01	0.10 ± 0.08	0.08 ± 0.05	0.24 ± 0.01
SPM8	0.91 ± 0.03	0.90 ± 0.02	0.89 ± 0.03	0.06 ± 0.05	0.05 ± 0.01	0.14 ± 0.06
ITDS	0.90 ± 0.05	0.88 ± 0.05	0.88 ± 0.04	0.07 ± 0.03	0.06 ± 0.02	0.12 ± 0.05
Proposed	0.94 ± 0.01	0.92 ± 0.01	0.90 ± 0.01	0.02 ± 0.01	0.02 ± 0.01	0.04 ± 0.01

$$DSC = \frac{2 \times TP}{2 \times TP + FP + FN} \qquad (6)$$

The VDR metric measures the volume difference between and the ground truth and the achieved segmentation results, defined a s

$$VDR = \frac{|FP-FN|}{TP + FN} \qquad (7)$$

where TP, FP and FN are the numbers of true positive, false positive and false negative voxels, respectively. A higher value of DSC and a lower value of VDR represent a better correspondence to the ground truth, which denotes a higher accuracy of the segmentation results.

Tables 1 and 2 shows the performance of the segmentation results for each method on the BrainWeb18 and IBSR18 datasets, respectively. As for the BrainWeb18 dataset, the proposed method provides the highest DSC values on CSF, GM and WM, followed by SPM8, FSL and ITDS. The ITDS method using traditional SLIC supervoxel method is sensitive to the noise in the images from the BrainWeb18 dataset. As for the IBSR18 dataset, the proposed method achieves best performance in segmentation of CSF and GM, and obtains comparable accuracy of WM segmentation compared with the other three methods. The ITDS can achieve better performance than the SPM8 and FSL for the low level of noise in the images of the IBSR18 dataset. The VDR value is quite lower than other three methods for the two datasets and especially for the IBSR18 dataset. This is because that the proposed method under-estimate the CSF tissue due to the small training number of supervoxels.

TIn the above experiments, the ratio of labels is set to 0.3 for each brain MRI image. We further investigate the

effect of the ratios for the segmentation accuracy in the proposed framework. The segmentation accuracies for each type of tissue are computed at the ratio of 0.02, 0.05, 0.1, 0.15, 0.2 and 0.3 for both the BrainWeb18 and IBSR18 dataset. Figures 3 and 4 illustrates the average DSC and VDR values of different volumes for the tissues of WM, GM and CSF at different ratio of known labels.

To further evaluate the effectiveness of the proposed supervoxel method, we compare the performance with the monSLIC and RSV method. All the methods generate about 4000 supervoxels, and same parameters are set with 30% labels with each types of tissues in the classification stage. For the BrainWeb datasets, the DSC values of results with the monSLIC method are 0.74, 0.71, 0.60 for WM, GM and CSF, and DSC values of results with the RSV method are 0.70, 0.72, and 0.69. For the IBSR datasets, the DSC values of results with the monSLIC method are 0.78, 0.84 and 0.53 for WM, GM and CSF, and DSC values of results with the RSV method are 0. 67, 0.78 and 0.40. Our method obtains better performance than other two popular supervoxels for the two datasets.

Discussion

The results on the two commonly utilized datasets demonstrated the effectiveness of the proposed brain tissue segmentation algorithm based on both qualitative and quantitative evaluations. The performance was achieved due to the appropriate supervoxels and the effective clustering approach. At first, a novel supervoxel method was developed to suppress the influence of noise in MRI to guarantee the boundaries of supervoxels to adhere well the brain tissue boundaries in image. Secondly, an effective semi-supervised clustering algorithm was

Table 2 Performance of segmentation results on the IBSR18 dataset

	DSC			VDR		
	WM	GM	CSF	WM	GM	CSF
FSL	0.87 ± 0.03	0.76 ± 0.03	0.53 ± 0.06	0.11 ± 0.13	0.23 ± 0.04	1.32 ± 0.37
SPM8	0.87 ± 0.01	0.80 ± 0.04	0.55 ± 0.06	0.06 ± 0.04	0.18 ± 0.04	1.11 ± 0.39
ITDS	0.86 ± 0.02	0.81 ± 0.03	0.60 ± 0.05	0.07 ± 0.06	0.16 ± 0.05	0.75 ± 0.38
Proposed	0.85 ± 0.01	0.87 ± 0.03	0.57 ± 0.08	0.08 ± 0.05	0.04 ± 0.03	0.17 ± 0.10

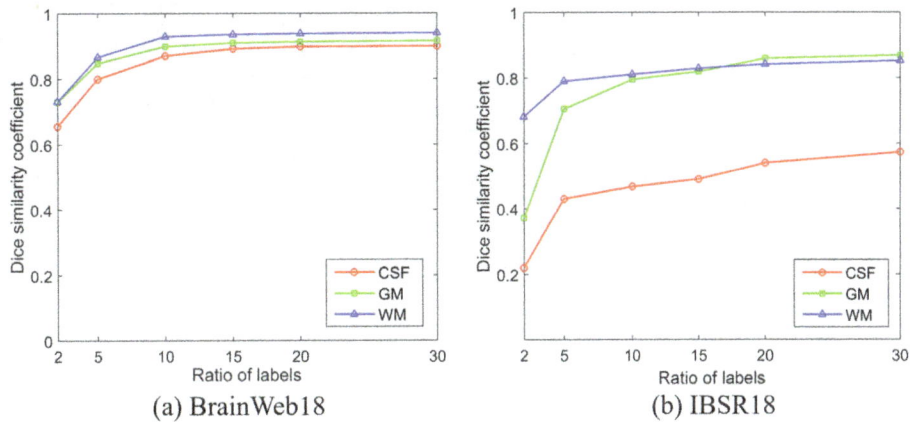

Fig. 3 Dice similarity coefficients of segmentation results for the BrainWeb 18 and IBSR 18 datasets using our proposed method with different ratio of labels

proposed based on graph filtering to classify the supervoxels into three types of tissues.

For the performance on the two datasets, there were dramatically decrease accuracy of CSF in the IBSR 18 compared with those from the BrainWeb18 dataset. There are two main reasons for such results. Firstly, the BrainWeb18 dataset is a simulated dataset, and the IBSR18 dataset is a real dataset. The BrainWeb 18 dataset can be easy segmented while it is more difficult for the IBSR18 dataset. Secondly, among the three tissues, CSF has a small number of voxels compared to GM and WM. The employed DSC and VDR values measure the overlapping ratio and volume difference between automatic segmentation results and ground truth. Therefore, a same number of wrong segmented voxels can lead to a larger decrease of the DSC values or a large increase of VDR values for CSF compared with the other two tissues.

For the supervoxel clustering, it is apparent that with a small ratio of labels, there was a relatively low

segmentation performance for all three tissues. Increasing the ratio of labels can obtain consistent increasing segmentation accuracy of all the three tissues. There was a slight improvement of performance when the ratio of labels is more than 0.15, which was sufficient enough to learn the intrinsic features of different types of tissues.

Conclusions

In this paper, we have proposed an effective algorithm for brain tissue segmentation from the MRI image based on supervoxel and graph filter. An effective supervoxel algorithm was proposed to suppress the noise influence in the MRI images. The supervoxels were then classified into three types of tissues integrating features using graph filter. Qualitative and quantitative evaluations on two widely utilized MRI datasets demonstrate the superior performance of the proposed approach compared to the state-of-art brain MRI segmentation algorithms.

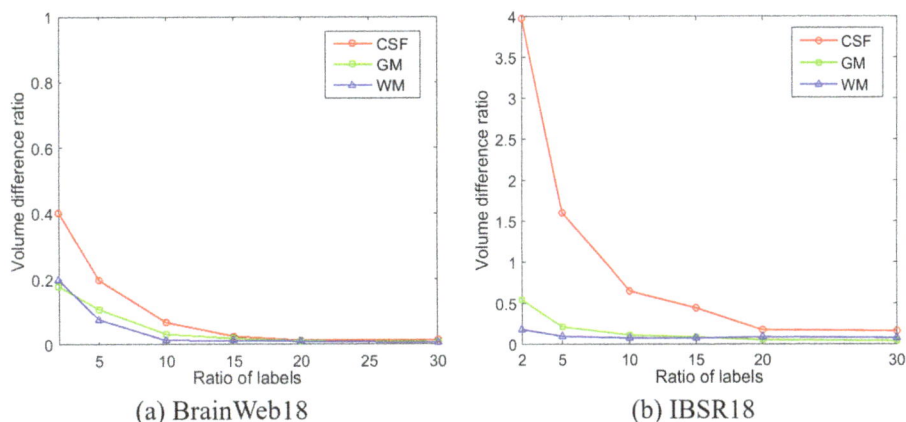

Fig. 4 Volume difference ratios of segmentation results for the BrainWeb 18 and IBSR 18 datasets using our proposed method with different ratio of labels

Abbreviations

CSF: Cerebrospinal fluid; DSC: Dice similarity coefficient; FSL: FMRIB Software Library; GM: Grey matter; IBSR: Internet Brain Segmentation Repository; INU: Intensity non-uniformity; MRI: Magnetic resonance imaging; RSV: Regularity preserved supervoxel; SLIC: Simple linear iterative clustering; SPM: Statistical Parametric Mapping; WM: White matter

Acknowledgements

We acknowledge Key Laboratory of Computer Network and Information Integration, Southeast University, Ministry of Education, Nanjing, People's Republic of China for providing us the computing platform.

Funding

The research is supported by grant BK20150650 Natural Science Foundation of Jiangsu Province, China and grant 31640028 National Natural Science Foundation of China. This work was supported in part by the State's Key Project of Research and Development Plan under Grants 2017YFC0107900, 2017YFC0109202, in part by the Fundamental Research Funds for the Central Universities and Short-term Recruitment Program of Foreign Experts (WQ20163200398).

Authors' contributions

YYK and HZS designed the proposed method. XPC and PZZ implemented this method. YC and JSW performed the experiments and the analysis of the results. All authors have been involved in drafting and revising the manuscript and approved the final version to be published. All authors read and approved the final manuscript.

Competing interests

The authors declare that they have no competing interests.

References

1. Yang G, Nawaz T, Barrick TR, Howe FA, Slabaugh G. Discrete wavelet transform-based whole-spectral and subspectral analysis for improved brain tumor clustering using single voxel MR spectroscopy. IEEE Trans Biomed Eng. 2015;62(12):2860–6.
2. Zheng H, Qu XB, Bai ZJ, Liu YS, Guo D, Dong JY, et al. Multi-contrast brain magnetic resonance image super-resolution using the local weight similarity. BMC Med Imaging. 2017;17(6):1–13.
3. Wang SH, Zhang Y, Zhan TM, Phillips P, Zhang YD, Liu G, et al. Pathological brain detection by artificial intelligence in magnetic resonance imaging scanning. Prog Electromagn Res. 2016;156:105–33.
4. Sauwen N, Acou M, Sima DM, Veraart J, Maes F, Himmelreich U, et al. Semi-automated brain tumor segmentation on multi-parametric MRI using regularized non-negative matrix factorization. BMC Med Imaging. 2017;17(29):1–14.
5. Kong Y, Shi L, Hui SC, Wang D, Deng M, Chu WC, et al. Variation in anisotropy and diffusivity along the medulla oblongata and the whole spinal cord in adolescent idiopathic scoliosis: a pilot study using diffusion tensor imaging. AJNR Am J Neuroradiol. 2014;35(8):1621–7.
6. Magnoni S, Mac Donald CL, Esparza TJ, Conte V, Sorrell J, Macri M, et al. Quantitative assessments of traumatic axonal injury in human brain: concordance of microdialysis and advanced MRI. Brain. 2015;138(Pt 8):2263–77.
7. Deng Y, Ren ZQ, Kong YY, Bao F, Dai QH. A hierarchical fused fuzzy deep neural network for data classification. IEEE Trans Fuzzy Syst. 2017;25(4):1006–12.
8. Wang S, Phillips P, Yang J, Sun P, Zhang Y. Magnetic resonance brain classification by a novel binary particle swarm optimization with mutation and time-varying acceleration coefficients. Biomed Tech (Berl). 2016;61(4):431–41.
9. Wang S, Zhang Y, Liu G, Phillips P, Yuan TF. Detection of Alzheimer's disease by three-dimensional displacement field estimation in structural magnetic resonance imaging. J Alzheimers Dis. 2016;50(1):233–48.
10. Li C, Huang R, Ding Z, Gatenby JC, Metaxas DN, Gore JC. A level set method for image segmentation in the presence of intensity inhomogeneities with application to MRI. IEEE Trans Image Process. 2011;20(7):2007–16.
11. Greenspan H, Ruf A, Goldberger J. Constrained Gaussian mixture model framework for automatic segmentation of MR brain images. IEEE Trans Med Imaging. 2006;25(9):1233–45.
12. Yang X, Fei B. A multiscale and multiblock fuzzy C-means classification method for brain MR images. Med Phys. 2011;38(6):2879–91.
13. Song Z, Tustison N, Avants B, Gee J. Adaptive graph cutrs with tissue priors for brain MRI segmentation. IEEE Intern Sympo Biomed Imaging. 2006:762–5.
14. Artaechevarria X, Munoz-Barrutia A, Ortiz-de-Solorzano C. Combination strategies in multi-atlas image segmentation: application to brain MR data. IEEE Trans Med Imaging. 2009;28(8):1266–77.
15. Fan Y, Huchuan L, Ming-Hsuan Y. Robust superpixel tracking. IEEE Transact Image Process. 2014;23(4):1639–51.
16. Deng Y, Bao F, Deng XS, Wang RP, Kong YY, Dai QH. Deep and structured robust information theoretic learning for image analysis. Ieee T Image Process. 2016;25(9):4209–21.
17. Li ST, Lu T, Fang LY, Jia XP, Benediktsson JA. Probabilistic fusion of pixel-level and Superpixel-level hyperspectral image classification. Ieee T Geosci Remote. 2016;54(12):7416–30.
18. Mahapatra D, Schueffler P, Tielbeek J, Makanyanga J, Stoker J, Taylor S, et al. Automatic detection and segmentation of Crohn's disease tissues from abdominal MRI. IEEE Trans Med Imaging. 2013;32(12):2332-47.
19. Wu W, Chen AY, Zhao L, Corso JJ. Brain tumor detection and segmentation in a CRF (conditional random fields) framework with pixel-pairwise affinity and superpixel-level features. Int J Comput Assist Radiol Surg. 2014;9(2):241–53.
20. Kong Y, Deng Y, Dai Q. Discriminative clustering and feature selection for brain MRI segmentation. IEEE Signal Processing Letters. 2015;22(5):573–7.
21. Soltaninejad M, Yang G, Lambrou T, Allinson N, Jones TL, Barrick TR, et al. Automated brain tumour detection and segmentation using superpixel-based extremely randomized trees in FLAIR MRI. Int J Comput Assist Radiol Surg. 2017;12(2):183–203.
22. Amoroso N, Errico R, Bruno S, Chincarini A, Garuccio E, Sensi F, et al. Hippocampal unified multi-atlas network (HUMAN): protocol and scale validation of a novel segmentation tool. Phys Med Biol. 2015;60(22):8851–67.
23. Morra JH, Tu Z, Apostolova LG, Green AE, Avedissian C, Madsen SK, et al. Validation of a fully automated 3D hippocampal segmentation method using subjects with Alzheimer's disease mild cognitive impairment, and elderly controls. NeuroImage. 2008;43(1):59–68.
24. Kwan RK, Evans AC, Pike GB. MRI simulation-based evaluation of image-processing and classification methods. IEEE Trans Med Imaging. 1999;18(11):1085–97.
25. Cocosco C, Kollokian V, Kwan R, Pike G, Evans A. Brainweb: online interface to a 3D MRI simulated brain database. NeuroImage. 1997;5:425.
26. Shi J, Malik J. Normalized cuts and image segmentation. IEEE Trans Pattern Anal Mach Intell. 2000;22(8):888–905.
27. Comaniciu D, Meer P. Mean shift: a robust approach toward feature space analysis. IEEE Trans Pattern Anal Mach Intell. 2002;24(5):603–19.
28. Lehmann F. Turbo segmentation of textured images. IEEE Trans Pattern Anal Mach Intell. 2011;33(1):16–29.
29. Achanta R, Shaji A, Smith K, Lucchi A, Fua P, Süsstrunk S. SLIC Superpixels compared to state-of-the-art Superpixel methods. IEEE Trans Pattern Anal Mach Intell. 2012;34(11):2274–82.
30. Heinrich MP, Simpson IJ, Papiez BW, Brady SM, Schnabel JA. Deformable image registration by combining uncertainty estimates from supervoxel belief propagation. Med Image Anal. 2016;27:57–71.
31. Tian Z, Liu L, Zhang Z, Fei B. Superpixel-based segmentation for 3D prostate MR images. IEEE Trans Med Imaging. 2016;35(3):791–801.
32. Verma N, Cowperthwaite MC, Markey MK. Superpixels in brain MR image analysis. Conf Proc IEEE Eng Med Biol Soc. 2013;2013:1077-1080.
33. Coupe P, Manjon JV, Gedamu E, Arnold D, Robles M, Collins DL. Robust Rician noise estimation for MR images. Med Image Anal. 2010;14(4):483–93.
34. Holzer M, Rene D. Over-segmentation of 3D medical image volumes based on monogenic cues. Computer vision winter workshop. 2014. p. 35–42.
35. Fu HZ, Cao XC, Tang D, Han YH, Xu D. Regularity preserved Superpixels and Supervoxels. IEEE Transact Multimedia. 2014;16(4):1165–75.
36. Chen Y, Shi LY, Feng QJ, Yang J, Shu HZ, Luo LM, et al. Artifact suppressed dictionary learning for low-dose CT image processing. IEEE Trans Med Imaging. 2014;33(12):2271–92.
37. Chen Y, Budde A, Li K, Li YS, Hsieh J, Chen GH. A platform-independent method to reduce CT truncation artifacts using discriminative dictionary representations. Med Phys. 2017;44(1):121–31.
38. Sandryhaila A, Moura JMF. Discrete signal processing on graphs: graph filters. IEEE International Conference on Acoustics, Speech and Signal Processing. 2013. 6163–6.

25

Use of ^{18}F-sodium fluoride bone PET for disability evaluation in ankle trauma

Tae Joo Jeon[1], Sungjun Kim[2], Jinyoung Park[3], Jung Hyun Park[3,5]* and Eugene Y. Roh[4]

Abstract

Background: There are no objective and accurate rating tools for permanent impairment of traumatized ankles. The purpose of this study is to assess the role of 18F-Sodium fluoride (18F-NaF) positron emission tomography-computed tomography (PET/CT) bone scans in evaluating patients with limited ankle range of motion (ROM) after trauma.

Methods: 18F-NaF PET/CT was performed in 121 patients (75 men, 46 women; mean age: 45.8) who had ROM < 70% of normal after trauma affecting ankles. Metabolic target volume (MTV), the sum of voxels with standardized uptake value (SUV) > 2.5 was automatically obtained from the 3D volume that included the ankle joint. The maximum & mean SUV (SUVmax & SUVmean), and the total lesion activity (TLA) were measured.

Results: The median period from injury to performing 18F-NaF PET/CT was 290 days. The causes of injury were as follows: fracture ($N = 95$), Achilles tendon rupture ($N = 12$), and ligament injury ($N = 12$). Hot uptake in the ankle was seen in 113 of 121 patients. The fracture group had higher SUVmax, SUVmean, and TLA values than the non-fracture group. More limited ROM correlated with higher hot-uptake parameters (SUVmax, SUVmean, TLA). In subgroup analysis, the same correlations were present in the fracture, but not in the non-fracture group.

Conclusions: 18F-NaF PET/CT can provide considerable information in impairment evaluations of limited ankle ROM, particularly in fracture around the ankle. Thus, 18F-NaF bone PET/CT may provide an additional option as an objective imaging tool in disability assessment after ankle injury.

Keywords: Ankle injuries, Disability evaluation, PET-CT, Positron emission tomography, Range of motion

Background

Limitation of range of motion (ROM) in the ankle is common after ankle trauma, even after the time has passed for maximum medical improvement (MMI). Ankle stiffness causes difficulties in walking and restrictions in the activities of daily living, which is worse when it is accompanied by pain. The objective and accurate rating of permanent impairment is very important in workers' compensation programs or automobile insurance, to determine an appropriate level of financial compensation [1, 2]. However, the impairment of ROM in the ankle joint is difficult to evaluate because it is based on direct observations, such as the patients' own activities, which can be subjective and are easily influenced by pain or by their motivations to improve, rather than on objective measurement [3]. Radiologic studies performed immediately after injury are helpful to provide information about the severity of the trauma; however, after achieving MMI, it is impossible to find a correlation between the functional impairment of the ankle joint (pain or limitation of ROM) and the latest objective radiologic assessments (simple plain radiography, computerized tomography [CT], or magnetic resonance imaging).

Impairment of the ankle joint, such as contracture or limitation of ROM, can occur after traumatic injury; its

* Correspondence: RMPJH@yuhs.ac
[3]Department of Rehabilitation Medicine, Gangnam Severance Hospital, Rehabilitation Institute of Neuromuscular Disease, Yonsei University College of Medicine, Seoul, South Korea
[5]Department of Rehabilitation Medicine, Gangnam Severance Hospital, Yonsei University College of Medicine, 211 Eonjuro, Gangnam-gu, Seoul 06273, South Korea
Full list of author information is available at the end of the article

pathomechanism may be explained by the concept of posttraumatic osteoarthritis (PTA) [4]. Ankle PTA after intra-articular injury could be related to the initial articular cartilage and subchondral bone damage, inadequate reduction of joint surfaces, or complications in the healing process [4–6]. Extra-articular injuries not involving joint structures could also cause end-stage ankle PTA by chronic instability or the long-term effects of posttraumatic malalignment [4, 7]. Furthermore, fibrosis of the soft tissue can play a role in post-traumatic joint contractures [8]. Posttraumatic Immobilization induces limitation of ROM by disuse osteoporosis and reversible bone loss with increased osteoclastic bone resorption in the mechanically unloaded bone [9]. However, to date, no biomarker has been available to represent ROM of the joint after injury.

Bone scanning using ^{18}F-sodium fluoride (18F-NaF) was performed by Blau et al. in 1962, [10] but this was rapidly replaced by technetium-99 m (^{99m}Tc)-labeled bone imaging agents after the introduction of gamma cameras equipped with a thallium-doped sodium iodide (NaI [Tl]) crystal. However, as positron emission tomography (PET) cameras came into use, interest in 18F-NaF bone scanning has renewed [11]. The uptake mechanism of 18F-NaF and ^{99m}Tc-labeled diphosphonate is essentially the same, involving chemisorption, and the amount of bone accumulation depends on blood flow and the exposed bone surface [12]. However, negligible plasma protein binding, and the rapid blood and renal clearance of NaF permits earlier image acquisition after tracer administration. Therefore, 18F-NaF bone scanning has several advantages, such as enabling high spatial resolution, attenuating correction, allowing 3D tomographic imaging, as well as hybrid PET/CT imaging [11, 13]. Similar to ^{99m}Tc agents, 18F-NaF has been mainly used for evaluation of bone metastasis; however, these high resolution tomographic images, with their corresponding CT images, are also very useful for evaluation of benign joint disease, such as enthesopathy, degenerative joint disease, and osteophytosis [14].

Impairment of ankle ROM after trauma has commonly been evaluated by physical examination by a doctor or therapist, which is subjective, rather than objective quantitative evaluation of images. In this study, the role of 18F-NaF bone PET/CT in the evaluation of impairment in trauma patients with limited ankle ROM was assessed.

Methods

Patients

Between September 2013 and March 2017, 121 patients (75 men and 46 women, mean age: 45.8 years; range: 17–75 years) were recruited into the study (Table 1); these patients had limited ankle ROM at least 6 months

after traumatic injury affecting their ankles. The etiology of injury varied: 1) fracture with intra-articular involvement of the tibiotalar joint, 2) fracture without intra-articular involvement, 3) ligament injury, 4) Achilles tendon rupture, and 5) others. These individuals attended the outpatients' clinic of a university hospital for an evaluation of the impairment of their ankles. For the impairment rating, the ROM of the ankle joint was measured according to "*AMA Guides to the Evaluation of Permanent Impairment*" [15]. Images of the ankles were obtained by plain radiography and 18F-NaF PET/CT. The study was approved by the institutional review board of our institute, and written informed consent was obtained from all study participants.

18F-NaF bone PET/CT imaging

18F-NaF bone PET/CT imaging was conducted in accordance with *SNM practice guidelines for Sodium F-18 Fluoride PET/CT bone scan 1.0* [16]. Patient fasting was not required, and 5.18 MBq/kg (0.14 mCi/kg) of 18F-NaF was injected. Regional PET with non-contrast-enhanced CT for attenuation correction was performed consecutively, 60 min after the injection of 18F-NaF, by means of a dedicated PET/CT system (Biograph mCT; Siemens Healthcare, Munich, Germany). The parameters for CT were 120 kVp, effective mAs controlled by Care Dose 4D software, 0.5-s gantry rotation, and 0.6-mm collimation. The kernel for CT reconstruction was the B60f sharp-type. 18F-NaF PET images so acquired were reconstructed using True X and time of flight (TOF), ultra-high definition (HD)-PET.

Imaging analysis

18F-NaF PET/CT images of 121 patients with limited ROM of the ankle were reviewed using the dedicated software for PET/CT workstation (Syngo VE32B, Siemens AG). Metabolic target volume (MTV), the sum of voxels with a standardized uptake value (SUV) > 2.5 was automatically obtained from the 3D volume that included the

Table 1 Demographic data of 121 patients

Sex	
Male	75
Female	46
Mean Age (range)	45.8 (17–75)
Etiology of Injury	
Fracture with intra-articular involvement of the tibiotalar joint	54
Fracture without intra-articular involvement	41
Ligament injury	12
Achilles tendon rupture	12
Others	3

ankle joint. MTV represented the active extent of trauma-related joint disease, similar to the metabolic tumor volume that is widely used in the oncology field. Within these MTVs, maximum and mean SUV (SUVmax and SUVmean) were measured. The total lesion activity (TLA) was also determined; this concept was adopted from total lesion glycolysis (TLG), and was the product of the SUVmean and MTV. These parameters express additional information about disease activity in terms of disease extent, represented by MTV [17].

Statistical analysis

Data were analyzed using SPSS 23.0 statistical software (SPSS Inc., Chicago, IL). An independent t-test was used to compare hot-uptake parameters of 18F-NaF PET/CT between the fracture group and non-fracture group. The relationship between ankle ROM and hot-uptake parameters of 18F-NaF PET/CT was analyzed using Pearson's correlation coefficient. $P < .05$ was considered to indicate statistically significant differences.

Results

The median period from injury to performing 18F-NaF PET/CT was 290 days (range: 180–2396). The causes of injury were as follows: fracture ($N = 95$; tibia, and/or fibular, and/or calcaneus), Achilles tendon rupture ($N = 12$), complex regional pain syndrome ($N = 2$), ligament injury ($N = 12$, anterior talofibular ligament, and/or calcaneofibular ligament, and/or deltoid ligament). Quantitative

analysis of 18F-NaF PET/CT revealed that 113 of 121 patients had hot uptake (SUVmax > 2.5) in the ROI (region of interest) of the ankle, whereas the remaining 8 did not. All 8 patients who did not show hot uptake were in the non-fracture group. Representative cases are presented in Figs. 1 and 2.

The SUVmax (13.31 ± 9.42 vs. 5.33 ± 3.24, $p < .01$), SUVmean (5.92 ± 4.94 vs. 3.07 ± 1.68, $p < .05$), and TLA (268.03 ± 349.76 vs. 73.05 ± 106.20, $p < .05$, Table 2) values were higher in the fracture than in the non-fracture group. The fracture group also showed a tendency for higher values in MTV than non-fracture group without statistical significance ($p = .068$). A more limited ROM of the ankle was correlated with higher hot-uptake parameters of 18F-NaF PET/CT: SUVmax ($\rho = -0.335$, $p < .01$), SUVmean ($\rho = -0.343$, $p < .01$), MTV ($\rho = -0.252$, < 0.05), and TLA ($\rho = -0.305$, $p < .01$, Table 3). In a subgroup analysis, the fracture group revealed similar results: SUVmax ($\rho = -0.336$, $p < .01$), SUVmean ($\rho = -0.354$, $p < .01$), and TLA ($\rho = -0.292$, $p < .05$), whereas these tendencies were not observed in the non-fracture group (Table 3).

Discussion

According to our retrospective study of 18F-NaF PET/CT findings, most patients with limited ROM after ankle trauma ($113/121 = 93.4\%$) showed hot uptake around the ankle joint. However, several cases ($8/26 = 30.8\%$) in the non-fracture group did not reveal hot uptake on PET/CT, and even if some hot uptake was observed, there

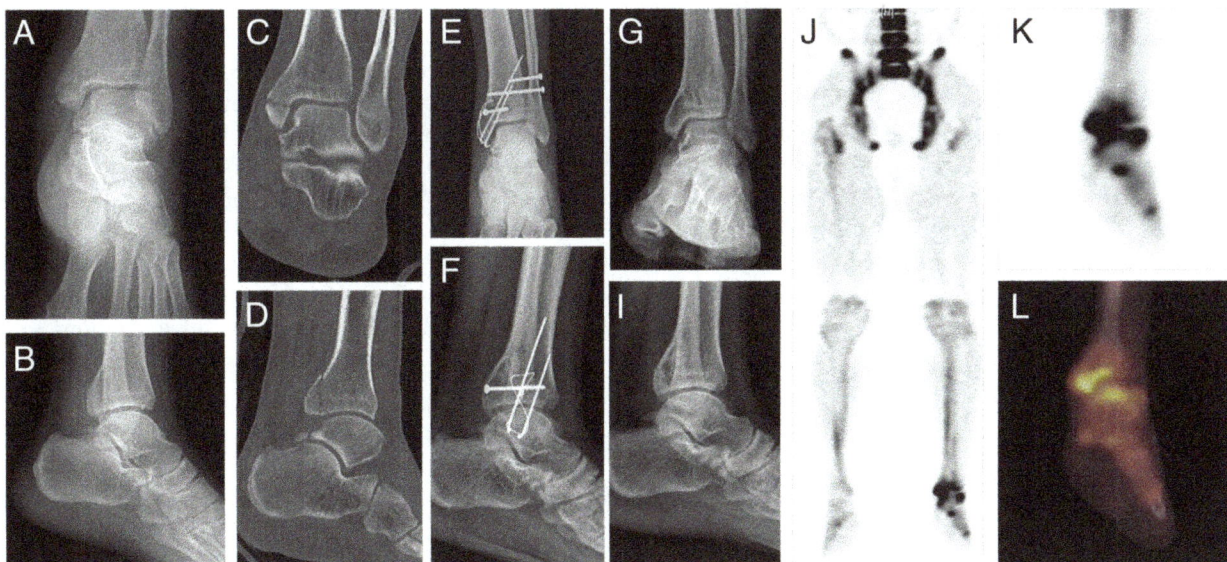

Fig. 1 Radiological and ^{18}F-Sodium fluoride (18F-NaF) positron emission tomography-computed tomography (PET/CT) images of a 37-year-old male patient who had a fracture of the left medial and posterior malleolus of the tibia. **a-d** Initial images of plain radiographs and computed tomography (CT); **a** ankle anterior-posterior view, **b** ankle lateral view, **c** ankle CT coronal view, **d** ankle CT lateral view. Note that the fracture involved the talocrural (tibiotalar) joint. **e, f** Plain radiographs after internal fixation with a metal pin. **g-i** Plain radiographs performed at 17 months after injury presents pin removal status and osteoporotic changes around the ankle joint, but does not provide any information about the degree of ankylosis in the ankle. **j-l**) 18F-NaF PET/CT shows hot uptake around the talocrural joint near the initial fracture area

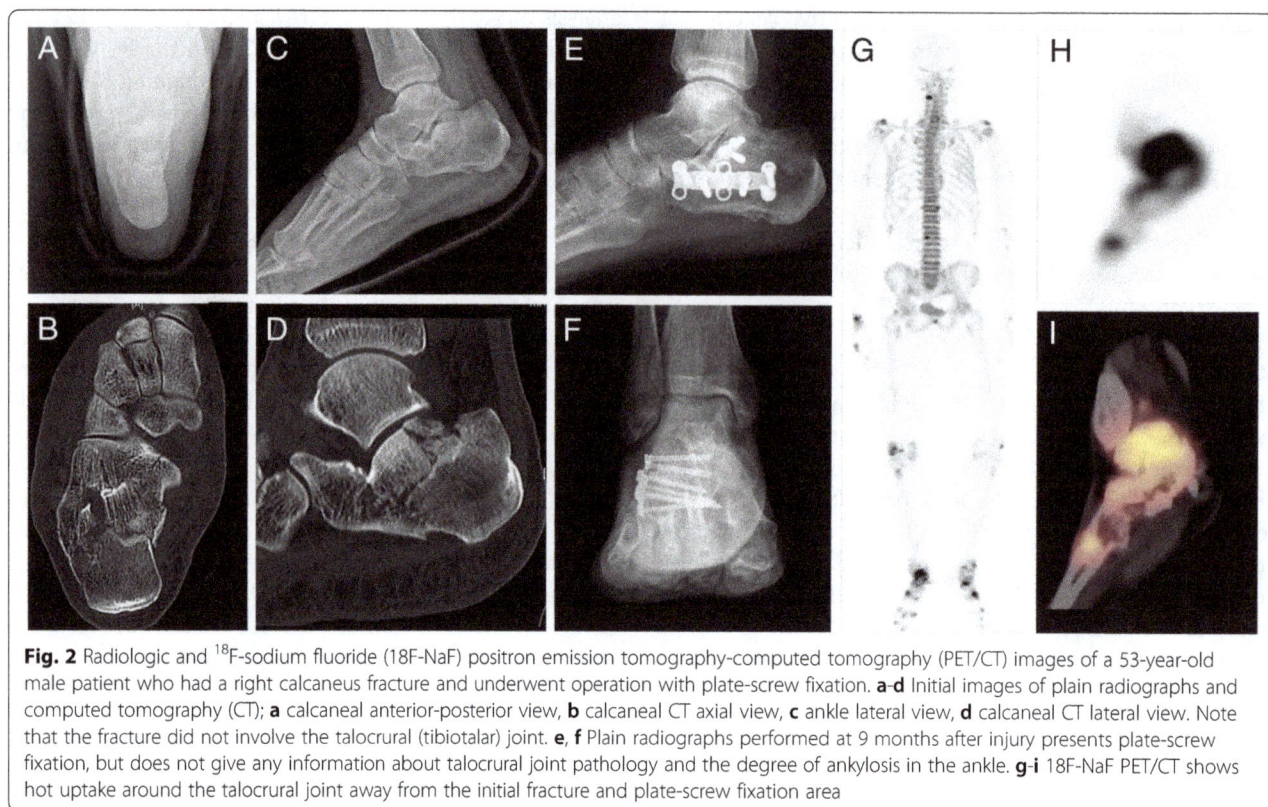

Fig. 2 Radiologic and ^{18}F-sodium fluoride (18F-NaF) positron emission tomography-computed tomography (PET/CT) images of a 53-year-old male patient who had a right calcaneus fracture and underwent operation with plate-screw fixation. **a-d** Initial images of plain radiographs and computed tomography (CT); **a** calcaneal anterior-posterior view, **b** calcaneal CT axial view, **c** ankle lateral view, **d** calcaneal CT lateral view. Note that the fracture did not involve the talocrural (tibiotalar) joint. **e, f** Plain radiographs performed at 9 months after injury presents plate-screw fixation, but does not give any information about talocrural joint pathology and the degree of ankylosis in the ankle. **g-i** 18F-NaF PET/CT shows hot uptake around the talocrural joint away from the initial fracture and plate-screw fixation area

was no statistical significant correlation between the degree of hot uptake and the limitation of ankle ROM (Table 3). In contrast, 100% patients in the fracture group ($N = 95$) showed hot uptake around the ankle joint, and the quantitative parameters (SUVmax and SUVmean, but not MTV) were statistically significantly correlated with the limitation of ankle ROM (Table 3). Therefore, it can be assumed that the "intensity" of hot uptake was more relevant than the "spread" of hot uptake. These results suggest that 18F-NaF bone PET/CT can be an objective imaging tool for evaluating ankle joint disability in patients with ankle fracture.

In our study, higher hot uptake parameters of 18F-NaF PET/CT were correlated with more limited

ROM of the ankle joint. As 18F-NaF is a bone imaging agent, the higher uptake of this agent in patients with greater immobility and soft tissue rigidity requires some explanation. Tatsuya et al. reported arthroscopic mobilization of the wrist by removing a septum that was assumed to have developed after trauma [8]. They reported that this septum could not be detected by plain radiographs, magnetic resonance image, or CT. Moreover, they reported that arthroscopic surgery could not restore the full ROM, and that immature chondrocytes were observed around the fibers. Furthermore, the joint contracture could be produced by altered length-tension relationships and neuromuscular mechanisms after fractures [18]. During the period of ankle fixation, some

Table 2 Comparison of hot uptake parameters of 18F-NaF PET/CT between the fracture group and the non-fracture group

	Fracture ($N = 95$)	Non-fracture ($N = 26$)	p-value
SUVmax	13.31 ± 9.42	5.33 ± 3.24	0.001
SUVmean	5.92 ± 4.94	3.07 ± 1.68	0.017
MTV	52.40 ± 67.09	22.86 ± 29.72	0.068
TLA	268.03 ± 349.76	73.05 ± 106.20	0.019

Values represent the mean ± standard deviation
18F-NaF PET/CT, 18-Fluorine sodium fluoride bone positron emission tomography-computed tomography; *MTV* metabolic target volume, *SUVmax* maximum standardized uptake value, *SUVmean* mean standardized uptake value, *TLA* total lesion activity

Table 3 Correlation coefficient between ankle ROM and hot uptake parameters of 18F-NaF PET/CT

	Total ($N = 121$)	Fracture ($N = 95$)	Non-fracture ($N = 26$)
SUVmax	− 0.335**	− 0.336*	− 0.102
SUVmean	− 0.343**	− 0.354**	− 0.059
MTV	− 0.252*	− 0.223	− 0.317
TLA	− 0.305**	− 0.292*	− 0.265

Values represent Pearson's correlation coefficient. * $P < 0.05$, ** $P < 0.01$
18F-NaF PET/CT, 18-Fluorine sodium fluoride bone positron emission tomography-computed tomography; *MTV* metabolic target volume, *ROM* range of motion, *SUVmax* maximum standardized uptake value, *SUVmean* mean standardized uptake value, *TLA* total lesion activity

changes in neuromuscular conditions occur due to immobilization to protect against overstretching of the fragile musculature around the ankle joint [18]. In light of these findings about soft tissue contracture after joint trauma, the higher bone uptake of 18F-NaF in the patients with greater ROM limitation may be attributable to greater immobility caused by tighter contracture. Greater immobility is expected to cause more disuse osteoporosis. Disuse osteoporosis involves reversible bone loss, associated with increased osteoclastic bone resorption in the mechanically unloaded bone [9]. The bones affected by disuse osteoporosis are associated with eventually greater turnover of bones and show a high radiopharmaceutical uptake reflecting osteoblastic activity [19]. Greater joint contracture is therefore expected to cause more disuse osteoporosis, and consequently more osteoblastic activities which are represented as radiopharmaceutical uptake in 18F-NaF PET/CT [14, 20]. Increased osteoblastic activities may cause hypertrophic sclerosis which leads pseudoarthroses and chronic disability.

Fluorodeoxyglucose (FDG) PET/CT indicates the tissue glucose metabolic rate, and thus, when it is performed for trauma-related arthritis, it mainly reflects the inflammatory process in the soft tissue in the joint [21]. However, FDG uptake is not sensitive for detection of bone formation or periosteal bone reaction. Although conventional bone scintigraphy is known to have high sensitivity for detection of bone reaction, its resolution is not high and exact localization of hot-uptake lesions is not possible [22]. Recently, SPECT/CT using ^{99m}Tc-labeled agents is available in some hospitals, but has relatively low image resolution and a long scan-time. Therefore, we evaluated the use of 18F-NaF bone PET/CT to validate bone reaction in the complicated bony structure of the ankle, because of its high resolution and sensitivity, as well as its ability to allow exact lesion localization.

Trauma involving the ankle joint can occur anywhere, such as work-related injury, a road traffic accident, or slipping in a public area. Although patients typically have significant improvement after appropriate initial treatment, they often still have residual physical impairment several years after the injury [23–25]. Because these cases can be related to medicolegal or various compensation issues, objective evaluation of permanent impairment is very important. Although ROM appears to be a suitable method for evaluating impairment of the ankle joint [26, 27], it may be subject to variation, because patients may complain of pain during motion at different times during the examination, and may be deliberately uncooperative and inconsistent. With such inconsistency, ROM assessment cannot be used as a valid parameter in impairment evaluations [26]. Under these

conditions, 18F-NaF bone PET/CT findings could be used as useful information for increasing the reliability of impairment evaluations. The results of our study suggest that hot uptake of 18F-NaF bone PET/CT reflects greater impairment, even if the ankle ROM assessment is somewhat inconsistent. However, it should not be concluded that less hot uptake of 18F-NaF during bone PET/CT indicates deception by the patients during impairment evaluation.

Our study had some limitations. Because this study was a pilot study, no control group was employed, which may be considered a limitation. A no-ROM limitation group, even after ankle injury, would facilitate understanding of the role of 18F-NaF bone PET/CT in permanent impairment evaluation. However, it is very difficult to recruit patients who have no physical impairment several months after ankle injury, as they would usually not visit the hospital regularly and there would be no reason to undergo expensive imaging examinations, such as PET/CT. The numbers between the fracture group and non-fracture group were much differed in this study (95 vs. 26). The reason for this is that the study was not a prospective study, and it is the patients in fracture group are more likely to have a disability because the impact of accident may be greater than non-fracture group. Moreover, we did not consider the effect of other factors that may affect hot uptake of 18F-NaF bone PET/CT, such as age, sex, and amount of physical activity of the patients. Further evaluation was not performed for several conditions or factors that could affect bone metabolism, such as diabetes mellitus, osteoporosis, and the use of steroids. Further studies are necessary to accumulate more 18F-NaF bone PET/CT data in the context of ankle injury in order to establish a cut-off value for adjudication of permanent impairment.

Conclusions

18F-NaF PET/CT can provide considerable information in impairment evaluations of limited ankle ROM, particularly in patients with fracture around the ankle joint. Therefore, it can be assumed that the "intensity" of hot uptake was more relevant than the "spread" of hot uptake.

Abbreviations
18F-NaF: ^{18}F-sodium fluoride; ^{99m}Tc: Technetium-99 m; CT: Computerized tomography; FDG: Fluorodeoxyglucose; HD: Ultra-high definition; MMI: Maximum medical improvement; MTV: Metabolic target volume (MTV); NaI (Tl): Thallium-doped sodium iodide; PET: Positron emission tomography; PTA: Posttraumatic osteoarthritis; ROM: Limitation of range of motion; SUV: Standardized uptake value; TLA: Total lesion activity;; TLG: Total lesion glycolysis; TOF: Time of flight (TOF)

Authors' contributions
TJJ and JHP contributed to the study design, data collection, data analysis, interpretation of data, writing of the manuscript and revision of the

manuscript. SJK contributed to data analysis, interpretation of data, writing of the manuscript and revision of the manuscript. JYP contributed to data analysis, writing of the manuscript and revision of the manuscript. EYR contributed to interpretation of data and revision of the manuscript. All authors read and approved the final manuscript.

Competing interests

Each author certifies that he or she has no commercial associations (eg, consultancies, stock ownership, equity interest, patent/licensing arrangements, etc) that might pose a competing interest in connection with the submitted article.

Author details

[1]Department of Nuclear Medicine, Gangnam Severance Hospital, Yonsei University College of Medicine, Seoul, South Korea. [2]Department of Radiology, Gangnam Severance Hospital, Yonsei University College of Medicine, Seoul, South Korea. [3]Department of Rehabilitation Medicine, Gangnam Severance Hospital, Rehabilitation Institute of Neuromuscular Disease, Yonsei University College of Medicine, Seoul, South Korea. [4]Division of PM&R, Department of Orthopaedic Surgery, Stanford University School of Medicine, Stanford, CA 94063, USA. [5]Department of Rehabilitation Medicine, Gangnam Severance Hospital, Yonsei University College of Medicine, 211 Eonjuro, Gangnam-gu, Seoul 06273, South Korea.

References

1. Parziale JR. Disability evaluation of extremity fractures. Phys Med Rehab Clin. 2001;12(3):647–58.
2. Spieler EA, Barth PS, Burton JF, Himmelstein J, Rudolph L. Recommendations to guide revision of the guides to the evaluation of permanent impairment. Jama. 2000;283(4):519–23.
3. Harper JD. Determining foot and ankle impairments by the AMA fifth edition guides. Foot Ankle Clin. 2002;7(2):291–303.
4. Horisberger M, Valderrabano V, Hintermann B. Posttraumatic ankle osteoarthritis after ankle-related fractures. J Orthop Trauma. 2009;23(1):60–7.
5. Heim D, Niederhauser K, Simbrey N. The Volkmann dogma: a retrospective, long-term, single-center study. Eur J Trauma Emerg Surg. 2010;36(6):515–9.
6. Van Den Bekerom MP, Haverkamp D, Kloen P. Biomechanical and clinical evaluation of posterior malleolar fractures. A systematic review of the literature. J Trauma Acute Care Surg. 2009;66(1):279–84.
7. Milner S, Davis T, Muir K, Greenwood D, Doherty M. Long-term outcome after tibial shaft fracture: is malunion important? JBJS. 2002;84(6):971–80.
8. Hattori T, Tsunoda K, Watanabe K, Nakao E, Hirata H, Nakamura R. Arthroscopic mobilization for contracture of the wrist. Arthroscopy. 2006; 22(8):850–4.
9. Takata S, Yasui N. Disuse osteoporosis. J Med Investig. 2001;48(3/4):147–56.
10. Blau M, Nagler W, Bender M. Fluorine-18: a new isotope for bone scanning. J Nucl Med. 1962;3.
11. Wong KK, Piert M. Dynamic bone imaging with 99mTc-labeled diphosphonates and 18F-NaF: mechanisms and applications. J Nucl Med. 2013;54(4):590–9.
12. Czernin J, Satyamurthy N, Schiepers C. Molecular mechanisms of bone 18F-NaF deposition. J Nucl Med. 2010;51(12):1826–9.
13. Grant FD, Fahey FH, Packard AB, Davis RT, Alavi A, Treves ST. Skeletal PET with 18F-fluoride: applying new technology to an old tracer. J Nucl Med. 2008;49(1):68–78.
14. Jadvar H, Desai B, Conti PS. Sodium 18 F-fluoride PET/CT of bone, joint, and other disorders. Semin Nucl Med. 2015;1:58–65.
15. Cocchiarella L, Andersson G. Guides to the evaluation of permanent impairment: American Medical Association; 2001.
16. Segall G, Delbeke D, Stabin MG, Even-Sapir E, Fair J, Sajdak R, Smith GT. SNM practice guideline for sodium 18F-fluoride PET/CT bone scans 1.0. J Nucl Med. 2010;51(11):1813–20.
17. Lee P, Weerasuriya DK, Lavori PW, Quon A, Hara W, Maxim PG, Le Q-T, Wakelee HA, Donington JS, Graves EE. Metabolic tumor burden predicts for disease progression and death in lung cancer. Int J Radiat Oncol Biol Phys. 2007;69(2):328–33.
18. Chesworth BM, Vandervoort AA. Comparison of passive stiffness variables and range of motion in uninvolved and involved ankle joints of patients following ankle fractures. Phys Ther. 1995;75(4):253–61.
19. McCarthy EF. Histopathologic correlates of a positive bone scan. Semin Nucl Med. 1997;4:309–20.
20. Uchida K, Nakajima H, Miyazaki T, Yayama T, Kawahara H, Kobayashi S, Tsuchida T, Okazawa H, Fujibayashi Y, Baba H. Effects of alendronate on bone metabolism in glucocorticoid-induced osteoporosis measured by 18F-fluoride PET: a prospective study. J Nucl Med. 2009;50(11):1808–14.
21. Zhuang H, Codreanu I. Growing applications of FDG PET-CT imaging in non-oncologic conditions. J Biomed Res. 2015;29(3):189.
22. Van den Wyngaert T, Strobel K, Kampen W, Kuwert T, van der Bruggen W, Mohan H, Gnanasegaran G, Delgado-Bolton R, Weber W, Beheshti M. The EANM practice guidelines for bone scintigraphy. Eur J Nucl Med Mol Imaging. 2016;43(9):1723–38.
23. Bhandari M, Sprague S, Hanson B, Busse JW, Dawe DE, Moro JK, Guyatt GH. Health-related quality of life following operative treatment of unstable ankle fractures: a prospective observational study. J Orthop Trauma. 2004;18(6):338–45.
24. Nilsson G, Jonsson K, Ekdahl C, Eneroth M. Outcome and quality of life after surgically treated ankle fractures in patients 65 years or older. BMC Musculoskelet Disord. 2007;8(1):127.
25. Nilsson G, Nyberg P, Ekdahl C, Eneroth M. Performance after surgical treatment of patients with ankle fractures—14-month follow-up. Physiother Res Int. 2003;8(2):69–82.
26. Association AM. Guides to the evaluation of permanent impairment, vol. 2001. 5th ed. Chicago: AMA Press. p. 533–8.
27. Krause DA, Cloud BA, Forster LA, Schrank JA, Hollman JH. Measurement of ankle dorsiflexion: a comparison of active and passive techniques in multiple positions. J Sport Rehabil. 2011;20(3):333–44.

Computer-aided evaluation of inflammatory changes over time on MRI of the spine in patients with suspected axial spondyloarthritis

Evgeni Aizenberg[1*], Rosaline van den Berg[2], Zineb Ez-Zaitouni[2], Désirée van der Heijde[2], Monique Reijnierse[1], Oleh Dzyubachyk[1] and Boudewijn P.F. Lelieveldt[1,3]

Abstract

Background: Evaluating inflammatory changes over time on MR images of the spine in patients with suspected axial Spondyloarthritis (axSpA) can be a labor-intensive task, requiring readers to manually search for and perceptually align a set of vertebrae between two scans. The purpose of this study was to assess the feasibility of computer-aided (CA) evaluation of such inflammatory changes in a framework where scans from two time points are fused into a single color-encoded image integrated into an interactive scoring tool.

Methods: For 30 patients from the SPondyloArthritis Caught Early (SPACE) cohort (back pain ≥ 3 months, ≤ 2 years, onset < 45 years), baseline and follow-up MR scans acquired 9–12 months apart were fused into a single color-encoded image through locally-rigid image registration to evaluate inflammatory changes in 23 vertebral units (VUs). Scoring was performed by two expert readers on a (−2, 2) scale using an interactive scoring tool. For comparison of direction of change (increase/decrease) indicated by an existing reference, Berlin method scores ((−3, 3) scale) of the same MR scans from a different ongoing study were used. The distributions of VU-level differences between CA readers and between the CA and Berlin methods (sign of change scores) across patients were analyzed descriptively. Patient-level agreement between CA readers was assessed by intraclass correlation coefficient (ICC).

Results: Five patients were excluded from evaluation due to failed vertebrae segmentation. Patient-level inter-reader agreement ICC was 0.56 (95% CI: 0.22 to 0.78). Mean VU-level inter-reader differences across 25 patients ranged (−0.04, 0.12) with SD range (0, 0.45). Across all VUs, inter-reader differences ranged (−1, 1) in 573/575 VUs (99.7%). Mean VU-level inter-method differences across patients ranged (−0.04, 0.08) with SD range (0, 0.61). Across all VUs, inter-method differences ranged (−1, 1) in 572/575 VUs (99.5%).

Conclusions: Fusion of MR scans of the spine from two time points into a single color-encoded image allows for direct visualization and measurement of inflammatory changes over time in patients with suspected axSpA.

Keywords: Axial Spondyloarthritis, Magnetic resonance imaging, Inflammation, Comparative visualization, Image registration

* Correspondence: E.Aizenberg@lumc.nl
[1]Department of Radiology, Leiden University Medical Center, P.O. Box 9600, 2300 RC Leiden, The Netherlands
Full list of author information is available at the end of the article

Background

Evaluating inflammatory changes over time on magnetic resonance (MR) images of the spine in patients with suspected axial Spondyloarthritis (axSpA) can be a labor-intensive task. Depending on the rheumatologic scoring method that is used, readers are often required to assess a set of vertebral units (VUs) in several slices [1, 2], manually searching for and perceptually aligning the vertebrae between two scans. It would be of great benefit to have a computer-aided (CA) method capable of automatically localizing and labeling the VUs and spatially aligning scans from two time points, so voxel-wise intensity differences could be visualized in a single image.

CA methods involving alignment between multiple images for voxel-wise analysis have been extensively applied in the fields of neuroimaging and radiation therapy. Examples include voxel-based morphometry for comparison of local concentration of gray matter between subjects [3], analysis of multi-subject diffusion data for studying brain connectivity [4], and adaptive radiotherapy [5]. These studies have demonstrated that CA alignment of medical images can aid clinicians with automated biomarker quantification and treatment replanning based on anatomical changes that occur over time.

Spatial alignment of scans from two time points compensates for patient posture differences between scanning sessions and allows to overlay the two images for visual assessment of changes over time. This is done by computing a spatial coordinate mapping between corresponding locations in the two scans, a process known as image registration [6]. Generally, this mapping involves a geometrically non-rigid correspondence between voxels. This may cause physically implausible deformations in rigid anatomical structures, such as bones. An efficient solution to this problem was proposed by Dzyubachyk et al. [7] and applied to comparative visualization of whole-body MR scans in patients with multiple myeloma lesions. The highlight of this approach is that, following a global alignment of two time points, a locally rigid (rotation and translation only) alignment is derived for selected regions of interest (ROIs) within bones. This ensures that bone rigidity is preserved in the final alignment.

In the work presented here, we applied the framework of Dzyubachyk et al. [7] to comparative visualization of MR images of the spine in patients with suspected axSpA. The aim of our study was to assess the feasibility of CA evaluation of axSpA inflammatory changes in the spine. This included fusion of scans from two time points into a single color-encoded image vividly distinguishing areas of increase versus decrease in inflammation over time, automatic labeling of VUs, and an interactive scoring module whose entry fields are activated/deactivated in synchronization with the VU selected by the reader in the image.

Methods

Patients

A total of 30 patients from the SPondyloArthritis Caught Early (SPACE) cohort were included in this feasibility study. The SPACE cohort has been described extensively before [8]. In short, the SPACE cohort is an ongoing cohort started in January 2009, including patients aged 16 years and older with chronic back pain ($\geq$ 3 months, $\leq$ 2 years, onset < 45 years). All patients underwent a diagnostic work-up at baseline, consisting of history taking, physical examination, laboratory tests, and imaging (MR imaging (MRI) and plain radiographs). Patients fulfilling the Assessment of SpondyloArthritis (ASAS) axSpA criteria [9, 10] and patients with possible axSpA were included for follow-up visits after 3 and 12 months (including MRI). Possible axSpA was defined as the presence of at least one specific SpA-feature with a high positive likelihood ratio (LR+ above 6) or at least two less specific SpA-features (LR+ below 6), but not fulfilling the ASAS axSpA criteria [10, 11].

MRI sequences

Patients underwent MRI of the complete spine in two stages (upper and lower spine) on a 1.5T MR system (Philips Medical Systems, The Netherlands). The acquired sequences were Short Tau Inversion Recovery (STIR) with repetition time (TR) 2500 msec, echo time (TE) 60 msec, inversion time 165 msec, acquisition matrix 304×300, echo train length (ETL) 25, number of averages 3 and T1-weighted Turbo Spin-Echo (TR 550/ TE 10, acquisition matrix 512×305, ETL 5, number of averages 3). Imaging was performed in the sagittal plane with a field of view of 380×380 mm, slice thickness of 4 mm, and a slice gap of 0.4 mm.

Vertebrae localization/segmentation/labeling

For each patient, 23 VUs were automatically localized, segmented, and labeled. A VU is defined as the region between the mid-points of two adjacent vertebral bodies. For example, VU1 consists of the lower endplate of vertebra C2 and the upper endplate of vertebra C3. Hence, VU levels 1–23 cover 24 vertebral bodies (C2–S1). Localization and segmentation were carried out using atlas-based segmentation [12]. The atlas set consisted of 11 patients from the SPACE cohort (no overlap with patients included in evaluation). For each atlas patient, 24 vertebral bodies (C2 to S1) were manually outlined in the slice closest to the mid-sagittal plane and the two adjacent slices (a total of three slices). The procedure was carried out separately for upper and lower spine images, producing a total of two manually segmented images per atlas patient. We chose to approximate each vertebral body with a simple polygonal region within the vertebral borders, taking the cortex as an anatomical boundary. This choice was motivated by the fact that for successful locally rigid alignment of two time points it is preferable to have a ROI estimate that under-segments the bone, rather than an estimate that spills over into inherently non-rigid neighboring soft tissue.

The first phase of atlas-based segmentation consisted of image registration between each of the 11 atlas patients and the target patient being segmented. Image registration was performed using the Elastix software package [13, 14]. After spatially mapping vertebrae ROIs from every atlas image onto the target image, a majority vote was applied across all mappings to determine whether a voxel was part of the background or of one of the vertebrae.

Labeling of vertebrae voxels in the upper spine image was done sequentially from top to bottom, over connected components, with the top-most connected component receiving the label "C2," the following "C3," etc. Similarly, labeling in the lower spine image was sequentially from bottom to top, with the bottom-most connected component receiving the label "S1," the following "L5," etc. We used a 26-connected neighborhood definition for connectivity in 3D. Connected components less than 20 voxels in size were considered to be noise and were removed.

Locally rigid inter-time point alignment

In what follows, let us consider a pair of MR scans of a single patient and, without loss of generality, refer to one of the scans as "Time Point 1 (TP1)" and the second scan as "Time Point 2 (TP2)." According to the framework proposed by Dzyubachyk et al. [7], locally rigid alignment of two images is derived from a global non-rigid alignment of this image pair. We used the Elastix software package [13, 14] to globally align TP2 to TP1. The registration yielded a deformation field specifying for each physical

position in TP1 the corresponding physical position in TP2. Next, for each VU, the landmark transform [15] was used to estimate a locally rigid alignment between the VU region in TP1 (specified by the atlas-based segmentation result) and the corresponding physical region in TP2 (specified by the deformation field) [7]. This ensured that spatial correspondence between voxels within the VU in TP1 and TP2 was restricted to translation and rotation, preserving bone rigidity.

It is important to note that the described method can be equivalently applied in the reverse direction, by globally aligning TP1 to TP2, and subsequently using VU segmentations from TP2. Thus, in order to align two scans in a locally rigid manner, it is sufficient to segment and label vertebrae in one of the two scans.

Color-encoded fusion of time points

After locally aligning two time points on the VU level, differences in intensity (e.g. inflammation) between corresponding voxels were visualized through color-encoded fusion of the two scans. First, intensity values of TP1 were color-mapped to orange color space (RGB triple {255,128,0}), and intensity values of TP2 were color-mapped to light blue color space (RGB triple {0,127,255}). The fusion image was then obtained by voxel-wise superposition of the two color-mapped images [7]. Since orange and light blue are complementary colors, areas where no changes occurred between the two time points (TP2 intensity = TP1 intensity) are displayed in shades of gray. On the other hand, an increase in inflammation over time (TP2 intensity > TP1 intensity) is displayed in shades of light blue (Fig. 1). In the opposite case, a decrease in inflammation over time (TP2 intensity < TP1 intensity) is displayed in shades of orange. In addition to its complementary nature, the

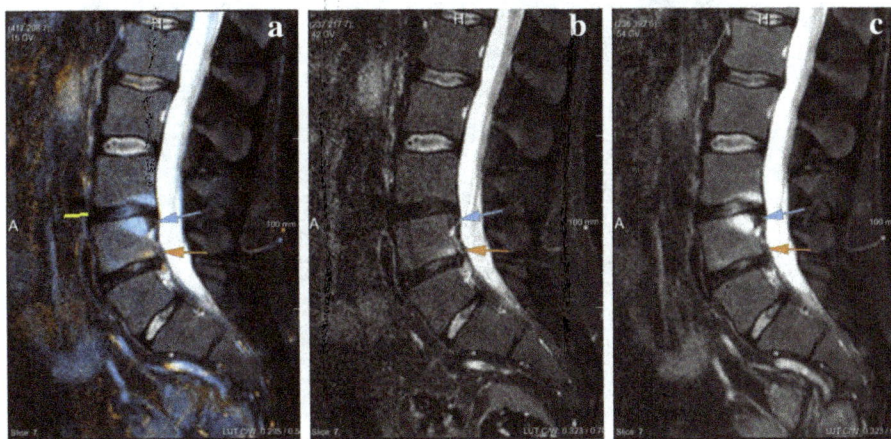

Fig. 1 Color-encoded fusion of two MR scans of the same subject acquired at two different time points. Inflammation increase (blue arrow) in VU21 and decrease (orange arrow) in VU22 in the second time point (**c**) compared to first time point (**b**) are displayed in blue and orange, respectively, in the color-encoded fusion image (**a**). In this example, the locally rigid alignment is applied to VU21, indicated by the yellow line in (**a**)

choice of orange and light blue is motivated by the fact that these two colors can be perceived even by readers with color vision deficiency [7]. No intensity standardization was applied to original images prior to color-encoded fusion.

Evaluation of inflammatory changes

Two experienced readers (RvdB and ZEZ) independently evaluated inflammatory changes between MR scans of the spine (STIR only), acquired 9–12 months apart, directly from the color-encoded fusion image. The choice of using only STIR images for CA scoring was motivated by our focus on inflammatory lesions and the fact that automatic alignment of T1 images to STIR images requires additional image registration steps, which would introduce additional sources of error. The readers were blinded to the original images and their time order, as well as patient and clinical characteristics. Each VU was assigned a score ranging from –2 (dramatic decrease of inflammation), via 0 (no change), to +2 (dramatic increase of inflammation), reflecting net change in the degree of inflammation within the VU. Navigation through the images and evaluation were carried out using an interactive software tool that we implemented in MeVisLab 2.7.1 (MeVis Medical Solutions, Germany) [16]. The tool consists of two windows: the comparative visualization module (Fig. 2) and the scoring module (Fig. 3).

For comparison of direction of change (increase/decrease) indicated by an existing reference, Berlin method [1] scores of the same pair of MR scans from a different ongoing SPACE cohort study at our institution were used. The MR scans (STIR and T1) were independently evaluated by two experts (MdH and PACB) according to the Berlin method [1], yielding status scores for each of

the time points. Each VU was assigned a score ranging from 0 to 3 reflecting the fraction of bone volume affected by bone marrow edema: 0, normal; 1, < 25% VU edematous; 2, 25–50%; 3, > 50%. The readers were blinded to the time order of the images, as well as patient and clinical characteristics. Changes in inflammation over time were calculated as differences in status scores after de-blinding the time order of the MR scans.

Statistical analysis

For each of the 23 VU levels, the distributions of VU-level inter-reader and inter-method differences across patients were analyzed descriptively. For inter-reader differences, the VU-level difference was computed between change scores assigned to the VU by the two CA readers. For inter-method differences, the focus was on the direction of change indicated by each method, and therefore, VU-level difference was computed between the sign of the CA change score (mean of two readers) and the sign of the Berlin change score (mean of two readers), where the sign function takes the value –1 in case of negative change, +1 in case of positive change, and 0 in case of no change.

Agreement between CA readers was assessed on the patient level (change summed across VUs of each patient) by computing intraclass correlation coefficient (ICC, two-way mixed, single measures, absolute agreement definition). The statistics were computed using MATLAB R2015b (The MathWorks, Inc., USA) and IBM SPSS Statistics 23 (IBM Corporation, USA).

Results

In 18/30 patients, atlas-based segmentation provided satisfactory segmentation and correct labeling of all 23

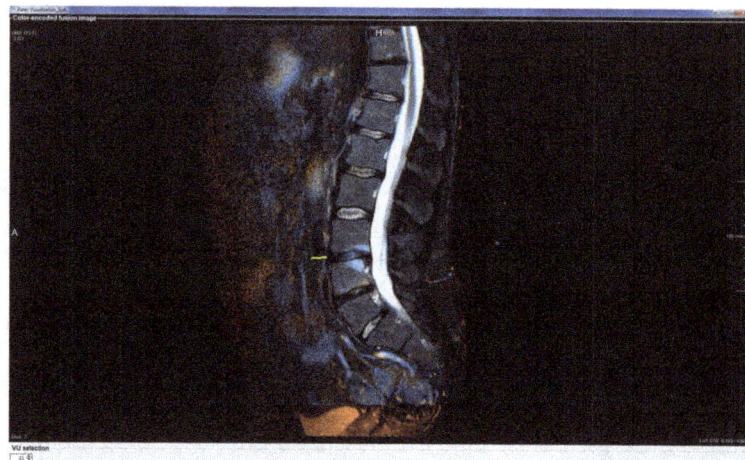

Fig. 2 Comparative visualization module. The module displays the color-encoded fusion image and allows the user to specify the VU of interest in the VU selection field at the bottom left of the window, which will trigger locally rigid alignment of two time points for that VU. A visual indication for the position of the VU in the image is provided to aid navigation (yellow line next to VU 21)

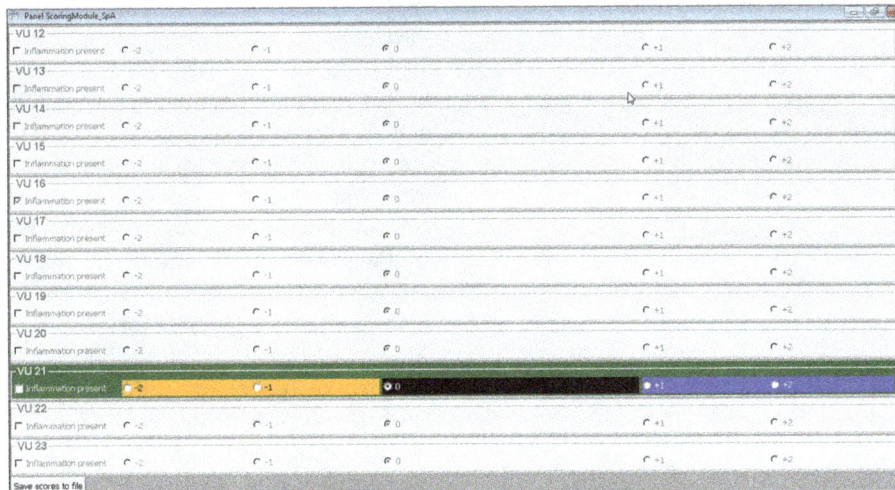

Fig. 3 Scoring module. The module acts as an interactive scoring sheet, consisting of 23 panels representing the VUs. Every panel contains a group of option buttons (only one of the options can be selected) through which the reader assigns a change score to the VU, as well as a checkbox to indicate the presence of inflammation in cases of no net change. Only one VU panel is active at any given moment. The choice of VU in the comparative visualization module activates the corresponding panel in the scoring module, while deactivating panels of the remaining 22 VUs. This ensures that one VU is not mistaken for another while filling out the interactive scoring sheet

VUs in at least one of the time points (as explained above, in order to align two scans in a locally rigid manner, it is sufficient to segment and label vertebrae in one of the two scans). In seven patients, failure to segment the lowest vertebra in the upper spine image and/or the highest vertebra in the lower spine image, resulted in lack of segmentation for one VU (frequently corresponding to the levels Th9–Th11). The segmentations for these VUs were added by manual correction. Five patients were excluded from further evaluation due to inaccurate alignment with atlas images that led to missing vertebrae segmentations and incorrect labeling of VUs. Thus, a total of 25 patients (and hence 575 VUs) were evaluated. Baseline patient characteristics and descriptive statistics of Berlin and CA scores at baseline and over time are presented in Table 1. As demonstrated by baseline characteristics, it should be pointed out that most patients had low levels of inflammation.

Inter-reader differences between CA readers

VU-level differences between CA readers' change scores are shown in Fig. 4a. Mean VU-level differences across patients ranged from –0.04 to 0.12 with standard deviation (SD) range (0, 0.45). Most differences were observed in the lower thoracic spine and the lumbar spine. In 21/23 VU levels, differences ranged between –1 and 1 across all patients. In 2/23 VU levels, a difference of 2 was observed in one patient. In total, across all patients, VU-level differences ranged (–1, 1) in 573/575 VUs (99.7%). On the patient level, the ICC between the two CA readers was 0.56 (95% confidence interval (CI): 0.22 to 0.78), indicating moderate agreement between readers.

Inter-method differences between CA and Berlin methods

VU-level differences between the direction of change indicated by the CA and Berlin methods are shown in Fig. 4b. Mean VU-level differences across patients ranged from –0.04 to 0.08 with SD range (0, 0.61). Most differences were observed in the lower thoracic spine and the lumbar spine. In 21/23 VU levels, differences ranged between –1 and 1 across all patients. In 1/23 VU levels, a difference of 2 (positive Berlin change, negative CA change) was observed in one patient. In 1/23 VU levels, a difference of –2 (negative Berlin change, positive CA change) was observed in one patient. In total, across all patients, VU-level differences ranged (–1, 1) in 572/575 VUs (99.5%). Differences of precisely –1 or 1 (change detected only by one of the two methods) were observed in 40/575 VUs, and among those in 33/40 VUs the change was detected by the CA method while Berlin score indicated zero change. Figure 5 shows examples of VU-level differences between the two methods.

Discussion

In this study, we assessed the feasibility of CA evaluation of inflammatory changes on MR scans of the spine in patients with suspected axSpA. Readers agreed that a key advantage of CA evaluation is that fusion of two scans acquired at different time points into a single color-encoded image allows for direct visualization and measurement of inflammatory changes, as opposed to derivation of change scores from status scores that measure presence and extent of lesions separately for each time point. The results indicate that in nearly all VUs of all patients, VU-level differences between CA

Table 1 Baseline patient characteristics and descriptive statistics of Berlin and CA scores of the 25 patients evaluated in the study

Baseline patient characteristics

Characteristic	Patients (n = 25)
Age at inclusion in years, mean (SD)	31.7 (8.3)
Male, n (%)	12 (48)
Duration of back pain in months, mean (SD)	14.4 (8.0)
BP, n (%)	19 (76)
HLA-B27 positivity, n (%)	15 (60)
Elevated CRP, n (%)	6 (24)
Sacroiliitis on MRI (ASAS definition), n (%)	8 (32)
Sacroiliitis on radiograph, n (%)	3 (12)
Positive MRI (ASAS definition), n (%)	2 (8)
ASAS classification positive, n (%)	14 (56)

Berlin and CA scores descriptive statistics

Variable	Berlin method (reader 1/reader 2)	CA method (reader 1/reader 2)
VU-level score at baseline, median (range)	0 (0, 1) / 0 (0, 1)	NA
VU-level score at follow-up, median (range)	0 (0, 1) / 0 (0, 1)	NA
Patient-level score at baseline, median (range)	0 (0, 5) / 0 (0, 3)	NA
Patient-level score at follow-up, median (range)	1 (0, 5) / 0 (0, 4)	NA
Change in VU-level score, median (range)	0 (−1, 1) / 0 (−1, 1)	0 (−1, 2) / 0 (−2, 2)
Change in patient-level score, median (range)	0 (−2, 3) / 0 (−1, 2)	0 (−3, 3) / 0 (−11, 5)

readers and between the CA and Berlin methods were bounded between −1 and 1, ensuring that scores do not offer opposing opinions on the direction of inflammatory change (increase versus decrease). The fact that most differences occurred in the lower thoracic spine and the lumbar spine is consistent with the observation that most inflammatory activity in the spine of early disease patients takes place in these regions [17, 18]. The majority of non-zero differences between the CA and Berlin scores were observed when change was detected by the CA method while zero change was indicated by the Berlin method. These quantitative results support our qualitative observation that small gradual changes in an existing lesion are often not reflected in Berlin status scores, but can be readily visualized and measured by the CA method.

The moderate inter-reader patient-level agreement and difference in the range of readers' scores suggest that the CA grading scale may be defined too loosely with

respect to affected bone volume, making the score more susceptible to subjective interpretation of the degree of change. Readers pointed out that a challenging aspect of the CA method is estimation of net inflammatory change in VUs with multiple inflammatory lesions. For example, one such VU exhibited increase in one quadrant, while exhibiting decrease in another quadrant. The two readers had different opinions as to which change was stronger, resulting in opposing scores and thus a mean change of zero. One way to overcome such discrepancies would be to score change separately for each of the four quadrants, akin to scoring in the Spondyloarthritis Research Consortium of Canada (SPARCC) method [2].

For the purpose of this feasibility study, we made a deliberate decision to measure change based only on the color-fused image, while blinding readers to the original images. However, the readers noted that in daily practice it would be helpful to have the original images (STIR and T1) available next to the color-fused image, as this would contribute to a more informative scoring decision. The color-fused image could then be used as a map that directs the reader's attention to locations of potential inflammatory changes, while the original images would be used to make the final judgement about the type and degree of observed change. The reader would still benefit from locally rigid alignment between the two time points while assessing original images, since the two scans will be aligned such that the VU of interest has identical viewing points in both images. Another feature that would enhance user experience is stitching of upper and lower spine images into a single image. This would offer a more natural workflow, without the need to load two separate images for every patient. A simultaneous view of the complete spine would also facilitate a more holistic assessment of disease activity.

This study has several important limitations. The SPACE cohort consists only of early disease patients with low levels of inflammation, making it harder to study inflammatory changes, since changes were infrequent. Another limitation is that it was not possible to provide patient-level inter-method agreement statistics, as the scoring methodology and scale range are different, and this would result in uninterpretable results. However, the CA method was not designed with the aim of replicating the Berlin method, but rather as an independent scoring framework. It is of interest to compare the responsiveness of the two methods by quantifying sensitivity to change in a population with treatment and placebo patient groups, as was previously done for other scoring methods [19]. Assessing responsiveness after an effective intervention could provide information on differences in the psychometric characteristics of the two scoring methods. This could be addressed in a follow-up study. The definition of the CA change score should also

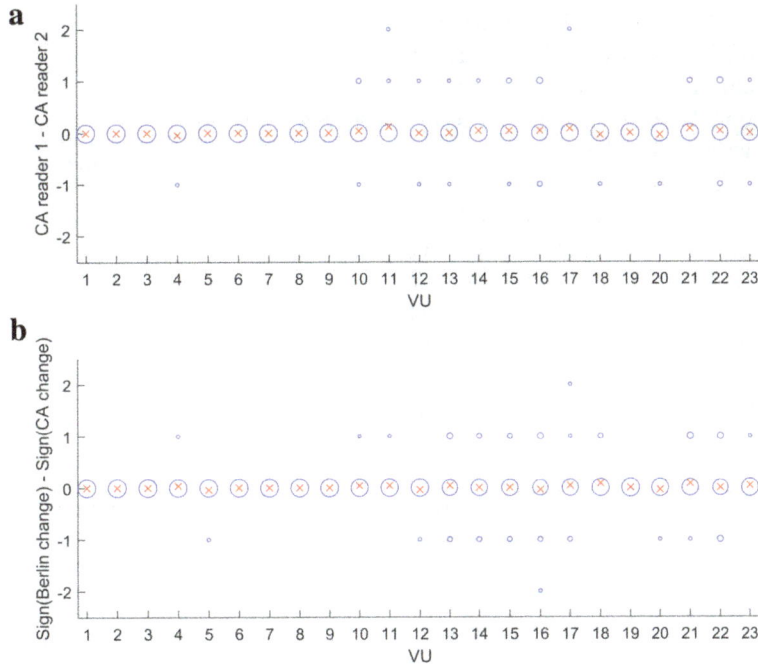

Fig. 4 VU-level difference between CA readers' change scores (**a**) and VU-level difference between sign of CA and Berlin change scores (**b**). Exact difference values are shown in blue (size of bubble data points is proportional to the occurrence of the difference value across 25 patients). Mean VU-level differences across 25 patients are shown in red

provide clear guidelines for the case of degenerative lesions to avoid discrepancies with existing methods that do not score these lesions (Fig. 5). The lack of intensity standardization prior to color-encoded fusion is a potential source of error. However, we should note that standardization is also not applied in the long-established procedure of Berlin method scoring. We sought to explore

the feasibility of color-encoded fusion without additional image post-processing steps that are not present in the Berlin method workflow. Future studies should indeed investigate the effect of intensity standardization on change scores of both methods. An additional limitation is that CA scoring was performed only using STIR images. This differs from the common clinical approach of confirming

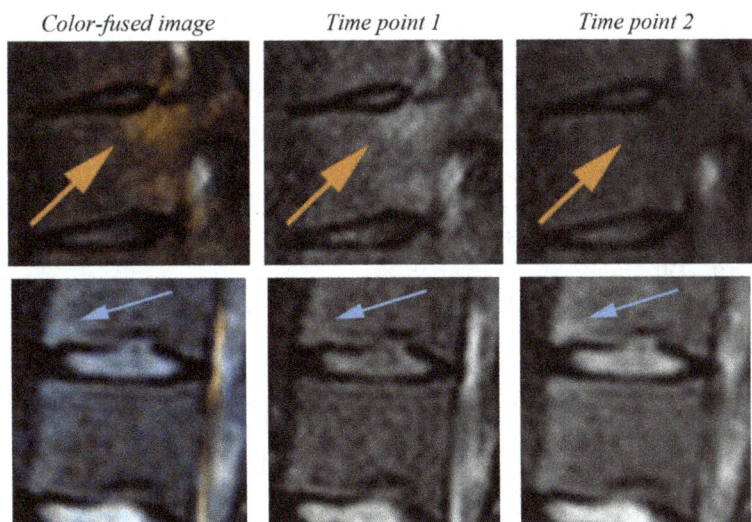

Fig. 5 Examples of VU-level inter-method differences. Top row: lesion area (orange arrow) received a CA change score of −1, but a Berlin change score of 0, because of being considered a degenerative lesion (status scores = 0). Bottom row: lesion area (blue arrow) received a CA change score of 1, but a Berlin change score of 0, because of zero Berlin status scores

inflammatory lesions observed in STIR images as low intensity areas in T1 images. Inclusion of T1 images may improve the robustness of the scoring method. Furthermore, it might allow visualization of changes in structural lesions, such as fatty lesions. Finally, it should be recognized that since 5/30 patients had to be excluded due to failed segmentation and 7/30 segmentations had to be manually adjusted, the method is not yet sufficiently robust to be used in practice. We should stress, however, that this study did not attempt to solve the problem of vertebrae segmentation in MRI. Our goal was to explore the prospect of CA assessment of patients with suspected axSpA and thereby provide yet another stimulus for development of robust vertebrae segmentation methods for MRI.

Although this study does not focus on the topic of vertebrae segmentation, we can note potential directions for improving the atlas-based segmentation framework used in this study. To ensure the applicability of this segmentation framework to a variety of MRI acquisition protocols and scanners, it would be helpful to construct an atlas consisting of sub-atlases of MR images acquired under similar echo/repetition times and magnetic field strengths. Then, prior to segmenting a target image, the system would automatically identify the most appropriate sub-atlas based on acquisition parameters recorded in the image's DICOM data. Additional improvement in segmentation might be achieved by operating with stitched images of the spine, as opposed to separate upper/lower spine images. We have observed that in some cases segmentation was successful in one part of the upper/lower pair but failed in the other. Therefore, we hypothesize that the more easily matched spine region can "pull" the second spine region into its correct position in the target image when stitched.

Conclusions

This feasibility study has demonstrated that fusion of MR scans of the spine from two time points into a single color-encoded image allows for direct visualization and measurement of inflammatory changes over time in patients with suspected axSpA. A future study, with similar design to that of Lukas et al. [19], should assess the performance of the CA method in patients with a wide range of activity at baseline and follow-up, quantifying inter-reader reliability, sensitivity to change, and time needed to score each set of MR images. This would also provide a comprehensive comparison of the CA method to the Berlin and SPARCC methods.

Abbreviations
ASAS: Assessment of SpondyloArthritis; axSpA: axial SpondyloArthritis; CA: Computer-aided; CI: Confidence interval; DICOM: Digital Imaging and Communications in Medicine; MR: Magnetic resonance; MRI: Magnetic resonance imaging; RGB: Red, Green, Blue; ROI: Region of interest;

SD: Standard deviation; SPACE: SPondyloArthitis Caught Early; SPARCC: Spondyloarthritis Research Consortium of Canada; STIR: Short Tau Inversion Recovery; TE: Echo time; TP1: Time Point 1; TP2: Time Point 2; TR: Repetition time; VU: Vertebral unit

Acknowledgements
We would like to thank Manouk de Hooge and Pauline A. C. Bakker for the Berlin method scoring of the patients in this study. We also thank Freek de Bruin for the insightful discussions that helped advance this study.

Funding
This research was supported by the Dutch Technology Foundation STW, under grant number 10894. STW is part of the Netherlands Organization for Scientific Research (NWO), which is partly funded by the Dutch Ministry of Economic Affairs.

Authors' contributions
All authors were involved in drafting the article or revising it critically for important intellectual content, and all authors approved the final version to be published. *Study conception and design:* EA, RvdB, OD, MR, DvdH, BPFL. *Acquisition of data:* RvdB, ZEZ, DvdH, MR. *Analysis and interpretation of data:* EA, RvdB.

Competing interests
The authors declare that they have no competing interests.

Author details
[1]Department of Radiology, Leiden University Medical Center, P.O. Box 9600, 2300 RC Leiden, The Netherlands. [2]Department of Rheumatology, Leiden University Medical Center, P.O. Box 9600, 2300 RC Leiden, The Netherlands. [3]Intelligent Systems Department, Delft University of Technology, Mekelweg 4, 2628 CD Delft, The Netherlands.

References
1. Haibel H, Rudwaleit M, Brandt HC, Grozdanovic Z, Listing J, Kupper H, et al. Adalimumab reduces spinal symptoms in active ankylosing spondylitis: clinical and magnetic resonance imaging results of a fifty-two-week open-label trial. Arthritis Rheum. 2006;54:678–81.
2. Maksymowych WP, Inman RD, Salonen D, Dhillon SS, Krishnananthan R, Stone M, et al. Spondyloarthritis research consortium of Canada magnetic resonance imaging index for assessment of spinal inflammation in ankylosing spondylitis. Arthritis Rheum. 2005;53:502–9.
3. Ashburner J, Friston KJ. Voxel-based Morphometry—the methods. NeuroImage. 2000;11:805–21.
4. Smith SM, Jenkinson M, Johansen-Berg H, Rueckert D, Nichols TE, Mackay CE, et al. Tract-based spatial statistics: Voxelwise analysis of multi-subject diffusion data. NeuroImage. 2006;31:1487–505.
5. Wang H, Dong L, O'Daniel J, Mohan R, Garden AS, Ang KK, et al. Validation of an accelerated "demons" algorithm for deformable image registration in radiation therapy. Phys Med Biol IOP Publishing. 2005;50:2887–905.
6. Rueckert D, Schnabel JA. Medical Image Registration. Berlin Heidelberg: Springer; 2010. p. 131–54.
7. Dzyubachyk O, Blaas J, Botha CP, Staring M, Reijnierse M, Bloem JL, et al. Comparative exploration of whole-body MR through locally rigid transforms. Int J Comput Assist Radiol Surg. 2013;8:635–47.
8. van den Berg R, de Hooge M, van Gaalen F, Reijnierse M, Huizinga T, van der Heijde D. Percentage of patients with spondyloarthritis in patients referred because of chronic back pain and performance of classification criteria: experience from the Spondyloarthritis caught early (SPACE) cohort. Rheumatology (Oxford). 2013;52:1492–9.
9. Rudwaleit M, Landewé R, van der Heijde D, Listing J, Brandt J, Braun J, et al. The development of assessment of SpondyloArthritis international society classification criteria for axial spondyloarthritis (part I): classification of paper patients by expert opinion including uncertainty appraisal. Ann Rheum Dis. 2009;68:770 6.

10. Rudwaleit M, van der Heijde D, Landewé R, Listing J, Akkoc N, Brandt J, et al. The development of assessment of SpondyloArthritis international society classification criteria for axial spondyloarthritis (part II): validation and final selection. Ann. Rheum. Dis. BMJ Publishing Group Ltd Eur League Against Rheumatism. 2009;68:777–83.

11. Rudwaleit M, van der Heijde D, Khan MA, Braun J, Sieper J. How to diagnose axial spondyloarthritis early. Ann Rheum Dis BMJ Publishing Group Ltd and Eur Leag Against Rheumatism. 2004;63:535–43.

12. Rohlfing T, Brandt R, Menzel R, Russakoff DB, Maurer CRJ. Quo vadis, atlas-based segmentation? Handb. Med. Image Anal. - Vol. III Regist. Model. 2005. p. 435–486.

13. Klein S, Staring M, Murphy K, Viergever MA, JPW P. Elastix: a toolbox for intensity-based medical image registration. IEEE Trans Med Imaging. 2010; 29:196–205.

14. Aizenberg E. Elastix parameters for atlas-based segmentation of vertebral bodies [Internet]. 2016. Available from: http://elastix.bigr.nl/wiki/index.php/Par0042. Accessed 12 Apr 2016.

15. Horn BKP. Closed-form solution of absolute orientation using unit quaternions. J Opt Soc Am A. 1987;4:629.

16. MeVisLab [Internet]. Available from: http://www.mevislab.de.

17. Althoff CE, Sieper J, Song I-H, Haibel H, Weiß A, Diekhoff T, et al. Active inflammation and structural change in early active axial spondyloarthritis as detected by whole-body MRI. Ann. Rheum. Dis. BMJ Publishing Group Ltd Eur Leag Against Rheumatism. 2013;72:967–73.

18. Lorenzin M, Ortolan A, Frallonardo P, Vio S, Lacognata C, Oliviero F, et al. Spine and sacroiliac joints on magnetic resonance imaging in patients with early axial spondyloarthritis: prevalence of lesions and association with clinical and disease activity indices from the Italian group of the SPACE study. Reumatismo. 2016;68:72.

19. Lukas C, Braun J, van der Heijde D, Hermann K-GA, Rudwaleit M, Østergaard M, et al. Scoring inflammatory activity of the spine by magnetic resonance imaging in ankylosing spondylitis: a multireader experiment. J Rheumatol. 2007;34:862–70.

27

CT texture features are associated with overall survival in pancreatic ductal adenocarcinoma – a quantitative analysis

Armin Eilaghi[1,6], Sameer Baig[1], Yucheng Zhang[1], Junjie Zhang[1], Paul Karanicolas[2], Steven Gallinger[3,4,5], Farzad Khalvati[1] and Masoom A. Haider[1*]

Abstract

Background: To assess whether CT-derived texture features predict survival in patients undergoing resection for pancreatic ductal adenocarcinoma (PDAC).

Methods: Thirty patients with pre-operative CT from 2007 to 2012 for PDAC were included. Tumor size and five texture features namely uniformity, entropy, dissimilarity, correlation, and inverse difference normalized were calculated. Mann–Whitney rank sum test was used to compare tumor with normal pancreas. Receiver operating characteristics (ROC) analysis, Cox regression and Kaplan-Meier tests were used to assess association of texture features with overall survival (OS).

Results: Uniformity ($p < 0.001$), entropy ($p = 0.009$), correlation ($p < 0.001$), and mean intensity ($p < 0.001$) were significantly different in tumor regions compared to normal pancreas. Tumor dissimilarity ($p = 0.045$) and inverse difference normalized ($p = 0.046$) were associated with OS whereas tumor intensity ($p = 0.366$), tumor size ($p = 0.611$) and other textural features including uniformity ($p = 0.334$), entropy ($p = 0.330$) and correlation ($p = 0.068$) were not associated with OS.

Conclusion: CT-derived PDAC texture features of dissimilarity and inverse difference normalized are promising prognostic imaging biomarkers of OS for patients undergoing curative intent surgical resection.

Keywords: Texture Features, Pancreatic Ductal Adenocarcinoma, Overall Survival Prediction, Dissimilarity, Inverse Difference Normalized

Background

Cancers are phenotypically heterogeneous and their pattern of spatial heterogeneity varies with time [1]. Tumor heterogeneity is thought to be a key factor in the development of therapeutic resistance [2]. Tumor genomics from needle biopsy may be reflective of only a portion of the cancer's characteristics. However, imaging has the distinct advantage of being non-invasive and providing an overview of the entire tumor. Therefore, imaging has increasingly been used to capture spatial heterogeneity of tumors [3]. The in-depth feature analysis of tumor sites has been brought into the "omics" terminology, called *radiomics*, which is defined as the high-throughput extraction of image features from radiographic images [1, 4, 5]. Imaging features can be derived from standard of care modalities such as contrast-enhanced computed tomography (CT), magnetic resonance imaging (MRI) and positron emission tomography (PET) without modification of the acquisition protocols making them less cost prohibitive [6–8]. For example, texture features from grey level co-occurrence matrices (GLCM) [9], which generate second-order statistical features have been used and improved [10] to quantify spatial texture of objects. There is an abundance of literature suggesting GLCM and other texture traits [11] are significantly associated with overall survival in lung [12], breast [13] and hepatic [14] carcinomas. However, to our

---

* Correspondence: masoom.haider@sunnybrook.ca
[1]Department of Medical Imaging and Sunnybrook Research Institute, Sunnybrook Health Sciences Center, University of Toronto, 2075 Bayview Ave., Room Rm AG 46, Toronto M4N 3 M5, ON, Canada
Full list of author information is available at the end of the article

best knowledge, there is paucity of studies to date about the potential prognostic value of CT texture features in pancreatic ductal adenocarcinoma (PDAC) [15].

PDAC has the lowest 5-year overall survival (OS) rate of any epithelial carcinoma at 7.7% [16] and surgical resection, applicable to < 30% cases [17], is the only potential cure [18] increasing OS to about 15–20% for resected cases [19]. More recently, neoadjuvant therapy has been introduced with the hope of extending survival for patients with resectable disease, allowing resection in patients with initially unresectable disease and selecting patients with different natural histories and chemosensitivities [20]. Since contrast-enhanced CT imaging is routinely used [21] for assessing resectability, staging and assessment of disease progression [22], a CT-derived quantitative imaging biomarker of OS could potentially provide a window into prognosis of PDAC.

The purpose of this study was to assess whether radiomic features from pre-operative contrast-enhanced CT in resectable PDAC patients were associated with overall survival. We hypothesized that pre-selected texture features are associated with the OS in resectable PDAC patients.

Methods
Patients
This retrospective study was approved by Sunnybrook Health Sciences Centre Research Ethics Board (reference number 400–2015). Written informed consent was waived.

Patients were identified from a database of all pancreatic resections performed at our institution. We included 30 consecutive patients who underwent curative intent surgical resection during 2007–2012, had pre-operative contrast-enhanced CT available for analysis (on average, one month prior to surgery). Cases of PDAC associated with an intra-ductal papillary mucinous neoplasm where excluded from this analysis. Also, patients who died within 3 months after surgery were excluded as the outcome may be significantly influenced by post-operative complications. Out of 30 patients, only 3 had gone under neoadjuvant therapy.

Image acquisition
Patients underwent contrast-enhanced CT with a biphasic pancreas protocol. Positive oral contrast was given to patients starting 1 h before the scan time followed by 500 cc of water prior to scan. Pancreatic cancer boundaries were most consistently seen in the portal venous phase of acquisition so this was selected for region of interest (ROI) selection in this cohort. Intravenous contrast (Iohexol) (100–120 cc) at a rate of 4.0–5.0 cc per second was administered with automatic power injection. Scan resolution for the biphasic protocol was as follows; Pancreatic phase: helical 0.625 mm × 0.625 mm through pancreas, manual bolus tracking scanning triggered at 150 Hounsfield unit (HU)

threshold; Portal phase: helical 0.625 mm × 0.625 mm through liver with 70 s delay; pitch was 0.984:1. CT images were reconstructed with 5 mm interval. Detector width was 40 mm and kV was 140 kVp for Pancreatic phase and 120 kVp for Portal phase. Examination was performed on a 64 row multidetector helical CT (GE Medical Systems, LightSpeed VCT, GE Healthcare).

Image analysis
For each primary cancer site, a ROI was drawn on all the slices with a visible tumor on the portal venous phase using an in-house developed contouring tool (Pro-CanVAS) [23]. ROIs were reviewed by a radiologist blinded to patient outcome. A ROI was also drawn to encompass normal pancreas on all slices that included tumor and 3 slices above and/or below the tumor depending on the location of tumor. In all cases, some hypointensity or relative contrast difference existed between background pancreas and the tumor. In cases where tumor boundary was not clear, boundary definition was facilitated by the presences of pancreatic or common bile duct cut-off and review of pancreatic phase images. A typical example of the contouring for two sample cases are presented in Fig. 1.

Tumor size plus five GLCM texture features [24] were preselected and calculated using an in house Matlab script (Mathworks Inc., USA, version 8.5.0.197613 - R2015a). GLCM feature set is one of the best known tools for texture analysis [25]. To calculate GLCM features, we used the bounding box around the ROIs annotated by the radiologist as the kernel, excluding the pixels in the bounding box located outside the ROI. The GLCM offset was set to be 1 pixel for the spatial relationship between adjacent pixels. Preselected features included entropy, dissimilarity, uniformity, correlation, and inverse difference normalized; selected based on previous literature suggesting high prognostic value in lung, colorectal, and prostate cancers [26–32]. In brief, these texture features provide a second order method for representing the conditional joint probabilities of all combination of grey levels. In brief, the probability measure can be defined as:

$$\Pr(x) = \{(Cij|(\delta, \theta)\}$$

Where δ and θ are interpixel distance and orientation, respectively. Cij, the co-occurrence probability between grey levels i and j, is defined as:

$$C_{ij} = \frac{P_{ij}}{\sum_{i,j=1}^{G} P_{ij}}$$

Pij is the number of occurrences of grey levels i and j within the given window, given a certain (δ, θ) pair, and G is the quantized number of grey levels.

Survival Time: 6 months
Tumour size: 2.22 cm^2
Dissimilarity: 12.97
Inverse Difference Normalized : 0.9756

Survival Time: 71 months
Tumour size: 1.72 cm^2
Dissimilarity: 20.22
Inverse Difference Normalized: 0.9627

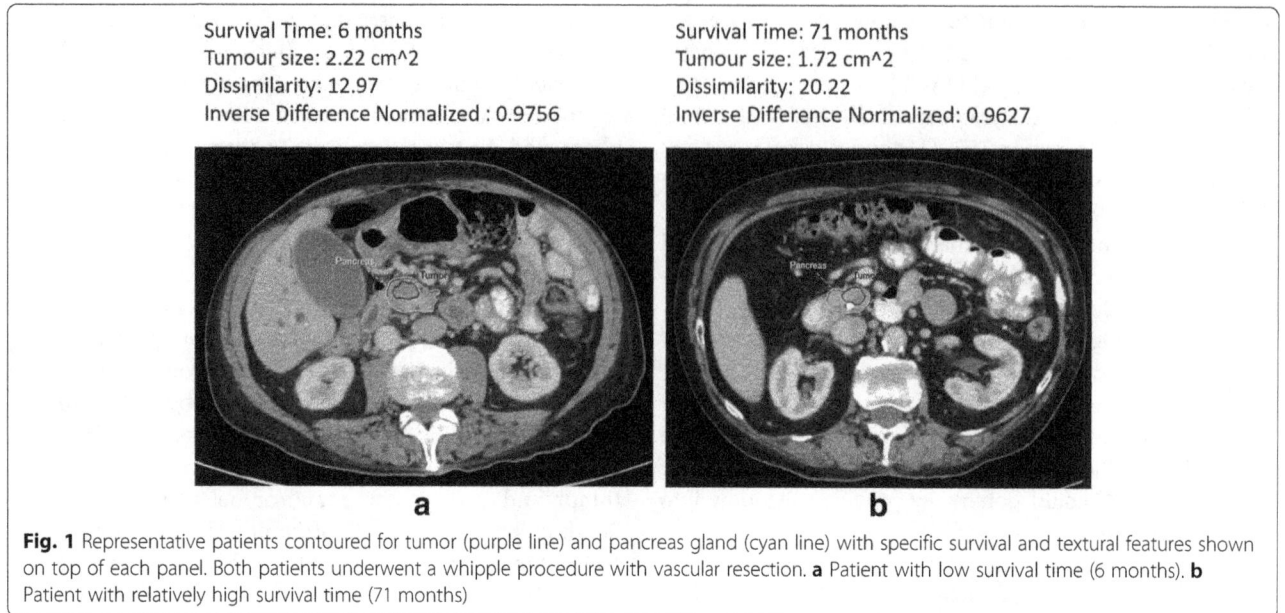

a　　　　**b**

Fig. 1 Representative patients contoured for tumor (purple line) and pancreas gland (cyan line) with specific survival and textural features shown on top of each panel. Both patients underwent a whipple procedure with vascular resection. **a** Patient with low survival time (6 months). **b** Patient with relatively high survival time (71 months)

The sum in the denominator thus represents the total number of grey level pairs (i,j) within the window. Statistics were applied to the co-occurrence matrix following [24] as presented in Table 1. Voxels with HU < −10 and > 500 were filtered from analysis in all cases to remove the fluid and stents placed before the preoperative CT [33]. Excluding voxels with HU < −10 is crucial because fat both surrounds and interdigitates between lobules of pancreatic tissue. This will produce significant texture effect in pancreatic tissue based on a process independent of cancer and more related to fatty infiltration which can be quite variable based on age and metabolic status of the patient. When contouring the pancreas, the radiologists can find it difficult to be so precise as to eliminate every voxel of fat at the margin thus small changes in contour at a fat boundary where contrast enhanced

tissue and non-contrast enhanced fat will have large variations in HU could produce erroneous texture measurements. We based the choice of -10HU on published thresholds for intralesional fat detection for angiomyolipoma which is a fat containing renal tumor [34]. Values of features from the largest cross section of the tumor were calculated across slices in which each ROI appeared. These values were used for the statistical analysis.

Statistical analysis

The texture features in tumor and normal pancreas were compared using a Mann–Whitney rank test. A Wald test

Table 1 Grey level co-occurrence texture features. All summations are over all (i,j) pairs

Parameter	Mathematical definition
Uniformity	$\sum_{i,j=1}^{G} C_{ij}^2$
Entropy	$\sum_{i,j=1}^{G} C_{ij}\, logC_{ij}$
Dissimilarity	$\sum_{i,j=1}^{G} C_{ij}\, |i-j|$
Inverse Difference Normalized	$\sum_{i,j=1}^{G} \frac{C_{ij}}{1+|i-j|^2/G^2}$
Correlation	$\sum_{i,j=1}^{G} \frac{(i-\mu x)(j-\mu y)C_{ij}}{\sigma x \sigma y}$

Table 2 Demographic information of studied cohort

Age (years)	Mean ± Standard deviation	69 ± 8
Sex	Female/Male/Total	13/17/30
Vascular resection	Yes/No/Total	15/15/30
Size (cm2)	Mean ± Standard Deviation	2.13 ± 1.88
Grade	G1/G2/G3/Total	3/19/8/30
Nodes Sampled (Per Patient)	Mean ± Standard Deviation	25 ± 11
Patients with Negative/ Positive Nodes	N0/N1	6/24
Margin	R2/R1/R0	0/16/14
Survival Time (months)	Mean ± Standard Deviation	31 ± 25

Nodes Sampled is the number of nodes taken from each patient. Patients with Negative Nodes is the number of patients whose sampled nodes were all negative. Patients with Positive Nodes is the number of patients who had at least one positive sampled node

Table 3 Comparison of normal and tumor tissues (Entries in bold were significant)

Texture feature	Tumor tissue median (interquartile range)	Normal tissue median (interquartile range)	Tumor vs Normal comparison p-value (Rank sum test)
Uniformity	0.181 (0.165–0.192)	0.210 (0.189–0.225)	**<0.001**
Entropy	{−0.758 (−0.987-0.681)} × 10^{-3}	{−0.611 (−0.746-0.508)} × 10^{-3}	**0.009**
Dissimilarity	0.286 (0.249–0.311)	0.270 (0.223–0.304)	0.530
Correlation	0.393 (0.267–0.464)	0.486 (0.430–0.591)	**<0.001**
Inverse Difference Normalized	0.859 (0.845–0.877)	0.866 (0.849–0.889)	0.511
Mean Intensity	55.988 (41.099–62.617)	70.255 (60.452–81.506)	**<0.001**

with Cox regression model was used to test for associations between each texture feature and survival. A two-sided p-value of less than 0.05 was considered statistically significant. Receiver operating characteristics (ROC), including area under the curve (AUC), was used to study the prognostic value of each texture parameter. The medians were used for Kaplan-Meier plots. Data management and statistical analysis were conducted using IBM SPSS Statistics package (version 23, SPSS Inc., Chicago, IL, USA).

Results

The demographic information of the cohort is shown in Table 2. Tumor region and the normal pancreas were used for analysis. The median (interquartile range) of HU was 71 (61–82) and 57 (41–63) in normal pancreas and tumor, respectively ($p < 0.001$). The HU was significantly higher in normal tissue than tumor regions in all patients ($p < 0.001$) for the portal venous phase. Tumor was significantly different than normal pancreas, as shown in Table 3; uniformity ($p < 0.001$), entropy ($p = 0.009$), and correlation ($p < 0.001$). However, the difference in dissimilarity ($p = 0.530$) and inverse difference normalized ($p = 0.511$) were not significant.

Wald-test in Cox regression analysis on tumor texture parameters showed dissimilarity (coefficient = −0.1292, p-value = 0.045) and inverse difference normalized (coefficient = 71.81, p-value = 0.046) were significantly associated with OS as shown in Table 4. Kaplan-Meier plots of cumulative survival for significant tumour features are provided in Fig. 2. Also, size of the tumor (coefficient = 0.000627, p-value = 0.611) and the average intensity of the tumor (coefficient = −0.011, p-value = 0.366) were not significantly associated with OS. Other tumor texture features were not significantly associated with survival with the coefficients and p-values as follows: uniformity (coefficient = −105.5, p-value = 0.334), entropy (coefficient = 0.324, p-value = 0.330), correlation (coefficient = 4.013, p-value = 0.068).

Among the studied features, dissimilarity (AUC = 0.716) and inverse difference normalized (AUC = 0.716) showed maximal predictive value for predicting OS. AUC for uniformity, entropy, and correlation were 0.560, 0.569, and 0.680, respectively. Table 5 represents details of the ROC analysis.

Figure 3 shows the histogram of two significant features namely dissimilarity and inverse difference normalized. This figure also illustrates the distribution of survival across the features values.

Discussion

In our study, we used GLCM textural analysis from venous phase contrast-enhanced CT and found that dissimilarity and inverse difference normalized were associated with OS in a cohort of resectable PDAC patients. These features provided a stronger association with OS than tumor intensity and tumor size.

We found that less inverse difference normalized and greater dissimilarity are associated with longer OS. As texture analysis has not been used in the context of resectable PDAC, there were no studies to compare our findings. However, we can compare our results with other studies that followed a similar hypothesis in other types of cancer. Our findings are consistent with previous radiomic studies for lung,

Table 4 Cox regression for survival analysis using texture features and size of tumor (Entries in bold were significant)

Parameter	B value	Standard error	Wald	p-value
Uniformity	−105.5	109.2	0.93	0.334
Entropy	0.3240	0.333	0.95	0.330
Dissimilarity	**−0.1292**	**0.065**	**4.01**	**0.045**
Correlation	4.013	2.195	3.34	0.068
Inverse Difference Normalized	**71.81**	**36.04**	**3.97**	**0.046**
Tumor Size	0.000627	0.00123	0.26	0.611
Tumor Intensity	−0.011	0.013	0.82	0.366

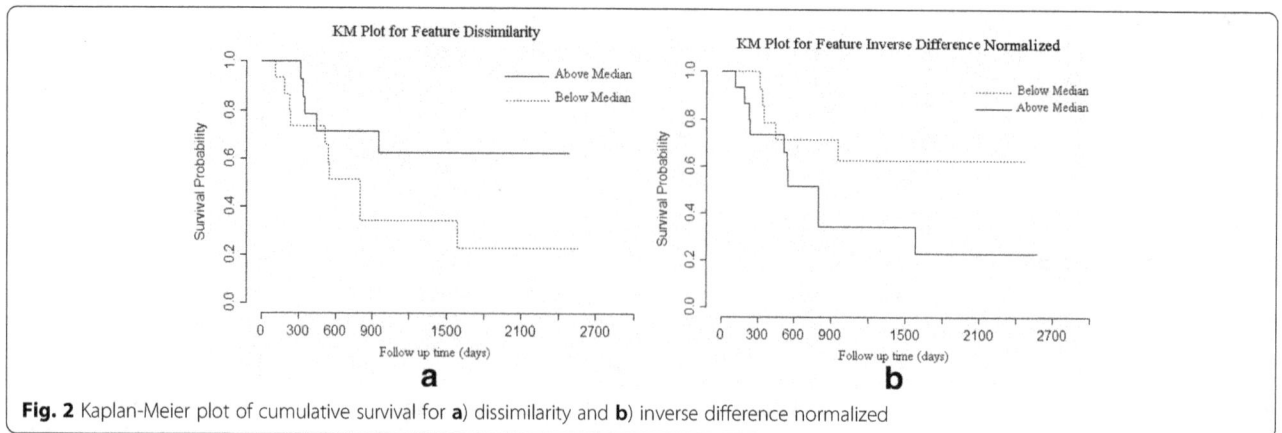

Fig. 2 Kaplan-Meier plot of cumulative survival for **a**) dissimilarity and **b**) inverse difference normalized

breast, and other cancer site. Different studies have also shown that dissimilarity feature extracted from ROIs in PET/CT has a positive correlation with survival time for non-small cell lung cancer [35, 36] and Multi–Cancer site patient cohorts [37]. It is important to note that the underlying meaning of imaging texture cannot be reduced to a mean regional intensity but is estimated from the probability of the occurrence of a specific pattern of intensities which can explain why mean intensity was not associated with survival outcome in our study and others. Such texture features may not be readily visible on standard grey scale images.

Given the challenging management of PDAC which presents late and is highly lethal, it is hoped that gathering clues of factors associated with overall survival from CT could augment the ability for treatment decision making [38] and aid in prognosticating treatment scenarios. Our findings show that with minimal cost and with no additional imaging burden, textural feature analysis of routine contrast-enhanced CT imaging before surgery may provide useful information for PDAC patients undergoing curative intent surgical resection. Our results show that textural analysis is more strongly

associated with OS than tumor size. Such informed decision may help in identifying therapeutic plan for patients, for example, considering targeted adjuvant or neoadjuvant treatments in some patients with predicted poor prognosis. On the other hand, it may help in identifying patients with very poor prognosis who are unlikely to benefit from surgery; in these patients chemotherapy or radiation may be the optimal treatment modality [39]. Certainly for clinical application in personalized medicine, a wider repertoire of treatment options with better survival is a fundamental challenge in this nearly uniformly lethal disease. As our understanding of imaging biomarkers continues to unfold, it is hoped that this may provide more insight into the likely benefit of new therapeutic regimes in subpopulations of patients.

This study has limitations. The small sample size limits our ability to perform a multivariate analysis and thus additional stratification based on tumor extent such as resectable versus borderline resectable stratification could not be evaluated. Despite a relatively small sample size, we found strong association of the textural features with OS. The findings of this study encourage investigating the association of a wider range of radiomic features

Table 5 Receiver operating characteristic analysis of texture features and size for predicting survival outcome (Entries in bold were found significant)

Parameter	Sensitivity	Specificity	AUC	Threshold	95% CI	p-value
Uniformity	0.6	0.4	0.560	0.002	0.230–0.650	0.576
Entropy	0.6	0.533	0.569	5.901	0.360–0.778	0.520
Dissimilarity	**0.667**	**0.733**	**0.716**	**16.311**	**0.528–0.903**	**0.044**
Correlation	0.533	0.733	0.68	0.610	0.484–0.875	0.093
Inverse Difference Normalized	**0.667**	**0.733**	**0.716**	**0.969**	**0.528–0.903**	**0.044**
Tumor Size	0.533	0.533	0.538	154.761	0.326–0.750	0.724
Tumor intensity	0.533	0.533	0.524	58.462	0.313–0.736	0.820

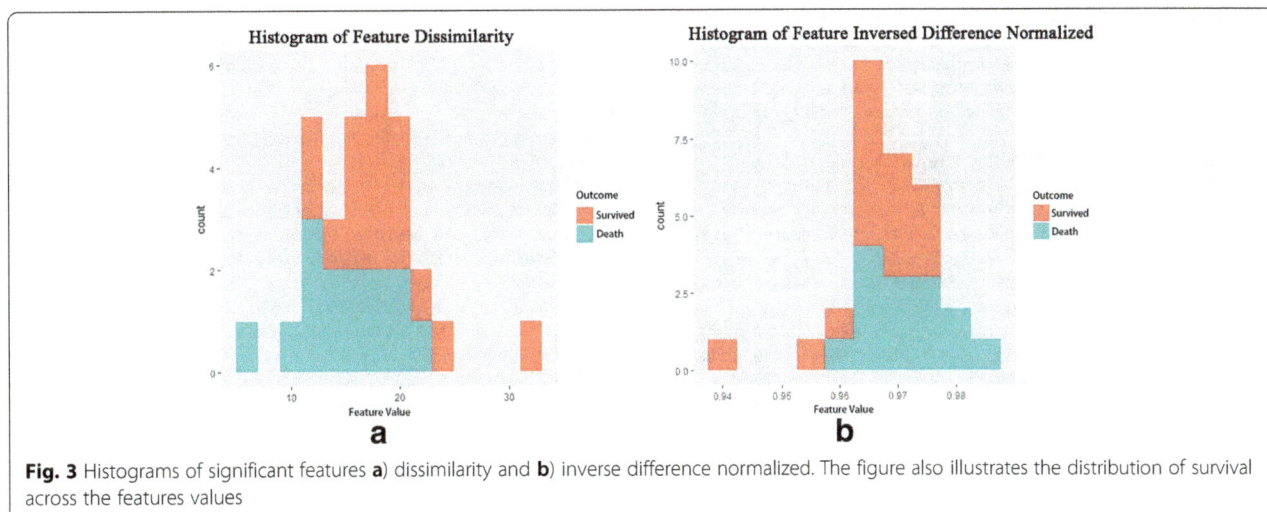

Fig. 3 Histograms of significant features **a**) dissimilarity and **b**) inverse difference normalized. The figure also illustrates the distribution of survival across the features values

with survival and intermediate factors such as radiogenomics in a larger sample size. Also the reported findings should be verified independently in future studies. Further work is also needed to address the repeatability of these quantitative imaging biomarkers as part of a biomarker validation process [40]. There is always a risk of achieving statistically positive results by chance with small sample sizes. We have tried to restrict the number of features being evaluated by choosing features that have already been shown to be prognostic in a variety of other adenocarcinomas [12, 26]. The fact that some of the texture features associated with OS match those in other adenocarcinomas is encouraging. Finally, there is a lack of understanding on the underlying relationship of texture features and histology, genomics and proteomics of PDAC which requires further work.

Conclusions

CT-derived PDAC texture features of dissimilarity and inverse difference normalized are promising prognostic imaging biomarkers of OS for patients undergoing curative intent surgical resection.

Abbreviations
AUC: Area under the curve; CT: Computed tomography; GLCM: Grey-level co-occurrence matrix; HU: Hounsfield unit; MRI: Magnetic resonance imaging; OS: Overall survival; PDAC: Pancreatic ductal adenocarcinoma; PET: Positron emission tomography; ROC: Receiver operating characteristics; ROI: Region of interest

Acknowledgements
Authors would like to thank Mr. Stephen Tasker for his insights about the acquisition protocol.

Funding
This research was conducted with the support of the Ontario Institute for Cancer Research (PanCuRx Translational Research Initiative) through funding provided by the Government of Ontario (Ministry of Research and Innovation).

Authors' contributions
AE, FK, and MAH contributed to the design and implementation of the concept. AE, SB, PK, SG, and MAH contributed in collecting and reviewing the data. AE, JZ, and FK contributed to the design and implementation of quantitative feature extraction modules. AE, YZ, FK, and MAH contributed to the statistical analysis of the data. All authors contributed to the writing and reviewing of the paper. All authors read and approved the final manuscript.

Competing interests
The authors declare that they have no competing interest.

Author details
[1]Department of Medical Imaging and Sunnybrook Research Institute, Sunnybrook Health Sciences Center, University of Toronto, 2075 Bayview Ave., Room Rm AG 46, Toronto M4N 3 M5, ON, Canada. [2]Department of Surgery, Sunnybrook Health Sciences Center, University of Toronto, Toronto, ON, Canada. [3]PanCuRx Translational Research Initiative, Ontario Institute for Cancer Research, Toronto, ON, Canada. [4]Lunenfeld-Tanenbaum Research Institute, Mount Sinai Hospital, Toronto, ON, Canada. [5]Hepatobiliary/pancreatic Surgical Oncology Program, University Health Network, Toronto, ON, Canada. [6]Mechanical Engineering Department, Australian College of Kuwait, Kuwait City, Kuwait.

References
1. Lambin P, Rios-Velazquez E, Leijenaar R, Carvalho S, Van Stiphout RGPM, Granton P, et al. Radiomics: Extracting more information from medical images using advanced feature analysis. Eur J Cancer. 2012;48(4):441–6.
2. Marusyk A, Polyak K. Tumor heterogeneity: Causes and consequences. Biochim Biophys Acta - Rev Cancer. 2010;1805(1):105–17.
3. Davnall F, Yip CSP, Ljungqvist G, Selmi M, Ng F, Sanghera B, et al. Assessment of tumor heterogeneity: an emerging imaging tool for clinical practice? Insights Imaging. Springer Berlin Heidelberg; 2012;3(6):573–89
4. Aerts HJ, Velazquez ER, Leijenaar RT, Parmar C, Grossmann P, Carvalho S, et al. Decoding tumour phenotype by noninvasive imaging using a quantitative radiomics approach. Nat Commun. 2014;5:4006.
5. Hwang I, Park CM, Park SJ, Lee SM, McAdams HP, Jeon YK, et al. Persistent Pure Ground-Glass Nodules Larger Than 5 mm. Invest Radiol. 2015;50(11):798–804.
6. Koo HJ, Sung YS, Shim WH, Xu H, Choi C-M, Kim HR, et al. Quantitative Computed Tomography Features for Predicting Tumor Recurrence in Patients with Surgically Resected Adenocarcinoma of the Lung. Rubin DL, editor. PLoS One. Public Library of Science; 2017;12(1):e0167955
7. Ahn SY, Park CM, Park SJ, Kim HJ, Song C, Lee SM, et al. Prognostic Value of Computed Tomography Texture Features in Non–Small Cell Lung Cancers Treated With Definitive Concomitant Chemoradiotherapy. Invest Radiol. 2015;50(10):719–25.

8. Chae H, Park CM, Park SJ, Lee SM, Kim KG, Goo JM. Computerized texture analysis of persistent part-solid ground-glass nodules: differentiation of preinvasive lesions from invasive pulmonary adenocarcinomas. Radiology. 2014;273(1):285–93. Available from: http://pubs.rsna.org/doi/10.1148/radiol.14132187?url_ver=Z39.88-2003&rfr_id=ori:rid:crossref.org&rfr_dat=cr_pub%3dpubmed.

9. Haralick RM, Shanmugam K, Dinstein I. Textural Features for Image Classification. IEEE Trans Syst Man Cybern. IEEE; 1973;3(6):610–21

10. Sebastian B, Unnikrishnan A, Balakrishnan K. Grey level co-occurrence matrices: generalisation and some new features. Int J Comput Sci Eng Inf Technol. 2012;2(2):610–21.

11. Ohanian PP, Dubes RC. Performance evaluation for four classes of textural features. Pattern Recognit. Pergamon; 1992;25(8):819–33

12. Coroller TP, Grossmann P, Hou Y, Rios Velazquez E, Leijenaar RTH, Hermann G, et al. CT based radiomic signature CT-based radiomic signature predicts distant metastasis in lung adenocarcinoma. Radiother Oncol. 2015;114:345–50.

13. Zhu Y, Li H, Guo W, Drukker K, Lan L, Giger ML, et al. Deciphering Genomic Underpinnings of Quantitative MRI-based Radiomic Phenotypes of Invasive Breast Carcinoma. Scientific Reports. 2015;5:17787. Available from http://dx.doi.org/10.1038/srep17787.

14. Hesketh RL, Zhu AX, Oklu R. Radiomics and circulating tumor cells: personalized care in hepatocellular carcinoma? Diagn Interv Radiol. 2015;21(1):78–84.

15. Stark AP, Sacks GD, Rochefort MM, Donahue TR, Reber HA, Tomlinson JS, et al. Long-term survival in patients with pancreatic ductal adenocarcinoma. Surgery. 2016;159(6):1520–7. doi: 10.1016/j.surg.2015.12.024.

16. National Cancer Institute. SurveiNIH llance, Epidemiology and End Results Program. 2016.

17. Landry J, Catalano PJ, Staley C, Harris W, Hoffman J, Talamonti M, et al. Randomized phase II study of gemcitabine plus radiotherapy versus gemcitabine, 5-fluorouracil, and cisplatin followed by radiotherapy and 5-fluorouracil for patients with locally advanced, potentially resectable pancreatic adenocarcinoma. J Surg Oncol. 2010;101(7):587–92.

18. Ferrone CR, Pieretti-Vanmarcke R, Bloom JP, Zheng H, Szymonifka J, Wargo JA, et al. Pancreatic ductal adenocarcinoma: long-term survival does not equal cure. Surgery. 2012;152(3 Suppl 1):S43–9.

19. Winter JM, Cameron JL, Campbell KA, Arnold MA, Chang DC, Coleman J, et al. 1423 pancreaticoduodenectomies for pancreatic cancer: A single-institution experience. J Gastrointest Surg. 2006;10(9):1199. -210-1.

20. Gillen S, Schuster T, Meyer zum Büschenfelde C, Friess H, Kleeff J. Preoperative/Neoadjuvant Therapy in Pancreatic Cancer: A Systematic Review and Meta-analysis of Response and Resection Percentages. Seiler C, editor. PLoS Med. Public Library of Science; 2010;7(4):e1000267.

21. Tamm EP, Bhosale PR, Lee JH. Pancreatic Ductal Adenocarcinoma: Ultrasound, Computed Tomography, and Magnetic Resonance Imaging Features. Semin Ultrasound CT MR. 2007;28(5):330–8.

22. Diehl SJ, Lehmann KJ, Sadick M, Lachmann R, Georgi M. Pancreatic cancer: value of dual-phase helical CT in assessing resectability. Radiology. 1998;206(2):373–8.

23. Zhang J, Baig S, Wong A, Haider MA, Khalvati F. A Local ROI-specific Atlas-based Segmentation of Prostate Gland and Transitional Zone in Diffusion MRI. J Comput Vis Imaging Syst. 2016;2(1):610–21.

24. Clausi DA. An analysis of co-occurrence texture statistics as a function of grey level quantization. Can J Remote Sens. 2002;28(1):45–62.

25. Tahir MA, Bouridane A, Kurugollu F. An FPGA Based Coprocessor for GLCM and Haralick Texture Features and their Application in Prostate Cancer Classification. Analog Integr Circuits Signal Process. Kluwer Academic Publishers; 2005;43(2):205–15.

26. Ganeshan B, Panayiotou E, Burnand K, Dizdarevic S, Miles K. Tumour heterogeneity in non-small cell lung carcinoma assessed by CT texture analysis: A potential marker of survival. Eur Radiol. 2012;22(4):796–802.

27. Ng F, Ganeshan B, Kozarski R, Miles KA, Goh V. Assessment of Primary colorectal cancer heterogeneity by Using Whole-Tumor Texture analysis: Contrast-enhanced CT Texture as a Biomarker of 5-year Survival. Radiology. 2013;266(1):177–84. doi: 10.1148/radiol.12120254.

28. Cameron A, Khalvati F, Haider M, Wong A. MAPS: A Quantitative Radiomics Approach for Prostate Cancer Detection. IEEE Trans Biomed Eng. 2016;63(6):1145–56.

29. Khalvati F, Wong A, Haider MA. Automated Prostate Cancer Detection via Comprehensive Multi-parametric Magnetic Resonance Imaging Texture Feature Models. BMC Med Imaging. BMC Medical Imaging; 2015;15(1):27. Available from: https://bmcmedimaging.biomedcentral.com/articles/10.1186/s12880-015-0069-9.

30. Yogesan K, Jorgensen T, Albregtsen F, Tveter KJ, Danielsen HE. Entropy - Based Texture Analysis of Chromatin Structure i n Advanced Prostate Cancer. Cytometry. 1996;24:268–76.

31. Wu H, Sun T, Wang J, Li X, Wang W, Huo D, et al. Combination of radiological and gray level co-occurrence matrix textural features used to distinguish solitary pulmonary nodules by computed tomography. J Digit Imaging. 2013;26(4):797–802. doi: 10.1007/s10278-012-9547-6.

32. Wang H, Guo X-H, Jia Z-W, Li H-K, Liang Z-G, Li K-C, et al. Multilevel binomial logistic prediction model for malignant pulmonary nodules based on texture features of CT image. Eur J Radiol. 2010;74(1):124–9.

33. Mathur A, Hernandez J, Shaheen F, Shroff M, Dahal S, Morton C, et al. Preoperative computed tomography measurements of pancreatic steatosis and visceral fat: prognostic markers for dissemination and lethality of pancreatic adenocarcinoma. HPB (Oxford). Elsevier; 2011;13(6):404–10

34. Westphalen AC. Diagnosis of renal angiomyolipoma with CT hounsfield unit thresholds. Radiology. 2012;262(1):370–1.

35. Lovinfosse P, Janvary ZL, Coucke P, Jodogne S, Bernard C, Hatt M, et al. FDG PET/CT texture analysis for predicting the outcome of lung cancer treated by stereotactic body radiation therapy. Eur J Nucl Med Mol Imaging. 2016;43(8):1453–60.

36. Tixier F, Hatt M, Valla C, Fleury V, Lamour C, Ezzouhri S, et al. Visual Versus Quantitative Assessment of Intratumor 18 F-FDG PET Uptake Heterogeneity: Prognostic Value in Non – Small Cell Lung Cancer. J Nucl Med. 2014;55(8):1235–41.

37. Hatt M, Majdoub M, Vallières M, Tixier F, Cheze-Le Rest C, Groheux D, et al. 18 F-FDG PET Uptake Characterization Through Texture Analysis: Investigating the Complementary Nature of Heterogeneity and Functional Tumor Volume in a Multi–Cancer Site Patient Cohort. J Nucl Med. 2015; 56(1):38–44. Available from: http://jnm.snmjournals.org/content/56/1/38.abstractN2.

38. Lennon A, Wolfgang C, Canto M, Klein A. The early detection of pancreatic cancer: what will it take to diagnose and treat curable pancreatic neoplasia? Cancer Res. 2014.

39. Moertel CG, Frytak S, Hahn RG, O'Connell MJ, Reitemeier RJ, Rubin J, et al. Therapy of locally unresectable pancreatic carcinoma: A randomized comparison of high dose (6000 rads) radiation alone, moderate dose radiation (4000 rads + 5-fluorouracil), and high dose radiation + 5-fluorouracil. The gastrointestinal tumor study group. Cancer. Wiley Subscription Services, Inc., A Wiley Company; 1981;48(8):1705–10.

40. Chung AG, Kumar D, Shafiee MJ, Chung AG, Khalvati F, Haider M a., et al. Discovery Radiomics for Computed Tomography Cancer Detection. arXiv. 2015;1–7. Available from: http://arxiv.org/abs/1509.00117.

28

Radial scars/complex sclerosing lesions of the breast: radiologic and clinicopathologic correlation

Su Min Ha[1], Joo Hee Cha[2]* ⓘ, Hee Jung Shin[2], Eun Young Chae[2], Woo Jung Choi[2], Hak Hee Kim[2] and Ha-Yeon Oh[3]

Abstract

Background: We investigated the radiologic and clinical findings of radial scar and complex sclerosing lesions, and evaluated the rate of pathologic upgrade and predicting factors.

Methods: From review of our institution's database from January 2006 to December 2012, we enrolled 82 radial scars/complex sclerosing lesions in 80 women; 51 by ultrasound guided core needle biopsy, 1 by mammography-guided stereotactic biopsy, and 38 by surgical excision. The initial biopsy pathology revealed that 53 lesions were without high risk lesions and 29 were with high risk lesions. Radiologic, clinical and pathological results were analyzed statistically and upgrade rates were calculated.

Results: Of the 82 lesions, 64 (78.0%) were surgically excised. After surgical excision, two were upgraded to DCIS and two were upgraded to lesions with high risk lesions. The rate of radial scar with high risk lesions was significantly higher in the surgical excision group (11.1% vs. 42.2%, $p = 0.015$), which also demonstrated larger lesion size (10.7 ± 6.5 vs. 7.1 ± 2.6 mm, $p = 0.001$). The diagnoses with high risk lesions on final pathological results showed older age (52.9 ± 6.0 years vs. 48.4 ± 6.7 years, $p = 0.018$).

Conclusions: Radial scars with and without high risk lesions showed no statistically significant differences in imaging, and gave relatively low cancer upgrade rates.

Keywords: Radial scar, Complex sclerosing lesion, Mammography, Ultrasound, Surgical management

Background

Radial scar is characterized by stellate configuration of a fibroelastic core with entrapped ducts and lobules, and is also referred to as complex sclerosing lesion (CSL) [1]. Radial scar/CSL is diagnosed at image-guided biopsy with an incidence ranging from 0.6 to 3.7% [2, 3]. Despite being uncommon, radial scars remain important in patient management because their radiologic appearance overlaps that of invasive carcinoma and their diagnosis is challenging for radiologists [4], with the potential to be misinterpreted by pathologists as low grade invasive ductal or tubular carcinoma [5]. Radial scars can be indistinguishable from invasive carcinoma on radiologic appearance alone, often presenting as a spiculated mass or architectural distortion [6, 7]. Once diagnosis has been made with core biopsy, management is controversial because of the intrinsic malignant potential of radial scars and their coexistence with breast cancer and other high risk lesions. Radial scar is one of the proliferative categories that can coexist alongside other proliferative high risk lesions, including atypia, with each contributing to the overall upgrade rate to malignancy at excision [8–10]. As both radiology and pathology are imperfect for predicting associated malignancy, the prudence of surgical excision versus conservative management remains debatable.

Radial scar/CSL is associated with atypical proliferative lesions and has been suggested as early stage development of invasive carcinoma. The radiologically detected

---

* Correspondence: jhcha@amc.seoul.kr
[2]Department of Radiology, Research Institute of Radiology, University of Ulsan College of Medicine, Asan Medical Center, 88 Olympic-Ro 43 Gil, Songpa-Gu, Seoul 05505, Republic of Korea
Full list of author information is available at the end of the article

radial scar associated malignancy rate ranged from 10.0 to 41.0% on excision [11]. However, recent studies with carefully performed correlations between radiological and pathology findings suggest that upgrade to carcinoma on core biopsy occurs in less than 2.0% [12–15]. Furthermore, most of the lesions upgraded from radial scar are ductal carcinoma in situ (DCIS) or low grade ductal or tubular type [12, 13, 15]. The short-term follow-up of radial scars that were not excised has shown no upgrades [13, 15–18]. Thus, some insist that a subset of patients with radial scars may safely forego excision, especially in the absence of coexisting high risk lesions or other indications for excision [14, 18]. Miller et al. [15] reported an upgrade rate to invasive carcinoma of less than 1% at surgical excision of radial scar, with or without associated high risk lesions, and also revealed that the radiologic appearances of a mass or architectural distortion on mammography or ultrasound (US) are more likely to be upgraded than calcifications. Brenner et al. [16] conducted a study on one of the largest cohorts and reported an upgrade rate of 5% from a median 38 months of follow-up or by surgery, and suggested that excision of radial scar can be avoided when there is no high risk lesion on core biopsy, more than 12 biopsy specimens have been collected, and the histologic and mammographic findings are concordant. With regard to MRI of radial scar, MRI has a 97.6–100.0% negative predictive value for differentiating between benign and malignant radial scar lesions [19–23]. With the emergence of digital breast tomosynthesis, increased screening examinations, and advanced MRI, many biopsies are now performed on lesions in their earlier stages and with a smaller size, and an increasing number of mammographically occult radial scars have been detected by US, with 15.7% to 39.0% of radial scars without atypia being diagnosed [2, 24, 25]. The objective of this study was to evaluate patients with radial scar/CSL with or without high risk lesions according to management strategy such as surgical excision or follow-up of at least 5 years, comparing associated malignancy, and to identify clinical, radiologic (mammography, US, and MRI), and pathologic features predictive of upgrade.

Methods
Study population
Our institutional review board approved this retrospective study, and the requirement for informed consent was waived. The database of our institution was retrospectively reviewed for image-guided biopsy and breast surgery occurring between January 2006 to December 2012 to identify patients with a diagnosis of radial scar/CSL with or without high risk lesions (i.e., atypical epithelial hyperplasia, lobular neoplasia, papilloma, or atypical papilloma). Radial scar was defined as a lesion of 1.0 cm or smaller, while CSL was defined as a lesion larger than

1.0 cm. We excluded patients who were initially diagnosed with ipsilateral breast cancer or those who were followed-up for a period of less than 5 years without having undergone surgery. Finally, we enrolled 82 radial scars/CSLs in 80 women; 51 were diagnosed by US-guided core needle biopsy, one by mammography-guided stereotactic biopsy, and 38 by surgical excision.

At initial diagnosis, 53 of the lesions were considered to be without high risk lesions and 29 lesions were considered as being accompanied by high risk lesions. Of the 53 radial scars/CSLs without high risk lesions, 37 lesions (69.8%) were surgically excised and 16 lesions (30.2%) were not excised but underwent imaging follow-up of at least 5 years. Of the 29 radial scars/CSLs with high risk lesions (15 atypical epithelial hyperplasia, 7 atypically papilloma, 7 papilloma), 27 lesions (93.1%) were surgically excised and two lesions (6.9%) were not excised but underwent imaging follow-up.

We recorded whether lesions were detected during screening or diagnostic examination, and whether patients were asymptomatic or symptomatic.

An upgrade was defined as occurring when the surgical pathology was changed from 1) a lesion without high risk to a high risk lesion, DCIS, or invasive carcinoma, and 2) from lesions with high risk to DCIS or invasive carcinoma.

Imaging technique and biopsy methods
Mammography was performed using a full-field digital mammogram unit (Senographe DS or Senographe Essential scanner, both from Generic Electric Medical System, Milwaukee, WI, USA). Two standard imaging planes were used, the mediolateral oblique and craniocaudal views.

Whole-breast US was performed using an IU22 unit (Philips Medical System, Bothell, WA, USA) equipped with a 50 mm linear array transducer with a bandwidth of 5–12 MHz. At our institution, the scanning technique for bilateral whole-breast US is standardized as follows: scanning is performed in a transverse and sagittal orientation, with the inner breast in a supine position and the outer breast in a supine oblique position with the patient's arm raised above her head. The pectoralis muscle has to be seen on all images to ensure that the entire breast is examined. Each lesion is documented with an image of its longest dimension and an orthogonal measurement.

Dynamic contrast-enhanced MRI was performed on a 1.5 T scanner (Magnetom Avanto, Siemens Medical Solutions, Erlangen, Germany) using a dedicated 18-channel phased-array breast coil. The standard breast MRI protocol included the following pulse sequences: 1) an axial two-dimensional T2-weighted short tau inversion recovery (STIR) turbo spin-echo pulse sequence (repetition time/echo time/time interval (TR/TE/TI), 6700/74/150 ms; field of view (FOV) 300 × 300 mm; matrix size, 448 × 448; slice thickness, 5 mm); 2) pre and post-contrast-enhanced fat-saturated axial three-dimensional T1-weighted fast low angle shot volume interpolated breath-hold examination (FLASH VIBE) pulse sequences (TR/TE, 5.2/2.4 ms; FOV 340 × 340 mm; matrix size, 384 × 384; slice thickness, 0.9 mm). The six dynamic sequences (one unenhanced and five contrast-enhanced acquisitions with a temporal resolution of 59 s) were acquired before and after injection of contrast medium.

US-guided core needle biopsy was performed with a 14-gauge dual action semi-automatic core biopsy needle (Stericut with coaxial guide, TSK Laboratory, Tochigi, Japan), and a minimum of five core samples were obtained. Biopsies of mammographic findings such as asymmetry, architectural distortions, and calcifications without a corresponding US finding were performed with a stereotactic technique involving 11-gauge vacuum probes (Mammotome; Ethicon Endo-Surgery, Cincinnati, OH) on an upright stereotactic digital unit, using a Senographe Essential stereotaxic machine (General Electric Medical Systems, Milwaukee, WI).

All surgical excision was performed after US or mammography-guided wire localization, with specimen mammography being performed in cases of mammography-guided wire localization.

Analysis of imaging findings

Mammography, US, and MRI were retrospectively reviewed (without regard to the initial clinical reporting) by two radiologists with 6 and 17 years of clinical experience in breast imaging, respectively. Each radiologist was blind to the readings of the other radiologist. When a discrepancy occurred, the two radiologists reviewed the case together and reached a consensus. Imaging features were described and assessed according to the American College of Radiology (ACR) BI-RADS 5th edition [26].

On mammography, lesions were classified into mass, calcification, mass with calcification, architectural distortion, architectural distortion with calcification, and asymmetry. For a mass, the shape was described as oval, round, or irregular, and the margin as circumscribed, obscured, microlobulated, indistinct, or spiculated. For calcifications, the distribution was analyzed as diffuse, regional, grouped, linear, or segmental, and the morphology as amorphous, coarse heterogeneous, fine pleomorphic, or punctate.

On US, the shape of each mass was described as oval, round, or irregular; the orientation as parallel or non-parallel; the margin as circumscribed, indistinct, angular, microlobulated, or spiculated; and the echo pattern as anechoic, hyperechoic, complex cystic and solid, hypoechoic, isoechoic, or heterogeneous. Posterior features were classified as no posterior feature, posterior enhancement,

posterior shadowing, or a combination. The visibility of any calcification on US was also assessed.

On breast MRI for mass lesions, the margins were described as circumscribed, irregular, or spiculated, and the shape as oval, round, or irregular. The internal enhancement of each mass was classified as homogeneous, heterogeneous, rim, or dark internal septation enhancement. For non-mass lesions, the distributions were described as focal, linear, segmental, regional, multiple regions, or diffuse, while the pattern of enhancement was classified as homogeneous, heterogeneous, clumped, or clustered ring. The enhancement kinetic curve was described as Type 1 (persistent enhancement), Type 2 (plateau), or Type 3 (peak early enhancement followed by delayed washout).

Statistical analysis

The characteristics of the patients and findings of the lesions, including upgrade rates, are summarized using number and percentage. Clinical characteristics and imaging findings were compared between lesions that underwent surgical excision ($n = 64$) and lesions that underwent follow-up ($n = 18$), with Student's t-tests being used for continuous variables and χ^2 tests for categorical variables. Lesions were also grouped according to the final pathological diagnosis (performed by surgical excision or follow-up of at least 5 years) as radial scar without high risk lesions ($n = 49$) or radial scar with high risk lesions ($n = 33$), and were compared using Student's t-test or a Mann-Whitney test for continuous variables, and Fisher's exact test for categorical variables. Calculations for statistical analyses were performed using SPSS software (version 23.0, IBM Corp., Armonk, NY, USA). A P-value of less than 0.05 was considered to indicate a statistically significant difference between groups.

Results

Of the 82 lesions, 64 (78.0%) were surgically excised and 18 (22.0%) were not excised (Fig. 1). During the 5-year follow-up of the non-excised 18 lesions, there was no imaging or clinical change suggestive of an upgrade. However, two DCIS lesions (3.1%) were identified among 64 lesions that were surgically excised. In comparison with the follow-up group, the surgical excision group had a significantly higher percentage of radial scars/CSLs with high risk lesions (11.1% vs. 42.2%, $p = 0.015$) and contained lesions with a larger mean size (7.1 ± 2.6 mm vs. 10.7 ± 6.5 mm, $p = 0.001$). There were more patients with a contralateral breast malignancy such as invasive ductal cancer ($n = 7$, 70.0%), DCIS ($n = 1$, 10.0%), or tubular carcinoma ($n = 2$, 20.0%) in the operated-on group, but not statistically significant ($p = 0.576$) and were mostly screen detected without symptoms in both groups (100% and 92.2%, $p = 0.581$).

Out of all the 82 lesions in 80 patients, mammography was performed on 73 (89.0%), US on 82 (100.0%), and

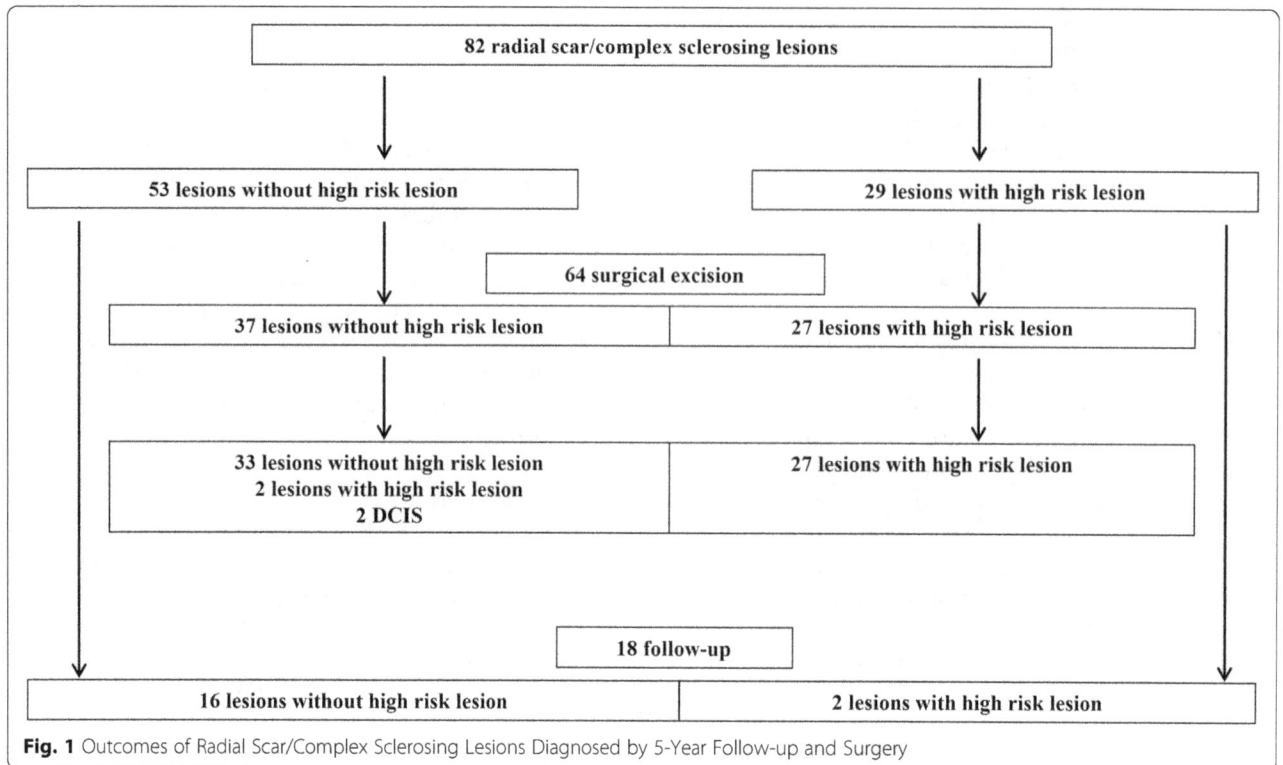

Fig. 1 Outcomes of Radial Scar/Complex Sclerosing Lesions Diagnosed by 5-Year Follow-up and Surgery

MRI on 13 (15.9%). Analysis of the imaging findings from mammography, US, and MRI, including the BI-RADS category, revealed no statistically significant differences between the surgical excision and follow-up groups. In both groups, masses on mammography (eleven mass only and six mass with calcification) had a mostly irregular shape (14/17, 82.4%), spiculated margin (10/17, 58.8%), and were hyperdense (10/17, 58.8%), while calcifications (four calcification only, six mass with calcification, and three architectural distortion with calcification) had a predominantly amorphous morphology (8/13, 61.5%) with regional (7/13, 53.8%) distribution. One lesion manifested as an architectural distortion only, and one as an asymmetry on mammography. On US, 79 lesions were seen as masses. Masses had mostly irregular shape (52/79, 65.8%), indistinct margin (34/79, 43.0%), and hypoechogenicity (69/79, 87.3%), without associated posterior features (62/79, 78.5%) or calcification (76/79, 96.2%). On MRI performed on thirteen lesions, six lesions (46.2%) were not seen, six lesions (46.2%) manifested as mass, and one lesion (7.6%) as non-mass enhancement. Six masses were irregular (3/6, 50%) with irregular margin (4/6, 66.7%) homogeneous enhancement (5/6, 83.3%) and showed Type 3 kinetic curve (5/6, 83.3%), and one non-mass lesion showed regional, homogeneous enhancement with Type 3 kinetic curve.

In the comparison between radial scars/CSLs with and without high risk lesions on final pathological results

(Table 1), there was a greater mean age in the group with high risk lesions (52.9 ± 6.0 years; range, 33–62 years vs. 48.4 ± 6.7 years; range, 38–63 years, $p = 0.018$). There were no differences in lesion size (9.8 ± 5.9 mm vs. 10.0 ± 6.2 mm, $p = 0.887$), symptoms ($p = 0.643$), or associated malignancy in the contralateral breast ($p = 0.717$), and the findings of mammography, US and MRI (Additional file 1: Table S1).

Four cases (4.8%, 4/82) that were detected on the screening examination and diagnosed as radial scars/CSLs without high risk lesions on core needle biopsy were upgraded to high risk ($n = 2$) or DCIS ($n = 2$) after surgical excision (Table 2). The two lesions (size 1.0 cm and 1.9 cm) that were upgraded to DCIS were both occult on mammography and seen as hypoechoic masses on US, with one of these lesions appearing as non-mass enhancement with Type 3 kinetic curve on MRI (Fig. 2). The two lesions (size 5 mm and 8 mm) that were upgraded to high risk lesions (atypical ductal hyperplasia and atypical papilloma, respectively) were both hypoechoic masses on US (Fig. 3).

Discussion

The radial scar manifests as an architectural distortion with long thin spicules radiating from an often radiolucent central area [27]. This spiculated radiologic finding mimics malignancy and is difficult to differentiate from tubular carcinoma [28], and surgical excision has

Table 1 Comparisons between Radial Scars/Complex Sclerosing Lesions with and without High Risk Lesions on Final Pathological Results

Characteristics		Radial scar/CSL without high risk (n = 49)	Radial scar/CSL with high risk (n = 33)	P-value
Mean age		48.4 ± 6.7	52.9 ± 6.0	0.018
Follow-up		16 (32.7)	2 (6.1)	0.004
Operation		33 (67.3)	31 (93.9)	
Symptom	–	45 (91.8)	32 (97.0)	0.643
	+	4 (8.2)	1 (3.0)	
Size (mm)		9.8 ± 5.9	10.0 ± 6.2	0.887
Contralateral breast malignancy[a]		5 (10.9)	5 (15.2)	0.717

Data indicate the number of lesions, *Numbers in parentheses* indicate percentages
CSL complex sclerosing lesion, *DCIS* ductal carcinoma in situ
[a]include *DCIS*, invasive ductal carcinoma, and tubular carcinoma

been generally recommended [29, 30]. Linda et al. agreed that the mammographic and US features of lesions diagnosed as radial scars are not predictive of the absence or presence of associated malignancy [2]. In our study, we also failed to find any radiologic features helpful for differentiating between radial scar/CSLs with and without associated high risk lesions or malignancy.

Reported upgrade rates after surgical excision have ranged from 0.0 to 40.0% because of heterogeneous study populations; a mixture of isolated radial scar with or without atypia, core and surgical excision biopsies, small sample sizes, and no comparisons between who did and did not undergo surgery [18]. Without there being any established malignancy upgrade rates or malignancy expectancy, a 2011 survey of practicing breast surgeons showed that 76.0% would recommend surgery for radial scar/CSL diagnosed on needle biopsy [31]. Similar surveys of radiologists performed at the American Roentgen Ray Society annual meetings in 2010 and 2011 showed that most radiologists would recommend surgical excision, with rates of 89.0% and 73.0%, respectively [32]. However, recent studies with careful correlations between radiology and pathology suggest that upgrade to carcinoma occurs in less than 2.0%, and advocate imaging follow-up rather than

surgical excision for radial scars without high risk lesions [12–15]. Moreover, Park et al. recently reported 0.0% upgrade rate to high risk lesions or malignancy in mammographically occult radial scar/CSL diagnosed by biopsy in asymptomatic patients [33]. At the excision of both mammographically evident and occult lesions, the malignancies associated with radial scars are frequently low- or intermediate-grade DCIS, or grade 1 or 2 invasive carcinoma [2, 24, 25]. Invasive cancers in radial scars are low grade, and their biological profiles (positivity for estrogen and progesterone receptors, low proliferative index) are favorable [34]. Similarly, in our study in which 3.1% (2/64) of surgically excised lesions were upgraded to DCIS after excision, which were occult on mammography. With the low upgrade rate and favorable histopathological prognosis, conservative management with US follow-up may be recommended, rather than prompt surgical management.

Radial scar/CSL has been associated with both age and lesion size; lesions smaller than 6–7 mm or in women under the age of 40 are not correlated with cancer, but patients over 50 years of age with lesions greater than 2 cm are at a slightly higher risk [35]. Upstaging in our study was noted with radial scars/CSLs larger than 1.0 cm, and a statistically significant older age was also

Table 2 Clinical, Radiologic, and Pathologic Data of those Radial Scars/Complex Sclerosing Lesions Upgraded after Excision

Case	Initial pathology on core biopsy	Size (mm)	Mammography	Ultrasound	MRI	Final pathology after surgical excision
1	Radial scar	5	Occult	Oval hypoechoic mass, parallel, indistinct	N/A	Radial scar with atypical ductal hyperplasia
2.	Radial scar	8	Irregular, indistinct, hyperdense mass	Irregular, non-parallel, angular, hypoechoic mass, with posterior enhancement	N/A	Radial scar with atypical papilloma
3.	Complex sclerosing lesion	19	Occult	Oval, parallel, circumscribed, hypoechoic mass	Non-mass lesion with regional, homogeneous enhancement and Type 3 kinetic curve	DCIS
4.	Radial scar	10	Occult	Irregular, non-parallel, indistinct, hypoechoic mass,	N/A	DCIS

DCIS ductal carcinoma in situ, *MRI* magnetic resonance imaging

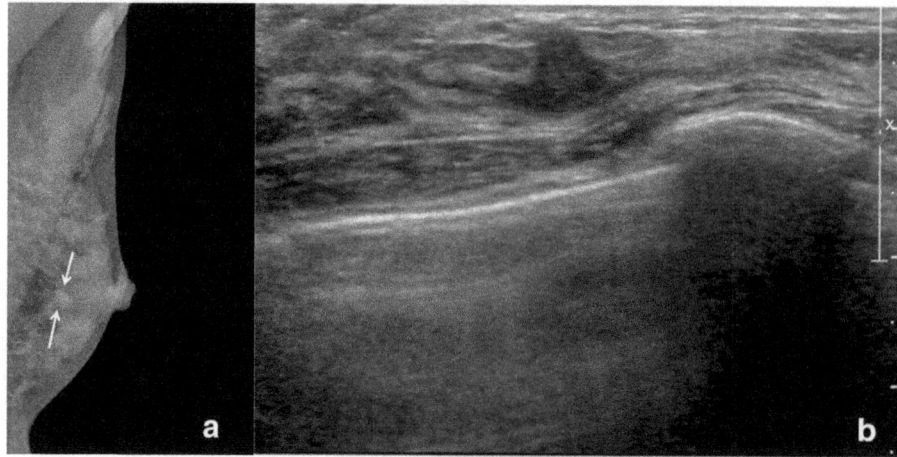

Fig. 2 A radial scar on ultrasound guided core needle biopsy and upgraded to radial scar with atypical ductal hyperplasia after surgical excision. **a** On mammography, there is an irregular, indistinct, hyperdense mass (arrow). **b** On ultrasound, there is an irregular, non-parallel, angular, hypoechoic mass

observed in radial scars with high risk lesions. Several risk factors have been found to be associated with upstaging of radial scar, including older age (> 50 years), postmeno-pausal status, larger size on radiography, and the presence of atypical hyperplasia [24]. High risk lesions such as atyp-ical hyperplasia are generally considered to be subject to high rates of malignancy underestimation, and thereby warrant surgical excision. [36–38]. Previous studies dem-onstrated that radial scars with associated high risk lesions had a higher rate of upgrade to invasive or noninvasive breast cancer [16, 24]. When radial scar is found with high risk lesion, the frequency of upgrade averages 26.0%, which compares with a rate of 7.5% for those without [39]. Several previous studies have described the use of large-gauge vacuum-assisted needle, and have suggested that if there is no association with atypia and radiologic and histologic findings are concordant, further surgery is not required [16]. However, other studies have not shown sig-nificant difference in upgrade rates between vacuum-assisted biopsy devices of differing sizes [40]. Knowledge on the outcomes of radial scars that did not undergo sur-gery is important for making decisions on optimal man-agement. In our study, none of the un-excised lesions that were followed for at least 5 years resulted in any subse-quent malignant lesions. This is consistent with previous study in which there were no malignant lesions during a follow-up period of up to 11 years [41], although the study excluded any atypical proliferative lesions. Resetkova et al.

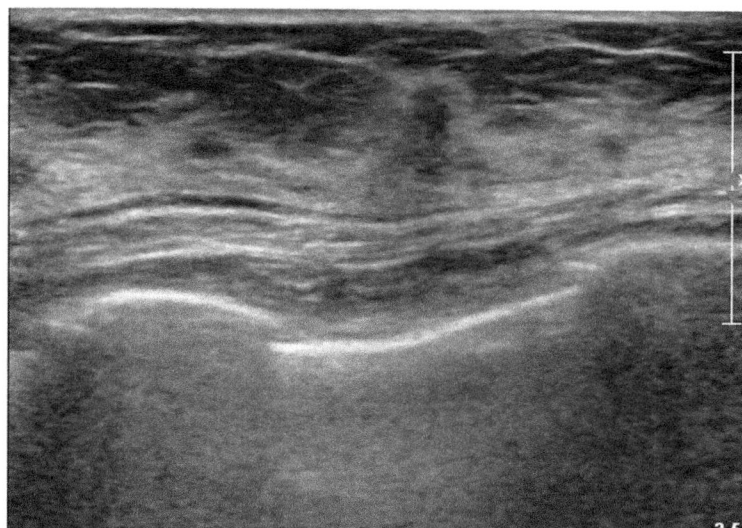

Fig. 3 A radial scar on ultrasound- guided core needle biopsy and upgraded to ductal carcinoma in situ after surgical excision. Ultrasound shows an irregular, non-parallel, indistinct, and hypoechoic mass

[18] also reported no subsequent carcinoma at a median follow-up of 29 months in patients who did not have radial scar excised.

Our study has limitations. It is a retrospective study and has relatively small sample size. Further prospective study with larger population should validate this claim. Also, there was a substantial proportion of US-guided biopsy and one case of mammography-guided biopsy, any meaningful statistical analysis regarding needle size with upgrade rate could not be carried out. Lastly, due to few cases examined on mammography and MRI, this may introduce bias to the imaging finding interpretations.

Conclusions

In conclusion, radial scar with or without high risk lesions was associated with a low upgrade rate (3.1%) to DCIS on surgery or 5 year follow-up, with no lesions being upgraded to invasive carcinoma. Therefore, excision of radial scars to diagnosis of carcinoma is not warranted. With the emergence of more sophisticated imaging modalities and an increasing number of screening examinations, the question of how to manage these lesions has arisen as a clinical dilemma. In the future, the management of patients with radial scars should be refined according to clinical data, radiologic findings, and the coexistence of high risk lesions, to minimize unnecessary interventions. Radial scar/CSL with associated high risk lesions or larger lesions may undergo surgical excision to maximize the early detection of coexistent invasive carcinoma, evaluate the presence of high risk lesions, and provide guidance on chemoprevention to reduce the future cancer risk.

Abbreviations

CSL: Complex sclerosing lesion; DCIS: Ductal carcinoma in situ; MRI: Magnetic resonance imaging; US: Ultrasound

Acknowledgements

Not applicable.

Funding

The author(s) received no financial support for the research, authorship, and/or publication of this article.

Authors' contributions

J.H.C and S.M.H analyzed and interpreted the patient clinical and imaging data and made consensus. S.M.H was a major contributor in writing and revising the manuscript. H.J.S, E.Y.C, H.H.K, and W.J.C acquired and interpreted imaging data of patients, involved in revising the manuscript and approved the final version by ensuring the integrity of the work. H.Y.O analyzed the interpretation of overall data more subjectively, revised the contents and approved the final version ensuring possible questions related to the final version work.

Competing interests

The authors declare that they have no competing interests.

Author details

[1]Department of Radiology, Research Institute of Radiology, Chung-Ang University Hospital, Chung-Ang University College of Medicine, 84 Heukseok-Ro, Dongjak-Gu, Seoul 06973, Republic of Korea. [2]Department of Radiology, Research Institute of Radiology, University of Ulsan College of Medicine, Asan Medical Center, 88 Olympic-Ro 43 Gil, Songpa-Gu, Seoul 05505, Republic of Korea. [3]Department of Radiology, Kangwon National University Hospital, 200-722 Baengnyeong-Ro 156, Chuncheon-Si, Republic of Korea.

References

1. Eusebi V, Millis RR. Epitheliosis, infiltrating epitheliosis, and radial scar. Semin Diagn Pathol. 2010;27(1):5–12.
2. Linda A, Zuiani C, Furlan A, Londero V, Girometti R, Machin P, Bazzocchi M. Radial scars without atypia diagnosed at imaging-guided needle biopsy: how often is associated malignancy found at subsequent surgical excision, and do mammography and sonography predict which lesions are malignant? Am J Roentgenol. 2010;194(4):1146–51.
3. Sohn VY, Causey MW, Steele SR, Keylock JB, Brown TA. The treatment of radial scars in the modern era--surgical excision is not required. Am Surg. 2010;76(5):522–5.
4. Meyer JE, Christian RL, Lester SC, Frenna TH, Denison CM, DiPiro PJ, Polger M. Evaluation of nonpalpable solid breast masses with stereotaxic large-needle core biopsy using a dedicated unit. Am J Roentgenol. 1996;167(1): 179–82.
5. Rabban JT, Sgroi DC. Sclerosing lesions of the breast. Semin Diagn Pathol. 2004;21(1):42–7.
6. Cohen MA, Sferlazza SJ. Role of sonography in evaluation of radial scars of the breast. AJR Am J Roentgenol. 2000;174(4):1075–8.
7. Cawson JN, Nickson C, Evans J, Kavanagh AM. Variation in mammographic appearance between projections of small breast cancers compared with radial scars. J Med Imaging Radiat Oncol. 2010;54(5):415–20.
8. Braakhuis BJ, Tabor MP, Kummer JA, Leemans CR, Brakenhoff RH. A genetic explanation of Slaughter's concept of field cancerization: evidence and clinical implications. Cancer Res. 2003;63(8):1727–30.
9. Chai H, Brown RE. Field effect in cancer-an update. Ann Clin Lab Sci. 2009; 39(4):331–7.
10. Cohen MA, Newell MS. Radial scars of the breast encountered at Core biopsy: review of histologic, imaging, and Management Considerations. AJR Am J Roentgenol. 2017;209(5):1168–77.
11. Fasih T, Jain M, Shrimankar J, Staunton M, Hubbard J, Griffith CD. All radial scars/complex sclerosing lesions seen on breast screening mammograms should be excised. Eur J Surg Oncol. 2005;31(10):1125–8.
12. Conlon N, D'Arcy C, Kaplan JB, Bowser ZL, Cordero A, Brogi E, Corben AD. Radial scar at image-guided needle biopsy: is excision necessary? Am J Surg Pathol. 2015;39(6):779–85.
13. Donaldson AR, Sieck L, Booth CN, Calhoun BC. Radial scars diagnosed on breast core biopsy: frequency of atypia and carcinoma on excision and implications for management. Breast. 2016;30:201–7.
14. Matrai C, D'Alfonso TM, Pharmer L, Drotman MB, Simmons RM, Shin SJ. Advocating nonsurgical Management of Patients with Small, incidental radial scars at the time of needle Core biopsy: a study of 77 cases. Arch Pathol Lab Med. 2015;139(9):1137–42.
15. Miller CL, West JA, Bettini AC, Koerner FC, Gudewicz TM, Freer PE, Coopey SB, Gadd MA, Hughes KS, Smith BL, et al. Surgical excision of radial scars diagnosed by core biopsy may help predict future risk of breast cancer. Breast Cancer Res Treat. 2014;145(2):331–8.
16. Brenner RJ, Jackman RJ, Parker SH, Evans WP 3rd, Philpotts L, Deutch BM, Lechner MC, Lehrer D, Sylvan P, Hunt R, et al. Percutaneous core needle biopsy of radial scars of the breast: when is excision necessary? Am J Roentgenol. 2002;179(5):1179–84.
17. Becker L, Trop I, David J, Latour M, Ouimet-Oliva D, Gaboury L, Lalonde L. Management of radial scars found at percutaneous breast biopsy. Can Assoc Radiol J. 2006;57(2):72–8.
18. Resetkova E, Edelweiss M, Albarracin CT, Yang WT. Management of radial sclerosing lesions of the breast diagnosed using percutaneous vacuum-assisted core needle biopsy: recommendations for excision based on seven years' of

experience at a single institution. Breast Cancer Res Treat. 2011;127(2):335–43.

19. Linda A, Zuiani C, Furlan A, Lorenzon M, Londero V, Girometti R, Bazzocchi M. Nonsurgical management of high-risk lesions diagnosed at core needle biopsy: can malignancy be ruled out safely with breast MRI? AJR Am J Roentgenol. 2012;198(2):272–80.

20. Pediconi F, Occhiato R, Venditti F, Fraioli F, Napoli A, Votta V, Laghi A, Catalano C, Passariello R. Radial scars of the breast: contrast-enhanced magnetic resonance mammography appearance. Breast J. 2005;11(1):23–8.

21. Razek AA, Gaballa G, Denewer A, Nada N. Invasive ductal carcinoma: correlation of apparent diffusion coefficient value with pathological prognostic factors. NMR Biomed. 2010;23(6):619–23.

22. Razek AA, Lattif MA, Denewer A, Farouk O, Nada N. Assessment of axillary lymph nodes in patients with breast cancer with diffusion-weighted MR imaging in combination with routine and dynamic contrast MR imaging. Breast cancer. 2016;23(3):525–32.

23. Abdel Razek AA, Gaballa G, Denewer A, Tawakol I. Diffusion weighted MR imaging of the breast. Acad Radiol. 2010;17(3):382–6.

24. Andacoglu O, Kanbour-Shakir A, Teh YC, Bonaventura M, Ozbek U, Anello M, Ganott M, Kelley J, Dirican A, Soran A. Rationale of excisional biopsy after the diagnosis of benign radial scar on core biopsy: a single institutional outcome analysis. Am J Clin Oncol. 2013;36(1):7–11.

25. Nassar A, Conners AL, Celik B, Jenkins SM, Smith CY, Hieken TJ. Radial scar/complex sclerosing lesions: a clinicopathologic correlation study from a single institution. Ann Diagn Pathol. 2015;19(1):24–8.

26. American College of Radiology. Breast imaging reporting and data system (BI-RADS). 5th ed. Reston Va: American College of Radiology; 2013.

27. Bianchi S, Giannotti E, Vanzi E, Marziali M, Abdulcadir D, Boeri C, Livi L, Orzalesi L, Sanchez LJ, Susini T, et al. Radial scar without associated atypical epithelial proliferation on image-guided 14-gauge needle core biopsy: analysis of 49 cases from a single-Centre and review of the literature. Breast. 2012;21(2):159–64.

28. Lopez-Medina A, Cintora E, Mugica B, Opere E, Vela AC, Ibanez T. Radial scars diagnosed at stereotactic core-needle biopsy: surgical biopsy findings. Eur Radiol. 2006;16(8):1803–10.

29. Berg WA. Image-guided breast biopsy and management of high-risk lesions. Radiol Clin N Am. 2004;42(5):935–46 vii.

30. Osborn G, Wilton F, Stevens G, Vaughan-Williams E, Gower-Thomas K. A review of needle core biopsy diagnosed radial scars in the welsh breast screening Programme. Ann R Coll Surg Engl. 2011;93(2):123–6.

31. Krishnamurthy S, Bevers T, Kuerer H, Yang WT. Multidisciplinary considerations in the management of high-risk breast lesions. Am J Roentgenol. 2012;198(2):W132–40.

32. Georgian-Smith D, Lawton TJ. Variations in physician recommendations for surgery after diagnosis of a high-risk lesion on breast core needle biopsy. Am J Roentgenol. 2012;198(2):256–63.

33. Park VY, Kim EK, Kim MJ, Yoon JH, Moon HJ. Mammographically occult asymptomatic radial scars/complex Sclerosing lesions at ultrasonography-guided Core needle biopsy: follow-up can be recommended. Ultrasound Med Biol. 2016;42(10):2367–71.

34. Mokbel K, Price RK, Mostafa A, Williams N, Wells CA, Perry N, Carpenter R. Radial scar and carcinoma of the breast: microscopic findings in 32 cases. Breast. 1999;8(6):339–42.

35. Sloane JP, Mayers MM. Carcinoma and atypical hyperplasia in radial scars and complex sclerosing lesions: importance of lesion size and patient age. Histopathology. 1993;23(3):225–31.

36. McGhan LJ, Pockaj BA, Wasif N, Giurescu ME, McCullough AE, Gray RJ. Atypical ductal hyperplasia on core biopsy: an automatic trigger for excisional biopsy? Ann Surg Oncol. 2012;19(10):3264–9.

37. Elsheikh TM, Silverman JF. Follow-up surgical excision is indicated when breast core needle biopsies show atypical lobular hyperplasia or lobular carcinoma in situ: a correlative study of 33 patients with review of the literature. Am J Surg Pathol. 2005;29(4):534–43.

38. Sohn V, Arthurs Z, Herbert G, Keylock J, Perry J, Eckert M, Fellabaum D, Smith D, Brown T. Atypical ductal hyperplasia: improved accuracy with the 11-gauge vacuum-assisted versus the 14-gauge core biopsy needle. Ann Surg Oncol. 2007;14(9):2497–501.

39. Sun J, Liu X, Zhang Q, Hong Y, Song B, Teng X, Yu J. Papillary thyroid carcinoma treated with radiofrequency ablation in a patient with hypertrophic cardiomyopathy: a case report. Korean J Radiol. 2016;17(4):558–61.

40. Eby PR, Ochsner JE, DeMartini WB, Allison KH, Peacock S, Lehman CD. Frequency and upgrade rates of atypical ductal hyperplasia diagnosed at stereotactic vacuum-assisted breast biopsy: 9-versus 11-gauge. Am J Roentgenol. 2009;192(1):229–34.

41. Hou Y, Hooda S, Li Z. Surgical excision outcome after radial scar without atypical proliferative lesion on breast core needle biopsy: a single institutional analysis. Ann Diagn Pathol. 2016;21:35–8.

29

MRI texture analysis in differentiating luminal A and luminal B breast cancer molecular subtypes

Kirsi Holli-Helenius[1*], Annukka Salminen[2], Irina Rinta-Kiikka[2], Ilkka Koskivuo[3], Nina Brück[3], Pia Boström[4] and Riitta Parkkola[5]

Abstract

Background: The aim of this study was to use texture analysis (TA) of breast magnetic resonance (MR) images to assist in differentiating estrogen receptor (ER) positive breast cancer molecular subtypes.

Methods: Twenty-seven patients with histopathologically proven invasive ductal breast cancer were selected in preliminary study. Tumors were classified into molecular subtypes: luminal A (ER-positive and/or progesterone receptor (PR)-positive, human epidermal growth factor receptor type 2 (HER2) -negative, proliferation marker Ki-67 < 20 and low grade (I)) and luminal B (ER-positive and/or PR-positive, HER2-positive or HER2-negative with high Ki-67 ≥ 20 and higher grade (II or III)). Co-occurrence matrix -based texture features were extracted from each tumor on T1-weighted non fat saturated pre- and postcontrast MR images using TA software MaZda. Texture parameters and tumour volumes were correlated with tumour prognostic factors.

Results: Textural differences were observed mainly in precontrast images. The two most discriminative texture parameters to differentiate luminal A and luminal B subtypes were sum entropy and sum variance ($p = 0.003$). The AUCs were 0.828 for sum entropy ($p = 0.004$), and 0.833 for sum variance ($p = 0.003$), and 0.878 for the model combining texture features sum entropy, sum variance ($p = 0.001$). In the LOOCV, the AUC for model combining features sum entropy and sum variance was 0.876. Sum entropy and sum variance showed positive correlation with higher Ki-67 index. Luminal B types were larger in volume and moderate correlation between larger tumour volume and higher Ki-67 index was also observed ($r = 0.499, p = 0.008$).

Conclusions: Texture features which measure randomness, heterogeneity or smoothness and homogeneity may either directly or indirectly reflect underlying growth patterns of breast tumours. TA and volumetric analysis may provide a way to evaluate the biologic aggressiveness of breast tumours and provide aid in decisions regarding therapeutic efficacy.

Keywords: magnetic resonance imaging (MRI), texture analysis (TA), breast cancer, invasive ductal carcinoma (IDC), volumetric analysis, prognostic factors

* Correspondence: kirsi.holli-helenius@pshp.fi
[1]Department of Medical Physics, Medical Imaging Centre and Hospital Pharmacy, Pirkanmaa Hospital District, Post Box 2000, 33521 Tampere, Finland
Full list of author information is available at the end of the article

Background

Breast cancer is known to be a heterogeneous disease that can be classified using several clinical and pathological features. Breast cancer classification may help in predicting clinical outcome, and it also has a significant role in targeting the treatment to those who are most likely to benefit. Different subtypes can be defined by using genetic array testing or approaches using immunohistochemical analyses [1]. Some of the most important factors that are related to prognosis are tumour size, histologic grade, nodal status, estrogen and progesterone receptors (ER, PR), human epidermal growth factor receptor type 2 (HER2) expressions and proliferation marker Ki-67 [2, 3]. Hormone receptor-positive breast cancers are usually classified into luminal A -like subtype and luminal B -like subtype with or without HER2 overexpression. The luminal A subtype is shown to express high levels of hormone receptor and has more favorable prognosis while, the luminal B-like subtype presents with a worse prognosis. The immunohistochemical surrogate of molecular subclasses of breast cancers proposed by the Saint Gallen Consensus Meetings [1, 4] is used to classify patients in different risk categories. In discriminating between luminal A and B subtypes, Ki-67 labeling index has been shown to be useful [5, 6]. In the era of personalized medicine, it is becoming more and more important to make a distinction between luminal A and luminal B cancers to ensure efficient treatment. The classification of molecular subtypes is done by means of genetic analysis, which is rather costly and requires specialized technical expertise. Therefore it might be beneficial to find a cost and time effective alternative means of classifying breast cancers into distinct molecular subtypes.

Breast MRI has a high sensitivity [7, 8] in diagnosing breast cancer but image interpretation still provides challenges. These challenges include misinterpretation due to technical factors [9] as well as hormonal status of the patient, difficulties in interpretation surgical [10, 11] or therapeutic interventions and [12], overlapping in the MRI appearance of some benign and malignant diseases and over-or underestimation of the lesions size [13, 14]. Breast MRI examinations generate a vast volume of image data and computer aided diagnosis systems such as texture analysis (TA) are developed to assist with lesion detection and classification. MR images contain pixel grey level variations which cannot be evaluated visually but could be detected with image analysis methods, such as TA. TA methods evaluate the spatial location and signal intensity characteristics of pixels in the images. It is a mathematical method that describes the grey level dependence between the image pixels. It offers a way to calculated mathematical values for texture features which can be used in characterizing the underlying structures of the observed tissues [15].TA has been studied as a one method to increase the specificity of breast MRI with promising results [16–20].

Breast tumors are usually heterogeneous in structure. Biopsy may often not be sufficient in assessing intratumoral heterogeneity since it does not always represent the complete phenotypic variation within a tumor. Therefore, a non-invasive method of assessing whole tumour heterogeneity might be beneficial [21]. Many studies have suggested that intra-tumoral heterogeneity can be quantified by using image texture analysis such as co-occurrence matrix (COM). Many researches have exploited texture features for distinguishing malignant from benign tumors from MR images [16–18, 22]. Though many researches had exploited COM texture features to quantify tumor heterogeneity for distinguishing malignant from benign tumors, only few very recent studies [20, 23, 24] have investigated COM feature correlation with pathological prognostic factors in invasive breast cancer. In a recent study by Sutton et al. [25] shape, texture and histogram based features were applied in differentiating breast cancer molecular subtypes with encouraging results. They divided the subtypes in ERPR+, ERPR-/HER2+ or triple negative. Since TA has proven to be potential tool in discriminating benign and malignant breast cancers, different histological types and even aid in discriminating different molecular subtypes we hypotized that it could even differentiate molecular subtypes luminal A and luminal B. Luminal A is associated with lower Ki-67 rate than subtype luminal B. Ki-67 on the other hand is associated with a higher expression of vascular endothelial growth factor in tumor cells [26] and thereby luminal B type cancers might show more heterogeneous textural appearance in MR images enabling the discrimination of the two types by the means of TA.

Larger tumors are generally associated with a poorer prognosis than smaller tumors, so tumour size can be considered as another important prognostic marker. Evaluating breast tumour size is important when determining cancer type and extent of subsequent surgical and oncological management. There are various methods to determine tumour size including palpation on physical examination and breast-imaging studies such as mammography, ultrasound, and MRI. Because of its superiority in assessing soft tissues, breast MRI is recommended to be performed also in cases where the actual tumour size cannot be estimated with other modalities [27]. In breast MR images the estimate of tumour size is usually done by measuring the largest diameter from a single slice. Volumetric analysis has also been proposed especially when studying the effectiveness of treatment [28].

Our aim was to further study the relationship between textural features and tumour volumes measured from breast MRI and molecular subtypes luminal A and B.

Since one significant difference between luminal A and luminal B subtypes is a higher cell proliferation rate in luminal B types, we studied correlation between textural features, tumour volume and Ki-67. We focused our study on analyzing precontrast MR images in contrast to many previous studies which have mainly focused on analyzing texture features from postcontrast images [16–18]. Many newly diagnosed breast cancer patients undergo breast MRI and if molecular subtypes could be reliably estimated from breast MRI and provide prognostic information in addition to diagnostic imaging, the utility of preoperative breast MRI would increase.

Methods
Patient population
From a total of 50 consecutive adult patients referred to the Department of Plastic and General Surgery, Turku University Hospital, Turku, Finland, 27 patients were chosen in this texture analysis study. Women were eligible to participate in the study if they were 18 years of age or older and if they had received a diagnosis of unilateral invasive ductal breast cancer based on complete mammography and ultrasound workup of both breasts and ultrasound-guided core needle biopsy. Preoperatively, all patients underwent routinely breast MRI. The study protocol was approved by the Ethical Review Committee of the Hospital District of the South-West Finland. All patients gave a written consent for the study. Exclusion criteria for texture analysis study were that images were taken with the same MR scanner using the same coil and imaging sequence, no visible artifacts on MR images or lesion size less than 7 mm. Luminal A subtype (15 / 27) was defined as being ER positive, HER2 negative, and Ki-67 low (< 20% cells positive) and luminal B (12/27) subtype as being ER positive,HER2 negative or positive, and Ki-67 high (≥ 20% cells positive). From total of 50 patient only 27 met our criteria. Eight patients were excluded for not being purely ductal carcinomas, 2 were not imaged with the same MR system, 4 were not ER positive, with 6 patients the lesion size was too small and 3 had visible artifacts on MR images.

Tumor Histology and Immunohistochemistry (IHC) analysis
Tumor type was determined on the core needle biopsy performed before chemotherapy or surgery. Four μm thick serial paraffin section were cut from tumour tissue and stained with haematoxylin and eosin. The breast cancer histology was assessed according to the World Health Organization classification [29] and tumour grading was based on the recommendations made by Elston and Ellis in 1991 [30]. Tumour grades are classified as: grade 1 is well-differentiated, grade 2 is moderately-differentiated and grade 3 is poorly-differentiated.

Immunohistochemical staining of needle core biopsies for estrogen and progesterone receptors (ER, PR), Ki-67 and HER2 were performed from subsequent sections. Four different ready-to-use rabbit monoclonal antibodies were used from Ventana Medical Systems/Roche Diagnostics: Estrogen Receptor (SPI, rabbit), Progesterone Receptor (IE2, rabbit), HER2 (4B5, rabbit) and Ki-67 (30–9, rabbit) with BenchMark XT immunostainer and *ultra*VIEW Universal DAB Detection Kit (Ventana/Roche, Tucson, Arizona, USA). The percentage of nuclei with immunoreactivity to ER, PR and Ki-67 was classified as continuous data from 0 to 100%. ER-positive and PR-positive cases showed staining in at least 10% of the tumour cell nuclei. Ki-67 was defined as low if ≤ 20% Ki-67 was detected and as high if > 20% Ki-67 was detected. HER2 expression was evaluated as membrane staining of invasive tumour cells and scored from 0 to 3. Carcinomas revealing 2+ or 3+ immunostaining were retested for HER2 gene amplification with chromogenic in situ hybridization (CISH) to determine HER2 positivity. Tumour size was taken to be the diameter of the largest focus in surgical specimens. Axillary lymph node status was achieved through sentinel lymph node biopsy or axillary lymph node dissections. Table 1 presents the lesion characteristics for the 27 invasive ductal, ER positive (luminal A and B types) cases that were entered into the texture analysis.

MRI acquisition
MR imaging was carried out on 1.5 T MRI scanner (Magnetom Avanto, Siemens Healthcare, Erlangen, Germany) using the following sequences: T2 weighted

Table 1 Lesion characteristics

Parameter	Patients (luminal A types)	Patients (luminal B types)
Histological type		
Invasive ductal	15	12
Histological grade		
grade 1	8	0
grade 2	7	5
grade3	0	7
Ki-67		
< 20	15	0
≥ 20	0	12
lymph node status		
negative	11	8
positive	4	4
diameter (mm)		
7 - 15 mm	9	4
≥ 15 mm	6	8

Ki-67, proliferation marker

fat saturated axial-, T1 weighted fat saturated dynamic-, T1 weighted non fat saturated series in dynamic phase and diffusion imaging. Images from T1 weighted non fat saturated dynamic sequence (1.5 T: TR/TE = 8.1 ms/ 4.72 ms, acquisition time: 8.56, FOV: 320 mm, matrix 448×448, slice thickness 1 mm, in-plane voxel size 0.7 mm, flip angle 25 deg., number of slices 144) were used in texture analysis and volumetric measurements. The first frame was acquired before injection of paramagnetic contrast agent (Gd, 0.1 mmol/kg body, Dotarem®), followed by 5 measurements. Un-enhanced images were subtracted from the contrast-enhanced images on a pixel-by-pixel basis, creating five subtraction series.

Image analysis
Texture analysis
The dynamic T1-weighted series for TA was chosen. We focused our analyses mainly on T1-weighted precontrast images but analyzed also the first sequence of T1-weighted postcontrast images for a comparison. Image slices were chosen on the basis of optimal representation of the largest tumour area.

Circular standard size regions of interest (ROI) of radius 5 pixels were positioned by hospital physicist with a special interest in developing quantitative radiology methods in clinical use. An experienced senior radiologist provided assistance for ROI settings. These regions of interest were placed into the area of the lesion where the enhancement was strongest in the first non-subtracted postcontrast image and same ROI placement was used also in precontrast images (Fig. 1). Standard size ROIs were used since a previous study has shown some texture features to be dependent on ROI size [31]. ROI size was chosen to ensure sufficient number of pixels for texture feature calculations and to fit all analyzed lesions to avoid partial volume effect. The grey level normalization of each standard circular ROI was performed using method which normalizes image intensities in the range $[\mu\text{-}3\sigma, \mu + 3\sigma]$, where μ is the mean grey level value and σ the standard deviation, to minimize the influence of contrast variation and brightness [32].

For TA we used a specialized program MaZda package version 4.6 (The Technical University of Lodz, Institute of Electronics). MaZda allows computation of texture parameters based on image histogram, co-occurrence matrix, run-length matrix, image gradients, autoregressive model and wavelet analysis [33]. In this study we used the 2D co-occurrence (COM) based parameters since, according to our experience, they have shown potential in breast MRI TA studies. The co-occurrence matrix is a second order histogram of an image and it relates into groups of pixels or pixel pairs. The basic element of grey level co-occurrence matrix is the count of the pixel pairs which have a certain grey level value in given direction and pixel distance. Rather than using

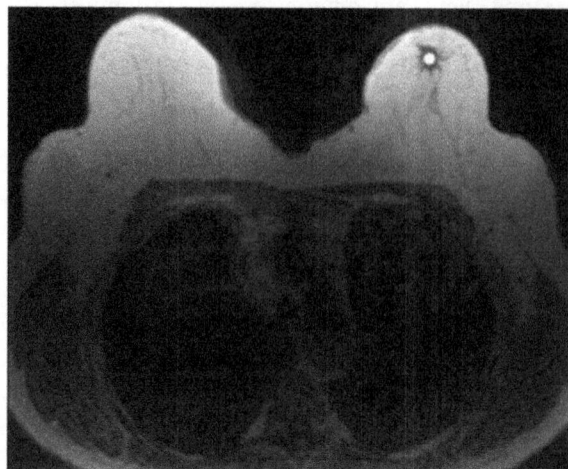

Fig. 1 Standard size circular region of interest (ROI) loaded over T1-weighted MR image in MaZda after image normalization. The tumour is grade 3 invasive ductal carcinoma in left breast

gray level co-occurrence matrix directly in texture analysis, the co-occurrence matrices can be converted into scalar measures of texture, which can be used to measure the textures of images and regions In total, 11 COM-based (angular second moment, contrast, correlation, sum of squares, inverse difference moment, sum average, sum variance, sum entropy, entropy, difference variance and difference entropy) were calculated with the distance of one pixel and in four directions (0°, 45°, 90°, and 135°). The four directional components of each parameter were averaged into one parameter in order to enhance the robustness of the method. Angular second moment is a measure image uniformity. This feature obtains a high value, when a grey level distribution in the image is either constant or periodic. Thus a higher value for this feature indicates that the image is homogenous. Also feature inverse difference moment measures image homogeneity. When inverse difference reaches high values, image can be considered to be smooth. Contrast measures the local variations in the image. The lowest contrast value can be obtained when the pixels have the same or very similar grey level values. Correlation measures the grey level linear dependencies in the image. It measures how well correlated one pixel is with its neighbor over the whole image. If an image has a large areas of similar intensities, correlation will be high. Sum of squares is the variance of the co-occurrence matrix and the values are somewhat similar to the values of histogram variance. Sum average gives the average of sums of two pixel values in the image of interest. The pixel pairs which are used in calculation are the ones used in forming the co-occurrence matrix, thus the sum average is not dependent on the direction or the on the pixel distance used in calculations. Entropy- based features indicate the complexity and randomness within the region of interest. Difference variance and difference entropy are based on differences calculated between two pixel values [33].

Tumour volume

Volumetric analysis was done with image postprocessing software ImageJ, which is a public domain, Java-based image processing program developed at the National Institutes of Health [34]. In all T1-weighted subtracted images tumour mass was manually outlined on the computer monitor. The area of tumour in each slice was multiplied by the slice profile, and total tumour volume was automatically calculated by summation of the adjacent volumes.

Statistical analysis

Statistical analysis was performed using commercially available software (SPSS, v. 22.0; Chicago, IL). Because of skewed distribution of the data, the independent Mann–Whitney U-test was used to determine whether the texture features calculated from pre- or postcontrast images were significantly differing between luminal A and luminal B cancers. To further evaluate how different and able to separate both groups TA parameters were, empirical ROC curves were generated for the parameters which presented significant differences between luminal A and luminal B types. The area under the curve (AUC) which measures how well a parameter can distinguish between two diagnostic groups (AUC close to 1 indicate a very informative test) was calculated. The texture features which proved to be statistically different between luminal A and B types and were not strongly correlated with each other were used as an entry in a binary logistic regression. Additional ROC curve was computed to assess the accuracy of a predictive model. ROC curves were used to identify optimal cutoff values in distinguishing luminal types. In order to assess the generalization error, leave-one-out cross validation (LOOCV) was performed. Spearman correlation was used to study how texture features correlated with Ki-67 or grade or volume. The values of r, 0–0.19 is regarded as very weak, 0.2–0.39 as weak, 0.40–0.59 as moderate, 0.6–0.79 as strong and 0.8–1 as very strong correlation. The resulting p-values less than 0.05 are considered to be statistically significant.

Results

Texture features and volumes between luminal A and luminal B

Luminal A and B types presented differing textural appearance. Most of the texture features calculated from precontrast images were significantly different. Postcontrast images however did not yield so promising results

(Table 2). Luminal types were also significantly differing in volume $(p = 0.041)$, luminal B types tended to be slightly larger.

The AUC obtained from the ROC curves were calculated for all significantly differing texture features and obtained values were near 0.7 in all analyses. The texture features sum entropy and sum variance presented the highest AUC (*Sum entropy, 0.828; Sum variance, 0.833*). These two features were used in a binary logistic regression as they did not have strong correlation with each other $(r = 0.447, p = 0.022)$. Additional ROC curve was computed to assess the accuracy of a predictive model with these two most discriminative texture parameters. The results of ROC curve analysis representing the complete data set for sum entropy, sum variance and the model combining these parameters are shown in Fig. 2 and Table 3. The combination of sum entropy and sum variance resulted in an AUC equal to 0.878 to correctly characterize luminal B type $(p = 0.001)$. For combination of these two parameters, a cutoff value of 0.497 resulted in a sensitivity of 91.7% and specificity of 86.7% to separate both groups. The diagnostic values barely decreased in the cross validation: The LOOCV resulted in 91.3% sensitivity and 86% specificity. Adding tumour volume in the prediction model did not yield any better outcome. As for comparison empirical ROC curves were generated also TA features calculated from postcontrast images, even though they did not statistically differ between luminal A and B types. The AUC obtained from the ROC curves were all under 0.5 (*Sum entropy, 0.327; Sum variance, 0.327*).

Correlations between texture features and prognostic features

There were 8 G1 lesions, 12 G2 lesions and 7 G3 lesions. A higher grade tumours showed tendency to be a slightly larger in volume $(p = 0.05)$. No notable correlations were observed in TA parameters calculated from pre- or postcontrast images between different grade tumours. Only one feature, difference variance, showed moderate negative correlation with tumour grade $(r = -0,469, p = 0.03)$ other correlation coefficients were all under 0.4 and p values over 0.05.

Moderate correlation between tumour volume and Ki-67 index was observed $(r = 0.499, p = 0.008)$, indicating that larger tumours had higher Ki-67 index. Most TA parameters calculated from precontrast images correlated with Ki-67 index. Sum entropy and sum variance both correlated with Ki-67 index (*sum entropy: r = 0.607, p = 0.001; sum variance: r = 0.5, p = 0.008*). Sum entropy also seemed to correlate positively with tumour volume $(r = 0.637, p < 0.001)$. Entropy-based TA features from postcontrast images seemed also correlated with Ki-67 index. However correlations were only moderate (sum

Table 2 Textural differences between luminal types A and B. Calculated from pre- and postcontrast images

		Precontrast		postcontrast	
	Texture feature	p-value	Higher value in group A/B	p-value	Higher value in group A/B
Texture difference between luminal A and luminal B	Angular second moment	**0.016**	luminal A	0.212	luminal A
	Contrast	**0.025**	luminal A	0.322	luminal A
	Correlation	**0.007**	luminal B	0.212	luminal B
	Sum of squares	0.126	luminal B	0.527	luminal B
	Inverse different moment	0.829	luminal A	0.118	luminal B
	Sum average	0.093	luminal B	0.595	luminal B
	Sum variance	**0.003**	luminal B	0.145	luminal B
	Sum entropy	**0.003**	luminal B	0.145	luminal B
	Entropy	**0.021**	luminal B	0.231	luminal B
	Difference variance	**0.007**	luminal A	0.595	luminal A
	Difference entropy	**0.021**	luminal B	0.118	luminal B

Significant p-values (p < 0.05) are given in bold face

entropy: $r = 0.447$, $p = 0.40$; entropy: $r = 0.391$, $p = 0.44$; diff entropy: $r = 0.5$, $p = 0.07$).

Discussion

We showed in this study that texture analysis could discriminate luminal A and luminal B types of ductal carcinomas. In this study we combined TA and tumour volumetric analysis in studying if we can differentiate the two ER positive cancers; luminal A and luminal B types. Malignant tumours possess more heterogeneous tissue architecture [35] and therefore might reflect a wider and more heterogeneous range of pixel values in MR images. Our hypothesis was that more aggressive

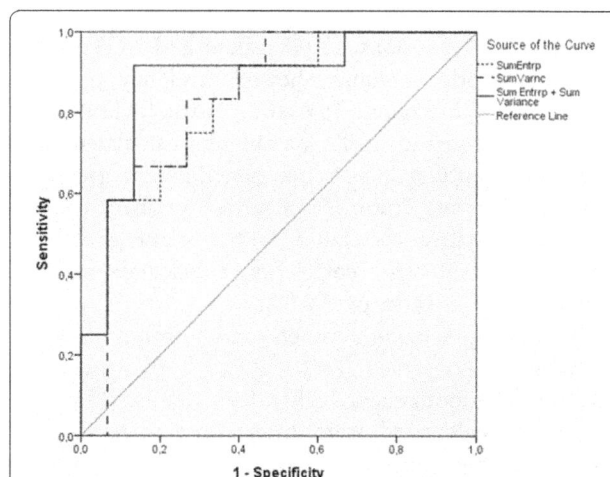

Fig. 2 ROC curves of texture analysis parameters in distinguishing between luminal A and luminal B types. Sum entropy (*dotline*), Sum variance (*dash line*), and predictive model combining sum entropy and sum variance (*solid line*) are shown. Diagonal line represents AUC of 0.50. The ROC curves represent the complete data set, please refer to text for LOOCV results. AUC values are given in Table 3.

cancers might also present greater degree of textural heterogeneity in the MR images.

Several calculated texture features from T1-weighted precontrast images were significantly different ($p < 0.05$) between luminal A and B types. Significantly differing features in our study; angular second moment, contrast, correlation, sum variance, sum entropy, difference variance and difference entropy are all one way or another, measures of heterogeneous textural appearance. According to our study luminal B type cancer have in fact more heterogeneous appearance in MR images than luminal A types. Especially entropy-based features or features representing heterogeneous and random textural patterns have also shown potential in discriminating benign and malignant breast tumours in breast MR images in previous studies [17–19]. Most previous studies have applied texture analysis in postcontrast MR images [16–20, 22]. By calculating texture features from postcontrast images one may captivate mostly the texture pattern caused by the spreading and distribution of the contrast media. One of our aims was specifically to study the textural appearances and differences between luminal A and B types in precontrast MR images, to reveal the underlying tissue architecture. In our study T1-weighted postcontrast images did not show significant textural differences between luminal A and B types. One possible reason for this might be ROI size, which was relatively small. The signal from the contrast media might have partially masked the real underlying texture pattern.

Luminal A and luminal B types showed also difference in tumour volume ($p = 0.041$). Luminal B types were larger in volume than luminal A types. Larger tumours tended to correlate positively with entropy based features (*entropy $r = 0.682$, $p < 0.001$ and sum entropy $r = 0.637$, $p < 0.001$*) and negatively with angular second

Table 3 ROC curve AUC values of texture features sum entropy, sum variance and their combination (precontrast images)

texture feature	AUC, Mean ± SD	p-value	AUC, Mean ± SD (LOOCV)
Sum entropy	0.828 ± 0.079	**0.004**	0.827 ± 0.065
Sum variance	0.833 ± 0.081	**0.003**	0.832 ± 0.076
Sum entropy + Sum variance	0.878 ± 0.72	**0.001**	0.876 ± 0.077

Significant p-values (p < 0.05) are given in bold face
AUC area under the curve, LOOCV leave-one-out cross validation

moment ($r = -0.65$, $p < 0.001$). Since entropy is a measure of randomness and heterogeneity of the studied region and correspondingly angular second moment represents homogeneity of the given region, it appeared that larger tumours are more heterogeneous and complex on their texture appearance. The Ki-67 index is correlated with a high mitotic count and recurrent disease [36]. In our study, a high Ki-67 index was related to higher values in entropy based features (*sum entropy: r = 0.607, p = 0.001*).

Since histologic grade is a characteristic feature when evaluating tumour aggressiveness, we studied also the effect of histological grade on tumour volume and texture features. A slightly greater tumour volume was observed in higher grade tumours. However, since only one texture feature correlated with tumour grade (*difference variance, r = −.419, p = 0.3*), we may think that tumour grade is not a dominant factor on revealed textural differences.

MRI texture analysis has been used in discriminating benign and malignant lesions [16] classifying the underlying breast cancer subtypes [20, 37] and also evaluating treatment response [38, 39]. There seems to be a growing interest in studying the potential of TA in shedding light to histopathologic features [20, 24, 40] and providing further information on the biologic aggressiveness of breast tumours. Tumour heterogeneity and its relationship with pathology have been studied [16, 20]. Ahmed et al. recently observed textural differences between triple negative breast cancers and other types in contrast-enhanced MRI [41] and in their work Bhooshan et al. showed that co-occurrence textural features measured in contrast-enhanced MRI could distinguish in situ ductal carcinoma and invasive ductal carcinoma, and also invasive ductal carcinoma with positive lymph node. The authors found that lesion heterogeneity, which can be presented using texture features, was an indicator of malignancy [42]. In a more recent study by Bhooshan et al. [43] applied texture analysis of DCE-MRI breast images with other computerized methods such as kinetic features in an attempt to distinguish between invasive ductal carcinoma lesions of Grade 1, Grade 2, and Grade 3 with very encouraging results.

According to our study the proliferation rate and, in some extend the size of the tumour, correlated with the texture features. Our previous study [31] has shown that

many, especially entropy-based features, are dependent of ROI size. Therefore in this study we used standard size and shape ROIs to eliminate the possible effect of ROI size to our texture measurements. Though it was not in fact an immense discovery that larger and higher grade tumours possess more heterogeneous textural appearance, it is an interesting finding that luminal A and B types proved to be different in volume and in texture. The study did not have a very large patient group due to the fact that we wanted to select homogeneous material. Nevertheless we were still able to identify statistically significant differences in textural features between luminal A and luminal B subtype. We acknowledge that the limitation of this study is the small sample size and texture features which were approaching significance also in T1-weighted postcontrast images may become statistically significant with a larger sample size. Features calculated from postcontrast images which did achieve smallest p-values were features which represent heterogeneous patterns and were in fact the same ones which did statistically differ in precontrast images (Table 2). It is necessary to also note that this study contained high number of comparisons and since p-values are not corrected for multiple comparisons there might be some false positive findings due to random variability. A future study of interest would be to further assess the performance of texture features especially with MR images without contrast media, with larger data set and proper classification analysis with an appropriate training set. Also the use of other MR sequences would be one of our future interests. Combining information from both T2-weighted and T1-weighted MR images for distinguishing different kind of breast lesions might be advantageous. Also another limitation of this preliminary study is that due to the small sample size we did not perform a separate validation set for the logistic regression model and the performance of the model remains somewhat unclear. A further evaluation of the model needs to be explored in future work on a larger data set and also combining magnetic resonance (MR) imaging kinetic and morphologic features to the analysis.

Conclusions

In conclusion, our results indicate that textural features of pre-contrast T1w images may be used for sub- typing of breast cancer. Texture features which measure randomness, complex or smoothness and homogeneity are the ones which seem to differentiate luminal A and luminal B types. These MR image texture features may either directly or indirectly reflect underlying growth patterns and, therefore, may prove useful in decisions regarding therapeutic efficacy and in the monitoring and follow-up of breast cancers during and after treatment. Differentiating between luminal A and luminal B breast cancers is nowadays important for treatment planning. The immunohistochemical classification of breast cancer as a clinical tool is supported because it can be used at a reasonable cost. However, biopsy represents just a small area of the tumour volume. Thus, a non-invasive analysis like TA offers a method to assess the whole tumour volume and could be of great value in assisting in treatment decision.

Abbreviations

CAD: Computer aided diagnosis; COM: Co-occurrence matrix; ER: Estrogen receptors; HER2: Human epidermal growth factor receptor type 2; MR: Magnetic resonance; MRI: Magnetic resonance imaging; Ki-67: Proliferation marker Ki-67; PR: Progesterone receptors; ROI: Regions of interest; TA: Texture analysis

Acknowledgements

This study was supported by grant from the research funding of the Pirkanmaa Hospital District, Tampere University Hospital.

Funding

Nothing to declare

Authors' contributions

KHH carried out to the design of the texture analysis study and analysis of the data. IK, PB, NB, RP collected the study data and participated in the design of the study. IR-K, AS participated in the design of the study. All authors read and approved the final manuscript.

Competing interests

The authors declare that they have no competing interests.

Author details

[1]Department of Medical Physics, Medical Imaging Centre and Hospital Pharmacy, Pirkanmaa Hospital District, Post Box 2000, 33521 Tampere, Finland. [2]Department of Radiology, Tampere University Hospital, Tampere, Finland. [3]Department of Plastic and General Surgery Turku University Hospital, Turku, Finland. [4]Department of Pathology, University of Turku and Turku University Hospital, Turku, Finland. [5]Department of Radiology, University of Turku and Turku University Hospital, Turku, Finland.

References

1. Goldhirsch A, Wood WC, Coates AS, Gelber RD, Thürlimann B, Senn HJ, Panel members. Strategies for subtypes–dealing with the diversity of breast cancer: highlights of the St. Gallen International Expert Consensus on the Primary Therapy of Early Breast Cancer 2011. Ann Oncol. 2011;22(8):1736–47. https://doi.org/10.1093/annonc/mdr304.

2. Györffy B, Hatzis C, Sanft T, Hofstatter E, Aktas B, Pusztai L. Multigene prognostic tests in breast cancer: past, present, future. Breast Cancer Res. 2015;17:11. https://doi.org/10.1186/s13058-015-0514-2.

3. Song YJ, Shin SH, Cho JS, Park MH, Yoon JH, Jegal YJ. The role of lymphovascular invasion as a prognostic factor in patients with lymph node-positive operable invasive breast cancer. J Breast Cancer. 2011;14(3): 198–203. https://doi.org/10.4048/jbc.2011.14.3.198.

4. Goldhirsch A, Winer EP, Coates AS, Gelber RD, Piccart-Gebhart M, Thürlimann B, Senn HJ. Personalizing the treatment of women with early breast cancer: highlights of the St Gallen International Expert Consensus on the Primary Therapy of Early Breast Cancer. Ann Oncol. 2013;24:2206–23.

5. Bustreo S, Osella-Abate S, Cassoni P, Donadio M, Airoldi M, Pedani F, Papotti M, Sapino A, Castellano I. Optimal Ki-67 cut-off for luminal breast cancer prognostic evaluation: a large case series study with a long-term follow-up. Breast Cancer Research and Treatment. 2016;157:363–71. https://doi.org/10. 1007/s10549-016-3817-9.

6. Cheang MC, Chia SK, Voduc D, Gao D, Leung S, Snider J, Watson M, Davies S, Bernard PS, Parker JS, Perou CM, Ellis MJ, Nielsen TO. Ki-67 index, HER2 status, and prognosis of patients with luminal B breast cancer. J Natl Cancer Inst 20. 2009;101(10):736–50. https://doi.org/10.1093/jnci/djp082.

7. Jansen S, Fan X, Karczmar G, Abe H, Schmidt R, Newstead G. Differentiation between benign and malignant breast lesions detected by bilateral dynamic contrast-enhanced MRI: A sensitivity and specificity study. Magnetic Resonance in Medicine. 2008;59(4):747–54.

8. Moy L, Elias K, Patel V, Lee J, Babb JS, Toth HK, Mercado CL. Is breast MRI helpful in the evaluation of inconclusive mammographic findings? AJR Am J Roentgenol. 2009;193(4):986–93. https://doi.org/10.2214/AJR.08.1229.

9. Ojeda-Fournier H, Choe KA, Mahoney M. Recognizing and Interpreting Artifacts and Pitfalls in MR Imaging of the Breast. RadioGraphics. 2007; 27:S147–64.

10. Millet I, Pages E, Hoa D, Merigeaud S, Curros Doyon F, Prat X, Taourel P. Pearls and pitfalls in breast MRI. Br J Radiol. 2012;85(1011):197–207.

11. Macura KJ, Ouwerkerk R, Jacobs MA, Bluemke DA. Patterns of enhancement on breast MR images: interpretation and imaging pitfalls. Radiographics. 2006;26(6):1719–34.

12. Turnbull LW. Dynamic contrast-enhanced MRI in the diagnosis and management of breast cancer. NMR Biomed. 2009;22(1):28–39. https://doi. org/10.1002/nbm.1273. Review.

13. Behjatnia B, Sim J, Bassett LW, Moatamed NA, Apple SK. Does size matter? Comparison study between MRI, gross, and microscopic tumor sizes in breast cancer in lumpectomy specimens. Int J Clin Exp Pathol 22. 2010;3(3):303–9.

14. Onesti JK, Mangus BE, Helmer SD. Breast cancer tumor size: correlation between magnetic resonance imaging and pathology measurements. Am J Surg. 2008;196:844–50.

15. Castellano G, Bonilha L, Li LM, Cendes F. Texture analysis of medical images. Clin Radiol. 2004;59(12):1061–9.

16. Gibbs P, Turnbull LW. Textural analysis of contrast-enhanced MR Images of the breast. Magn Reson Med. 2003;50(1):92–8.

17. Nie K, Chen JH, Yu HJ, Chu Y, Nalcioglu O, MY S. Quantitative analysis of lesion morphology and texture features for diagnostic prediction in breast MRI. Acad Radiol. 2008;15(12):1513–25.

18. Newell D, Nie K, Chen JH, Hsu CC, Yu HJ, Nalcioglu O, MY S. Selection of diagnostic features on breast MRI to differentiate between malignant and benign lesions using computer-aided diagnosis: differences in lesions presenting as mass and non-mass-like enhancement. Eur Radiol. 2010;20(4):771–81.

19. McLaren CE, Chen WP, Nie K, MY S. Prediction of malignant breast lesions from MRI features: a comparison of artificial neural network and logistic regression techniques. Acad Radiol. 2009;16(7):842–51.

20. Waugh SA, Purdie CA, Jordan LB, Vinnicombe S, Lerski RA, Martin P, Thompson AM. Magnetic resonance imaging texture analysis classification of primary breast cancer. Eur Radiol. 2016;26(2):322–30. https://doi.org/10. 1007/s00330-015-3845-6.

21. Davnall F, Yip CS, Ljungqvist G, Selmi M, Ng F, Sanghera B, Ganeshan B, Miles KA, Cook GJ, Goh V. Assessment of tumor heterogeneity: an emerging imaging tool for clinical practice? Insights Imaging. 2012;3:573–89. https:// doi.org/10.1007/s13244-012-0196-6.

22. Karahaliou A, Vassiou K, Arikidis NS, Skiadopoulos S, Kanavou T, Costaridou L. Assessing heterogeneity of lesion enhancement kinetics in dynamic contrastenhanced MRI for breast cancer diagnosis. Br J Radiol. 2010;83:296–309.

23. Pickles MD, Lowry M, Gibbs P. Pretreatment prognostic value of dynamic contrast-enhanced magnetic resonance imaging vascular, texture, shape, and size parameters compared with traditional survival indicators obtained from locally advanced breast cancer patients. Invest Radiol. 2016;51(3):177–85.

24. Chang RF, Chen HH, Chang YC, Huang CS, Chen JH, Lo CM. Quantification of breast tumor heterogeneity for ER status, HER2 status, and TN molecular subtype evaluation on DCE-MRI. Magn Reson Imaging. 2016;34(6):809–19.

25. Sutton EJ, JH O, Dashevsky BZ, Veeraraghavan H, Apte AP, Thakur SB, Deasy JO, Morris EA. Breast cancer subtype intertumor heterogeneity: MRI-based features predict results of a genomic assay. J Magn Reson Imaging. 2015; 42(5):1398–406.

26. Szabo BK, Aspelin P, Kristoffersen WM, Tot T, Bone B. Invasive breast cancer: correlation of dynamic MR features with prognostic factors. Eur Radiol. 2003; 13:2425–35.

27. Knuttel FM, Menezes GL, van den Bosch MA, Gilhuijs KG, Peters NH. Current clinical indications for magnetic resonance imaging of the breast. J Surg Oncol. 2014;110(1):26–31. https://doi.org/10.1002/jso.23655. Epub 2014 May 26

28. Partridge SC, Gibbs JE, Lu Y, Esserman LJ, Tripathy D, Wolverton DS, Rugo HS, Hwang ES, Ewing CA, Hylton NM. MRI measurements of breast tumor volume predict response to neoadjuvant chemotherapy and recurrence-free survival. AJR Am J Roentgenol. 2005;184(6):1774–81.

29. Ellis P, Schnitt S, Sastre-Garau X, Bussolati G, Tavassoli F, Eusebi V, Peterse J, Mukai K, Tabar L, Jacquemier J, Cornelisse C, Sasco A, Kaaks R, Pisani P, Goldgar D, Devilee P, Cleton-Jansen M, Borresen-Dale A, Van´t Veer L, Sapino A. WHO Classification of Tumours. In: Tavassoli FA, Devilee P, editors. Pathology and Genetics of Tumours of the Breast and Female Genital Organs. Lyon: IARC Press; 2003.

30. Elston CW, Ellis IO. Pathological prognostic factors in breast cancer. The value of histological grade in breast cancer: experience from a large study with long-term follow up. Histopathology. 1991;19:403–10.

31. Sikiö M, Holli KK, Harriso LC, Ruottinen H, Rossi M, Helminen M, Ryymin P, Paalavuo R, Soimakallio S, Eskola HJ, Elovaara I, Dastidar P. Parkinson's Disease Interhemispheric Textural Differences in MR Images. Acad Radiol. 2011;18(10):1217–24.

32. Castellano G, Bonilha L, Li LM, Cendes F. Texture analysis of medical images. Clin Radiol. 2004;59:1061–9.

33. Hajek M, Dezortova M, Materka A, Lerski R (ed) (2006). Texture analysis for magnetic resonance imaging. Med4publishing, Prague.

34. Rasband WS. ImageJ, U. S. National Institutes of Health, Bethesda, Maryland, USA, http://imagej.nih.gov/ij/, 1997-2014.

35. Hansen RK, Bissell MJ. Tissue architecture and breast cancer: the role of extracellular matrix and steroid hormones. Endocr Relat Cancer. 2000; 7(2):95–113.

36. Esteva FJ, Hortobagyi GN. Prognostic molecular markers in early breast cancer. Breast Cancer Res. 2004;6:109–18.

37. Holli K, Lääperi AL, Harrison L, Luukkaala T, Toivonen T, Ryymin P, Dastidar P, Soimakallio S, Eskola H. Characterization of breast cancer types by texture analysis of magnetic resonance images. Acad Radiol. 2010;17(2):135–41. https://doi.org/10.1016/j.acra.2009.08.012.

38. Michoux N, Van den Broeck S, Lacoste L, Fellah L, Galant C, Berlière M, Leconte I. Texture analysis on MR images helps predicting non-response to NAC in breast cancer. BMC Cancer 5. 2015;15:574. https://doi.org/10.1186/s12885-015-1563-8.

39. Teruel JR, Heldahl MG, Goa PE, Pickles M, Lundgren S, Bathen TF, Gibbs P. Dynamic contrast-enhanced MRI texture analysis for pretreatment prediction of clinical and pathological response to neoadjuvant chemotherapy in patients with locally advanced breast cancer. NMR Biomed. 2014;27(8):887–96. https://doi.org/10.1002/nbm.3132.

40. Yun BL, Cho N, Li M, Jang MH, Park SY, Kang HC, Kim B, Song IC, Moon WK. Intratumoral heterogeneity of breast cancer xenograft models: texture analysis of diffusion-weighted MR imaging. Korean J Radiol. 2014;15(5):591–604. https://doi.org/10.3348/kjr.2014.15.5.591.

41. Ahmed A, Gibbs P, Pickles M, Turnbull L. Texture analysis in assessment and prediction of chemotherapy response in breast cancer. J Magn Reson Imaging. 2013;38(1):89–101.

42. Bhooshan N, Giger ML, Jansen SA, Li H, Lan L, Newstead GM. Cancerous breast lesions on dynamic contrast-enhanced MR images: computerized characterization for image-based prognostic markers. Radiology. 2010;254(3):680–90.

43. Bhooshan N, Giger M, Edwards D, Yuan Y, Jansen S, Li H, Lan L, Sattar H, Newstead G. Computerized three-class classification of MRI-based prognostic markers for breast cancer. Phys Med Biol. 2011;56(18):5995–6008.

30

Efficacy of sellar opening in the pituitary adenoma resection of transsphenoidal surgery influences the degree of tumor resection

Shousen Wang[*†], Yong Qin[†], Deyong Xiao and Liangfeng Wei

Abstract

Background: Endonasal transsphenoidal microsurgery is often adopted in the resection of pituitary adenoma, and has showed satisfactory treatment and minor injuries. It is important to accurately localize sellar floor and properly incise the bone and dura matter.

Methods: Fifty-one patients with pituitary adenoma undergoing endonasal transsphenoidal microsurgery were included in the present study. To identify the scope of sellar floor opening, CT scan of the paranasal sinus and MRI scan of the pituitary gland were performed for each subject. Intraoperatively, internal carotid artery injury, leakage of cerebrospinal fluid, and tumor texture were recorded, and postoperative complications and residual tumors were identified.

Result: The relative size of sellar floor opening significantly differed among the pituitary micro-, macro- and giant adenoma groups, and between the total and partial tumor resection groups. The ratio of sellar floor opening area to maximal tumor area was significantly different between the total and partial resection groups. Logistic regression analysis revealed that the ratio of sellar floor opening area to the largest tumor area, tumor texture, tumor invasion and age were independent prognostic factors. The vertical distance between the top point of sellar floor opening and planum sphenoidale significantly differed between the patients with and without leakage of cerebrospinal fluid.

Conclusion: These results together indicated that relatively insufficient sellar floor opening is a cause of leading to residual tumor, and the higher position of the opening and closer to the planum sphenoidale are likely to induce the occurrence of leakage of cerebrospinal fluid.

Keywords: Sellar opening, Hypopituitarism, Pituitary adenoma, Transsphenoidal surgery, Degree of tumor excision, Complication

Background

Pituitary adenoma [1], tumors at in the pituitary gland, represent from 10% to 25% of all intracranial neoplasms, and the estimated prevalence rate in the general population is approximately 17% [2, 3]. In the clinical practice, neurosurgeons commonly adopted endonasal transsphenoidal microsurgery for the resection of pituitary adenoma,

which showed satisfactory treatment effects with minor injuries. However, accurately identifying the intraoperative localization of sellar floor is always challenging in the clinical practice, due to the limited space in the surgical operation, anatomical variations of sphenoid sinus, as well as its adjacent structures, including conchal sphenoidal sinus, sphenoidal sinus separation (e.g., multiple, horizontal or slanting), flat sellar floor, and Onodi cell. Inaccurate identifications of sellar floor would induce the unsuccess of the operation [4]: (1) if the localization of sellar floor deviated frontally, it would occur error entries into the posterior ethmoidal sinus and tuberculum sellae; (2) if the localization of

* Correspondence: wshsen@126.com
†Equal contributors
Department of Neurosurgery, Fuzhou General Hospital, Fujian Medical University, No. 156 Xi'erhuanbei Road, Fuzhou 350025, People's Republic of China

sellar floor deviated bilaterally, it would probably lead to the injuries of the cavernous segment of the internal carotid artery (CSICA), as well as the injuries of cranial nerves in cavernous sinus, thus resulting in intraoperative massive hemorrhage, and several post-operation clinical symptoms, e.g., ambiopa; (3) if the localization of sellar floor deviated posteriorly, it would cause injuries to the brain stem. Thus, it has been proposed to develop individualized approach to identify the location of sellar floor based on the three-dimensional reconstruction (3-DR) of the relevant anatomical landmarks in the operation, with advantages of allowing for simplifying the process, improving the direction sense, increasing the positioning accuracy, and shortening the operation time.

With the precise localization of sellar floor, it is of vital importance to properly incise the bone and dura matter, to guarantee the satisfactory treatment of the endonasal transsphenoidal microsurgery for the resection of pituitary adenoma. Conventionally, the scope of the sellar floor opening in the endonasal transsphenoidal microsurgery would not exceed the tuberculum sellae and the sellar- clivus point frontally and posteriorly respectively, and close to the medial wall of the cavernous sinus. Abe et al. [5] applied the bone window CT scanning parallel to the transsphenoidal approach to help determine the lateral boundaries of sellar opening, which showed good operative performance. However, these are generalized boundaries and scopes across patients, it still remains unclear about individualized sellar floor opening procedure, as well as the potential factors affecting the sellar floor opening.

The majority of studies discussing the influencing factors of pituitary adenoma excision focused on the clinical characterizations of the tumor [6–8], e.g., the size, texture, invasiveness and orientation of the tumor, with the factors regarding the scope and positioning of sellar floor opening remaining unclearly. Indeed, Mattozo et al. [9] and Alahmadi et al. [10] conducted transsphenoidal excision of the residual pituitary adenoma under microscope and endoscope, and concluded that insufficiency of sphenoidal sinus anterior wall and sellar floor opening of the previous surgery are the major causes of residual tumor. However, several drawbacks existed in these studies leading to the inaccurate conclusions, including (1) they were descriptive studies based on the subjective experience of the researchers, without the solid demonstrations; (2) with the long intervals between the two consecutive surgeries, there may be the enlargement and migration of the residual tumors, as well as bone ossifications of the anterior wall of the sphenoid sinus and sellar defects. In addition, Wei et al. [11] reported that excessive sellar floor opening probably causes injury of pituitary gland and leakage of cerebrospinal fluid. Wang et al. [12] hypothesized that larger

sellar floor opening enlarged the surgical field, aggravated mechanical irritation to adjacent structures, and led to the incidence of posterior pituitary gland injury and diabetes insipidus.

Based on these understanding, the present study aims to comprehensively and quantitatively assess the relationship between sellar floor opening (scope and position) and intraoperative/postoperative complications (e.g., leakage of cerebrospinal fluid, diabetes insipidus and hypopituitarism).

Methods

Patients

Fifty-one patients ((22 males and 29 females, aging from 19 to 75 years with average of 46.7 ± 12.6 years) with pituitary adenoma, undergoing endonasal transsphenoidal surgeries in the Department of Neurosurgery of Fuzhou Genera Hospital from March 2014 to March 2015 were included in the present study. Inclusion criteria were (1) complete medical data including preoperative and postoperative CT scan of paranasal sinus, and MRI of pituitary gland, hormone levels at preoperative 3 days and postoperative 1 week; (2) all surgeries completed by one single physician; (3) all clinical data provided by one single medical center (i.e., Fuzhou Genera Hospital); (4) the diagnosis of pituitary adenoma validated by immunohistochemical staining. Exclusion criteria were (1) a history of pituitary adenoma surgery or radiotherapy; (2) a history of sphenoidal sinus trauma, surgical trauma or malignant tumor.

According to the clinical data of patients, 44 patients suffered from headache, 21 patients with visual field defects, 2 patients with acromegaly, and 10 patients with amenorrhea-galactorrhea syndrome. Physical examination revealed that 1 patient presented declining sexual function, 1 patient with stuffy nose, 1 patient with palpitation, and 1 patient with chest distress. According to the immunohistochemical staining analysis [13], 13 patients with null-cell adenoma, 15 patients with prolactin (PRL) adenoma, 1 patient with growth hormone (GH) adenoma, 11 patients with plurihormonal adenoma, 7 patients with gonadotropic tumor, 1 patient with thyroid stimulating hormone (TSH) adenoma, and 3 patients with adrenocorticotropic hormone (ACTH) adenoma. According to the tumor diameter, the patients were divided into the micro-, macro-, and giant-adenoma groups [14], which were respectively defined as follow: (1) micro-adenoma with tumor diameter less than 10 mm; (2) macro-adenoma with tumor diameter between 10 and 30 mm; (3) giant-adenoma with tumor diameter larger than 30 mm. As a result, 2 patients had microadenoma, 35 patients had macroadenoma, and 14 patients had giant adenoma.

CT and MRI scan

At 1 week before and after surgeries, CT plain scan of paranasal sinus was performed separately using 256-slice spiral CT scanner (Discovery Ultra, GE Corporation). Scan parameters were consecutive scan along with the axis position, layer thickness of 0.625 mm with an interval of 0.625 mm, scan time of 1.2 s, FOV of 250 mm × 250 mm, and matrix of 512 × 512. All patients received CT scan in a supine position. Infraorbital line was regarded as the base line. Scan area ranged from the mandible to the upper frontal sinus. With multiple planar reconstruction (MPR) reconstructed using CT reconstruction software, the three-dimensional image models of the sella turcica were calculated in the environment of Mimics 15.0 software (Materialise Inc., Belgium).

At 1 week before and after surgeries, T1WI, T2WI, and T1WI contrast-enhanced MRI was performed separately using 3.0 T MRI system (Trio Tim, SIE corporation). MRI parameters were: layer thickness of 1.0 mm, FOV 250 mm × 250 mm, matrix 256× 256 and scan time of 6 min. Contrast-enhanced MRI was performed via intravenous injection of Gd-DTPA at a dosage of 0.2 mmol/kg body weight at a flow speed of 3.6 ml/s. Using INFINITT software (Seoul, South Korea), the localization of tumor were identified from the adjacent tissues. The maximal tumor diameter and the tumor area (S) of each layer were calculated automatically in coronal position. All tumors were divided into micro-, macro- and giant –adenoma (as illustrated in Fig. 1), and the tumor volume was calculated [15].

Based on the method proposed by Knosp et al. [16] the degree of tumor invasiveness was classified into

grades from 0 to 4: (1) grade 0, the tumor margin did not pass the tangent of the medial aspects of the supra- and intracavernous ICA; (2) grade 1, the tumor margin did not pass a line between the cross-sectional centers of the carotid arteries, the so-called "intercarotid line"; (3) grade 2, the tumor margin extended beyond the intercarotid line, but does not extend beyond or tangent to the lateral aspects of the intra- and supracavernous ICA; (4) grade 3, the tumor margin extended lateral to the lateral tangent of the intra- and supracavernous ICA; (5) grade 4, the CSICA was completely encased by tumor tissues. If the Knosp classification grade higher than 3, the tumors were defined as the invasive pituitary adenoma.

Evaluation of pituitary gland function by measuring blood levels of hormones

Hormone levels were measured at 8 a.m. of 2 days after admission and postoperative 7 days. The venous blood samples were collected for chemiluminescence analysis (Siemens ADVIA Centaur XP automatic electrochemical luminescence analyzer, Germany). The hormones of GH, ACTH, free triiodothyronine (FT3), free thyroxine (FT4), estradiol (E2), testosterone (T), TSH, PRL, follicle stimulating hormone (FSH), luteotropic hormone (LH), cortisol and insulin-like growth factor 1 (IGF-1), were measured and summarized in Table 1.

Patients were diagnosed as hypopituitarism for hypofunction of anyone axis, such as pituitary gland-thyroid axis, growth hormone axis, adrenal cortex axis or gonad axis [17]: (1) hypofunction of adenohypophysis-gonad axis were identified as testosterone level lower than normal range for male patients; serum FSH/LH lower than normal range for female patients at menopause; decreased level of estradiol accompanied by normal or decreased levels of FSH and LH for the female at non-menopause, amenorrhoea or infrequent menstruation [5]; (2) hypofunction of adenohypophysis-thyroid axis were identified as serum level of FT4 lower than normal range accompanied by low or normal TSH level; (3) hypofunction of adenohypophysis-adrenal cortex axis were identified as cortisol level lower than normal reference value and normal ACTH or lower than normal reference value [18].

Surgical procedures

The surgical procedures via right single nostril-sphenoidal sinus approach, performed and recorded under camera-equipped surgical microscope, were completed by one single physician as follows. After disinfection, the cotton strips, soaked with 0.0067% adrenaline saline were, inserted into bilateral nasal cavities for 3 min, for nasal vasoconstriction and nasal cavity dilatation. An incision was made in the nasal septum (approximately 3 cm posterior to anterior

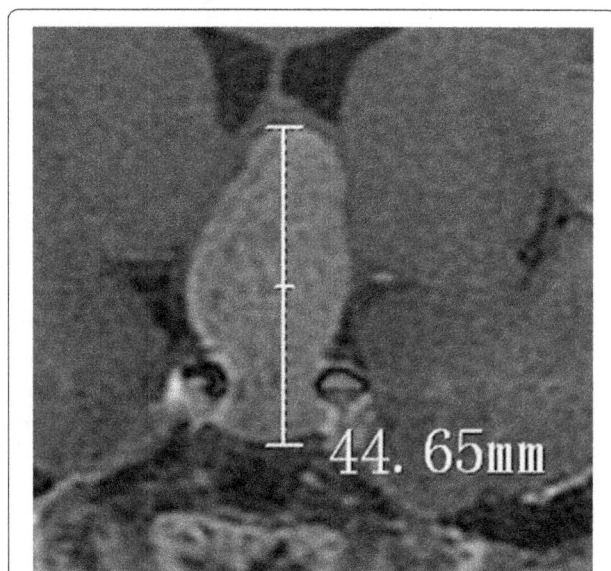

Fig. 1 Schematic diagram of the maximal tumor diameter evaluated by enhanced coronal MRI (44.65 mm represents the maximum diameter of this pituitary adenoma)

Table 1 Normal reference values of hormone levels

Hormones	Reference value
GH	<10 ng/mL for females, <1 ng/mL for males
ACTH	4.7-48.8 pg/mL
Cortisol	Blood sampling in the morning: 4.3-22.4 g/dL
	Blood sampling in the afternoon: 3.09-16.66 g/dL
FT3	3.5-6.5 pmol/L
FT4	11.5-22.7 pmol/L
TSH	0.35-5.5 μ IU/mL
FSH	2.5-10.2 mIU/mL at follicular stage; 3.4-33.4 mIU/mL at ovulatory stage
	1.5-9.1 mIU/mL at luteal stage; 23-116 mIU/mL at menopause stage
LH	1.9-12.5 mIU/mL at follicular stage; 8.7-76.3 mIU/mL at ovulatory stage
	0.5-16.9 mIU/mL at luteal stage; 15.9-116 mIU/mL at menopause stage
E2	15.9-144.2 pg/mL at follicular stage; 63.9-356.7 pg/mL at ovulatory stage
	55.8-214.2 pg/mL at luteal stage; 0-32.2 pg/mL at menopause stage
T	14-76 ng/dL
IGF-1	127-584 ng/mL for 18-20 years old; 116-358 ng/mL for 21-30 years old
	109-307 ng/mL for 31-40 years old; 94-267 ng/mL for 41-50 years old
	81-238 ng/mL for 51-60 years old; 69-212 ng/mL for 61-70 years old
PRL	2.5-10.2 mIU/mL at follicular stage; 1.8-20.3 ng/mL at ovulatory stage
	1.5-9.1 mIU/mL at luteal stage; 1.8-20.3 ng/mL at menopause stage
	2.8-29.2 ng/mL for non-pregnant women; 9.7-208 mIU/mL for pregnant women

naris). The surgical approach extended to the anterior wall of sphenoidal sinus between the right periosteum and perpendicular plate of ethmoid bone, with bilateral ostia of the sphenoid sinus exposed and the anterior wall of sphenoidal sinus removed. According to CT and MRI data of preoperative paranasal sinus, the position of sella turcica was comprehensively determined based upon the vomer, Onodi cell, sphenoidal sinus separation, and sellar protuberance. In addition, the regime of sellar floor opening was individualized designed according to tumor size, sella turcica, sphenoidal sinus, minimal distance between bilateral CSICA, etc. Following sellar floor opening, the opening scope of dura mater was determined to match with the bone opening as possible. With the resected tumor specimen prepared for pathological examination, the tumorous cavity was packed with gelatin sponge, fixed and sealed by medical glue. Then, one drainage tube of sphenoidal sinus was retained, and bilateral nasal cavities were filled with

vaseline gauze. At postoperative 1 day, the drainage tube was removed and the gauze was abandoned at 3 days after surgery. Intraoperatively, the incidence of ICA injury, leakage of cerebrospinal fluid and tumor texture were recorded for each patient. All tumor tissues were divided into the hard and soft tumor groups according to the criteria proposed by Yamamoto et al. [19].

Postoperative evaluations

The average amount of urine per hour and 24 h were recorded after surgery. Diagnostic criteria of diabetes insipidus: specific gravity of urine lower than 1.005; consecutive 2-h amount of urine more than 600 ml or amount of urine more than 2500 ml/d; requiring antidiuresis medication. All these criteria should be properly met when identified as diabetes insipidus. The endocrine secretion of pituitary gland was re-examined at the 7th postoperative day. The plasma levels of electrolytes were measured on a regular basis. CT scan of the paranasal sinus was conducted to identify the incidence of intracranial hemorrhage.

Multiple planar reconstruction was conducted after CT scan by using the Mimics 15.0 software (Materialise corporation, Belgium). Three-dimensional images of the sella turcica were calculated and constructed and then subject to dynamic partitioning. The bone opening area was calculated according to the equation as below. Area = π × (maximal transverse diameter/2) × (maximal vertical diameter/2) = $\pi/4$ × maximal transverse diameter × maximal vertical diameter. The plane with maximal vertical diameter was selected to quantitatively measure the vertical distance between the top point of sellar floor opening and planum sphenoidale, as illustrated in Fig. 2.

According to the MRI scanning, the incidence, size, and position of residual tumor were identified. Specifically, the degree of tumor excision was evaluated by calculating the ratio of preoperative to postoperative tumor size. For total tumor resection, no residual tumor could be noted by enhanced-MRI examination. For sub-total resection, the percentage of residual tumor size should be less than 10%, and 10%-40% for partial excision of the tumors [20].

To evaluate the effects of sellar floor opening, appropriate sellar floor opening was defined as no tumor residues were detected by postoperative MRI for patients undergoing total resection surgery. For the patients with residual tumors, appropriate sellar floor opening was defined if residual tumors were located in anterior cranial fossa, posterior cranial fossa or in the cavernous sinus, whereas insufficient opening was identified for those with residual tumors inside the sella.

If postoperative imaging reveals the residual suprasellar tumor, CT image of the paranasal sinus should be

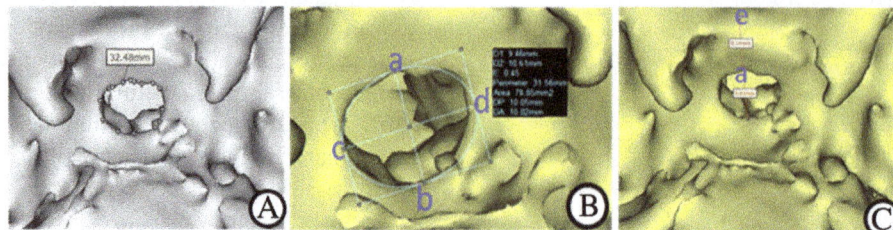

Fig. 2 CT 3-DR images revealing postoperative morphology of sellar floor and relevant parameters. **a**. postoperative morphology of sellar floor; **b**. ab = 9.45 mm as the maximal vertical diameter of sellar floor opening, cd = 10.62 mm as the maximal transverse diameter of sellar floor opening, Area: 78.85 mm² as the approximate opening area; **c**. ae = 9.14 mm as the vertical distance between the top point of sellar opening and planum sphenoidale

fused with MRI image of the pituitary gland, for the reconstruction of the sellar floor opening and residual tumor. In combination with tumor texture and morphology, comprehensive evaluations were made. If tumor texture was hard and/or in dumb-bell shape, sellar floor opening was defined as appropriate. If tumor texture was soft and wasn't in dumb-bell shape, sellar floor opening was defined as insufficient, with the tumor resected by enlarging sellar floor opening. If the degree of tumor excision cannot be enhanced by widening sellar floor opening, sellar floor opening was defined as appropriate.

All the surgical specimens were sent to the Department of Pathology of the medical center for pathological examination. Tumor tissues were fixed into 10% neutral formalin solution, paraffin embedding and sections for H.E staining, as well as staining of Syn, PRL, GH, ACTH, TSH, FSH, LH, etc. Positive outcome was obtained if above 10% of the cells were stained according to the diagnostic criteria of pituitary adenoma proposed by the WHO in 2004 [20].

Statistical analysis

The measured data, mentioned above, were analyzed in the SPSS 17.0 statistical software (SPSS Inc., Chicago, IL). Particularly, normally-distributed measurement data were expressed as mean ± standard deviation, whereas non-normally-distributed data were expressed as median + range interquartile (M + QR). To identify the differences between groups, qualitative data were statistically analyzed by chi-square test or Fisher exact test, whereas quantitative data were analyzed by independent sample t-test or Mann-Whitney U test. Linear relationship between two variables was analyzed by Pearson correlation analysis. Moreover, multivariate analysis was performed by logistic regression model. In these statistical analysis, $P < 0.05$ was considered as statistical significance.

Results

Tumor characteristics

Across the 51 patients, the course of diseases ranged from 3 days to 20 years (2.5 ± 4.0 years in average), the tumor diameter ranged from 0.8 to 4.3 cm, with an average of 2.4 ± 0.9 cm. The maximal tumor area in coronal position was measured in the range from 0.2 to 10.7 cm², with an average of 4.2 ± 2.6 cm². The tumor volume was in the range from 0.2 to 30.2 cm³, with an average of 7.4 ± 6.8 cm³. The morphology of tumor was summarized as follow: 12 patients with lobulated tumor, 2 patients with dumbbell-shaped tumor, and 37 patients with oval-shaped tumor. The invasiveness of the tumor was summarized as follow: 17 patients with Knosp classification grade 0, 7 patients with grade 1, 11 patients with grade 2, 9 patients with grade 3, and 7 patients with grade 4. The deviations of tumor were summarized as follow: 24 patients with midline deviations, 11 patients with left deviations, 16 patients with right deviations. In addition, there were 9 patients with MRI T2WI hypointense signal, 42 patients with isointense signal, and 15 patients complicated with cystic lesions in the tumor.

Intraoperative evaluations

For all patients, preoperative 3D CT reconstruction images were consistent with intraoperative observations of sphenoidal sinus separation. The sellar floor was rapidly localized under the guidance of sphenoidal sinus separation. No obvious complications induced by localization deviation were observed. Intraoperatively, 8 patients showed hard tumor texture, and 44 patients showed soft tumor texture. In addition, 11 patients presented leakage of cerebrospinal fluid, and no ICA injury was noted.

Postoperative evaluations

Across the 51 patients, 35 patients received total tumor resection, 9 patients received sub-total resection, and the other 7 patients received partial resection. In terms of residual tumor location, 5 patients had suprasellar tumor, 7 patients with cavernous sinus, 2 patients with suprasellar plus anterior cranial fossa, 2 patients with cavernous sinus and posterior fossa. The postoperative complications of patients were summarized as follow: 2 patients with intracranial hemorrhage, 3 patients with electrolyte disturbance, 17 patients with temporary diabetes insipidus, and 1 patient with cerebrospinal rhinorrhea.

Across the 51 patients, 15 patients with preoperative hypopituitarism were excluded for the following postoperative evaluation of pituitary function. The results of the remaining 36 patients showed that 13 patients developed hypopituitarism, i.e., 9 patients with gonad axis hypofunction alone, 2 patients with thyroid axis hypofunction, and 2 patients with thyroid axis complicated with gonad axis hypofunction, as illustrated in Table 2.

The area of sellar floor opening was (94.71+ 95.55) mm^2 vs. (151.00 + 118.38) mm^2 for the toral tumor resection (35 patients) and residual tumor group (16 patients) respectively, and the area of sellar floor opening was significantly smaller in the total tumor resection group than that in the residual tumor group ($Z = -2.274$, $P < 0.05$). In addition, the ratio of sellar floor opening area to maximal tumor area was 0.44 + 0.35 in the total resection group, significantly larger ($Z = -2.153$, $P < 0.05$) than those in the residual tumor group with ratio of 0.27+ 0.12.

Across the 51 patients, with the extent of tumor resection as dependent variable, and factors including patient's age, sex, tumor invasion, texture and the ratio of sellar floor opening area to maximal tumor area as independent variables, multi-factor analysis revealed that tumor invasion, tumor texture, age and the ratio of sellar floor opening area to maximal tumor area served can significantly predict the extent tumor resection ($p < 0.05$ for all variables), as illustrated in Table 3.

Across the 51 patients, there were 11 patients presenting cerebrospinal fluid leakage. The vertical distance between the top point of sellar floor opening and planum sphenoidal was summarized as 3.2 ± 2.1 mm vs. 7.9 ± 2.5 mm for the patients with and without cerebrospinal fluid

leakage respectively. In addition, there was significant differences between these two groups ($t = 5.704$, $P < 0.05$).

Across the 51 patients, 17 patients suffered from postoperative temporary diabetes insipidus. The sellar floor opening area in the diabetes insipidus group was 157.97 + 166.77 mm^2, which was not significantly different ($Z = -1.319$, $P > 0.05$) from those patients without diabetes insipidus (112.92 + 78.68 mm^2).

Across the 51 patients, 36 patients showed normal function of pituitary gland, and 13 patients showed hypopituitarism after surgery. In the hypopituitarism group, the sellar floor opening area was summarized 133.64 + 134.38 mm^2, which did not significantly differ from (73.79 + 86.85) mm^2 in their counterparts without hypopituitarism ($Z = -1.531$, $P > 0.05$).

Discussion

The present study adopted preoperative CT and MRI scan to identify the anatomical variations of sphenoid sinus and adjacent structures, and developed individualized opening strategies combined with the characteristics of tumor and sella turcica, minimal distance of bilateral CSICA and alternative parameters.

The effect of sellar floor opening was explicitly evaluated after the surgery. The majority of the patients displayed appropriate sellar floor opening, and only 2 patients displayed had insufficient sellar floor opening, which negatively influenced the extent of tumor resection. In addition, as revealed by the assessed relationship among multiple variables, i.e., sellar floor opening area, position, degree of tumor resection, intraoperative and postoperative complications, relative insufficiency of sellar floor opening is one of the factors influencing the residual pituitary adenoma. The higher sellar floor opening is more likely to induce the incidence of leakage of cerebrospinal fluid. In contrast, postoperative hypopituitarism is not significantly relevant with sellar floor opening area.

Mattozo et al. [9] and Alahmadi et al. [10] ever reported that sellar floor opening insufficiency is the major cause of residual tumor after the previous surgery. Nevertheless, the possibility of enlargement and migration of the residual tumors also may significantly increase due to relatively long interval between the consective two surgeries. Thus, the conclusion that sellar floor opening is associated with residual tumor, still remain untenable due to lack of solid evidence. Even early signs of errhysis, cataclysm and artificial materials for sellar reconstruction after surgery tend to affect the evaluation accuracy of residual tumors, several research groups [21, 22] insisted no statistical significance noted in terms of the detection rate of residual tumors for patients undergoing MRI between early and late stages. Consequently, postoperative early CT and MRI images were properly fused by two independent experienced physicians, which significantly improved

Table 2 Postoperative complication of 51 patients undergoing tumor resection

	N (percentages out of 51)
Degree of tumor resection	
Total resection	35 (68.6%)
Subtotal resection	9 (17.7%)
Partial resection	7 (13.7%)
Position of residual tumor	
Suprasellar region	5 (9.8%)
Cavernous sinus	7 (13.7%)
Suprasellar + anterior cranial fossa	2 (3.9%)
Posterior cranial fossa and cavernous sinus	2 (3.9%)
Postoperative complication	
Intracranial hemorrhage	2 (3.9%)
Electrolyte disturbance	3 (5.9%)
Temporary diabetes insipidus	17 (33.3%)
Cerebrospinal rhinorrhea	1 (2.0%)
Hypopituitarism	13 (36.1%)

Table 3 Logistic regression analysis of the influential factors of the degree of tumor resection

Factors	B	Standard error	Wald	df	P	Exp(B)
Ratio (sellar floor opening area to maximal tumor area)	6.269	2.711	5.348	1	0.021	528.15
Tumor invasion	−2.817	0.969	8.446	1	0.004	0.060
Gender	0.139	0.892	0.024	1	0.876	1.149
Age	−0.093	0.042	5.013	1	0.025	0.911
Tumor texture	−3.823	1.915	3.983	1	0.046	0.022

the evaluation accuracy. For tumors extending into the cavernous sinus and anterior cranial fossa, the tumors cannot be fully exposed and resected by conventional microscopic transsphenoidal surgery [23]. For suprasellar residual tumors, although the bone opening has been enlarged, it fails to fully resect the hard and dumbbell-shaped tumors. For such case, sellar floor opening is considered as an appropriate approach.

The sellar floor opening area of the micro- and macroadenoma groups was significantly smaller compared with that of the giant adenoma group. The sellar floor opening was positively correlated with tumor size, i.e., the larger pituitary adenoma was, the larger the sellar floor opening area was. Moreover, to enhance the exposure and resection of tumors, the sellar floor opening area should be enlarged accordingly. Compared with those in the total resection group, the sellar floor opening area in the sub-total resection group was significantly larger whereas the ratio of sellar floor opening area to maximal tumor area was considerably smaller. Importantly, multi-factor analysis revealed that the ratio of sellar floor opening area to maximal tumor area, tumor texture, invasion and patients' age act as independent prognostic factors of degree of tumor resection. These results together provide direct evidence that relative insufficiency of sellar floor opening is one of the factors leading to residual tumors.

Since the ratio of sellar floor opening area to maximal tumor area was calculated as (0.44 + 0.35) in the total resection group, it is likely that the total tumor resection can be completed when the ratio of sellar floor opening area to maximal tumor area up to 50%. With the sellar floor opening area excessively small, the degree of tumor resection would be reduced. With the sellar floor opening area excessively large, it is easy to induce ineffective sellar floor opening, resulting in unnecessary injuries. Considering that the limited sample size in the present study, further studies with more samples should be conducted to verify this hypothesis.

The large tumors likely to extending into anterior or posterior cranial fossa and cavernous sinus, cannot be fully exposed and removed by conventional opening via microscopic transsphenoidal approach, while hard tumors located at suprasellar region cannot be completely resected. The results of the present study also indicated

that the age of the patients could significantly influence the degree of tumor resection, probably because the tumors in elderly patients are large and have high invasiveness. In consistent with the obtained result in the present study that tumor texture and invasion can significant influence the tumor resection, Losa et al. [24] also proposed that that the cystic lesions of tumors are beneficial for total tumor resection, and several researchers suggest that the orientation of tumor extension and tumor morphology are both important factors of tumor resection.

Across the 51 patients, 2 patients presented small degree of tumor resection, probably resulting from insufficient tumor exposure and mechanical operation. Restricted visual field influences the evaluation on the sinking of diaphragma sella. The suprasellar tumor is mistakenly considered as diaphragma sella or partial sinking of diaphragma sella as complete sinking, leading to residual suprasellar tumors. In addition, compared with that in their counterparts without cerebrospinal fluid leakage, the vertical distance between the top point of sellar floor opening and planum sphenoidale was significantly shorter in patients with leakage of cerebrospinal fluid. It indicates that excessively high sellar floor opening probably is more likely to induce the leakage of cerebrospinal fluid during surgery.

Following the surgeries, approximately 33.3% of enrolled patients developed temporary diabetes insipidus, which is consistent with 15%-70% as reported by previous investigations [25]. As proposed by Wang et al. [26] during transsphenoidal surgery, enlargement of surgical scope is likely to induce injury to the neurohypophysis and its blood supply, eventually leading to the incidence of diabetes insipidus.

Transsphenoidal operation can stimulate or injure adenohypophysis tissues, resulting in the postoperative occurrence of hypopituitarism [15]. Zhou et al. [27] ever reported that 48% of patients presented hypopituitarism induced by surgical procedures. In this study, the incidence rate of hypopituitarism after surgery is 36.1%. Zada et al. [20] showed that male patients with relatively large tumors are more likely to show hypopituitarism after surgery, compared with alternative counterparts. Wei et al. [11] proposed that excessive resection of sellar floor bone probably causes injuries to adenohypophysis, thereby leading to the occurrence of hypopituitarism. Nevertheless, in this investigation, the risk of hypopituitarism is not significantly associated with the size of sellar floor opening.

With preoperative MRI conducted to accurately pinpoint the position of pituitary, intraoperative surgical procedures completed by experienced surgeons experienced in avoiding the risk of excessive traction and averted frequent use of electrocoagulation, the present study provided direct evidence that the enlargement of sellar floor opening effectively increasing the surgical field, allowed for properly distinguishing the tumors from the surrounding normal tissues, but not induce risks of injuries to the pituitary gland, hypothalamus and blood vessels.

There were two weaknesses in this preliminary study. First, in some patients, the residual tumor was located in the cavernous sinus. In clinical practice, some surgeons preferred not to resect tumor in the cavernous sinus. Thus, the residual tumor would be a certain factor if a tumor extends into the cavernous sinuses rather than a result affected by the size of the sella opening. Second, the correlation between the bony opening near the tuberculum sella and CSF leakage was not considered separately for micro and macroadenomas. The sella is likely to have arachnoid in its most rostral part in patients with small tumors, while macroadenomas can completely fill the sella and extend suprasellar; in this circumstance, a more rostral opening of the sellar floor would be much less likely to result in a breach of the arachnoid, and may help with tumor resection. In the future, we will conduct studies to further consolidate our findings by conducting more clinically useful correlation between the extent of bony opening and resection of all "surgically accessible" tumor (i.e., not in the cavernous sinus) and considering separately for micro and macroadenomas.

Conclusion

This paper indicated that residual tumor could be caused by relatively insufficient sellar floor opening and the occurrence of leakage of cerebrospinal fluid could be induced by choosing the opening position higher and closer to the planum sphenoidale.

Abbreviations
3-DR: Three-dimensional reconstruction; ACTH: Adrenocorticotropic hormone; CSICA: Cavernous segment of the internal carotid artery; E2: Estradiol; FSH: Follicle stimulating hormone; FT3: Free triiodothyronine; FT4: Free thyroxine; GH: Growth hormone; IGF-1: Insulin-like growth factor 1; LH: Luteotropic hormone; M + QR: Median + range interquartile; MPR: Multiple planar reconstruction; PRL: Prolactin; T: Testosterone; TSH: Thyroid stimulating hormone

Acknowledgements
None.

Funding
This work was supported by grants from The Nanjing Military Medical Science and Technology Innovation Key Fund Project (Funding No. 11Z034), and Fuzhou General Hospital Innovation Team Fund Project (Funding No. 2014CXTD07).

Authors' contributions
SSW participated in the design of the study and the clinical surgery. YQ and SSW carried out the clinical studies and the statistical analysis. DYX and SSW participated in the data acquisition and the data analysis. LFW and SSW conceived of the study, and participated in its design and coordination and helped to draft the manuscript. All authors read and approved the final manuscript.

Competing interests
The authors declare that they have no competing interests.

References
1. Budan RM, Georgescu CE. Multiple Pituitary Adenomas: A Systematic Review. Front Endocrinol. In Press. 2016.
2. Asa SL, Ezzat S. The cytogenesis and pathogenesis of pituitary adenomas. Endocr Rev. 1998;19:798–827.
3. Ezzat S, Asa SL, Couldwell WT, Barr CE, Dodge WE. The prevalence of pituitary adenomas: a systematic review. Cancer. 2004;101:613–9.
4. Ramakrishnan VR, Suh JD, Lee JY, O'Malley BW, Grady MS, Palmer JN. Sphenoid sinus anatomy and suprasellar extension of pituitary tumors. J Neurosurg. 2013;119:669–74.
5. Abe T, Asahina N, Kunii N, Ikeda H, Izumiyama H. Usefulness of bone window CT images parallel to the transnasal surgical route for pituitary disorders. Acta Neurochir. 2003;145:127–31.
6. Fayeye O, Shad A. A Giant pituitary adenoma: surgical excision via a staged endoscopic and open approach. World J Neuroscience. 2014;4:434–6.
7. Pratheesh R, Rajaratnam S, Prabhu K, Mani SE, Chacko G, Chacko AG. The current role of transcranial surgery in the management of pituitary adenomas. Pituitary. 2012;16:419–34.
8. Yu FF, Chen LL, Su YH, Huo LH, Lin XX, Liao RD. Factors influencing improvement of visual field after trans-sphenoidal resection of pituitary macroadenomas:a retrospective cohort study. Int J Ophthalmol. 2015;8:131–5.
9. Mattozo CA, Dusick JR, Esposito F, Mora H, Cohan P, Malkasian D, Kelly DF. Suboptimal sphenoid and seller exposure: a consistent finding in patients treated with repeat transsphenoidal surgery for residual endocrine-inactive macroadenomas. Neurosurgery. 2006;58:857–65.
10. Alahmadi H, Dehdashti AR, Gentili F. Endoscopic endonasal surgery in recurrent and residual pituitary adenomas after microscopic resection. World Neurosurg. 2012;77:540–7.
11. Wei Q, Li YJ, Shen CS, He JH, Qi JZ, Luo YC, Liang CY, Xu RX. Relationship of sphenoid intersinus septa with transsphenoidal resection of sellar area tumor. Chin J Neuromed. 2011;10:697–9.
12. Wang RZ, Yin J, Su CB, Ren ZY, Yao Y. Extended transsphenoidal operation for giant and invasive pituitary adenomas. Chin J Surg. 2006;44:1548–50.
13. Trouillas J, Roy P, Sturm N, Dantony E, Cortet-Rudelli C, Viennet G, et al. A new prognostic clinicopathological classification of pituitary adenomas: a multicentric case–control study of 410 patients with 8 years post-operative follow-up. Acta Neuropathol. 2013;126:123–35.
14. Juraschka K, Khan OH, Godoy BL, Monsalves E, Kilian A, Krischek B, Ghare A, Vescan A, Gentili F, Zadeh G. Endoscopic endonasal transsphenoidal approach to large and giant pituitary adenomas: institutional experience and predictors of extent of resectione. J Neurosurg. 2014;121:75–83.
15. Kinoshita Y, Tominaga A, Arita K, Sugiyama K, Hanaya R, Hama S, Sakoguchi T, Usui S, Kurisu K. Post-operative hyponatremia in patients with pituitary adenoma: post-operative management with a uniform treatment protocol. Endocr J. 2011;58:373–9.
16. Knosp E, Steiner E, Kitz K, Matula C. Pituitary adenomas with invasion of the cavernous sinus space: a magnetic resonance imaging classification compared with surgical findings. Neurosurgery. 1993;33:610–8.
17. Campero A, Socolovsky M, Torino R, Martins C, Yasuda A, Rhoton AL. Anatomical landmarks for positioning the head in preparation for the transsphenoidal approach: the spheno-sellarpoint. Br J Neurosurg. 2009;23:282–6.
18. Fleck SK, Wallaschofski H, Rosenstengel C, Matthes M, Kohlmann T, Nauc M, Schroeder HW, Spielhagen C. Prevalence of hypopituitarism after intracranial operations not directly associated with the pituitary gland. BMC Endocr Disord. 2013;13:51.

19. Yamamoto J, Kakeda S, Shimajiri S, Takahashi M, Watanabe K, Kai Y, Moriya J, Korogi Y, Nishizawa S. Tumor consistency of pituitary macroadenomas: predictive analysis on the basis of imaging features with contrast-enhanced 3D FIESTA at 3T. Am J Neuroradiol. 2014;35:297–303.
20. Zada G, Agarwalla PK, Mukundan JS, Dunn I, Golby AJ, Laws ER. The neurosurgical anatomy of the sphenoid sinus and sellar floor in endoscopic transsphenoidal surgery. J Neurosurg. 2011;114:1319–0.
21. Fatemi N, Dusick JR, Mattozo C, McArthur DL, Cohan P, Boscardin J, Wang C, Swerdloff RS, Kelly DF. Pituitary hormonal loss and recovery after transsphenoidal adenoma removal. Neurosurgery. 2008;63:709–19.
22. Mehta GU, Bakhtian KD, Oldfield EH. Effect of primary empty sella syndrome on pituitary surgery for Cushing's disease. J Neurosurg. 2014;21:518–26.
23. Bordo G, Kelly K, McLaughlin N, Miyamoto S, Duong HT, Eisenberg A, Chaloner C, Cohan P, Barkhoudarian G, Kelly DF. Sellar masses that present with severe Hyponatremia. Endocr Pract. 2014;20:1178–86.
24. Losa M, Mortini P, Barzaghi R, Ribotto P, Terreni M, Marzoli S, Pieralli S, Giovanelli M. Early results of surgery in patients with nonfunctioning pituitary adenoma and analysis of the risk of tumor recurrence. J Neurosurg. 2008;108:525–32.
25. Wichers-Rother M, Hoven S, Kristof R, Bliesener N, Stoffel-Wagner B. Non-functioning pituitary adenomas: endocrinological and clinical outcome after transsphenoidal and transcranial surgery. Exp Clin Endoc Diab. 2004;112:323–7.
26. Wang S, Lin S, Wei L, Zhao L, Huang Y. Analysis of operative efficacy for giant pituitary adenoma. BMC Surg. 2014;14:59.
27. Zhou ZC, Dou JT, Lv CH, Ba JM, Gu WJ. Investigation on evaluation of pituitary function after transsphenoidal ectomy of hypophysoma. Chin J End Met. 2012;28:542–5.

31

A consistency evaluation of signal-to-noise ratio in the quality assessment of human brain magnetic resonance images

Shaode Yu[1,2], Guangzhe Dai[1,3], Zhaoyang Wang[1,3], Leida Li[4], Xinhua Wei[5,6] and Yaoqin Xie[1*]

Abstract

Background: Quality assessment of medical images is highly related to the quality assurance, image interpretation and decision making. As to magnetic resonance (MR) images, signal-to-noise ratio (SNR) is routinely used as a quality indicator, while little knowledge is known of its consistency regarding different observers.

Methods: In total, 192, 88, 76 and 55 brain images are acquired using T_2^*, T_1, T_2 and contrast-enhanced T_1 (T_1C) weighted MR imaging sequences, respectively. To each imaging protocol, the consistency of SNR measurement is verified between and within two observers, and white matter (WM) and cerebral spinal fluid (CSF) are alternately used as the tissue region of interest (TOI) for SNR measurement. The procedure is repeated on another day within 30 days. At first, overlapped voxels in TOIs are quantified with Dice index. Then, test-retest reliability is assessed in terms of intra-class correlation coefficient (ICC). After that, four models (BIQI, BLIINDS-II, BRISQUE and NIQE) primarily used for the quality assessment of natural images are borrowed to predict the quality of MR images. And in the end, the correlation between SNR values and predicted results is analyzed.

Results: To the same TOI in each MR imaging sequence, less than 6% voxels are overlapped between manual delineations. In the quality estimation of MR images, statistical analysis indicates no significant difference between observers (Wilcoxon rank sum test, $p_w \geq 0.11$; paired-sample t test, $p_p \geq 0.26$), and good to very good intra- and inter-observer reliability are found (ICC, $p_{icc} \geq 0.74$). Furthermore, Pearson correlation coefficient (r_p) suggests that SNR_{wm} correlates strongly with BIQI, BLIINDS-II and BRISQUE in T_2^* ($r_p \geq 0.78$), BRISQUE and NIQE in T_1 ($r_p \geq 0.77$), BLIINDS-II in T_2 ($r_p \geq 0.68$) and BRISQUE and NIQE in T_1C ($r_p \geq 0.62$) weighted MR images, while SNR_{csf} correlates strongly with BLIINDS-II in T_2^* ($r_p \geq 0.63$) and in T_2 ($r_p \geq 0.64$) weighted MR images.

Conclusions: The consistency of SNR measurement is validated regarding various observers and MR imaging protocols. When SNR measurement performs as the quality indicator of MR images, BRISQUE and BLIINDS-II can be conditionally used for the automated quality estimation of human brain MR images.

Keywords: Signal-to-noise ratio, Consistency evaluation, Medical image quality assessment, Magnetic resonance imaging

* Correspondence: yq.xie@siat.ac.cn
[1]Shenzhen Institutes of Advanced Technology, Chinese Academy of Sciences, Shenzhen, China
Full list of author information is available at the end of the article

Background

Medical image quality is highly related to many clinical applications, such as screening, abnormality detection and disease diagnosis. Nowadays, various kinds of imaging modalities are daily used, such as computerized tomography (CT) and magnetic resonance (MR) imaging, not to speak of these devices under development [1–3]. At the same time, massive medical images are collected and used to support the clinical decision making in each day. Therefore, how to evaluate the medical image quality wins increasing attention [4, 5].

Medical image quality assessment (MIQA) is crucial in the equipment quality assurance [6–8], comparison of algorithms for image restoration [9–13], image interpretation [14–17] and disease diagnosis [18, 19]. These MIQA algorithms can be grouped into the full- and no-reference categories [19–23]. The full-reference algorithms require the access to the reference image, while it is often unavailable in the medical imaging domain. To tackle this problem, the images from advanced devices are used as the reference to validate the proposed methods with images from common devices [24, 25]. However, this kind of approaches leads to new obstacles due to uncontrollable motion and particularly the different imaging characteristics. Comparatively, no-reference MIQA algorithms are more useful and challenging, and no reference information can be borrowed [20, 23, 26].

As a quality indicator of medical images, signal-to-noise ratio (SNR) is widely used to evaluate the development of new hardware and image processing algorithms [19, 23, 26–31]. The most common approach for SNR measurement, known as a "two-region" approach, is based on the signal statistics in two separate regions of interest (ROIs) from a single image. One is the tissue ROI (TOI) which determines the signal and the other ROI is localized in the object-free region which measures the noise [27, 28, 32]. The quality comparison of medical images with SNR measurement is still difficult across studies [23]. Above all, SNR values might vary according to the delineation of ROIs. For specific purposes, different tissues are concerned. And regarding the same purpose, it is impossible to delineate an identical tissue region. Moreover, the quality of MR imaging acquisition is closely related to the magnetic field strength (1.5 T, 3 T, etc), imaging protocol (T_1, T_2, etc), field of view (FOV), reconstruction methods and other significant factors. Furthermore, medical imaging is prone to unavoidable noise and artifacts. Besides, a great challenge might come from the fact that there are diverse imaging characteristics across modalities. Therefore, a consistency evaluation of SNR measurement is helpful in the further comparison of medical image quality.

In this paper, we evaluate the reliability of SNR measurement regarding different observers. At the preliminary stage, this study is confined to human brain MR images and four MR imaging sequences are analyzed. To the best of our knowledge, the most similar work is [26], in which it conducted the correlation analysis between subjective evaluation and 13 full-reference models. These models are primarily used for natural image quality assessment (NIQA). However, the study is with poor generalization. First, the experiment was based on synthesized distortions on 25 reference MR images and the result might be not so convincing in regard to real-life medical images. Second, the study involved subjective estimation to score the image quality, which is time consuming and expensive. On contrary, in this study, 411 in vivo human brain MR images are collected and 2 observers are involved to localize the tissue regions of white matter (WM) and cerebral spinal fluid (CSF) as the TOI for SNR measurement. Most importantly, this study investigates the SNR consistency regarding different observers. After the reliability of SNR measurement is verified, 4 no-reference NIQA models are borrowed from the computer vision community to predict the MR image quality, and furthermore, the correlation between the predicted results and SNR values is explored. On the whole, this study might shed some light on automated objective MIQA with less time and expenditure.

Methods

Data collection

In total, 192 T_2^* weighted MR images of healthy brain, 88 T_1, 76 T_2 and 55 contrast enhanced T_1 (T_1C) weighted MR images of brain with cancerous tumors are collected. Participants were scanned with a 3.0 T scanner (Siemens, Erlangen, Germany) and an 8-channel brain phased-array coil was used.

Specifically, T_2^* weighted images are acquired using gradient-echo pulse sequence. Its time of repetition (TR) is 200 ms and time of echo (TE) varies from 2.61 ms to 38.91 ms with an equal interval of 3.3 ms. The flip angle is 15°, FOV is 220 × 220 mm², slice thickness is 3.0 mm and the resultant image matrix is 384 × 384. Note that the original purpose of multi-echo T_2^* weighted image acquisition is toward tissue dissimilarity analysis [12]. T_1, T_2 and T_1C weighted images are acquired using spin echo protocol with different TR and TE pairs (535 ms and 8 ms; 3500 ms and 105 ms; 650 ms and 9 ms). The flip angle is 15°, FOV is 220 × 220 mm² and slice thickness is 1 mm or 2 mm. The resultant image size of T_1 and T_1C weighted MR images varies from 512 × 432 to 668 × 512, while the matrix size of T_2 weighted MR images is ranged from 384 × 324 to 640 × 640.

Image pre-processing

To each image, pixel intensity is linearly scaled to [0, 255]. Then, two TOIs (WM and CSF) are outlined in addition to two air regions. A non-physician (observer A, OA) and a radiologist with more than 15-year experience (observer B, OB) are asked to determine ROIs manually. Since the observers work separately and independently, they agree on that the size of outlined ROIs should be as large as possible. Furthermore, to T_1, T_2 and T_1C weighted MR images, they also agree on that TOIs should be homogeneous and keep away from the tumor areas. The initial shape of each ROI is approximated with six points (the red sparkles in Fig. 1) and further refined by using a free-form curve-fitting method [33, 34]. The curve-fitting method takes the six points as the control points and Hermite cubic curve [35] is utilized for smooth interpolation between the points. In the end, outlined regions are as input to our in-house built algorithm with MATLAB (Mathworks, Natick, MA, USA) to measure the WM-based SNR (SNR_{wm}) and CSF-based SNR (SNR_{csf}) values. Note that the procedure is repeated on another day within 30 days for intra-observer reliability analysis.

Figure 1 shows T_2^* (A), T_1 (B), T_2 (C) and T_1C (D) weighted MR images. In each image, WM, CSF and AIR regions are in closed curves which are highlighted with pink, blue and yellow lines, respectively. Note that the red sparkles are primarily points localized by observers and images have been cropped for display purpose.

SNR measurement

Two approaches exist for SNR measurement. The most common one requires two separate ROIs from a single image [27, 28]. By taking the signal (S) to be the average intensity in a tissue ROI (μ_{TOI}) and the noise (σ) to be the standard deviation of the pixel intensity in a background ROI (σ_{AIR}), we can approximate the SNR value of the image as below,

$$SNR_{TOI} = \frac{S}{\sigma} = 0.655 \times \frac{\mu_{TOI}}{\sigma_{AIR}}. \tag{1}$$

Due to the Rician distribution of the background noise in a magnitude image, the factor of 0.655 arises because noise variations can be negative and positive [27, 28].

If the image is not homogeneous, the SNR measurement can be derived from the second approach [36, 37]. At first, a couple of images are acquired by consecutive scans and the MR device is equipped with identical imaging settings. And then, a difference image is derived by subtracting the images one from the other. Since the images are consecutively acquired on without any instability, the noise should be the only difference between the two original images. Taking the signal (S) as the mean pixel intensity value in a tissue ROI (μ_{oTOI}) on one original image and the noise as the standard deviation (σ) in the same ROI on the subtracted image (σ_{sTOI}), SNR can be estimated as

$$SNR_{TOI} = \frac{S}{\sigma} = \sqrt{2} \times \frac{\mu_{oTOI}}{\sigma_{sTOI}}, \tag{2}$$

where the factor of $\sqrt{2}$ arises because the standard deviation (σ) is derived from the subtraction image but not from the original image.

This study utilizes Eq. (1) to measure SNR values of MR images, since image homogeneity is warranted in this study. In addition, the second approach is commonly used for equipment quality assurance and requires scanning the object twice.

No-reference NIQA

Massive NIQA models are developed each year, while few models are used in the medical imaging community [38–40]. This study makes use of four automated no-reference NIQA methods to predict the MR image quality. The correlation analysis between SNR values

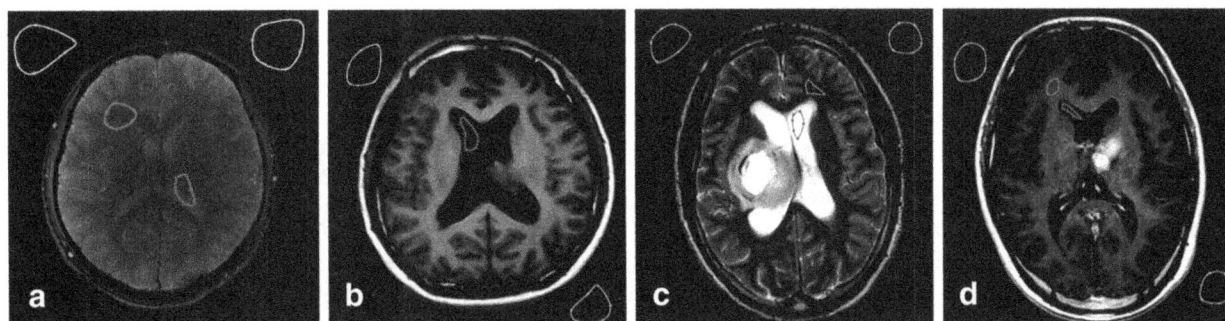

Fig. 1 Manual outline of tissue regions and air regions. **a**, **b**, **c**, **d** are T_2^*, T_1, T_2 and T_1C weighted MR images, respectively. **b**, **c**, **d** demonstrates one example of a subject. Primarily points localized by observers are noted with red sparkles. Outlined WM, CSF and AIR regions are in closed curves with pink, blue and yellow lines, respectively. Note that images have been cropped for display purpose

Table 1 The number of voxels in the outlined tissue regions

		T_2^*		T_1		T_2		T_1C	
		WM	CSF	WM	CSF	WM	CSF	WM	CSF
The first time	OA	423 (95)	381 (117)	558 (173)	614 (258)	609 (239)	889 (366)	523 (146)	704 (314)
	OB	**330** (72)	333 (138)	567 (181)	649 (318)	414 (174)	699 (288)	477 (156)	663 (272)
The second time	OA	382 (88)	378 (104)	530 (187)	626 (219)	589 (251)	853 (349)	505 (138)	692 (290)
	OB	357 (119)	342 (119)	582 (176)	663 (282)	447 (195)	721 (306)	480 (177)	686 (268)

and NIQA results aims to find potential no-reference NIQA models for MIQA applications.

Involved NIQA models utilize natural scene statistics (NSS) to estimate the general quality of natural images. Specifically, the blind image quality index (BIQI) [41] estimates the image quality based on the statistical features extracted in discrete wavelet transform (DWT). It requires no knowledge of the distortion types and can be extended to any kinds of distortions. The second indicator (BLIINDS-II) [42] is an improved version of blind image integrity notator using discrete cosine transform (DCT) statistics [38]. It adopts a general statistical model for score prediction. The third one, blind/referenceless image spatial quality evaluator (BRISQUE) [43], makes use of the locally normalized luminance coefficients and quantifies possible losses of "naturalness" which is a holistic measure of image quality. The last one is the natural image quality evaluator (NIQE) [44]. It builds a "quality-aware" selector that collects statistical features for natural image quality estimation.

These NIQA models are implemented with MATLAB (the Mathworks, Natick, MA, USA) and the codes provided by the authors are accessible online. The models are evaluated without modifications in this study. Full details of these algorithms can be referred to corresponding literature [41–44].

Experiment design

The experiment is divided into three steps. First, the overlapping ratio of manually outlined TOIs between and within observers are concerned and Dice index is employed. The index is defined as $d = 2 \times \frac{|X \cap Y|}{|X| + |Y|} \times 100\%$, where X and Y stand for the TOI, and the signal | | indicates TOI computed as the number of voxels in the region. The Dice index equal to 100% means the two TOIs are identical, while it equal to 0% indicates the two TOIs are absolutely non-overlapping.

Then, with respect to the same TOI in each imaging sequence, the inter-observer difference is assessed with Wilcoxon rank sum test [45, 46] and paired-sample t-test [47]. The statistical analysis is performed using R (http://www.Rproject.org) and a significance level is set as 0.05. Moreover, the test-retest reliability is evaluated

in terms of intra-class correlation coefficient (ICC, p_{icc}) using a two-way mixed-effects model [48]. The values of p_{icc} ranging from 0.81 to 1.00 suggest very good reliability and 0.61 to 0.80 good reliability.

In the end, the correlation between SNR values and NIQA results is analyzed by using Pearson correlation coefficient (r_p) [49]. Note that the values of r_p ranging from 0.81 to 1.00 indicate very strong or good correlation, while 0.61 to 0.80 good or strong correlation.

Results

Overlapped voxels in TOIs

Table 1 summarizes the number of voxels in TOIs in each MR sequence (the mean and standard deviation, $\mu \pm \sigma$). It is found that hundreds of voxels are outlined for SNR measurement and the minimum is 330±72.

Specifically, the overlapping ratio is described with Dice index as shown in Table 2. It indicates that less than 6% voxels are overlapped between and within observers in the manual delineation of TOIs.

Analysis of SNR values

Figure 2 shows the first-time measurement of SNR values by using Bland & Altman plots [50]. It is a scatter diagram of the differences plotted against the averages of two SNR observations. In each plot, the average and the

Table 2 Dice index for the overlapped percentage of voxels in the TOIs between and within observers

		WM		CSF		
		OB1	OB2	OA2	OB1	OB2
T_2^*	OA1	0.05	0.03	0.05	0.04	0.03
	OA2	0.03	0.04		0.03	0.03
	OB1		0.06			0.06
T_1	OA1	0.02	0.03	0.03	0.04	0.03
	OA2	0.03	0.03		0.01	0.02
	OB1		0.02			0.02
T_2	OA1	0.02	0.04	0.02	0.02	0.01
	OA2	0.03	0.03		0.03	0.02
	OB1		0.02			0.02
T_1C	OA1	0.02	0.02	0.03	0.02	0.03
	OA2	0.02	0.03		0.01	0.03
	OB1		0.04			0.02

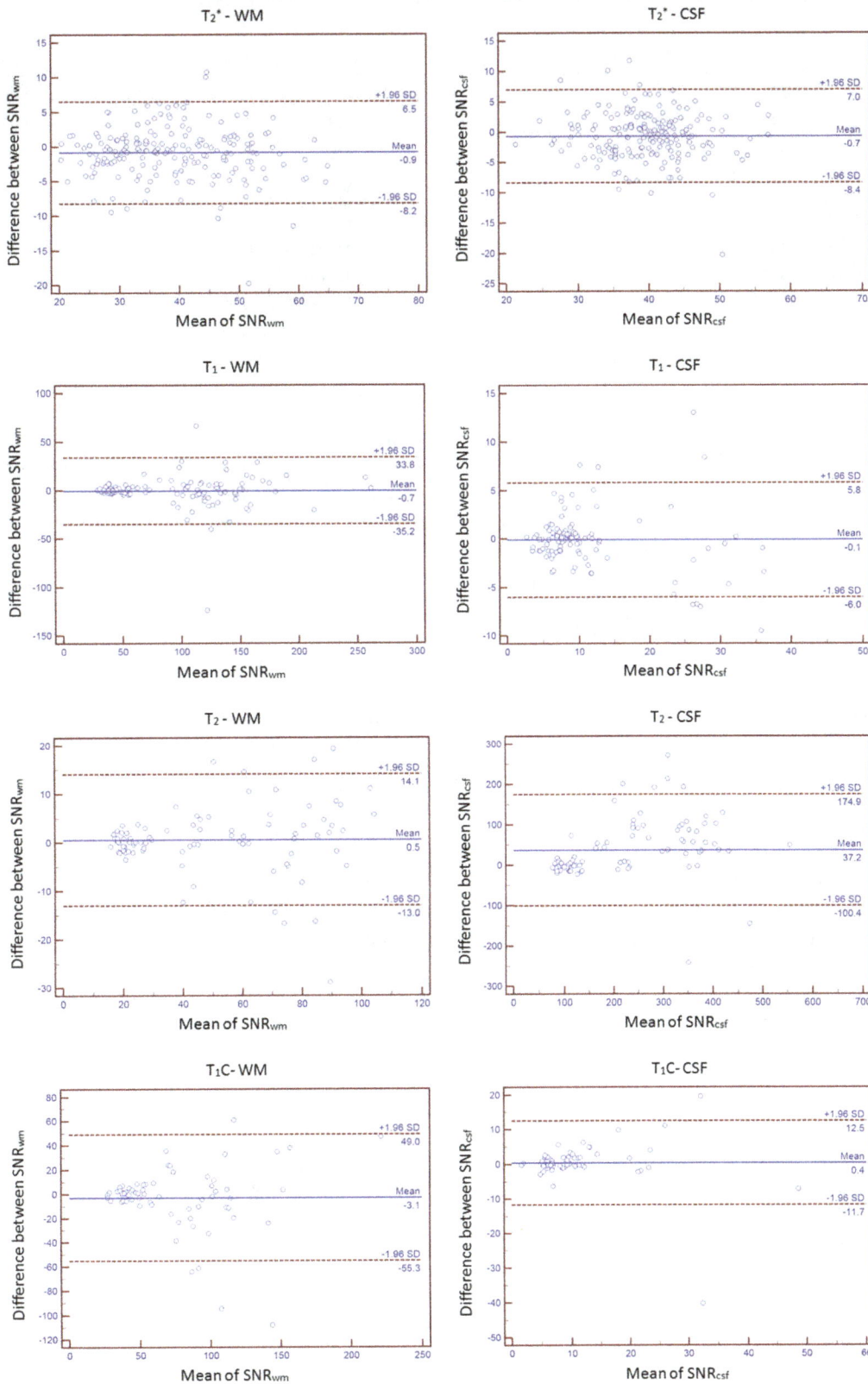

Fig. 2 Bland & Altman plots of SNR values. It presents the SNR values of the first time measurement. The left column represents SNR_{wm} values and the right shows SNR_{csf} values. The solid lines indicate the mean values of SNR measurements and the dashed lines indicate the 95% confident interval of the difference between observations

Table 3 Statistical analysis of SNR measure in each imaging sequence regarding different TOIs

| | | T2* | | T1 | | T2 | | T1C | |
		WM	CSF	WM	CSF	WM	CSF	WM	CSF
The first time	p_w	0.54	0.39	0.88	0.74	0.99	**0.11**	0.69	0.56
	p_p	0.41	0.30	0.98	0.59	0.94	**0.28**	0.77	0.46
The second time	p_w	0.57	0.33	0.92	0.75	0.95	**0.18**	0.72	0.58
	p_p	0.44	0.36	0.96	0.62	0.96	**0.26**	0.79	0.47

difference of SNR values can be perceived from the horizontal and the vertical axis respectively. In addition, horizontal lines are drawn at the mean difference between two SNR observations and at the limits of agreement. The latter is defined as the mean difference plus and minus 1.96 times the standard deviation (SD) of the SNR difference. The Bland & Altman plots show that more than 89% points are localized between the limits of agreement.

Inter-observer difference
Inter-observer difference of SNR observations is analyzed with Wilcoxon rank sum test (p_w) and paired-sample t test (p_p). Corresponding results are show in Table 3. Note that the minimum value is boldfaced in each test. It is observed that the minimal p_w is 0.11 and p_p is 0.26. It is also found that both p_w and p_p from SNR_{wm} are larger than those from SNR_{csf}, correspondingly.

Test-retest reliability
Table 4 lists the result of test-retest reliability. Note that ICC_1 and ICC_2 respectively stands for intra- and inter-observer correlation coefficient. As shown in the Table, very good intra-observer reliability of the experience radiologist (OB) is found ($p_{icc} \geq 0.81$). Similar results are found on the non-physician (OA) except that only good reliability is achieved for SNR_{csf} on T_2^* ($p_{icc} \geq 0.79$) and T_2 ($p_{icc} \geq 0.76$) weighted MR images. Furthermore, good to very good inter-observer reliability is found ($p_{icc} \geq 0.80$) but only good inter-observer reliability is found for SNR_{csf} in T_2^* weighted MR imaging sequence ($p_{icc} \geq 0.74$).

Correlation between SNR and NIQA
Table 5 shows the correlation coefficients (r_p) between mean SNR values of each TOI (two measurements each observer) and NIQA results. The bold-faced r_p values in red and blue denote $r_p \geq 0.60$. Specifically, to SNR_{wm},

BIQI, BLIINDS-II and BRISQUE on T_2^* ($r_p \geq 0.78$), BRISQUE and NIQE on T_1 ($r_p \geq 0.77$), BLIINDS-II on T_2 ($r_p \geq 0.68$), and BRISQUE and NIQE on T_1C ($r_p \geq 0.62$) images show strong correlation; while to SNR_{csf} values, BLIINDS-II correlates well on T_2^* ($r_p \geq 0.63$) and T_2 ($r_p \geq 0.64$) weighted MR imaging sequence.

Discussion
This paper has validated the consistency of SNR measurement in the quality assessment of human brain MR images. Moreover, the correlation between TOI-based SNR measurement and NIQA models has been analyzed. The study suggests that off-the-shelf NIQA models used in computer vision community are full of potential for automated and objective MIQA applications.

The consistency evaluation indicates that SNR measurement is reliable to different observers in each MR imaging sequence. In image pre-processing, TOIs are randomly localized. When no overlapping between TOIs, the Dice index would be zero. On average, TOIs are slightly overlapped by no more than 6% [Table 2], while the statistical analysis indicates that SNR values are not significantly changed between observers [Table 3]. That means independent localization of TOIs makes no difference to SNR measurement. Moreover, the test-retest reliability study suggests good to very good intra- and inter-observer reliability (Table 4). That might be the reason why SNR is widely used in clinical situations. And accordingly, a non-physician can independently perform the SNR measurement of MR images as good as an experienced physician does.

The correlation between SNR values and NIQA models shows that BLIINDS-II correlates well with SNR_{csf} on T_2^* and T_2 weighted MR images, since CSF presents relatively higher voxel intensity over other tissues that leads to the robust estimation of SNR_{csf}. In comparison to SNR_{csf}, more NIQA results are in good

Table 4 Intra- and inter-observer reliability in terms of intra-class coefficients between the non- and experienced physician

| | | T2* | | T1 | | T2 | | T1C | |
		WM	CSF	WM	CSF	WM	CSF	WM	CSF
Intra-observer reliability	OA	0.84	0.79	0.91	0.87	0.95	0.76	0.89	0.86
	OB	0.86	0.81	0.95	0.83	0.97	0.85	0.88	0.82
Inter-observer reliability	ICC2	0.81	0.74	0.92	0.80	0.90	0.81	0.85	0.83

Table 5 Correlation between TOI-based SNR values and no-reference NIQA results

	T2*				T1				T2				T1C			
	SNRwm		SNRcsf		SNRwm		SNRcsf		SNRwm		SNRcsf		SNRwm		SNRcsf	
	OA	OB	OA	OB	OA	OB	OA	OB	OA	OB	OA	OB	OA	OB	OA	OB
BIQI	**0.81**	**0.79**	0.55	0.57	0.16	0.11	0.15	0.13	0.18	0.25	0.07	0.29	0.36	0.33	0.08	0.12
BLIINDS-II	**0.78**	**0.80**	**0.72**	**0.63**	0.23	0.20	0.02	0.06	**0.72**	**0.68**	**0.73**	**0.64**	0.34	0.38	0.10	0.15
BRISQUE	**0.82**	**0.81**	0.56	0.52	**0.77**	**0.81**	0.18	0.22	0.45	0.37	0.52	0.28	**0.62**	**0.73**	0.33	0.36
NIQE	0.24	0.27	0.35	0.03	**0.82**	**0.84**	0.24	0.28	0.55	0.46	0.53	0.32	**0.63**	**0.72**	0.32	0.30

correlation with SNR_{wm} values, since WM is distinguishable in involved MR imaging sequences. Therefore, the authors suggest that tissue regions with higher intensities should function as the TOI in SNR measurement. On the whole, BRISQUE performs well as an automated no-reference NIQA model for the quality assessment of T_2^*, T_1 and T_1C weighted MR brain images, and BLIINDS-II is superior on assessing the quality of T_2^* and T_2 MR images independent of the TOI selection. Consequently, it is full of potential to modify NIQA models developed in the computer vision community for MIQA applications in the medical imaging domain [51]. It should be mentioned that the correlation of SNR values and predicted results is not very good ($r_p \leq 0.85$) and further improvement or modifications of existing NIQA models is needed.

SNR is frequently used as an image quality indicator in clinic. It is a local measure regarding the whole MR image. The SNR measurement can also be formulated from the global signal by using the whole object region as the tissue region. An overview of existing definitions of SNR measurement can be referred to [23]. More general and automated MIQA algorithms include using Shannon's theory to describe the image content and then to model the spatial spectral power density of the image as the quality indicator [21] or analyzing the background of magnitude images of structural brain to represent the image quality [52]. In particular, some researchers explore to bridge the gap between SNR measurement and diagnostic accuracy or detectability [9, 18]. These studies show superiority over the physical measure of image quality, since the ultimate goal of medical imaging aims at abnormality detection and disease diagnosis.

Conclusions

The consistency of SNR measurement is validated regarding different observers. The correlation between SNR measurement and NIQA models indicates that BRISQUE works well for automated MIQA of T_2^*, T_1 and T_1C weighted brain MR images, and BLIINDS-II is superior over T_2^* and T_2 weighted images independent

of the TOI selection. Our future work will focus on the connection of SNR measurement, NIQA models and MIQA applications.

Abbreviations

BIQI: Blind image quality index; BLIINDS-II: The improved version of blind image integrity notator using DCT statistics; BRISQUE: Blind/referenceless image spatial quality evaluator; CSF: Cerebral spinal fluid; CT: Computerized tomography; DCT: Discrete cosine transform; DWT: Discrete wavelet transform; FOV: Field of view; ICC_1: Intra-observer correlation coefficient; ICC_2: Inter-observer correlation coefficient; MIQA: Medical image quality assessment; MR: Magnetic resonance; NIQA: Natural image quality assessment; NIQE: Natural image quality evaluator; NSS: Natural scene statistics; OA: Observer A; OB: Observer B; ROI: Regions of interest; SD: Standard deviation; SNR: Signal-to-noise ratio; SNR_{csf}: CSF-based SNR; SNR_{wm}: WM-based SNR; T_1C: Contrast-enhanced T_1; TE: Time of echo; TOI: Tissue region of interest; TR: Time of repetition; WM: White matter

Acknowledgements

The authors would like to thank the editor, reviewers and Rached Belgacem from Institut Superieur des Technologies Medicales de Tunis (ISTMT) for their valuable advices that have helped to improve the paper quality.

Funding

This work is supported in part by grants from the National Key Research and Develop Program of China (2016YFC0105102), the Leading Talent of Special Support Project in Guangdong (Y77504), the Shenzhen Key Technical Research Project (JSGG20160229203812944), the National Science Foundation of Guangdong (2014A030312006) and the Beijing Center for Mathematics and Information Interdisciplinary Sciences; the National Natural Science Foundation of China (61471349), the Science and Technology Plan Projects of Guangdong Province (2015B020233004), the Shenzhen Basic Technology Research Project (JCYJ20160429174611494 and JCYJ20170818160306270); the National Natural Science Foundation of China (61771473 and 61379143), the Six Talent Peaks High-level Talents in Jiangsu Province (XYDXX-063) and the Qing Lan Project; and the Science and Technology Planning Project of Guangzhou (201804010032). The funding sponsors had no role in the design of the study; in the collection, analysis or interpretation of data; in the writing of the manuscript; nor in the decision to publish the results.

Authors' contributions

Conceived and designed the experiments: SY, LL, XW, YX Performed the experiments: GD, XW Analyzed the data: SY, GD, ZW Contributed reagents/materials/analysis tools: SY, XW Wrote the manuscript: SY Discussed and proof-read the manuscript: LL, XW, YX. All authors read and approved the final manuscript.

Competing interests

The authors declare that they have no competing interests.

Author details

[1]Shenzhen Institutes of Advanced Technology, Chinese Academy of Sciences, Shenzhen, China. [2]Shenzhen College of Advanced Technology, University of Chinese Academy of Sciences, Shenzhen, China. [3]Sino-Dutch Biomedical and Information Engineering School, Northeastern University, Shenyang, China. [4]School of Information and Control Engineering, Chinese University of Mining and Technology, Xuzhou, China. [5]Department of Radiology, Guangzhou First Peoples Hospital, Guangzhou Medical University, Guangzhou, China. [6]The Second Affiliated Hospital, South China University of Technology, Guangzhou, China.

References

1. Sandhu GY, Li C, Roy O, Schmidt S, Duric N. Frequency domain ultrasound waveform tomography: breast imaging using a ring transducer. Phys Med Biol. 2015;60(14):5381.

2. Ahmad M, Bazalova-Carter M, Fahrig R, Xing L. Optimized detector angular configuration increases the sensitivity of x-ray fluorescence computed tomography (XFCT). IEEE Trans Med Imaging. 2015;34(5):1140–7.

3. Zhang Z, Yu S, Liang X, Zhu Y, Xie Y. A novel design of ultrafast micro-CT system based on carbon nanotube: a feasibility study in phantom. Phys Med. 2016;32(10):1302–7.

4. Razaak M, Martini MG, Savino K. A study on quality assessment for medical ultrasound video compressed via HEVC. IEEE J Biomed Health Inform. 2014;18(5):1552–9.

5. Zhang L, Cavaro-M'enard C, Le Callet P, Ge D. A multi-slice model observer for medical image quality assessment. IEEE ICASSP. 2015;1:1667–71.

6. Jenkins CH, Xing L, Fahimian BP. Automating position and timing quality assurance for high dose rate brachytherapy using radioluminescent phosphors and optical imaging. Brachytherapy. 2016;15:28.

7. Firbank MJ, Coulthard A, Harrison RM, Williams ED. Quality assurance for MRI: practical experience. Br J Radiol. 2000;73(868):376–83.

8. Peltonen JI, Makela T, Sofiev A, Salli E. An automatic image processing workflow for daily magnetic resonance imaging quality assurance. J Digit Imaging. 2016;73(868):1–9.

9. Eck BL, Fahmi R, Brown KM, Zabic S, Raihani N, Miao J, Wilson DL. Computational and human observer image quality evaluation of low dose, knowledge-based CT iterative reconstruction. Med Phys. 2015; 42(10):6098–111.

10. Baselice F, Ferraioli G, Pascazio V. A 3D MRI denoising algorithm based on Bayesian theory. Biomed Eng Online. 2017;16(1):25.

11. Peng C, Qiu B, Li M, Guan Y, Zhang C, Wu Z, Zheng J. Gaussian diffusion sinogram inpainting for X-ray CT metal artifact reduction. Biomed Eng Online. 2017;16(1):1.

12. Yu S, Wu S, Wang H, Wei X, Chen X, Pan W, Hu J, Xie Y. Linear-fitting-based similarity coefficient map for tissue dissimilarity analysis in T_2^*-w magnetic resonance imaging. Chinese Physics B. 2015;24(12):128711.

13. Li H, Wu J, Miao A, Yu P, Chen J, Zhang Y. Rayleigh-maximum-likelihood bilateral filter for ultrasound image enhancement. Biomed Eng Online. 2017;16(1):46.

14. Zhang R, Zhou W, Li Y, Yu S, Xie Y. Nonrigid registration of lung CT images based on tissue features. Comput Math Methods Medicine. 2013;834192:1–7.

15. Yu S, Zhang R, Wu S, Hu J, Xie Y. An edge-directed interpolation method for fetal spine MR images. Biomed Eng Online. 2013;12(1):102.

16. Guo L, Wang H, Peng C, Dai Y, Ding M, Sun Y, Yang X, Zheng J. Non-rigid MR-TRUS image registration for image-guided prostate biopsy using correlation ratio-based mutual information. Biomed Eng Online. 2017;16(1):8.

17. Li X, Huang W, Rooney WD. Signal-to-noise ratio, contrast-to-noise ratio and pharmacokinetic modeling considerations in dynamic contrast-enhanced magnetic resonance imaging. Magn Reson Imaging. 2012;30(9):1313–22.

18. Cosman PC, Gray RM, Olshen RA. Evaluating quality of compressed medical images: SNR, subjective rating, and diagnostic accuracy. Proc IEEE. 1994; 82(6):919–32.

19. Cao Z, Park J, Cho ZH, Collins CM. Numerical evaluation of image homogeneity, signal-to-noise ratio, and specific absorption rate for human brain imaging at 1.5, 3, 7, 10.5, and 14T in an 8-channel transmit/receive array. J Magn Reson Imaging. 2015;41(5):1432–9.

20. Chow LS, Paramesran R. Review of medical image quality assessment. Biomed Signal Process Control. 2016;27:145–54.

21. Fuderer M. The information content of MR images. IEEE Trans Med Imaging. 1988;7(4):368–80.

22. Geissler A, Gartus T, Foki T, Tahamtan AR, Beisteiner R, Barth M. Contrast-to-noise ratio (CNR) as a quality parameter in fMRI. J Magn Reson Imaging. 2007;25(6):1263–70.

23. Welvaert M, Rosseel Y. On the definition of signal-to-noise ratio and contrast-to-noise ratio for fMRI data. PLoS One. 2013;8(11):77089.

24. Niu T, Zhu L. Scatter correction for full-fan volumetric CT using a stationary beam blocker in a single full scan. Med Phys. 2011;38(11):6027–38.

25. Liang X, Zhang Z, Niu T, Yu S, Wu S, Li Z, Zhang H, Xie Y. Iterative image-domain ring artifact removal in cone-beam CT. Phys Med Biol. 2017;62:5276–92.

26. Chow LS, Rajagopal H, Paramesran R. ANDI. Correlation between subjective and objective assessment of magnetic resonance (MR) images. Magn Reson Imaging. 2016;34(6):820–31.

27. Henkelman RM. Measurement of signal intensities in the presence of noise in MR images. Med Phys. 1985;12(2):232–3.

28. Kaufman L, Kramer DM, Crooks LE, Ortendahl DA. Measuring signal-to-noise ratios in MR imaging. Radiology. 1989;173(1):265–7.

29. Shokrollahi P, Drake JM, Goldenberg AA. Signal-to-noise ratio evaluation of magnetic resonance images in the presence of an ultrasonic motor. Biomed Eng Online. 2017;16(1):45.

30. Reeder SB, Wintersperger BJ, Dietrich O, Lanz T, Greiser A, Reiser MF, Glazer GM, Schoenberg SO. Practical approaches to the evaluation of signal-to-noise ratio performance with parallel imaging: application with cardiac imaging and a 32-channel cardiac coil. Magn Reson Med. 2005;54(3):748–54.

31. Chen S, Wu H, Wu L, Jin J, Qiu B. Compressed sensing MRI via fast linearized preconditioned alternating direction method of multipliers. Biomed Eng Online. 2017;16(1):53.

32. Murphy BW, Carson PL, Ellis JH, Zhang YT, Hyde RJ, Chenevert TL. Signal-to-noise measures for magnetic resonance imagers. Magn Reson Imaging. 1993;11(3):425–8.

33. Zhou W, Xie Y. Interactive contour delineation and refinement in treatment planning of image-guided radiation therapy. J Appl Clin Med Phys. 2014;15(1):4499.

34. Yu S, Wu S, Zhuang L, Wei X, Sak M, Neb D, Hu J, Xie Y. Efficient segmentation of a breast in B-mode ultrasound tomography using three-dimensional GrabCut (GC3D). Sensors. 2017;17(8):1827.

35. Lu L. A note on curvature variation minimizing cubic Hermite interpolants. Appl Math Comput. 2015;259:596–9.

36. Firbank MJ, Coulthard A, Harrison RM, Williams ED. A comparison of two methods for measuring the signal to noise ratio on MR images. Phys Med Biol. 1999;44(12):261.

37. Kellman P, McVeigh ER. Image reconstruction in SNR units: a general method for SNR measurement. Magn Reson Med. 2005;54(6):1439–47.

38. Saad MA, Bovik AC, Charrier C. A DCT statistics-based blind image quality index. IEEE Signal Process Lett. 2010;17(6):583–6.

39. Yu S, Wu S, Wang L, Jiang F, Xie Y, Li L. A shallow convolutional neural network for blind image sharpness assessment. PLoS One. 2017;12(5):e0176632.

40. Gu K, Li L, Lu H, Min X, Lin W. A fast reliable image quality predictor by fusing micro-and macro-structures. IEEE Trans Ind Electron. 2017;64(5):3903–12.

41. Moorthy A, Bovik A. A two-step framework for constructing blind image quality indices. IEEE Signal Process Lett. 2010;17(5):513–6.

42. Saad MA, Bovik AC, Charrier C. DCT statistics model-based blind image quality assessment. IEEE ICIP. 2011;1:3093–6.

43. Mittal A, Moorthy A, Bovik A. No-reference image quality assessment in the spatial domain. IEEE Trans Image Process. 2012;21(12):4695–708.

44. Mittal A, Soundararajan R, Bovik A. Making a "completely blind" image quality analyzer. IEEE Signal Process Lett. 2013;20(3):209–12.

45. Wilcoxon F. Individual comparisons by ranking methods. Biom Bull. 1945;1(6):80–3.

46. Kerby DS. The simple difference formula: an approach to teaching nonparametric correlation. Compr Psychol. 2014;3:11.

47. Zimmerman DW. A note on interpretation of the paired-samples t test. J Educ Behav Stat. 1997;22(3):349–60.

48. Lin HS, Chen YJ, Lu HL, Lu TW, Chen CC. Test–retest reliability of mandibular morphology measurements on cone-beam computed tomography-synthesized cephalograms with random head positioning errors. Biomed Eng Online. 2017;16(1):62.

Permissions

All chapters in this book were first published in MI, by BioMed Central; hereby published with permission under the Creative Commons Attribution License or equivalent. Every chapter published in this book has been scrutinized by our experts. Their significance has been extensively debated. The topics covered herein carry significant findings which will fuel the growth of the discipline. They may even be implemented as practical applications or may be referred to as a beginning point for another development.

The contributors of this book come from diverse backgrounds, making this book a truly international effort. This book will bring forth new frontiers with its revolutionizing research information and detailed analysis of the nascent developments around the world.

We would like to thank all the contributing authors for lending their expertise to make the book truly unique. They have played a crucial role in the development of this book. Without their invaluable contributions this book wouldn't have been possible. They have made vital efforts to compile up to date information on the varied aspects of this subject to make this book a valuable addition to the collection of many professionals and students.

This book was conceptualized with the vision of imparting up-to-date information and advanced data in this field. To ensure the same, a matchless editorial board was set up. Every individual on the board went through rigorous rounds of assessment to prove their worth. After which they invested a large part of their time researching and compiling the most relevant data for our readers.

The editorial board has been involved in producing this book since its inception. They have spent rigorous hours researching and exploring the diverse topics which have resulted in the successful publishing of this book. They have passed on their knowledge of decades through this book. To expedite this challenging task, the publisher supported the team at every step. A small team of assistant editors was also appointed to further simplify the editing procedure and attain best results for the readers.

Apart from the editorial board, the designing team has also invested a significant amount of their time in understanding the subject and creating the most relevant covers. They scrutinized every image to scout for the most suitable representation of the subject and create an appropriate cover for the book.

The publishing team has been an ardent support to the editorial, designing and production team. Their endless efforts to recruit the best for this project, has resulted in the accomplishment of this book. They are a veteran in the field of academics and their pool of knowledge is as vast as their experience in printing. Their expertise and guidance has proved useful at every step. Their uncompromising quality standards have made this book an exceptional effort. Their encouragement from time to time has been an inspiration for everyone.

The publisher and the editorial board hope that this book will prove to be a valuable piece of knowledge for researchers, students, practitioners and scholars across the globe.

List of Contributors

Edward Gilbert-Kawai and Jonny Coppel
University College London Centre for Altitude Space and Extreme Environment Medicine, UCLH NIHR Biomedical Research Centre, Institute of Sport and Exercise Health, 170 Tottenham Court Road, London W1T 7HA, UK

Daniel Martin
University College London Centre for Altitude Space and Extreme Environment Medicine, UCLH NIHR Biomedical Research Centre, Institute of Sport and Exercise Health, 170 Tottenham Court Road, London W1T 7HA, UK
Division of Neonatology, Erasmus MC-Sophia Children's Hospital, Wytemaweg 80, 3000 CB Rotterdam, Netherlands

Vassiliki Bountziouka
Statistical Support Service, Population, Policy and Practice Programme, Institute of Child Health, University College London, London, England

Can Ince
Department of Intensive Care, Erasmus MC University Hospital Rotterdam, 3000 Rotterdam, The Netherlands

Sylviane Dongmo Fomekong
Department of Radiology and Radiation Oncology, Faculty of Medicine and Biomedical Sciences, The University of Yaounde 1, Yaounde, Cameroon

Boniface Moifo
Department of Radiology and Radiation Oncology, Faculty of Medicine and Biomedical Sciences, The University of Yaounde 1, Yaounde, Cameroon
Radiology Department YGOPH, Yaounde Gynaeco-Obstetric and Pediatric Hospital, Yaounde, Cameroon

Jean Roger Moulion Tapouh and François Djomou
Department of Radiology and Radiation Oncology, Faculty of Medicine and Biomedical Sciences, The University of Yaounde 1, Yaounde, Cameroon
Yaounde University Teaching Hospital, Yaounde, Cameroon

Emmanuella Manka'a Wankie
Douala General Hospital, Douala, Cameroon

Weiguang Shao, Jingang Liu and Dianmei Liu
Department of Imaging Center, the Affiliated Hospital of Weifang Medical University, Weifang 261031, China

D. Góngora and M. A. Bobes
Key Laboratory for NeuroInformation of Ministry of Education, Center for Information in Medicine, University of Electronic Science and Technology of China, 2006, Xiyuan Ave, West Hi-Tech Zone, Chengdu 61000, China
Cuban Neuroscience Center, 190th Ave between 25th and 27th Ave, Havana 11300, Cuba

M. Domínguez
IDIBELL Bellvitge Biomedical Research Institute, Barcelona, Spain

Pablo Navarro and Ramón Fuentes
Research Center in Dental Sciences (CICO), Endodontic Laboratory, Dental School, Universidad de La Frontera, Temuco, Chile

Pablo Betancourt
Research Center in Dental Sciences (CICO), Endodontic Laboratory, Dental School, Universidad de La Frontera, Temuco, Chile
Integral Adultos Department, Dental School, Universidad de La Frontera, Claro Solar 115, Temuco, Chile

Gonzalo Muñoz
Dental School, Universidad de La Frontera, Temuco, Chile

Xin Zhou, Yuan Liu, Song Zhou, Xiao-Xing Fu, Xiao-Long Yu, Chang-Lin Fu, Bin Zhang and Min Dai
Department of Orthopedics, The First Affiliated Hospital of Nanchang University, Nanchang 330006, China
Artificial Joint Engineering and Technology Research Center of Jiangxi Province, Nanchang 330006, China

Yiming Gao, Brian Quinn, Usman Mahmood, Daniel Long, Yusuf Erdi and Jean St. Germain
Department of Medical Physics, Memorial Sloan Kettering Cancer Center, 1275 York Avenue, New York, NY 10065, USA

Lawrence T. Dauer
Department of Medical Physics, Memorial Sloan Kettering Cancer Center, 1275 York Avenue, Box 84, New York, NY 10065, USA
Department of Radiology, Memorial Sloan Kettering Cancer Center, 1275 York Avenue, New York, NY 10065, USA

Neeta Pandit-Taskar
Department of Radiology, Memorial Sloan Kettering Cancer Center, 1275 York Avenue, New York, NY 10065, USA

X. George Xu
Department of Mechanical, Aerospace, and Nuclear Engineering, Rensselaer Polytechnic Institute, Troy, NY 12180, USA

Wesley E. Bolch
J.Crayton Pruitt Family Department of Biomedical Engineering, University of Florida, Gainesville, FL 32611, USA

Michele Di Martino, Michele Anzidei, Fulvio Zaccagna, Luca Saba, Sandro Bosco, Massimo Rossi, Stefano Ginanni Corradini and Carlo Catalano
Sapienza, University of Rome, Rome, Italy

Jan Theopold, Kevin Weihs, Bastian Marquaß, Christoph Josten and Pierre Hepp
Department of Orthopedics, Trauma and Plastic Surgery, University of Leipzig, Liebigstrasse 20, 04103 Leipzig, Germany

Christine Feja
Institute of Anatomy, University of Leipzig, Liebigstrasse 13, 04103 Leipzig, Germany

Vassiliki Lyra and Georgios Lamprakopoulos
2nd Department of Radiology, Nuclear Medicine Section, National and Kapodistrian University of Athens, Attikon Hospital, 1 Rimini St., Athens 12462, Greece

Sofia N. Chatziioannou
2nd Department of Radiology, Nuclear Medicine Section, National and Kapodistrian University of Athens, Attikon Hospital, 1 Rimini St., Athens 12462, Greece
Nuclear Medicine Section, Biomedical Research Foundation Academy of Athens, BRFAA, 4 Soranou Efesiou St., Athens 11527, Greece

Maria Kallergi
Department of Medical Instruments Technology, Technological Educational Institution of Athens, TEI, 28 Ag. Spiridona St., Athens 12210, Greece

Emmanouil Rizos
2nd Department of Psychiatry, National and Kapodistrian University of Athens, Attikon Hospital, 1 Rimini St., Athens 12462, Greece

Astrid Ellen Grams, Alexander Bartsch, Sarah Honold and Elke Ruth Gizewski
Department of Neuroradiology, Medical University of Innsbruck, Anichstraße 35, A-6020 Innsbruck, Austria

Rafael Rehwald and Bernhard Glodny
Department of Radiology, Medical University of Innsbruck, Anichstraße 35, A-6020 Innsbruck, Austria

Christian Franz Freyschlag
Department of Neurosurgery, Medical University of Innsbruck, Anichstraße 35, A-6020 Innsbruck, Austria

Michael Knoflach
Department of Neurology, Medical University of Innsbruck, Anichstraße 35, A-6020 Innsbruck, Austria

Nobuyoshi Fukumitsu, Toshiyuki Terunuma, Toshiyuki Okumura, Haruko Numajiri, Yoshiko Oshiro, Kayoko Ohnishi, Masashi Mizumoto, Teruhito Aihara, Hitoshi Ishikawa, Koji Tsuboi and Hideyuki Sakurai
Proton Medical Research Center, University of Tsukuba, 1-1-1, Tennoudai, Tsukuba, Japan

Kazunori Nitta
Division of Radiology, Ibaraki Prefectural Central Hospital, 6528, Koibuchi, Kasama, Japan

Yunzhi Wang, Yuchen Qiu, Hong Liu and Bin Zheng
School of Electrical and Computer Engineering, University of Oklahoma, Norman, OK 73019, USA

Theresa Thai and Kathleen Moore
Health Science Center of University of Oklahoma, Oklahoma City, OK 73104, USA

Luca Pio Stoppino, Stefania Rizzi, Elsa Cleopazzo, Annarita Centola, Donatello Iamele, Christos Bristogiannis, Roberta Vinci and Luca Macarini
Division of Diagnostic Imaging, Department of Surgical Sciences, University of Foggia, Viale Luigi Pinto n.1, Foggia 71122, Italy

Nicola Della Valle
Division of Gastroenterology, Department of Surgical Sciences, University of Foggia, Viale Luigi Pinto n.1, Foggia 71122, Italy

Giuseppe Stoppino
Division of Gastroenterology, Department of Surgical Sciences, Azienda Sanitaria Locale Provincia di Foggia, Piazza della Libertà n.1, Foggia 71122, Italy

Mads Liisberg
Department of Cardiothoracic and Vascular Surgery, Odense University Hospital, Cardiovascular Centre of Excellence (CAVAC), Sdr. Boulevard 29, Afd. T - Forskerreden, 5000 Odense C, Denmark
Elitary Research Centre of Individualised Treatment of Arterial Diseases (CIMA), Odense University Hospital, Odense C, Denmark

Jes S. Lindholt
Department of Cardiothoracic and Vascular Surgery, Odense University Hospital, Cardiovascular Centre of Excellence (CAVAC), Sdr. Boulevard 29, Afd. T - Forskerreden, 5000 Odense C, Denmark
Elitary Research Centre of Individualised Treatment of Arterial Diseases (CIMA), Odense University Hospital, Odense C, Denmark
OPEN, Odense Patient data Explorative Network, Odense University Hospital, Odense C, Denmark

Axel C. Diederichsen
Elitary Research Centre of Individualised Treatment of Arterial Diseases (CIMA), Odense University Hospital, Odense C, Denmark
Department of Cardiology, Odense University Hospital, Odense C, Denmark
OPEN, Odense Patient data Explorative Network, Odense University Hospital, Odense C, Denmark

Niladri K. Mahato and Susan Williams
Ohio Musculoskeletal and Neurological Institute, Ohio University, Athens, OH 45701, USA
Department of Biomedical Sciences, Ohio University, Athens, OH 45701, USA

John Cotton
Ohio Musculoskeletal and Neurological Institute, Ohio University, Athens, OH 45701, USA
Department of Mechanical Engineering, Ohio University, Athens, OH 45701, USA

James Thomas
Ohio Musculoskeletal and Neurological Institute, Ohio University, Athens, OH 45701, USA
School of Rehabilitation and Communication Sciences, Ohio University, Athens, OH 45701, USA

Brian Clark
Ohio Musculoskeletal and Neurological Institute, Ohio University, Athens, OH 45701, USA
Department of Biomedical Sciences, Ohio University, Athens, OH 45701, USA
Department of Geriatric Medicine, Ohio University, Athens, OH 45701, USA

Stephane Montuelle
Department of Biomedical Sciences, Ohio University, Athens, OH 45701, USA

Wenxu Qi, Gongyu Lan and Qiyong Guo
Department of Radiology, Shengjing Hospital, China Medical University, Shenyang 110004, People's Republic of China

Song Gao
Morphology Teaching and Reasearch Section, Liaoning Vocational College of Medcine, Shenyang 110100, People's Republic of China

Caixia Liu and Xue Yang
Department of Obstetrics and Gynecology, Shengjing Hospital, China Medical University, Shenyang 110004, People's Republic of China

Zhaojun Li and Lianfang Du
Department of Ultrasound, Shanghai General Hospital, Shanghai Jiaotong University School of Medicine, No.100 Hai Ning Road, Hongkou District, Shanghai 200080, China

Yan Qin
Department of Urology, Shanghai General Hospital, Shanghai Jiaotong University School of Medicine, No.100 Hai Ning Road, Hongkou District, Shanghai 200080, China

Xianghong Luo
Department of Echocardiography, Shanghai General Hospital, Shanghai Jiaotong University School of Medicine, No.100 Hai Ning Road, Hongkou District, Shanghai 200080, China

Maria D'Amato
Department of Pneumology, "Federico II University", AO "Dei Colli" Monaldi Hospital, Via Domenico Fontana, 134, Naples, Italy

Gaetano Rea
Department of Radiology, AO "Dei Colli" Monaldi Hospital, Naples, Italy

Vincenzo Carnevale
Unit of Internal Medicine, "Casa Sollievo della Sofferenza" Hospital, IRCCS, San Giovanni Rotondo (FG), Italy

Maria Arcangela Grimaldi
Unit of Internal Medicine and Pneumology, "Casa Sollievo della Sofferenza" Hospital, IRCCS, San Giovanni Rotondo (FG), Italy

Anna Rita Saponara
Unit of Internal Medicine, Local Health Service, Potenza, Italy

Eric Rosenthal
Department of Internal Medicine, Hospital Archet 1, Nice, France

Michele Maria Maggi
Unit of Emergency Medicine, "Casa Sollievo della Sofferenza" Hospital, IRCCS, San Giovanni Rotondo (FG), Italy

Lucia Dimitri
Unit of Pathology, "Casa Sollievo della Sofferenza" Hospital, IRCCS, San Giovanni Rotondo (FG), Italy

Marco Sperandeo
Unit of Interventional and Diagnostic Ultrasound of Internal Medicine, "Casa Sollievo della Sofferenza" Hospital, IRCCS, San Giovanni Rotondo (FG), Italy

Ruigang Lu, Yan Zhang, Wei Zhao and Ruijun Guo
Department of Ultrasonography, Beijing Chao-Yang Hospital, Capital Medical University, Beijing 100020, China

Yuxin Meng
Department of Endocrinology, Beijing No. 6 Hospital, Beijing 100007, China

Xun Wang
Department of Otorhinolaryngology Head and Neck Surgery, Beijing Chao-Yang Hospital, Capital Medical University, Beijing 100020, China

Mulan Jin
Department of Pathology, Beijing Chao-Yang Hospital, Capital Medical University, Beijing 100020, China

Christina Baun, Kirsten Falch, Jeanette Hansen, Tram Nguyen, Poul-Flemming Høilund-Carlsen and Malene G. Hildebrandt
Department of Nuclear Medicine, University Hospital, Sdr. Boulevard 29, 5000 Odense C, Denmark

Oke Gerke
Department of Nuclear Medicine, University Hospital, Sdr. Boulevard 29, 5000 Odense C, Denmark
Centre of Health Economics Research, University of Southern Denmark, Odense, Denmark

Abass Alavi
University of Pennsylvania, Philadelphia, USA

Qian Zhang, Ju-fang Wang, Qing-qing Dong, Qing Yan, Xiang-hong Luo, Xue-ying Wu, Jian Liu and Ya-ping Sun
Department of Echocardiography, Shanghai General Hospital, Shanghai Jiao Tong University School of Medicine, No.100 Hai Ning Road, Shanghai 200080, China

Xin Qin
School of Biomedical Engineering, Xinxiang Medical University, Xinxiang 453003, China

Chang Wang, Qiongqiong Ren and Yi Yu
School of Biomedical Engineering, Xinxiang Medical University, Xinxiang 453003, China
Xinxiang City Engineering Technology Research Center of Neurosensor and Control, Xinxiang 453003, China

Youyong Kong, Xiaopeng Chen, Jiasong Wu, Pinzheng Zhang, Yang Chen and Huazhong Shu
Laboratory of Image Science and Technology, Key Laboratory of Computer Network and Information Integration, School of Computer Science and Engineering, Southeast University, Nanjing, People's Republic of China
International Joint Laboratory of Information Display and Visualization, Nanjing, People's Republic of China

Tae Joo Jeon
Department of Nuclear Medicine, Gangnam Severance Hospital, Yonsei University College of Medicine, Seoul, South Korea

Sungjun Kim
Department of Radiology, Gangnam Severance Hospital, Yonsei University College of Medicine, Seoul, South Korea

Jinyoung Park
Department of Rehabilitation Medicine, Gangnam Severance Hospital, Rehabilitation Institute of Neuromuscular Disease, Yonsei University College of Medicine, Seoul, South Korea

Jung Hyun Park
Department of Rehabilitation Medicine, Gangnam Severance Hospital, Rehabilitation Institute of Neuromuscular Disease, Yonsei University College of Medicine, Seoul, South Korea
Department of Rehabilitation Medicine, Gangnam Severance Hospital, Yonsei University College of Medicine, 211 Eonjuro, Gangnam-gu, Seoul 06273, South Korea

Eugene Y. Roh
Division of PM&R, Department of Orthopaedic Surgery, Stanford University School of Medicine, Stanford, CA 94063, USA

Evgeni Aizenberg, Monique Reijnierse and Oleh Dzyubachyk
Department of Radiology, Leiden University Medical Center, 2300 RC Leiden, The Netherlands

Boudewijn P. F. Lelieveldt
Department of Radiology, Leiden University Medical Center, 2300 RC Leiden, The Netherlands
Intelligent Systems Department, Delft University of Technology, Mekelweg 4, 2628 CD Delft, The Netherlands

Rosaline van den Berg, Zineb Ez-Zaitouni and Désirée van der Heijde
Department of Rheumatology, Leiden University Medical Center, 2300 RC Leiden, The Netherlands

Sameer Baig, Yucheng Zhang, Junjie Zhang, Farzad Khalvati and Masoom A. Haider
Department of Medical Imaging and Sunnybrook Research Institute, Sunnybrook Health Sciences Center, University of Toronto, 2075 Bayview Ave., Room Rm AG 46, Toronto M4N 3 M5, ON, Canada

Armin Eilaghi
Department of Medical Imaging and Sunnybrook Research Institute, Sunnybrook Health Sciences Center, University of Toronto, 2075 Bayview Ave., Room Rm AG 46, Toronto M4N 3 M5, ON, Canada
Mechanical Engineering Department, Australian College of Kuwait, Kuwait City, Kuwait

Paul Karanicolas
Department of Surgery, Sunnybrook Health Sciences Center, University of Toronto, Toronto, ON, Canada

Steven Gallinger
PanCuRx Translational Research Initiative, Ontario Institute for Cancer Research, Toronto, ON, Canada
Lunenfeld-Tanenbaum Research Institute, Mount Sinai Hospital, Toronto, ON, Canada
Hepatobiliary/pancreatic Surgical Oncology Program, University Health Network, Toronto, ON, Canada

Su Min Ha
Department of Radiology, Research Institute of Radiology, Chung-Ang University Hospital, Chung-Ang University College of Medicine, 84 Heukseok-Ro, Dongjak-Gu, Seoul 06973, Republic of Korea

Joo Hee Cha, Hee Jung Shin, Eun Young Chae, Woo Jung Choi and Hak Hee Kim
Department of Radiology, Research Institute of Radiology, University of Ulsan College of Medicine, Asan Medical Center, 88 Olympic-Ro 43 Gil, Songpa-Gu, Seoul 05505, Republic of Korea

Ha-Yeon Oh
Department of Radiology, Kangwon National University Hospital, 200-722 Baengnyeong-Ro 156, Chuncheon-Si, Republic of Korea

Kirsi Holli-Helenius
Department of Medical Physics, Medical Imaging Centre and Hospital Pharmacy, Pirkanmaa Hospital District, 33521 Tampere, Finland

Annukka Salminen and Irina Rinta-Kiikka
Department of Radiology, Tampere University Hospital, Tampere, Finland

Ilkka Koskivuo and Nina Brück
Department of Plastic and General Surgery Turku University Hospital, Turku, Finland

Pia Boström
Department of Pathology, University of Turku and Turku University Hospital, Turku, Finland

Riitta Parkkola
Department of Radiology, University of Turku and Turku University Hospital, Turku, Finland

Shousen Wang, Yong Qin, Deyong Xiao and Liangfeng Wei
Department of Neurosurgery, Fuzhou General Hospital, Fujian Medical University, No. 156 Xi'erhuanbei Road, Fuzhou 350025, People's Republic of China

Yaoqin Xie
Shenzhen Institutes of Advanced Technology, Chinese Academy of Sciences, Shenzhen, China

Shaode Yu
Shenzhen Institutes of Advanced Technology, Chinese Academy of Sciences, Shenzhen, China
Shenzhen College of Advanced Technology, University of Chinese Academy of Sciences, Shenzhen, China

Guangzhe Dai and Zhaoyang Wang
Shenzhen Institutes of Advanced Technology, Chinese Academy of Sciences, Shenzhen, China
Sino-Dutch Biomedical and Information Engineering School, Northeastern University, Shenyang, China

Leida Li
School of Information and Control Engineering, Chinese University of Mining and Technology, Xuzhou, China

Xinhua Wei
Department of Radiology, Guangzhou First Peoples Hospital, Guangzhou Medical University, Guangzhou, China
The Second Affiliated Hospital, South China University of Technology, Guangzhou, China

Index